PATHWAYS TO WELLNESS

PATHWAYS TO WELLNESS

Sherman R. Dickman, PhD
University of Utah

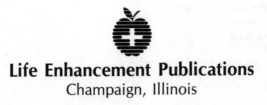

Life Enhancement Publications
Champaign, Illinois

Library of Congress Cataloging-in-Publication Data

Dickman, Sherman R., 1915–
  Pathways to wellness / Sherman R. Dickman
    p.   cm.
  Bibliography: p.
  Includes index.
  ISBN 0-87322-922-3
  1. Health.   I. Title
RA776.D468 1988   87-31667
613--dc 19   CIP

Developmental Editor: Sue Wilmoth, PhD
Production Director: Ernie Noa
Projects Manager: Lezli Harris
Copy Editor: Claire Mount
Assistant Editor: Julie Anderson
Typesetters: Sandra Meier and Yvonne Winsor
Text Design: Keith Blomberg
Cover Design: Hunter Graphics
Back Cover Photo: Reprinted with permission from
  the *Deseret News*. Photo by O. Wallace Kasteler.
Text Layout: Denise Peters
Printed By: Braun-Brumfield

ISBN: 0-87322-922-3

Printed in the United States of America

10 9 8 7 6 5 4 3 2 1

Life Enhancement Publications
A Division of Human Kinetics Publishers, Inc.
Box 5076, Champaign, IL 61820
1-800-342-5457
1-800-334-3665 (in Illinois)

To Tom
from whom I have learned so much

Acknowledgments

My completing this book was facilitated and made more pleasurable by the comments, suggestions, and encouragement of many people. I would like to thank Barbara Anderson, John Becker, David Bennett, Gerald Braza, Sue Breckenridge, George Briggs, Dick Burgess, Marion Cahoon, Joan Coles, Mary Dadone, Marion Dickman, Michael Dickman, Susan Dickman, Lee Ann Djelkans, Patricia Eisenman, John Endler, Kathy Englebert-Fenton, Betty Fife, John Gardner, Alex Glazer, Paul Hopkins, Steven Johnson, Linda Jara, Peggy Lee, Fred Linker, Trudy McMurrin, Gene Millhouse, Patty Reagan, Karen Reeds, Robert Ruhling, Mary Beth Sahami, Barbara Samuels, Jay Sharp, Gordon Short, Marvin Van Dilla, Sue Wallace, and Roger Williams.

I assume full responsibility for the statements and viewpoints expressed. I also thank Anne Kidd for patient typing and retyping the sometimes-scribbled notes of a first-time author, Anny LeFebvre for drawings, and Sue Wilmoth for editing.

Contents

CHAPTER 6: FOOD AND WELLNESS   179

CHAPTER 7: PHYSICAL FITNESS AND WELLNESS   251

Preface

Some years ago I began writing a book with the idea of explaining nutrition to the lay public. I felt well prepared for the task because I had been teaching the subject to freshman medical students for about 10 years. There has been great popular interest in nutrition—especially diet books—for the past 20 years or so. I had noticed at parties that, if I met new people and told them that I was a biochemist, they would remark that it must be a fascinating subject and walk away as soon as it was polite. But, if I told them I was a nutritionist, I was overwhelmed with questions, and answers, about diet, natural foods, additives, residues, and the dangers of sugar.

There were two things about my questioners that impressed me. First was their great interest in the subject, and second was their ignorance and naiveté about it. I was most appalled, however, by their inability to distinguish between what was sound—from a scientific standpoint—and the most outlandish balderdash, which they had read in some obscure magazine or heard from a friend. For example, I was told in all seriousness that wheat sprouts contain a magic vitamin called chlorophyll that rapidly disappears if the sprouts are not eaten raw. Another time, when I asked a person why he was opposed to eating red meat, he answered, "Because it contains fibers that are harder to digest than meat from fowl or fish." When I mentioned the effect of tenth normal hydrochloric acid ($0.1 N$ HCl) on the structure and digestibility of proteins, he was astounded to hear that the stomach contained an acid.

From the beginning, I had planned not to write just another book on nutrition, in which I told people to eat their vitamins and watch their waistlines. My book would be different! I defined my readers as intelligent people over 35, with little or no scientific background, who really wanted to learn more about managing their diets, but who were bewildered as to what to believe in the multitude of claims and counterclaims they have heard and read about. The conversations I had gave me the lead I was looking for. I came up with the title, *How to Tell Sense From Nonsense in Nutrition*. It was unique. Nothing like it had been written, and it would serve a very valuable function. I would explain the scientific approach to nutritional problems for people who could not tell what was sound from what was unsound.

It was a great idea, and I soon found out that I couldn't accomplish it. There were two major blocks to the objective. Scientists who wish to become knowledgeable on a subject can read reviews on it for summaries and go to the original literature if they wish to examine the data on which conclusions are based. In a practical sense, this direct approach is not open to the public. Laypeople don't have the background, expertise, or time to trace down the scientific basis, or lack of it, for a given statement. To complicate matters still further, what does one do when the experts disagree?

This realization led to the second block. The public is forced to rely on second- and third-hand sources of information. In addition, the public naively expects simple answers to complex questions. To be popular, the popularizers employed by the media are forced to oversimplify; to explain a disease process as though only one factor is involved; and finally, to bring a disease or condition home to the reader by utilizing anecdotal information. The popular press often downplays controversial material that might confuse the public.

What I had accomplished so far was to convince myself that health science popularizers are essential if the public is to stay informed. What I didn't understand for a long time was why the most popular books and magazines that discussed these questions were also the least trustworthy. I looked at them again trying to discover their secret. I found three devices that I believe explain their popularity. They all have an interesting style. They achieve interest partly by including anecdotal stories of the type: "How I Cured Myself of Blackheads Overnite by Taking Vitamin X_1." The implication was strong throughout these articles that, if something worked for the writer or for a client, it would also work for you. A single example sufficed to support a generalization. Secondly, the authors offer the hope that almost any disease can be prevented by dietary means and that, if one is so unfortunate as to come down with a disease anyway, cures are available.

The third device is like sleight of hand. Numerous chapters and articles are written with an antimedical bias. Here the implication is: "Your doctor will probably tell you that this won't work, but that's because he or she has been brainwashed by the American Medical Association." Am I unfair? The net result: Interesting articles on health and disease that are closer to fiction than to science.

Giving up the idea of writing a how-to book, I shortened the title to *Sense and Nonsense in Nutrition*. I wrote along this line for about 6 months when I came to a fork in the road. I had to make a decision between the role of nutrition in maintaining health in distinction to its role in prevention of disease. I chose the former. As a result, the title was lengthened to *Sense and Nonsense in Nutrition and Health*. Although I didn't recognize it at the time, the addition of the word *health* led to a major shift in emphasis. It transformed the book.

In the chapter on prevention of heart disease, for example, I found that, although nutrition was important, other factors, such as smoking, physical activity, and stress management, were also important. A balanced treatment required discussion of these nonnutritional factors. Somewhere in this shift of emphasis, *Sense and Nonsense* became irrelevant, and a new title emerged, *Nutrition, Disease Prevention, and Health*. This title seemed adequate for a time, but as I learned more about other factors that are involved in health maintenance, it seemed that the word *nutrition* in the title still reflected my initial emphasis and glossed over the other factors. This meant either adding exercise and attitude to the title or changing it completely in the direction of a holistic approach.

My final concern was with the word *health* in the title. It is quite ambiguous, and I was, of course, using it as meaning *good health* and not *poor health*. In addition, many people understand health as referring to the body rather than the mind. The relatively new term *wellness* does not suffer from these disadvantages and, in my interpretation, also includes a more positive psychological attitude than the word *health* connotes.

Finally, a word about the title, *Pathways to Wellness*. Most of the ideas and suggestions in the book are not new; neither are they very popular. The majority of the American public goes along its way—overeating, overdrinking, avoiding exercise, watching TV an average of 6 hours a day, popping pep pills for the blahs, and expecting the medical profession to cure any diseases it may have picked up along the way. How much of this behavior is due to ignorance, how much to personal discontent, and how much to the feeling that "it won't happen to me" is anyone's guess.

I think the public's behavior does demonstrate that it will not adopt a healthy lifestyle in order to live longer. In these years of the nuclear arms race, I can understand this attitude. The emphasis in *Pathways to Wellness* is not on longevity—the quantity of life—but on enjoyment—the quality of life. The thesis is frankly hedonistic. It is what I call responsible hedonism. Because hedonism implies a playboy attitude, a person who seeks perpetual fun, a ski-bum, a person into drugs, I qualify my use of the term as *responsible hedonism*. One should enjoy one's work, but if that is not possible, one should at least do it competently and seek enjoyment after hours.

I maintain that if you take responsibility for your own health and wellness, you will enjoy doing whatever you have to do, or like to do, to a greater extent than if you feel that you are a victim of the system, grossly overweight, or an incipient alcoholic, or if you think that walking the dog twice a day is sufficient exercise.

Wellness is not achieved automatically or as a by-product of healthful living. It must be sought by following healthful practices of nutrition and aerobic physical activity, by consciously employing stressor management techniques, and by recognizing the importance of evaluating one's own assumptions and value judgments.

I conceive of health and wellness as an indefinable, general objective. This view is strengthened by the World Health Organizations' definition of health as "a state of complete physical, mental, and social wellbeing, and not merely the absence of disease or infirmity" (p. 1). I submit that this definition of health is unattainable by any sensitive, socially conscious person in the world today, to say nothing of the billions of the underfed, underprivileged, and unfree.

However wellness may be defined or left undefined, it is dependent on at least three interdependent factors, which I refer to as positive attitudes, sound nutrition, and physical fitness (exercise). These three factors do not rest on bedrock but on two other variables that are labeled genetic endowment and environment. As you'll discover, genetic endowment covers a tremendous range of biological variability.

Environmental factors likewise exert a strong, continuous influence on a person's development from the time of conception. These factors interact with the genetic ones in such a complicated fashion that it is often impossible to assign a specific effect to one or the other.

The goal of wellness, however, is more inclusive than the prevention of disease. Wellness, to me, represents a positive orientation, an enjoyment of living over and beyond the absence of medically defined disease, and also over and beyond the satisfactions of stress management. In fact, wellness can be achieved in the presence of severe handicaps arising from hereditary deficiencies, birth accidents, or later disabilities. It would be misleading, however, to deny that normal people have a broader range of options than those who are handicapped.

This book is written for two types of people. The first group is comprised of adults who are interested in maintaining their health and are aware of their various risk factors and their control. Many people in this group with whom I have talked are following a recipe of healthy behavior composed of dos and don'ts that they are applying by rote. Although they may have read widely, they have little or no understanding of the scientific basis behind the recommendations that they are following, or their limitations, but would like to know more about these matters.

Over and above the possibility of increased longevity and prevention of disease, millions have discovered that a fitness lifestyle has added new dimensions to their enjoyment of living. From this perspective, the present interest in health–wellness is not a fad but is an indication that a significant percentage of the public has grasped and is acting in accordance with this observation. It is for these people that this book is written.

The other group includes professionals in the general area of health care: physicians, nurses, exercise physiologists, psychologists, nutritionists, aerobic dance instructors, fitness club managers and instructors, and dieticians—people who are expert in some area of health–wellness but would like a book that integrates their specialty with other aspects of health care.

An author who encourages readers to take responsibility for their lives and to pursue wellness as a goal has the obligation to inform them of some of the problems that they will face in this endeavor and to suggest possible tactics in solving them. The first three chapters take up these questions. The first chapter includes my conception of wellness as a basis for each reader to develop his or her own ideas on the subject. Some of the problems of living in a competitive, materialistic society are mentioned. Chapter 2 discusses the problems associated with acquiring information. Where are sources of reliable information? How do people distinguish the reliable from the unreliable? How do they handle controversial or contradictory information? How do people apply general information to their own situations? These are important questions without simple answers.

The objective of chapter 3 is to provide a platform for developing judgment on what to believe. The importance of recognizing assumptions—one's own as well as those of friends, teachers, authors, and pundits—is emphasized. Is it safe to assume that data obtained from an experiment with rats will apply to humans? Do you require proof to change a habit? Are you aware that generalizations from different types of scientific experiments vary widely in credibility?

Most of us have been brought up to desire certainty in our lives. We are sometimes dismayed when we find that scientific conclusions do not offer as much certainty as we had hoped. Many people give up on science and turn to quacks. People seeking certainty are sitting ducks for quacks. The way scientists deal with uncertainty is suggested as a model for nonscientists to handle this complex situation.

The next group of four chapters takes up the roles of psychological attitude, nutrition, and physical fitness in contributing to wellness. I attempt to show the interrelations of these areas, and I conclude that attitude determines motivation, which in turn strongly affects behavior. We do not act in a vacuum, however. Knowledge also affects specific behaviors. There is a large overlap between behaviors directed towards achieving wellness and those directed towards prevention of certain diseases.

Because there are far more data on the prevention of obesity, high blood pressure, and coronary heart disease than there are on achieving wellness, I discuss risk factors and their control in the prevention of these diseases in chapters 8, 9, and 10. In my view, people who have learned to manage risk factors without becoming hypochondriacs have taken a long step towards wellness.

The final chapter emphasizes the joy and benefits of the quest for wellness. I suggest that, if living can be considered as a game or as play, the feelings of wellness may appear more frequently than though one is consistently serious. It is in this sense that I offer the game of wellness index as a means of checking up on yourself. I suggest that you look it over—preferably rating yourself on a separate sheet of paper before reading the book, and then again afterwards. I agree with the Buddha's view of Nirvana: It is "enjoying life's tensions untensely" (Bahm, 1962, p. 74).

In a few more years, a generation that has been practicing a wellness lifestyle will reach retirement. These people will not settle for mere longevity. They will expect facilities and expertise in medical care, nutrition, and physical activity that will allow them to continue doing what they enjoy. The history of America is a record of progress. What had to be sold to one generation was accepted by the next and demanded by the third. It seems to me that the wellness lifestyle is in the second stage of this triad.

I consider the book as encouraging an exploration both of one's inner self and of how diet and aerobic exercise can positively affect your self-image and your outlook on living. The point of *Pathways to Wellness* is to emphasize that you can alter these factors to increase your chances for wellness and to enhance your enjoyment of life—if you choose to make the effort.

Sherman R. Dickman

Chapter

1

Wellness as an Objective

In the old days Public Health workers did
things for people—cleaning up water
supplies, restaurant food preparation, im-
munization against diseases. These were
effective measures against infective diseases, but now, we are dealing with
chronic diseases, and the results are related to what people do for themselves in
the way of eating, smoking, and exercise.
The goal of Public Health workers is to
get people to do things for themselves.
    Dr. Leona Baumgartner
    (cited in Ubell, 1972, p. 209)

This chapter will help you

- understand why taking personal responsibility for your own health is so important;
- appreciate the short-term and long-term
  benefits of the wellness lifestyle; and
- see yourself as a whole.

Wellness, Behavior, and Feedback

Wellness refers to a feeling, a conscious perception, an awareness by the
whole person that his or her components and processes are not only under
control but working together harmoniously as a unit. These feelings are
intensely personal and may be, at least temporarily, almost independent

1

of the state of the world. A person who desires some degree of wellness needs to understand its relation to behavior. Wellness is associated with behavior through thoughts. The relations of the three can be diagrammed as:

$$\text{WELLNESS} \rightleftharpoons \text{THOUGHTS} \rightleftharpoons \text{BEHAVIOR}$$

From the diagram we can understand that wellness leads to certain kinds or types of behavior and those behaviors, in turn, affect the degree of wellness. Even the most well-meaning person can commit a *faux pas*. Feedback from either inappropriate or appropriate behavior can be immediate and affect wellness to some degree.

Characteristics of Wellness

Wellness, in distinction to happiness, can and needs to be pursued as a conscious objective. It does not occur automatically with most people, and unless it is set up as a desirable objective, it cannot affect behavior in a consistent manner. A person may not be ill (i.e., have a disease), but also may not be well because wellness is primarily an attitude, a response to living. I distinguish wellness from narcissism, which is a preoccupation with the self and with personal desires that may lead to a neglect of interest in others and to ignoring problems beyond skin, family, and job.

A sense of humor—seeing one's activities in perspective—is a frequent trait of a well person. Such people are often socially active and do not let the state of the world get them down.

The condition of wellness is not static. A person does not achieve it and then relax, thinking that the mountain has been climbed and the struggle is over. I suspect that for most people wellness must be won anew each day. Because wellness depends on awareness of self, and awareness is constantly being interrupted by work, by concentration on almost anything but oneself, and by interpersonal relations, it frequently happens that when awareness returns wellness has gone. To regain it requires introspection and analysis of attitudes and actions that may have been responsible for losing it. Wellness is not like a punching bag that returns to a stable, fixed position when it is no longer being struck. Wellness results from a dynamic process.

A person who wants to maintain wellness is superficially acting like a radar apparatus, which is programmed to keep a moving object in the center of its screen. Both objectives require dynamic action. Both utilize feedback systems in accomplishing a goal. In a human, goal setting is much more complicated than the most sophisticated radar. What determines aspirations versus mere survival? A person's past and present activities and responsibilities, as well as how satisfactorily the person evaluates his or her relations to other people and society, are all involved. One reason that a wellness objective is difficult to achieve, but an exciting challenge to undertake, is that we become aware of the consequences of our actions in a context of sometimes conflicting desires. A trivial question like, "Should I eat another piece of pie?" requires a bit of thought beyond the initial desire to indulge oneself in a favorite dessert. The question needs to be related to all the personal factors mentioned above.

Adaptation and Change

It is quite obvious that the human species is unique in its ability to change and utilize the natural environment for its own benefit. These alterations were of relatively small magnitude until the technological revolution. In the last two centuries, however, these changes have become both more numerous and much larger in scope than ever before. Some of the consequences of these changes can be viewed as positive and others as negative. As with many value judgments, one's opinion is often influenced by one's economic stake in the consequences. It is worthy of emphasis to mention that the human species is now adapting to and utilizing manmade environmental factors that are of similar magnitude to some natural ones. The draining of the Zuider Zee and desalting of the soil is one example; building dams that enable the irrigation and cultivation of millions of acres is another.

Two major changes that are generally considered positive in the way people live in industrialized countries are (a) the lessening in the amount of physical (manual) labor required by most workers; and (b) the increases in the amount, quality, and diversity in the kinds of food that are available for most of the population. The decrease in physical work on a broad scale has resulted in a tremendous decrease in energy expenditure *by people*. The health consequences of these two changes have been profound. Overweight/obesity is becoming the norm.

A news item that was meant to be humorous was published a few years ago when Yankee Stadium was being renovated. Based on actual measurements of the average seat size of the fans, the stadium now contains some thousands fewer seats than when it was built approximately 70 years ago. Scientific data confirm that Johnny and Judy Public are significantly larger in midgirth than they were two generations ago. In this same time period, medical science has established that overweight/obesity is a major risk factor for a variety of chronic diseases that appear in middle age and later. Apart from its effect on longevity and the incapacitating effects of these diseases are the premature restrictions overweight/obesity places on pleasurable activities, both physical and mental. These restrictions are discussed in chapter 11.

The recognition of these disabilities and their causes has led health workers to a relatively new concept in public health. This idea is succinctly expressed as "taking personal responsibility for your own health." Avoiding excess fat storage is perhaps the keystone of this message.

There is something new under the sun! The longevity of middle-aged adults has been increasing in the U.S. in recent years. Personal responsibility for health is recognized as an important new factor in this encouraging trend. Personal responsibility for wellness can also increase one's enjoyment of those extra years.

Environmental Consequences of the Technological Revolution

There are two types of environmental factors that affect a person's health. One type of environmental factor includes those over which people can exert personal control if they choose. What and how much one eats and drinks, whether or not one smokes, are examples of this type. Personal habits have been shown to affect susceptibility to chronic diseases like atherosclerosis, hypertension, mid-onset diabetes, and cancer. Because of this relationship, these diseases have become known as the lifestyle diseases because so many of the contributing factors are under an individual's control.

However, the slogan, "taking responsibility for your own health," has implications beyond those that deal with personal habits. Discussing these implications takes us back to other consequences of the technological revolution. These consequences refer to the health effects of toxic products that have been spewed over the countryside of industrialized nations for many decades. The term *health effects* is not restricted to direct effects on human health. The Environmental Protection Agency was established to monitor the effects of widespread human activities on the whole environment. The reason for this broad scope was the recognition that the human species is part of an interdependent ecosystem. At present we do not know enough, and will probably not know enough in the foreseeable future, to make wise environmental decisions based solely on human wants.

The discovery of toxic wastes in many parts of the country has surprised and shocked many people. I consider the establishment of a *superfund* as a joint project of government and industry as a landmark progressive step for the control of toxic products and prevention of contamination of groundwater and aquifers in maintaining the public health. The actions of individual citizens at the local level have also been a prime moving force in initiating both local and national cleanup measures. I applaud those people who recognized a danger and took appropriate steps to publicize it and to end it. We dare not become complacent. It is dangerous to assume that government—federal or local—is routinely taking responsibility for the public's health. In my opinion, living in a democracy requires that citizens participate in decisions affecting the public health. Remember, you are part of the public.

Over 50 years ago, Freud wrote a thought-provoking book called *Civilization and its Discontents* (1930). Its focus was primarily on the psychological problems that arise from people living in cities. Freud arrived at a significant conclusion: The dissatisfactions of civilized peoples often outweigh the satisfactions. He spoke of two inevitable forces: the superior power of nature and the feebleness of our own bodies. In addition, the competition for wealth and influence, as well as other inadequacies of society, result in civilization's contributing to a great deal of the suffering and unhappiness of humans.

Even more basic that these reasons, however, were Freud's propositions that civilization has so restricted the aggressive instinct that we feel frustrated—and beyond that—suffer from a sense of guilt. Freud considered ". . . the sense of guilt as the most important problem in the development of civilization. The price we pay for our advance in civilization is a loss of happiness through the heightening of the sense of guilt" (p. 81). These frustrations lead to chronic anxiety, and most people become neurotic to some degree.

Freud was not very optimistic about the ability of people to overcome life's difficulties. He mentioned three palliative measures that are widely used to decrease suffering, and thereby increase happiness to some extent. The first is to make light of it and to ignore civilization as much as possible. This tactic amounts to following Voltaire's dictum to "cultivate one's garden."

The second measure is to engage in substitute activities that take one's mind off one's troubles for at least some hours a week. Active or passive interests in art, science, or sports accomplish this objective for millions. Developing an expertise in hobbies and crafts, helping others— creativity of any sort—can serve as an excellent diversion from guilt and anxiety.

In his third category, Freud commented on the role of intoxicants. Many people use alcohol or drugs as a convenient form of anesthetic. When things get too bad, they remove themselves from the conflicts and sufferings of their lives. In a brilliant passage, Freud suggested that "there must be substances in the chemistry of our own bodies which have similar effects (to intoxicants) for we know at least one pathological state, mania, in which a condition similar to intoxication arises without the administration of any intoxicating drug" (p. 25). Freud would have been much intrigued by the recent discovery of substances in the brain that act as painkillers and as natural opiates. They are called beta-endorphins, and their concentration in the blood has been found to increase after aerobic exercise (Carr et al., 1981).

The general use of painkilling drugs such as aspirin and tension relievers such as tranquilizers and antidepressants suggests the occurrence of anxiety and guilt in millions of Americans. It is interesting that Freud— and many American physicians—considered anxiety and depression solely as psychological problems. The widespread use of drugs by Americans— from aspirin to heroin—follows logically from this viewpoint.

Mind and Body

Freud's analysis of the problems that arise from people living together in civilized societies—and his description of people's attempts to deal with their unhappiness and guilt—is brilliant as far as it goes. In my reading of Freud, I have the distinct impression that he not only assumed that mind and body were separate entities but also attributed a person's mental health to the mind and ignored any contribution from the body or soma. Sulloway (1979) pointed out that Freud's original hypothesis concerning the origin of neuroses included a contribution from the soma, but after 1926 the hypothesis was modified and became based exclusively on phychic origins. Freud's long-term objective was to develop a science of the mind. In accomplishing this objective, he became trapped by his own genius and neglected the interplay between mind and body in affecting a person's psychological attitude.

The mind–body dichotomy is a prime example of a type of false dualism that has pervaded Western thought for centuries, and these assumptions have resulted in some serious, inaccurate analyses of the human condition. A holistic view of humans does not assume dualities. It emphasizes the unity of human beings and the interconnectedness and interdependencies of our various systems on each other.

For thousands of years, Eastern philosophers have advocated the unity of the individual—in modern terms, of the interactions between the physical entities, muscles, and other organs and the nervous system. These views are readily compatible with recent developments in science. The dualism of matter and energy was transcended by Einstein in the theory of relativity; and relativity now is accepted as a confirmed theory. The false dualism of mind and body likewise is now being recognized by many psychologists. Biological relativity suggests that mind and body are two aspects of the human life-force. They are so interconnected that one cannot be affected without affecting the other. Wellness includes recognizing this interplay among the systems: nervous, endocrine, and muscular. In addition, a well person has learned how to get these systems to work in unison.

Perhaps the dominant, nonhazardous, external factor in the application of technology during the past hundred years has been the gradual replacement of human energy by machines in accomplishing the hard physical labor of the world. This development has been extolled as progress in the popular press, and this conclusion has been endorsed by a public that has gained many material advantages from it. All human communities, including the medical profession, however, have been slow to realize the subtle, long-term effects of the machine age on the human organism.

Kraus and Raab (1961) in *Hypokinetic Disease* addressed directly the effects of physical activity. Half of the book is devoted to the effects of lack of exercise on the heart. In addition, they included obesity, back pain, and orthopedic disabilities such as muscle spasms, tenderness, muscle weakness, and stiffness in the list of hypokinetic diseases.

These authors point out that hard physical labor was the common lot of the human race as it evolved through the ages. As a result, we are not just adapted to physical activity, we require it for health. Modern humans may think that vigorous aerobic physical activity has been outmoded through the introduction of labor-saving devices, but we cannot escape from our evolutionary past. This fact remained hidden as long as the average life span was about 50 years. Now that it is over 70 in developed countries, a new conclusion has become obvious. Long-term wellness demands a certain minimum amount of regular aerobic activity.

It is significant that Kraus and Raab included certain emotional conditions in the group of hypokinetic diseases. Not many studies had been carried out in 1960 on the relationship between physical activity and emotional stability. They cited two early researchers in this area. Mary Alexander (1956) wrote *The Relationship Between the Muscular Fitness of the Well-Adjusted Child and the Non-Well-Adjusted Child*. She found a correlation between fitness and adjustment. Hawkins (1956) came to similar conclusions in *Exercise and Emotional Stability*.

Kraus and Raab (1961) reproduced some of Appleton's (1949) data on the relationship between fitness of West Point cadets and discharges from the Academy for psychiatric reasons. There were no discharges from the highest fitness group, whereas 13% of the lowest fitness group were discharged. In my opinion, the conclusions of Kraus and Raab support those espoused by Hindu philosophy for thousands of years. Swami (1946) reviewed the role of physical activity by Hindus in the attainment of emotional stability.

Another general approach to the diseases of civilization has been taken by Burkitt and Trowell (1975) in *Refined Carbohydrate Foods and Disease*. They observed that the Bantu who lived in South African villages and cities and had adopted the diets of Caucasians were subject to the same diseases as the whites, whereas Bantus who lived their traditional lifestyle and ate their traditional diets were not. These diseases include heart disease, stroke, hypertension, diabetes, diverticulosis, constipation, appendicitis, hiatus hernia, and certain types of cancer. They attributed this group of diseases to the lack of dietary fiber in the food of those who consumed diets high in highly processed products. No mention of differences in physical activity or differences of psychological stressors between the two groups was included. The book makes a case for lack of dietary fiber acting as a primary factor in inducing the diseases mentioned above. The book stresses the body approach to disease.

Striving to Be Whole

The wellness approach to the human condition embodies a holistic view of humans. It suggests that there are other alternatives to deal with the dissatisfactions of civilization than those mentioned by Freud, or the wholesale prescribing of tranquilizers by physicians. One of these alternatives is a properly designed exercise program for each person. A number of scientists (Jacobson, 1938; Schultz & Luthe, 1959; Whatmore & Kohli, 1974; Wolpe, 1973) have arrived at a common conclusion of the greatest importance. "This is the fact that anxiety cannot exist in the presence of deep muscle relaxation" (Gaarder & Montgomery, 1981, p. 19). Thus it appears that anxiety can be treated by methods that reduce muscle tension. I mention this development as an example of what holistic science can accomplish. These exciting research results suggest the possibility that exercise may actually abolish anxiety and its accompanying unhappiness rather than merely providing a diversion from them.

Since Freud wrote, chronic diseases have become the major killers and disablers of middle-aged and elderly Americans. Are unwell habits widespread because people are so distraught by the rat race and by their unsatisfactory relations with friends and family that they attempt to forget their problems in self-damaging behavior and in spectator-type amusements as Freud speculated many years ago? Are urban dwellers living longer but enjoying it less?

The Eastern holy man who emphasized meditation and awareness gave up family and work so that he could devote himself full-time to establishing his unity with nature. These people are respected for their wisdom, and it is considered a duty for ordinary people to give them food and money. Here in the West, we live by a different code. Our concept of wellness does not suggest withdrawal from everyday affairs. Rather, it is to engage in them but not to let the system get us down. Achieving serenity under these conditions is probably much more difficult than the objective of an Eastern holy man.

Eastern ideas are beginning to permeate Western culture. The wellness idea, for example, is an Eastern holistic conception camouflaged as a Western term. In its adoption by the West, wellness has already begun to change in meaning and interpretation. Its evolution will continue, and it would be presumptuous of me to try to set bounds to it or to suggest the direction it should take.

My general approach in the book has been not to lecture or tell people what to do, but to summarize specific topics as well as I am able with the idea that mature readers can make their own decisions about what activities they choose to engage in and risks they choose to take. There are some environmental factors and dangers, however, which, in the interest of the public, require governmental regulation. In discussing these issues, I depart from objectivity and encourage readers to engage in political and social activism of some sort. I feel deeply that we as individuals are limited in what we can do in maintaining a healthy environment and in working towards world peace. As citizens, however, we can accomplish a great deal by becoming informed and uniting our efforts.

Chapter

2

Problems With Interpreting Wellness Information

Give me a fish and I can eat today,
Teach me to fish and I can eat forever.
Native American Proverb

This chapter will help you

- recognize and control risk factors;
- formulate wellness goals; and
- evaluate media reports on health.

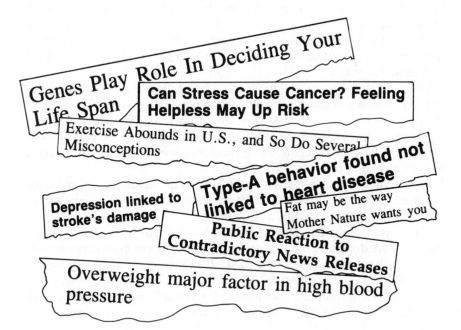

Genes Play Role In Deciding Your Life Span

Can Stress Cause Cancer? Feeling Helpless May Up Risk

Exercise Abounds in U.S., and So Do Several Misconceptions

Depression linked to stroke's damage

Type-A behavior found not linked to heart disease

Fat may be the way Mother Nature wants you

Public Reaction to Contradictory News Releases

Overweight major factor in high blood pressure

These eight headlines have contributed to the dilemma in which millions of Americans and other inhabitants of developed countries have found themselves in recent years. There is no doubt that people are interested in health matters and are aware that *risk factors* play an important role in the induction of certain diseases as well as in their prevention. To satisfy this interest, the media publicizes the results of health-related research as soon as it is published in the scientific press or is presented at scientific meetings. As the headlines demonstrate, the press releases are often inconsistent or confusing.

The public, however, has not been trained to evaluate controversial information and claims. As a result, many people have become confused and do not know what to believe on questions relating to health, nutrition, and fitness. The open reporting of health-related news items, which is one of the advantages and prerogatives of a free press, has had an unsettling and disturbing effect on the public it is supposed to benefit. Many people have turned to quacks and charlatans as sources of information because these people provide definite, simple answers to complicated medical questions. Other people have decided to ignore the whole area.

Multifactorial Diseases— Monofactorial Reporting

The risk factor concept that was developed for heart disease in the 1950s began a new phase in the history of medicine. Up to that point, diseases were considered to have a single cause; the vitamin deficiency diseases mentioned in the previous chapter, bacterial infections, most endocrine diseases like juvenile diabetes, gigantism, and so on—each was ascribed to a single agent.

The sex difference and the time lag set heart disease apart from the beginning. It attacked males preferentially to females, and although the first signs of the disease appeared in young men 18–25, the most common age for an unmistakable heart attack to occur was in the 40–50 year bracket. The 20- to 30-year lag allowed considerable leeway for environmental factors to play a role.

More than one factor was assumed early in the epidemiological investigations. Diet was implicated from the start, and hypertension, smoking, and a heart condition known as *left ventricular hypertrophy* (enlargement of the left ventricle of the heart) were soon added. In the past 35 years dozens of other possible risk factors have been investigated, and a few have been added to the list. (Risk factors for heart disease are discussed in detail in chapter 10.)

The end result has been that, although the public has heard about risk factors for heart disease, most people have but a vague understanding of how these factors relate to one another in the origin and development of the disease. Are some more important than the others? Does a person have to control them all in order to stay healthy?

I also want to mention that other chronic, noninfectious diseases like certain forms of cancer, mid-onset diabetes, hypertension, and obesity have been added to the list of multifactorial diseases. A new type of statistics has been developed to handle the complicated mathematics of analyzing the dose-response relationship between variations in individual factors and the incidence of a disease.

This successful approach—and I want to emphasize that in a number of diseases it has been very successful—has raised a very tough problem for health science popularizers. How can one deal with complexity and still keep an article interesting? The usual solution has been to oversimplify the conclusions of many investigations in favor of emphasizing one factor at a time. The headlines at the beginning of this chapter illustrate the point.

In this book I plan not to take the road of oversimplification. In the chapters on multifactorial diseases, I will discuss each risk factor individually, but in the summary I will attempt to show how the factors may interact and increase the risk. Living is a risky business, and learning to recognize and control risk factors can be an interesting and important part of reducing the risk.

Another aspect of epidemiological research that I believe has not been sufficiently emphasized to the public is that the results are statistical; the conclusions do not apply to individuals. Many persons would like an assurance that, if they stop smoking, eat less fat, and adopt a healthy lifestyle, they will live longer, achieve inner peace, and so forth. No such assurance can be given, although for impact, articles imply that the reader will personally benefit. Children's behavior is often controlled by their parents with promises and rewards for being good. Is it necessary to beguile American adults in the same fashion?

Diet and Disease: Overpublicized?

For the past 30 years diet has often been branded as the major cause of heart attacks—the biggest killer disease in the U.S. In recent years the influence of diet on the incidence of certain types of cancer has also been publicized. Diet has been implicated as the causative factor in a variety of other diseases ranging from hypoglycemia at one extreme to diabetes at the other. A number of books linking diet to arthritis and to hyperactivity in children have sold well. I could produce a much longer list of supposedly diet-related diseases, but I think the ones mentioned are sufficient to make the point.

In my view, an unhealthy diet as the major causative factor of many diseases has been overemphasized to the public by the media and occasionally by scientific organizations that should know better. This opinion is reinforced by many books and magazines dealing with nutrition and disease. In this connection, *Dietary Goals for the U.S.*, published by the U.S. Senate Select Committee (1977), has given many people the impression that if they eat right they will remain healthy. This conclusion is not only an erroneous oversimplification, it is also dangerous. I consider it dangerous because it undervalues the roles of exercise and attitude in weight control and in maintaining wellness. The dietary goals are OK, but standing alone they overemphasize the role of nutrition in disease prevention.

In addition, I think that the emphasis on prevention of disease such as heart disease or cancer when one is old misses the mark. Most healthy young people whom I have talked to find it hard to imagine themselves aged, sick, and infirm. The illusion that "it can't happen to me" is strong, and it prevents them from overcoming their unhealthy habits. They keep postponing their change in lifestyle or forget about it until middle age—when it may be too late.

Wellness and Enjoying Life

Americans do need wellness goals. They should include exercise goals and attitude goals as well as dietary ones. Furthermore, I suggest that all these goals stress the advantages of a healthy lifestyle on a short-term basis. I make the basic assumption that, in general, people who keep themselves fit enjoy their lives more than those who don't. There are many individuals who, by themselves or as part of an experimental group, provide evidence that adopting a healthy lifestyle results in an increase in the enjoyment of life, as well as retaining the long-term benefits. In my opinion, it is these conclusions that should be emphasized to the public. Eating—but not overeating—a nutritious diet would, of course, be included in this publicity. Don't consider a healthy lifestyle as part of an old-age pension that will pay off when you retire. The benefits start immediately, and you should feel them in a month or two. After that, enjoyment is compounded.

The growing holistic health movement in the U.S. stresses the unity of the individual, but unfortunately much of the holistic literature that I have read contains an antiscientific bias. It has borrowed too much from Eastern philosophy that is nonanalytical, and not enough from the Western scientific tradition that is strong in analysis and weak in integration, especially as applied to people. There is no a priori reason why the two viewpoints cannot be unified while recognizing the limitations of each. This synthesis is one objective of this book.

The Safety of the American Food Supply

The American food supply has been attacked in a variety of ways. In *The Taste of America*, Hess and Hess (1977) claim that mass production methods have decreased the taste quality of many of our foods. Or consider this quotation from Adelle Davis' popular book, *Let's Get Well* (1965). She writes, "When possible, therefore, obtain medically certified raw milk and butter; fertile eggs, poultry grown on the ground rather than on wire; pressed vegetable oils; fresh, stone-ground flours and corn meal; and fruits and vegetables produced on humus-rich soils without chemical fertilizers or poison sprays" (p. 405). This one statement raises suspicions about the safety of almost the entire American food supply.

The possible dangers of certain food additives have also been widely publicized. Many of them, such as nitrites, BHT (butylated hydroxytoluene), and even fluoride—which is added to many municipal water supplies—have been branded as carcinogens. These claims worry many people.

In an effort to allay the public's anxiety over food additives, the Food and Drug Administration (FDA) has publicized its role as the monitor of the safety of the American food supply. The information about food additives as well as other nutritional facts has been increased on the labels of packaged foods. As an example, consider the list of ingredients in a widely used nondairy coffee whitener (Michael Lewis Co.): "Corn syrup solids, partially hydrogenated vegetable oils (may contain one or more of the following: coconut oil, cottonseed oil, soybean oil, palm kernel oil, palm oil or safflower oil), lactose, sodium caseinate, dipotassium phosphate, sodium silicoaluminate, artificial colors, mono- and diglycerides, lecithin, BHA, and propyl gallate, and citric acid to preserve freshness of oil, and artificial flavor."

My point in reproducing this long list is not to criticize the FDA. I think that informative labeling is a step in the right direction. But I also think that not only are these names unintelligible to most people but also the technical terms put off and frighten them. The lay public has no idea why their coffee whitener has so many constituents, what their functions are, and whether some may act as carcinogens. A list of ingredients such as this has value only insofar as it can be understood and applied by the audience to which it is addressed.

These examples illustrate the problems the public faces: Contradictory information published by the media, authoritarian statements by well-known authors, and a large volume of technical information that is unintelligible to most people because they do not possess a sufficient scientific background to understand it.

The Role of Controversy in Scientific Research

Many nonscientists believe that the progress of science is calm, smooth, and sure. It isn't. The controversies that appear in the press are merely the cone of the volcano. As I'll mention more fully in the next chapter, science progresses by means of testable hypotheses. The process of testing involves challenging the reproducibility of experimental results, noting differences in the interpretation of results, and, finally, checking the validity of conclusions by inventing new testable hypotheses. Controversy can, and usually does, appear at every stage in the process of discovering new knowledge. For example, controversy has played an essential role in increasing knowledge on the development of atherosclerosis. In the past 20 years, an international research effort has pared the number of suggested risk factors from several hundred to less than 10 in 1986. During this entire period, controversy served as the hone that continuously sharpened the cutting edge of the research effort. To emphasize this point, I'll cite an example of a controversy and mention how it might be publicized in the press.

The following title is from *Medical Tribune* (Jan. 3, 1979), a newspaper that summarizes recent advances in medicine for physicians and medical students: "Do lowered lipids, diet really reduce coronary risk? Has the reduction of dietary cholesterol intake been proven an effective technique for combatting heart disease?" (p. 3). These questions were debated at a meeting of the American Heart Association Conference on coronary risk factors.

As reported in the article, Dr. Ahrens, Professor of Medicine at Rockefeller University, challenged the lipid hypothesis. He argued that "while it is generally acknowledged that risk increases with higher cholesterol levels, it's never been really proven that by lowering the cholesterol level we also reduce risk."

Dr. William Castelli, Director of Laboratories for the Framingham Heart Study, was in sharp opposition. "Every study that has used diet to lower lipids has lowered heart disease. Every aspect of the atherosclerotic lesion is reversible" and so, on they went.

This example of strong disagreement between expert scientists in the field of heart disease is not unusual. On the contrary, controversy among health and nutrition scientists is common. It has occurred for many years and undoubtedly will continue for many more. In fact, I consider rational controversy to be healthy. Sharp critique tightens logic and exposes weak assumptions in the body of an argument.

Reporting on Science for the Public

A reporter attending the conference on Diet and Heart Disease that I mentioned above could not include many facts in his article. There were few that were acceptable to both sides of the argument. About all that a competent reporter could do would be to summarize the controversial points and the reasoning behind each scientist's position.

But suppose a reporter attends a lecture or a press conference called by only one expert? There is generally no exchange of views under these conditions, and the reporter can only summarize the one side that has been presented. On some other day, at some other place, another expert may present his or her views, which may be diametrically opposed to those of the first. These, too, are duly reported. Laypeople have trouble dealing with publicity announcements. They have no basis for drawing sound conclusions from scientific controversies or from contradictory claims. They are stopped at the very beginning: The facts are not at their disposal.

Here we arrive at a crucial distinction between the situation of the scientist and that of the nonscientific public. *The basic facts on nutrition and health are not readily available to most people.* This restriction is not due to any plot or conspiracy to keep the public uninformed. People have neither been trained nor do they have the time or interest to read the original literature, seek out the facts, and draw their own conclusions. Actually, the information is available for anyone who wants to read it.

The situation leads to the second distinction between the scientist and the public. The reviews and summarizing articles on nutrition and health that are written for the layperson may or may not have been written by an expert. In a country with a free press, there is no restriction on who can or cannot write books or articles. Publishers, who make the decisions on what they publish, often decide not on the basis of the author's expertise but on the basis of an article's interest to an audience and whether it conforms to the position of the publication. This situation, which is not likely to change, leads to the public's being exposed to a continuing stream of misinformation.

The writing of popular articles on nutrition and health involves summarizing the scientific literature in terms that the public can understand. This important endeavor is, at best, difficult, and at worst, impossible. I say impossible, because the public seems to want or is thought to want by popularizers and publishers definite conclusions about whatever subject is being covered. People expect to have learned facts from having read an article. Popularizers of science satisfy this desire by sometimes providing conclusions when none are warranted. Popularizers of nutrition apparently believe that the public would be confused if both sides of a question were presented, and so, many articles and talks contain presifted facts that lead to a foregone conclusion. Many people, after reading a well-written article of this type, are unaware that they have been duped.

J.I. Rodale maintained to the end of his life that massive doses of vitamin E would prevent heart attacks. In reading his book *Your Diet and Your Heart* (1970), one would never guess that many careful experiments had been performed to check the claim (of Dr. Shute) and that the results were uniformly negative. Dr. Shute was so convinced of the soundness of the vitamin E hypothesis that he refused to conduct controlled experiments because they would be unethical.

Scientists Have Learned to Live With Uncertainty

The research areas of individual scientists usually cover a very small portion of a particular specialty. To keep up with their general fields, scientists must read the literature. In accomplishing this objective, they have a number of options. If they have sufficient interest and expertise, they can go to the original literature, look at the data, and draw their own conclusions. As another alternative, they can read one or more reviews of a subject, each written by an expert. They can also refer to advanced monographs, symposia summaries, and other books for additional information. An easy and popular method for a scientist to keep up with a field is to attend meetings and talk with other scientists who are experts in it. But in developing areas of research, none of these sources of information may give them a definite, conclusive answer.

Scientists are as opinionated on technical matters as artists on art, or stockbrokers on the meaning of the latest trend in the market. But scientists—as well as many other trained experts—have learned to withhold judgment on a controversial topic until the data are all in, which means until there are sufficient experimental data to conclusively favor one generalization or conclusion over the alternatives. In some instances, this process may take years. No matter what their beliefs outside of their scientific specialty, in their field competent scientists have learned to live with uncertainty.

The Public Also Needs to Learn to Live With Uncertainty

A serious difficulty stems from the public's belief that experts demonstrate that they really are experts by presenting their material in an authoritarian manner. How else can one explain the widespread popularity of such authors as Adelle Davis, David Reuben, or Robert Atkins? In the writings of these authors, the line between authority, dogmatism, and bias is frequently obscured. A fact is stated as either right or wrong, a conclusion as true or false.

In this connection, an examination of the three words—author, authority, and authoritarian—is interesting. A person demonstrates that he or she is an authority by becoming an author and writing in an authoritarian style.

The distinction between authoritarian and authoritative helps illustrate my point. Authoritarian writers demand submission to authority. Their style is very positive. Situations are summarized as true or false; complicated questions are oversimplified as in the quotation from Adelle Davis. The scientific credibility of such authors is low because their subjectivity is high. I have the impression from some books—names available on request—that the author has formed an opinion in advance, collected references that support this conclusion, and ignored those that do not support it.

Authoritative writers, in contrast, are consciously as objective as possible. They discuss the pros and cons of each side dispassionately. Their credibility is high because, with their help, a reader can evaluate the different sides of a complicated argument.

To make matters worse, our educational system is based on authority and authoritarianism. A good student is often defined as one who learns the facts set before him or her and who can manipulate them to draw conclusions in a logical fashion. A person who has not had experience in distinguishing facts from evidence, evaluating facts, and establishing to what extent a hypothesis is proved, is a sitting duck for a quack, no matter how adept the person may be at drawing logical inferences from the accepted facts he or she may be given. It is for these reasons that I have come to the conclusion that the public is trapped. The odds are high against anyone not trained in health and nutrition becoming accurately knowledgeable by reading the popular literature.

Because the results of scientific research are being popularized by the news media almost immediately after publication in scientific journals, people need to adopt the attitude of the scientist towards new information—mull it over, think about it, discuss it with others, do anything they want with it, *but don't believe it.* Don't accept it as reliable until it has been checked and rechecked by other competent scientists. Even then, allow about a 1% chance that it might be disproved.

Patient, logical people may choose to wait for a consensus among the scientists, even though that may take years. Such people may be dead before anyone can say, "The facts on heart diseases are. . . ." Others may ignore the whole area and pay no attention to controversial questions such as the relation of diet to heart disease. Some people may prefer one side of the question to the other and follow a diet or regimen as though that conclusion were proved.

Fortunately, there are still other alternatives. One is somehow to find a sound book or source of information on the subject. A number of these are listed at the end of the chapter. A difficulty with books is that they may provide accurate information at the time they were written, but they soon become outdated. A book is like a floating signpost in a river. The sandbar it points to was 10 miles upstream.

Another alternative is to read this book. It attempts to be authoritative rather than authoritarian. My plan is to introduce you to some of the controversies in the area of health and nutrition by presenting not just a consensus and suggesting that you follow it but both sides and the reasoning and assumptions behind each position. It assumes a level of interest and sophistication in the reader that will make the usual type of oversimplification unnecessary. It is written for an audience who will be intrigued, and possibly amused as well, when it sees how widely the experts disagree, as the example above on diet and heart disease illustrates.

I recognize that this book contains blind spots and will become outdated as rapidly as any other. I hope, however, that the approach used here will catch on and be improved on by other authors so that the public interest may continue to be served.

Personal Responsibility: The Challenge to the Individual

Taking personal responsibility for your own health and wellness in the latter half of the twentieth century and beyond has two aspects. The first is acquiring accurate information, and the other is putting it into practice in your own life. Action without knowledge is usually futile if not dangerous, but knowledge without action is sterile.

In our free society there is almost too much information out there. I am referring to the information explosion that comes from scientific research and the media's attempts to publicize the latest results to an interested public. In my view, people have a right to know—they paid for the research, and much of it has the objective of helping them to live healthier, longer lives. Yet, along with summaries of the latest research from prestigious institutions are other accounts of research that was poorly planned and improperly executed. How does a nonscientist distinguish one from the other? One of my main objectives is to help you make such distinctions.

Although this book is not limited to nutrition, I purposely used many nutritional examples in this chapter to give it a focus and to demonstrate how complicated and controversial the subject appears to be. In later chapters I will also review the subjects of stress, weight control, and exercise. I can tell you now that they will not be any simpler. An author covering this wide a range of subjects for laypeople has two general alternatives in how he plans to treat the material. The most popular method is to summarize the present knowledge in each subject as accurately as possible. In this approach authors use their expertise in arriving at a fair summary of the subject and presenting it as simply as possible. Readers of this type of book are not usually informed of how the information was obtained, how definite the conclusions are, or to what qualifications they are subject. Later, I will mention a number of recent books that accomplish this objective well.

In contrast, this book will attempt to go behind the scenes and will discuss how knowledge is generated in scientific research, how knowledge is evaluated, and how conclusions may become a topic of stringent debate due to lack of consensus. The objective is to help you, the reader, draw your own conclusions and to encourage you to put them into practice. If the book has a message, it is that wellness is an ideal well worth pursuing. The whole book amounts to a challenge to go for it!

The Challenge to Act

It is my impression that most humans in industrialized countries are unwell to some extent. For evidence in support of this conclusion, I offer all those who engage in self-destructive activities: the overweight, the smokers, the heavy drinkers, the Type A personalities, compulsive overachievers, and others. The author of a book on wellness is faced with a dilemma. How can he encourage readers to take up and participate in activities that are not familiar to them, in the hope of attaining a state of well-being that they have never experienced—at least as adults? I respect and admire those who accept my suggestions as a challenge. They are engaged in nothing less than an act of faith. They are heirs to Columbus, setting forth on uncharted seas into an unknown universe. I feel lucky to be included in their company.

In the next chapter I'll discuss the degrees of certainty that one can place in different kinds of experimental data. Some types of research, by their very nature, cannot furnish results that provide a high degree of reliability.

The answers to many questions cannot be proved. Even proved conclusions are modified by time, as more is discovered about their connections to other aspects of the system of which they are a part. The wise person learns to accept the uncertainties of conclusions. Modifications of the diet—or other personal activity—should be approached cautiously with these reservations in mind.

Summary

This chapter has addressed the questions of belief and decision making. Whom can we trust to give us sound information on health questions? On what basis do we decide whom to believe? Besides these questions, we are also faced with making a decision between contradictory claims. How do we decide when we are not too familiar with the subject?

Most of us were raised to distinguish between two alternatives. We are being presented with three, four, or more risk factors for a number of diseases. Complexity has replaced simplicity. We are confused. The risk factor concept has thrown certainty out the window. Everyone is at risk to some extent. We need to adopt the attitude of many professionals who play the odds. They have learned to live with uncertainty.

The risk concept has also publicized the fact that many risk factors are under an individual's control. It is now widely recognized that each person needs to accept responsibility for his or her own health—like it or not. Friends and physicians may advise, but in the final analysis, it is we who must live with consequences of our own behavior. How can we learn these skills before it is too late?

Appendix A
Quotations to Be
Evaluated for Soundness

I have two objectives in listing these nine quotations on sugar. The first is to demonstrate that there is no correlation between soundness and the number of sources an author may cite. Secondly, contradictory statements such as these are common in the nutrition literature with the exception of #4, which is anecdotal. There is little or no basis for choice unless you know a great deal about nutrition.

1. Davis (1965): "Persons suffering from atherosclerosis often have a particularly high intake of refined sugar" (p. 57). Author cites two sources.
2. Deutsch (1976): "It is important to distinguish between the genuine scientific concerns and the irrational condemnation of sugar as poisonous, which it is not" (p. 151). Author cites no sources.
3. Wurtman (1979): "There is, however, nothing inherently dangerous about sugar despite the claims of some people who write books saying that it causes psychiatric problems" (p. 38). Author cites two sources.
4. Solomon (1976): "12% of the people who see me do not handle carbohydrates properly. You might complain about being excessively tired, having a fast-racing heart, sweating, feeling weak and anxious, and 'not thinking straight' after eating carbohydrates—especially sugar, cookies, candy, cakes, soda pop, and ice cream. The more you gobble the more you want—and the worse you feel. I call people with these symptoms, 'Carboholics' " (p. 95). Author cites no sources.
5. Donsbach (1976): "One of the little-known deleterious effects of refined sugar is its effect on protein digestion. Sugar, depending on its concentration, inhibits or retards the action of proteolytic enzymes. Sweet foods (such as desserts) should not be eaten at the same time as protein foods" (p. 64). Author cites no sources.
6. Atkins (1977) "Sugar appears to be a bigger cause of heart disease than either cholesterol or fat" (p. 248). Author cites no sources.
7. Atkins (1977) "Refined carbohydrates are responsible for higher insulin levels, and insulin causes increased amounts of gastric acids and enzymes" (p. 263). Author cites two sources.
8. Hoffer (1977): "Junk food is any food adulterated with sucrose, starch, or white flour" (p. 85). Author cites no sources.
9. Dickman (in chapter 6 of this book): "I am not one of those who consider sugar and sweeteners as poisons or as contributing directly to heart disease, cancer, and diabetes . . . Sugar sweeteners [,however,] do lower nutrient density of the diet . . . [They increase] the risk of becoming obese" (p. 196). Author cites no sources.

Chapter

3

Science, Certainty, and Wellness

The essence of knowledge is, having acquired it, to apply it.
Confucius

The essence of incomplete knowledge is, being aware of it, to apply it cautiously.
S.R. Dickman

This chapter will help you

- understand the importance of assumptions and value judgments as they affect human behavior;
- realize that scientific knowledge has limitations—it does not offer certainty;
- become aware that research conclusions in health sciences vary in their degree of credibility; and
- appreciate that government policies on public health questions include political and economic considerations as well as scientific ones.

What has science to do with wellness? Why should anyone concerned with wellness read a chapter with *science* and *certainty* in the title? Why would an author expect his readers to be interested in this subject? My objective in this chapter is to demonstrate that the way scientists think can be used as a model by anyone: artist, stockbroker, or housewife. You may think this claim rather preposterous. My justification for making it is that scientists are forced by their peers to conform to four general rules. These four rules are: to reason logically, to become aware of assumptions, to allow one's work to be subject to criticism by one's peers, and to be scrupulously honest. Conforming to this standard by a scientist is not easy, even with peer pressure as the motivating force. Yet this type of behavior is part of my description of how well persons think and act. They think and act this way voluntarily. Here, I will compare the thought processes of scientists to those of other intelligent people.

The Role of Assumptions

The thinking processes of scientists and intelligent members of the public are amazingly similar. This important fact is obscured by the jargon of scientific specialties and the use of mathematics by scientists as a special language for handling relationships. One reason for the similarity is that everyone, including both scientists and the lay public, utilizes assumptions. Most educated people today, no matter what their backgrounds, assume that nature is regular and not capricious, and that there will be oxygen in their next breath. Scientists assume that they can learn more about nature by carrying out experiments. Readers of this book assume that they can increase their degree of wellness by working at it.

One important characteristic of scientific assumptions is their consistency. The laws of thermodynamics are thought to apply to every process on this earth without exception. Occasionally a biologist will publish a paper in which the claim is made that either the First Law or the Second Law does not hold. This is a serious claim because, if exceptions occurred in biological systems, the consequences would be most profound. For example, some years ago a book was published with the provocative title, *Calories Don't Count* (Taller, 1961). It created quite a stir and became a best-seller. The thesis was that on a high-unsaturated fat diet people could continue to overeat and yet lose weight. This idea is contradictory to the First Law of thermodynamics and thus, if correct, would have upset most of the postulates in chemistry and physics. It turned out that the diet decreased appetite, and weight loss could be explained without invalidating thermodynamics.

Inconsistent assumptions are also a threat to wellness. Assumptions are like hidden springs that feed into a lake. If one of them is wrong, invalid, or inconsistent with another, the effects are like a single poisoned spring that contaminates the whole lake. All of a person's thinking is influenced by an inconsistent assumption, and his or her health and wellness can be adversely affected by it. For example, a person who believes (assumes) that blacks are inferior to whites may have no choice but to be treated by a black physician in an emergency room after an accident.

Because of his or her prejudice, the person may ignore the advice of the doctor and suffer serious consequences.

Rigidity of belief is not conducive to good science or wellness, for often the rigidity stems from one or more untested, unconscious assumptions. I am not espousing an antiassumption position. In my view, assumptions are as necessary in daily living as they are in science. I do advocate, however, that well persons become aware of their assumptions, in both general and specific situations. If people examined their mistakes in judgment, they would be surprised to note how many of these errors came about because of an invalid assumption.

The scientific literature is filled with hypotheses and speculations based on new and original experiments. Many scientific papers present the assumptions as well as the results and conclusions of the author(s) to other specialists for criticisms and comments. The well person acts similarly. In discussing general topics with friends, assumptions should be discussed as openly and critically as the accuracy of facts. Awareness of one's assumptions helps keep the road of learning free from rocky detours and dead ends. Continual learning is essential for the maintenance of wellness. I hope that readers will understand that hopes for certainty in health matters are assumptions that are inconsistent with those of science. A path to wellness will be blocked until this inconsistency is resolved.

Like it or not, we are living in an age when science and technology affect most aspects of our lives. Just as a matter of self-defense, nonscientists should know something about how science works. Ignorance of the principles of science weakens the foundation on which a wellness program can be built. Everyone should realize the variations in the degree of certainty furnished by various types of scientific experiments. Everyone should be aware of the role of probability in dealing with cause and effect. To make these topics concrete, this chapter will discuss the importance of assumptions in nutritional research by the use of examples. In addition, I will show how the degree of certainty of nutritional conclusions varies with the type of experiment.

There is a twofold reason for using examples from nutritional research in explaining the relations of assumptions, facts, hypotheses, and the degree of certainty of conclusions in scientific research. The first is that the role of nutrition as a causative factor in a number of diseases has been probed more deeply than any other single variable. Secondly, by focusing on one important area such as nutrition, I can emphasize similarities and differences among different types of research protocols. My hope is that, after this much exposure to a single area, you will acquire a better idea of how science works than if I chose examples from a variety of science specialties.

Should you modify your diet to decrease its saturated fat content when the experiments on heart disease only provide a degree of credibility of 50% for this conclusion? What additional information is needed to answer this question? Your life may depend on what answer you accept.

Some wellness advocates assert that the maintenance of wellness requires an ongoing awareness and accurate assessment of the external world. I am suggesting that a critical assessment of your internal world—your logic, your value judgments, and your assumptions—is equally essential. Familiarity with the principles of scientific reasoning will be helpful in your wellness endeavors.

For these reasons, I am introducing this chapter with a list of my own assumptions and value judgments in the field of nutrition and health. Reading these will give you some idea of what kind of person I am and what you may expect in terms of specific biases and overall viewpoint in the chapters to follow. In addition, you should find hints that may help you to increase your own wellness.

Some Assumptions and Value Judgments of S.R. Dickman
(in no particular order)

1. That the primary motive of the food industry is profit. Any innovations, benefits, or health-promoting effects to the public are the results of competition for the consumer's dollars.

2. That, except in cases of outright malnutrition (undernutrition), psychological factors are as important as nutritional ones as causative factors of many so-called "nutritional diseases."

3. That aerobic physical activity (exercise) equivalent to a minimum of a brisk walk of 3 miles a day, three times a week, is essential in health maintenance.

4. That we differ sufficiently as individuals to justify a skeptical attitude towards any and all nutritional advice that is based on one person's experience.

5. That each of us should learn enough about health matters to take personal responsibility for our own health. "A person is a physician or a fool at forty."

6. That people's capacity to deceive themselves equals or exceeds the power of others to deceive them.

7. That all human intellectual systems, including science, have limitations.

8. That "natural is better" and similar slogans should be taken as propositions to be examined rather than as axioms.

9. That a risk/benefit analysis should precede the addition of substances to foods.

10. That a person who has not begun to probe his or her assumptions is living with a stranger.

Differences Between
Conventional and Scientific Certainty

Humans love certainty and security. There are practical reasons for these hopes. Our species originated and has lived for millions of years in a world full of dangers. A person, or a whole tribe, could be wiped out by any number of natural disasters such as earthquakes, volcanoes, tidal waves, plagues, and famines. A list of past and present personal dangers would occupy pages. Early man invented gods and spirits who were held responsible for these disasters as well as for wars and personal misfortunes. Prayer and sacrifices probably originated in order to appease the gods and to request that safety and certainty be provided to the faithful.

Humans also love explanations of events. The enormous complexity of religious systems bears witness to the attempts to create explanations for good and for evil. For many people alive today, these thought systems provide the explanations and rationale for personal fortune and misfortune. No matter what forms and beliefs these systems include, the objective is the same: to provide certainty to man in an uncertain, dangerous world.

The ancient Greeks developed rationalism—a view of the world and how it works based on reason. These ideas lay dormant, however, until the Renaissance, when the foundations of modern science were stated. Science provides explanations of natural events, but it does not rely on mysticism to answer the questions it is incapable of answering. From its inception, the backbone of science has been composed of two parts: the framing of hypotheses to explain an event or a process, and the devising of experiments to test hypotheses. If the hypothesis is supported, other experiments are designed to find out under what conditions the hypothesis holds and under which ones it does not. This process amounts to recognizing new problems and modifying the hypotheses to fit each one. Scientific research furnishes hypotheses and/or proofs of varying degrees of certainty.

Here we come to one of the cornerstones that distinguishes science from other human endeavors. A scientific hypothesis must be susceptible to being disproved. Popper (1968) called this requirement the principle of falsifiability. Two important consequences flow from this principle. The first is that a scientific statement or hypothesis is never considered proved in an absolute sense, but it can be disproved, but again not absolutely. Secondly, if a hypothesis cannot be subjected to an experimental test, at least in principle, it is not considered scientific.

These qualifications on the nature of scientific proof place *100% certainty* as outside the realm of science. It also follows that the phrase *the search for truth*, if truth is taken as something immutable and final, is a misleading overstatement. The goals of science are a bit more modest: Science is concerned with stating falsifiable generalizations that are based on reproducible experiments or on inferences from observations. Scientific knowledge is subject to change. It can be modified with time.

I am not implying that nonscientific statements are necessarily wrong or false. It is important, however, to distinguish those statements that have a scientific basis from those that do not. For example, millions of people accept conclusions based on faith as true in an absolute sense. History is replete with examples of wars and controversies in which each side claimed that their conclusions were based on absolute truth. Such assertions leave little room for discussion or compromise.

To me, one of the strengths of the scientific method is that it avoids the trap of absolutism. As you will see, science is filled with controversies —but they ultimately get settled without bloodshed. In this book I will refrain from claiming that anything I write or refer to is true or certain in an absolute sense.

Observations, Facts, and Generalizations

Each of us makes thousands of observations every day. I think it is important to distinguish observations from facts because observations depend on the sensitivity of our sense perceptions and our interpretations of them. The interpretations depend on our assumptions, past history, state of health, and so on, and thus are not an objective description of reality. If our observation of a specific incident is freely confirmed by one or more people, it approaches factual status. In this view, facts depend on a consensus. Similarly, raw data obtained in a laboratory should be considered as observations until confirmed in a subsequent independent experiment, or preferably by another research group. In science, too, facts depend on a consensus among scientists.

However, there is an important difference between scientific facts and ordinary facts. In science, facts are seldom discovered in a random fashion. Instead, the scientist makes planned observations for the purpose of confirming or disconfirming a hypothesis. Most scientific facts originated as hypotheses. A hypothesis amounts to a prediction that can be checked by an experiment. If the prediction is not confirmed by the results, it is discarded and another hypothesis is substituted. In many experiments, the confirmed hypotheses and the conclusions are identical and can be stated as facts.

Another important difference between scientific facts and ordinary facts is that scientific experiments include what are called controls. For example, if the experiment's objective was to study the effect of X rays on the mutation rate of fruit flies, a control would include a number of fruit flies that were not X-rayed but were otherwise treated the same as the experimental group. The number of mutations of the control group would then be compared to those in the X-rayed group. Counting gives quantitative results so that the differences in the number of mutations, if any, are immediately apparent. Secondly, by the use of statistics, the scientists can calculate the probability that the results were due to chance. Probability—abbreviated *p-value*—is extremely important in calculating the results of complicated, long-term experiments of epidemiology.

As you are probably aware, experiments with humans usually contain more uncontrolled factors than those with animals, and without sophisticated statistical methods, it would be very difficult if not impossible to separate the influence of the various factors. Unfortunately, the entire field of statistics has a bad name. Expressions like "You can prove (or disprove) anything with statistics" and "There are liars, damn liars, and statisticians" abound. In an attempt to simplify statistical conclusions, the popular press or organizations with an axe to grind have sometimes misrepresented statistical conclusions.

For a fact to become well established in science, it must be confirmed by another scientist. This confirmation may take a year or more. In the meantime, scientists in that field of research do not sit on their hands and wonder who will confirm a given fact and when. If it is crucial to their own research, they will repeat the experiment themselves. An alternative is for interested scientists to attend a meeting or phone the author(s) who published the new fact and decide for themselves whether they accept it.

An important tool that scientists use to help them judge the reliability of new facts is whether the publication appeared in a refereed journal. Such journals contain articles that have been critically examined by specialists in a particular area of science like biochemistry, physics, or epidemiology. Conclusions that appear in refereed journals are usually confirmed later, and are often quoted by other scientists as facts before independent confirmation occurs. James Bonner has called such facts "factlets."

Nonrefereed journals may contain sound articles or others that were refused by a refereed journal because the experiments were sloppy, lacked proper controls, or contained conclusions that were not warranted on the basis of the facts presented. The general public has no way of ascertaining if an author of a popular article may be quoting facts or factlets, observations that have appeared in nonrefereed journals or statements from a book that may have no experimental basis. Many striking statements have appeared in the popular press that were downright errors and were never accepted by scientists in the field. The following statement is an example of this type of error: Low concentrations of fluoride, as that added in fluoridated water, can cause cancer. Because of all these safeguards, scientific facts are usually considered more reliable than ordinary facts.

The conclusion of an experiment states a generalization. The generalization may be narrow or very broad. For example, you may hypothesize that a certain brand of kitchen matches will burn twice if they are rubbed a certain way. The experiment includes striking 12 of these matches two times each in this specified way. Result: No match lights twice. Conclusion: The hypothesis was invalid with regard to the matches tested. The generalization is quite narrow. It refers only to the matches tested and does not exclude the possibility that other matches might light twice if struck in a certain way.

Now let's look at a broader generalization. Consider the conclusion: All objects fall if dropped. This generalization was universally accepted until it was found that when balloons were filled with hot air, they rose. One experiment divided one broad generalization into two broad generalizations.

Self-Fulfilling Prophecies and Other Complications of Deriving Facts From Observations

The difficulty of establishing facts from everyday experiences or observations has plagued the human race for thousands of years. What type of behavior was used to convict a woman as a witch in the seventeenth century? What actions or thoughts provided sufficient evidence to convict a person as a traitor in Stalinist Russia?

These questions raise the possibility that facts are not isolated bits of information that have meaning independent of the people or culture that are interpreting them. With humans, facts are often related to motives and expectations, and these associations usually lead to a loss of objectivity. The following two examples illustrate how objectivity can be lost: the first demonstrates how objectivity can be lost through expectations of events and experiences; the second demonstrates how memory for facts can be altered by environmental factors.

Chinese Restaurant Syndrome (CRS)—Fact or Figment?

In 1968 a Chinese physician named Kwok (1968) wrote a letter to the *New England Journal of Medicine* in which he described certain symptoms that he had experienced 15 to 20 minutes after eating Chinese food. The symptoms of the syndrome are now regarded as facial pressure, a burning sensation over the upper trunk, and chest pain. Kwok suggested four possible causes for Chinese Restaurant Syndrome (CRS): soy sauce, the wine in which the food was cooked, the high salt content of the food, and monosodium glutamate (MSG). The first three were soon eliminated, and investigations centered on MSG, which is used extensively as a flavor enhancer in Chinese restaurants. There are about 3 g of MSG in a 200-ml serving of wonton soup, and about 30% of subjects are affected by this quantity of MSG (Gore, 1982). In one series of studies, 55 of 56 subjects complained of symptoms after ingesting 12 g of MSG (Schaumburg, Byck, Gerstl, and Mashman, 1969).

One interesting aspect of the syndrome is that placebo-controlled trials do not agree. Gore (1982) mentions that some investigators have observed CRS in about 30% of the subjects tested, whereas other investigators have found very few. Experimental subjects who have not heard of the syndrome and do not know they are ingesting MSG in an experiment are unlikely to develop the symptoms. Gore also mentions that one of the chief investigators who had obtained positive results now admits that other substances than MSG may give rise to the syndrome (Kenney, 1980). These include matzo and split pea soup in kosher delicatessens, mustard, tea, and a species of poison fish. Present evidence casts considerable doubt as to whether CRS actually exists as a physiological response to a specific substance. CRS remains an enigma—a possible hoax.

But wait! The story isn't over yet. Two papers published in 1984 (Cochran & Cochran, 1984; Folkers, et al., 1984) are casting new light on the old syndrome. Dr. Cochran describes how his three-year-old daughter giggled, talked baby talk and expressed other "inappropriate behavior" after eating wonton soup (Cochran & Cochran, 1984). The symptoms disappeared after 40 minutes. This type of behavior had not occurred in the absence of eating wonton soup. One of the child's parents has had the classic symptoms of CRS after eating wonton soup. This report suggests a hereditary aspect to the syndrome and tends to discredit the self-fulfilling-prophecy hypothesis.

Folkers et al. (1984) attempted to link up CRS with a deficiency of pyridoxine (vitamin B_6). A derivative of this vitamin functions as a coenzyme in the metabolism of many amino acids. They screened students for vitamin B_6 activity and chose 27 who exhibited a deficiency. These 27 were challenged with MSG and a placebo. Twelve showed CRS symptoms, and 15 did not. The respondents were given pyridoxine and a placebo for 12 weeks in a double-blind study and were then retested. Of the nine who had received the vitamin, eight no longer showed symptoms, while all of the three who had received placebo showed the symptoms again. The authors concluded that MSG metabolism is affected by vitamin B_6 acting as a coenzyme for an enzyme that removes MSG. I suspect that the last words on CRS have yet to be written.

The Validity of Eyewitness Testimony

The difficulty of establishing facts from experience is a well-known complication of ascertaining what actually happened in activities as varied as riots or courts of law. Elizabeth Loftus (1975) investigated the variations in eyewitness testimony in experimental situations with students at the University of Washington. She has found that what people think they have observed is strongly influenced by what questions are asked of them about the event sometime after it has occurred.

For example, students were shown a 3-minute videotape that depicted the disruption of a class by eight demonstrators. The noisy confrontation resulted in the demonstrators leaving the classroom. Following the videotape, two questionnaires were distributed, each containing 19 filler questions and one key question. Half the students were asked, "Was the leader of the 4 demonstrators who entered the classroom a male?" The other half were asked, "Was the leader of the 12 demonstrators who entered the classroom a male?" The students responded by circling "yes" or "no."

A week later the students were given a list of 20 new questions about the disruption, which contained the key question, "How many demonstrators did you see entering the classroom?"

Ten percent of each group of students responded with the same number that they had been given in their question a week previously. Of the others, the ones who had been given the "12"-question responded with an average value of 8.5; and the ones given the "4"-question responded with an average value of 6.7 ($p < .05$). The experiment demonstrated that a false presupposition can affect a student's answer about a quantitative fact. The consensus was not sufficiently large to establish what the facts were. Well people learn to be nondogmatic when reporting their observations of past events to others.

Complications in Interpreting Facts

Some scientific distinctions are occasionally published directly in the popular press. A recent example comes from Newsweek (Gelman, Hager, Thomas, & Canin, 1985) in a report on the cancer found in President Reagan's colon. The article mentioned that there are five layers in the colon wall and cancers are classified according to how many layers they have penetrated. As one pathologist put it, "it's like a line call in tennis." The cells just barely touch the line—is it in the layer or out? Newsweek continues, "The results were a bit ambiguous; it was left to Dr. Rosenberg, the chief pathologist, to make the final determination."

In another follow-up article on President Reagan's cancer, Kolata (1985) describes some of the uncertainties surrounding the diagnosis. In March the President had four tests for blood in his stool. Two were negative; two were positive. He then had six more tests. All were negative. Yet, as later events demonstrated, he had a malignant tumor growing in his colon at the time the tests were carried out. This deficiency in the test has given rise to an active debate as to whether it is worthwhile. The American Cancer Society, for example, recommends that everyone over age 50 have an annual examination for blood in the stool. Some physicians think that the results obtained are not worth the effort.

The problems are due to what are called false negatives and false positives. False negatives occurred with President Reagan. He had a growing cancer that the tests did not reveal. These occur in 20%–30% of people. Another difficulty comes from false positives. The test shows blood in the stool when none is actually present. Meats, fresh fruit and fish, and vitamin C supplements produce false positives. They are so common that only 5%-10% of people who have positive tests actually have cancer. The stool test itself is relatively inexpensive. The problems are concerned with what should be done after a positive test is found.

First-rate medical practice requires that all positive tests be followed by sigmoidoscope exams and barium enemas or by colonoscopes. These procedures cost in the range of $200 to $600 not counting physicians' fees. If all people over 50 with positive tests were to have this type of follow-up, the cost would run about a billion dollars a year. Is it worth it? Dr. David Eddy of Duke University states, "There is a conceptual issue here—how certain do you have to be before you say it is beneficial?" (Kolata, 1985, p. 637). On the other hand, Dr. John Bailar of Harvard University remarks, "I can't say that screening is of no value. What I can say is that I think the chance of substantial value is not great enough to recommend widespread screening at present" (Kolata, 1985, p. 637). Kolata (1985) concludes, "The debate over the value of screening has no easy answers—only difficult questions" (p. 637).

These examples make the point that some facts are softer than others, and predictions based on them are likewise less certain than those based on less ambiguous facts. This qualification in no way impugns the competence of the people involved. It merely states the limitations of the state of the art in that specialty. Some sciences, like epidemiology, by the nature of the subject matter and the kind of data that can be obtained, contain a higher proportion of soft facts than the hard sciences like chemistry. This distinction becomes of practical importance in applying the results and conclusions of large-scale epidemiological experiments to populations. Before discussing these complicated questions, I think it will be useful to look at a series of classical experiments on scurvy in which the relations of hypotheses, facts, conclusions, and generalizations are clearly evident. To illustrate how scientists approach problems and devise experiments to help solve them, I'll briefly describe the disease known as scurvy and relate how science has been able to explain its occurrence and hence its treatment.

A Brief History of Scurvy

Scurvy was known and feared in Northern Europe since prehistoric times. It was so rare in Mediterranean countries, however, that the Greeks did not have a word for it. The disease usually appeared in late winter or early spring and disappeared during the summer months. As with most serious afflictions of mankind, there were numerous hypotheses to explain its mysterious comings and goings. Because northern peoples spent most of the winter indoors, scurvy was thought to be due to the air becoming unclean. Likewise, because many members of one family would acquire the disease, it was thought to be infectious. Scurvy was also attributed to a poison in food or water.

Scurvy was not common on ships until the long voyages of discovery began. At this time, it became a very serious problem. For example, on his famous trip around the world in 1519–1522, Magellan lost 9/10 of his crew to the disease.

The use of fresh fruits for the cure of scurvy was apparently discovered accidentally by the Dutch in the 16th century. According to one account, the crew of a ship that was carrying citrus fruits came down with scurvy. The men who ate the fruit were miraculously cured. This cure was lost and rediscovered many times in the next few centuries. Numerous anecdotes such as this one probably flourished in Renaissance Europe. Many dietary cures for scurvy were suggested, but most of them were ineffectual.

The Lind Experiment

In 1753, Dr. James Lind of the British Royal Navy carried out what was probably the first controlled experiment in nutrition, and one of the oldest in all of science. He divided scorbutic sailors into six groups. One group served as a control and continued on the standard scorbutic diet. The other five groups each received one additional food or liquid as follows: sea water, diluted sulfuric acid, cider, vinegar, or citrus fruits. The results were striking: The group receiving citrus fruits recovered quickly, those receiving cider slowly, and the others remained scorbutic.

The significance of the Lind experiment does not lie in the originality of the therapies he tested. They had all been suggested as curative at one time or another in isolated observations. Lind's brilliance lay in his including a control group against which the others could be compared. The results proved, for the first time, that citrus fruits cured scurvy promptly while the other dietary additions did not.

The Lind experiment illustrates the power of the scientific approach to questions in a variety of ways. It established a number of facts. First of all, it proved that scurvy was a dietary disease, and by the same token it excluded infections and foul air as causes. Secondly, it demonstrated that citrus fruits but not the other suggested remedies cured scurvy in the sailors involved in the experiment. From this fact, the generalization was drawn that citrus fruits would cure scurvy in *all* humans, and by inference would also protect against the disease. These predictions were soon substantiated.

The strength of the Lind conclusion stems from the fact that only one item in the diet of each group was altered. Here, we have an example of a one-variable experiment, or at least a close approximation of one. The reason I need to qualify my statement is that Lind used humans as subjects, and humans differ from one another. In this experiment they reacted similarly, but in other experiments, especially quantitative ones, they do not.

Even rats that have been inbred for 30 generations do not react exactly alike. It is for this reason that each variable in an experiment is studied with a group of animals and the results are averaged. If the variation from one animal to another is relatively small, averaging the results is perfectly legitimate and can lead to sound conclusions.

Becoming aware of the number of variables in an experiment is essential in science. In the Lind experiment, the basic diets of all the subjects were the same. If they had been different, Lind could not have been as certain as he was that the results were due to the variables he was studying.

The Statistical Basis of Cause

The results of a clear-cut, one-variable experiment allow us to come as close as humanly possible to speaking of cause and effect. In a philosophical sense, these two terms are metaphysical abstractions, which are outside the realm of scientific investigation. The eighteenth-century philosopher David Hume recognized the complications of employing the terms cause and effect and suggested that they be replaced with statistical statements about the frequency and consistency of events. This suggestion has been slowly adopted by scientists, but the terms *cause* and *effect* are still in common use by the general public and most philosophers today. Because the use of cause and effect often results in confusion and in senseless arguments, I shall use them as seldom as possible, but I will point out when they have been misused.

A committee that was concerned with the safety of food additives (Select Committee on GRAS Substances, 1977) formulated the following statement:

"Cause" in the interpretation of biological data, therefore, is a decision based on statistical considerations to the effect that B follows A sufficiently often that one is able to predict with a high probability that the same sequence will continue to occur. (p. 2535)

The use of the term *cause* also implies that the linkage between the two events has a rational explanation. This explanation is often called the *mechanism of action* and is subject to change as more is learned about the topic. For example, Lind had obtained a correlation between certain foods and the cure or lack of cure of scurvy. He could not explain why citrus fruits cured the disease and the other foods did not. He could only speak of the *antiscorbutic principle* or similar term in citrus fruits.

The important role that creative ideas play in suggesting experiments is illustrated in the next development. By 1900, a number of scientists had demonstrated that a diet composed solely of proteins, fats, and carbohydrates was incapable of keeping animals healthy for very long. F.G. Hopkins (1906) utilized these observations to suggest that adequate diets should contain a hitherto unrecognized class of substances, which he called *accessory food substances*. These, he said, were required to prevent a new category of diseases which he termed *vitamin-deficiency diseases*. Scurvy and rickets were given as examples of this type of disease. These were exciting hypotheses and opened up new vistas of research.

The replacement of the term *antiscorbutic principle* by *antiscorbutic substance* was almost revolutionary. Chemists are adept at isolating substances. They don't do so well with principles. In a relatively few years, ascorbic acid (vitamin C) was isolated and its structure determined.

The use of the word *statistical* in the statement on cause quoted above is also worth emphasis. To my knowledge, all humans who have been tested require ascorbic acid in their diets. But in guinea pigs, who also require ascorbic acid, Ginter (1976) has found a few who thrived without it. Lind's simple experiment with a few sick sailors started a trail of research that is continuing today. We can say that vitamin C is essential for the prevention of scurvy with as much certainty as we can state any nutritional fact. But even so, we can't state it with absolute certainty. It is possible that there may be other causes of scurvy than a lack of vitamin C. Some few people may react similarly to the exceptional guinea pigs and not require it. Scientists have learned to keep an open mind to alternative explanations as causes of diseases. Real-life situations seldom present health specialists with simple problems.

The proof that the antiscorbutic substance was actually ascorbic acid had to await its isolation and purification. Then the crucial experiment could be carried out: If the pure compound was fed to scorbutic guinea pigs, would it result in the disappearance of all the symptoms? It did. Thus, at the end of the research on the isolation of the active compound, we find a one-variable experiment almost as important as Lind's. Fortunately, both experiments gave unequivocal results. I say fortunately because there was no way of predicting that all the symptoms of scurvy would be removed by the administration of just one chemical. If any of the symptoms had remained, the search would have continued for a second or an nth vitamin.

In fact, there were some reports that capillary fragility, which is one of the symptoms of scurvy, was decreased by feeding one or more substances with the chemical name of bioflavonoids to scorbutic guinea pigs.

In these experiments, it was necessary to have four groups of animals. One received no dietary additions, another ascorbic acid alone, the third bioflavonoids alone. The fourth group received both test substances. For a time this family of substances was called vitamin P to denote its effect of decreasing capillary permeability.

I mention these experiments in this much detail, not because they are a hot item in 1988, but to show that an experiment in which two variables are suspected requires four groups, compared to two in a one-variable experiment. As I'll mention later, it also demonstrates how long an inaccurate conclusion can be maintained in the popular press.

If three variables are being tested, 8 test groups are required; four variables require 16 groups, and so on. In other words, the experiments become quite large and complicated when three or more variables are being studied. As the number of groups increases, the chances for error also increases. Such experiments have been accomplished with animals, but assembling a sufficiently large number of humans of similar age, sex, and so on, and who will comply with the long-term dietary restrictions of a three-variable experiment, is a truly Herculean task. For these reasons, there is a negative correlation between the number of variables and degree of credibility in the results of human nutritional experiments.

The Use of Statistical Methods

In complicated experiments with several variables the data must be calculated and evaluated by statistical methods. The degree of proof and the probability of the results being reproducible are invariably lower than in experiments with fewer variables. One of the major factors responsible for this lower degree of certainty of the results in complicated experiments is the variation within the groups. A significant result with a particular variable must exceed the random variation of the control groups by a minimum amount. These differences can be calculated by statistical methods and provide estimates of the degree of confidence we can place in the differences as being due to chance. Because of the complex interactions among the variables in multivariable experiments, it is generally impossible to speak of cause–effect relationships or of proof. The scientist/nutritionist/epidemiologist learns to draw conclusions as suggestions, correlations, and probabilities.

In epidemiological research, it is common to see the expressions $p < .05$ or $p < .01$, meaning that the probability that the results are due to chance is less than 5% and 1%, respectively. These values are widely accepted among scientists as denoting significant differences; however, it is clearly understood that this convention is arbitrary. It is also important to realize that an epidemiological result of $p < .01$ does not furnish as high a degree of confidence as a one-variable experiment in which the results are 99% reproducible. In the statistical calculation of p, the results are substituted in an equation that is thought to fit the experimental situation. *Assumptions* are involved in this substitution, and generally it is not possible to check or evaluate all of them. In contrast, in many one-variable experiments the degree of reproducibility is usually obtained from the data of repeated experiments. The necessity of matching the assumptions of the experiment with those of a statistical equation is usually unnecessary.

Credibility of Health Science Experiments

We should not ignore conclusions from complex experiments because their relative certainty is not as high as from a one-variable experiment. Most epidemiological research falls in this category, and some very valuable conclusions have come out of this type of work. I've implied above that experiments in which two or more variables are being studied are more complicated than a one-variable experiment. Complicated experiments usually furnish less conclusive results than simple experiments. In Table 3.1, I have listed six major categories of human health science experiments and studies in order of increasing number of variables and have included my estimates of the relative certainty of the conclusions furnished by each type. In my usage, the terms *relative credibility, relative validity,* and *degree of certainty* are interchangeable.

The categories have considerable practical significance. As we shall see in the discussion of the diet–heart controversy in chapter 10, credibility of results is the crux of the argument about what degree of proof is necessary before dietary recommendations by the U.S. government to the public are justified. For readers who find this kind of material hard going, I suggest skimming over this discussion the first time through. I refer to these categories frequently in later chapters, and at those places you can refer back to this chapter and gradually pick up the distinctions I make here and why they are important.

One-Variable Human Nutritional Experiments

In the most rigidly controlled types of experiments, human subjects (generally student volunteers) live in a closed environment with no direct contact with the outside world. Their food is provided; their exercise is monitored; their blood and excreta are frequently sampled and analyzed; they are not allowed to smoke or drink alcohol unless these are experimental variables. Their recreation is generally limited to reading or watching TV. In short, the conditions resemble an animal experiment as closely

Table 3.1   Credibility of Different Types of Health Science Experiments

Type of Study	Relative Certainty of Conclusions If Applied to Other Groups*	
	Experimental	Observational
	%	%
1. One-variable, all other factors held constant	90-99	—
2. Two-variable to multivariable, environment held constant	80-90	—
Epidemiological[a]		
3. Prospective:		
Cohort studies	60-80	50-70
Intervention studies		
4. Retrospective:		
Case-control studies	40-60	30-50
Ecological		
5. Correlation between per capita consumption of something and incidence of a disease	—	1-15
6. Descriptive: Patterns of disease occurrence in populations	—	1-15
Individual		
7. Personal experiment or observation:		
Anecdotal	0-1[b]	0-1[b]

*The gross estimates in percent are my own judgments and have no theoretical basis. I have listed the relative validity of each type semiquantitatively, so that readers may acquire some idea of the tremendous variation that is represented.

[a]Assume $p < .05$.

[b]If applied to another person.

as possible. Some of these experiments go on for months. They are very expensive to carry out, and for this reason the number of subjects is generally quite low. The RDA (recommended dietary allowance) for ascorbic acid, for example, is based on two experiments involving a small number of adult men.

Under these experimental conditions, variables can be controlled quite closely, and the experiments come as near the ideal one-variable experiment as possible. Nutritionists place a great deal of confidence in the results, and the conclusions approach classical proof. The major variables in these experiments are human variation, both genetic and in the past history of the subjects. These variations are reduced by averaging the results. Please note that the one-variable experiment, the kingpin of the scientific approach to knowledge, does not provide 100%, or absolute, certainty.

Epidemiological Studies

MacMahon and Pugh (1970) have classified epidemiology as predominantly an observational science. Some epidemiological nutritional studies, however, have involved dietary intervention tactics, which justify placing them in the experimental column. In the research reported by Hall et al. (1972), for example, a diet low in saturated fat and cholesterol and moderate in total fat and carbohydrates was eaten by a number of middle-aged men, some of whom were obese. After 1 year on the diet, significant decreases in serum triglycerides and cholesterol were found. In this experiment the subjects served as their own controls.

In general, experimental epidemiological studies contain fewer uncontrolled variables than the observational type, and prospective studies fewer than retrospective. As a consequence, the credibility of the results is higher in experimental, prospective studies than in observational, retrospective ones. For purposes of simplification, I have not shown this distinction in Table 3.1.

Both prospective and retrospective studies are used widely in nutritional epidemiological research. In the prospective type, a population is selected—preferably on a random basis—at the beginning of the experiment. The experimental diet is either provided directly or suggested by the scientists but selected by the subjects; in some cases, it is even the usual diet of the subjects. In this latter case, typical meals may be analyzed for certain components, or the composition estimated from food tables. The subjects may be followed for years, and a wide variety of diseases or conditions may be measured. The important Framingham diet–heart study, which was initiated in 1948, is an example of this type of observational research.

Retrospective studies, on the other hand, usually examine a population after something has happened, such as heart attacks or the appearance of tumors in the subjects. They are then questioned as to their diets and lifestyles during a period preceding the onset of disease. These studies usually include more uncontrolled variables than prospective studies. Retrospective studies are by their very nature observational.

The key factor in long-term nutritional experiments is, of course, the accuracy of the measurement of the diet. Because it is practically impossible to measure the chemical composition of each and every meal and snack over a long period, estimates are made from food composition tables, computer data bases, or occasional analyses. The quantity of food eaten is also an important and difficult variable to measure. The subjects may be asked to write down everything they have eaten or drunk during the previous 24 hours. More frequently, they rely on memory. Errors crop up in either situation. Nutritionists have found, for example, that merely writing down one's food intake at the time affects what one eats! This technique is used in some weight reduction schemes.

Memory has been found to be a notoriously inaccurate method of recalling what foods and serving sizes were eaten yesterday or even today. In addition, for the many people who eat out frequently, it is practically impossible to answer simple questions like what fat the eggs were fried in, how much salt was in the soup, or how much sugar was in the oriental spareribs. Sorenson and Lyon (1979) have discussed some of the problems of obtaining accurate data in nutritional epidemiology.

Because of these recognized inaccuracies, the results and conclusions of any single experiment in nutritional epidemiology are suspect. Confidence is increased only when a number of studies, differing in time, place, genetic background of subjects, and dietary habits, tend to confirm each other. These questions have been discussed by Stamler (1978) in an excellent summary of the connection between diet and heart disease.

Each of the four categories of experiments listed above has its strong points and its limitations. One-variable human experiments, for example, yield results in which we have a high degree of confidence. Yet these experiments are limited because they use only a few subjects, for a short time, under laboratory conditions. Strictly speaking, the generalizations are limited to the experimental conditions. If one asks, "What would be the effect of changing the fiber content of the diet, or of allowing a certain amount of alcohol to be consumed?" no direct answer is forthcoming unless variations in fiber or alcohol were part of the experiment. Interested scientists can estimate or assume what the effects of a given change may be, but that's what they remain—educated guesses—unless a new experiment that includes the change is carried out.

The epidemiological experiments in Categories 3 and 4 of Table 3.1 have the advantage of taking place in the real world, often with thousands of average people as subjects; but as I've mentioned, there are always large question marks surrounding the actual food consumed. Small but significant changes in lifestyle can also occur in long-term experiments. These, and many other unmeasured variables, set limits on the extent of applicability of the conclusions to other populations.

Comparing these different experimental types is like comparing a string quartet to a symphony orchestra. Each has its place; each its advantages and disadvantages. Tschaikovsky knew what he was doing when he scored the *1812 Overture* for full symphony orchestra, including cannons. Likewise, nutritionists know their objectives when they set up large-scale epidemiological experiments. It is doubtful that the risk factors for heart disease could have been discovered in laboratory experiments with human subjects.

I also wish to emphasize that within each category there are wide variations in the quality of the research results. Many factors influence quality.

The accuracy with which the diet is monitored and analyzed is an example of an important factor. An experiment involving 5 people is of lower quality than one with 50, which, in turn, is lower than one with 500—other things being equal. A nutritional or other lifestyle experiment that lasts 1 month is of lower quality than one that lasts 1 year, and so on. If the habits of the control group change in a long-term epidemiological experiment, its quality is lowered. This unfortunate change—from a scientific viewpoint—occurred in the multiple risk factor intervention trial (MRFIT), which is discussed in chapter 10.

Unfortunately, the information that people acquire through popular articles or books does not usually include an assessment of the quality of the research or an estimate of the credibility of the conclusions by scientists. I believe that this assessment is part of the responsibility of popular writers. They should mention both the strong and weak points of a particular piece of research so that readers get an idea about the quality of the research. Are people so gullible that they must be spoon-fed as though all experiments are perfect and all conclusions certain? I assume that many readers of this book are no longer that naive.

Ecological: Per Capita Consumption and Disease Incidence

Correlations of this type are called ecological because they relate some factor in the environment such as people's diet or income or other variable to some other factor—often disease incidence. The data are generated solely by observational methods rather than experimental. Consumption of almost anything can be calculated on a per capita basis and correlated with almost anything else. This is the type of study that is frequently cited as humorous because the correlation found cannot possibly be based on a functional or realistic relationship. Examples are the correlation between the lengths of women's skirts and the health of the economy, or that of the consumption of bananas in England and the number of automobile accidents. The world is full of correlations; some of them humorous as the two above, some of them interesting. The trick is to identify meaningful correlations and, beyond that, to trace the connections between them.

In any free-living population, the number of unmeasured variables is so large that correlations are incapable of proving anything. The conclusions from observations need to be stated as suggestions or indications. Despite these limitations, studies of this type often have provided leads in the design of more controlled studies, which have led to more conclusive results. For example, during World War II the diets in many European countries were severely restricted in fats and meat. Malmros (1950) was among the first to point to a correlation between the drop in per capita consumption of fats and the sharp decrease in heart disease during the war years in these countries. Epidemiologists followed up on this lead with a series of studies to test the diet-heart hypothesis in various parts of the world (Keys, 1970). Much of our present knowledge of the nutritional factors influencing heart disease has grown from this work.

The descriptive ecological category covers situations about which even less is known. For example, black people in the same economic bracket and geographical location as whites often have a higher incidence of hypertension. Why? What is the reason that Japanese men have the highest rate of stomach cancer and the lowest rates of prostate and bladder cancer in the world (Cairns, 1978)? Data of this type serve as springboards for research.

Individual Experiments: Anecdotal Information

The results of what happens to individuals when they alter their diets, take a pill of some type, or change their exercise habits are frequently used by their friends as the basis for a similar change. It seems reasonable that if a friend has doubled her vitamin C intake or is into jogging and "never felt better" that we might, too. But, there are a number of reasons why the conclusions from individual experiments usually do not furnish generalizations that apply to other people.

In the first place, the friend might have felt better, for the day or two that she did feel better, if she had taken nothing, or if she had taken a sugar pill. Most people are so variable in their feelings that utilizing them as a measure of an effect is as sound as building a house on quicksand. Experience has demonstrated over and over again that conclusions from data of this type, based only on the feelings of the person who altered something, have little carryover to other people. In the second place, even if the friend benefited on a long-term basis from the change, her genetic background, life history, and diet are unique, so that, again, what happened to her is not very likely to apply to other people.

Another limitation of individual experiments comes from the type of data that is generated. A person, after taking the latest fad-type pill for a week, may tell a friend, "I've never felt better in my life," "I have more energy than I've had for years," or "I don't feel tired anymore." These subjective remarks may accurately describe the feelings of the person who experienced them, but they are not general facts; they are private observations and should not be used as generalizations.

Facts and Observations: General and Personal

The distinction between personal observations and general facts is an important one. One of the objectives of science is the discovery and reporting of general facts. In scientific usage a fact is an event, result, or process that has been confirmed by a different person than the one who first published it.

The word *published* is noteworthy in this definition. A scientific experiment remains an observation until it is published and confirmed. At times new observations from more than one laboratory are published in the same journal; with others, confirmation may take years; sometimes a result is confirmed by other scientists and not confirmed by still others. This situation can result in strong controversy until the reasons for the discrepancies are sorted out.

For example, in the Lind experiment, the conclusion of the experiment could be stated as, *Scurvy could be cured by eating a certain minimum of citrus fruits.* This statement became a fact as soon as the conclusion was verified with other subjects. General facts and hypotheses are closely linked. The obvious next step from the Lind conclusion that citrus fruits would cure scurvy was the hypothesis that eating them would prevent scurvy. The hypothesis became a fact as soon as the experiment was published and confirmed.

Most private observations apply only to one person and cannot be verified by someone else, in contrast to general ones. Examples are "I have a headache," or "I feel great!" Here we run into a complication. Some types of headaches affect brain waves and can be confirmed by a technologist with the proper equipment. Other types of headaches do not affect brain waves. Thus, some private observations are verifiable and others are not.

Even feelings can serve to produce general facts under some conditions and when consensus approaches 100%. Tom Wolfe (1968) in *The Electric Kool-Aid Acid Test* tells the story of Ken Kesey and others who were being tested at Stanford University for the effects of LSD. The scientists were interested in physiological effects such as blood pressure, temperature, pulse rate, and so on. Kesey and friends kept telling the scientists of their hallucinations after receiving the drug, but their tales were ignored. It remained for other investigators to discover the hallucinogenic effects of LSD.

Another example came from research on pellagra many years ago. One of the symptoms of advanced pellagra is a type of dementia or loss of touch with reality. The feelings are severe enough to affect behavior, which can be observed by others. Because some nutritional deficiencies affect attitudes and behavior in many ways, it is sometimes difficult to draw a line between where private observations end and general facts begin.

An Interesting Published, Personal Experiment

Consider this interesting example. In her book, *Diet for Life*, Francine Prince (1981) describes how her husband determined his optimum intake of each of 14 vitamins. Harold Prince was recovering from a heart attack from which he had almost died; thus he probably began his experiment at a much lower energy level than if he had been well. His wife, Francine, a gourmet cook, was tempting him to eat a healthy diet with all her culinary ability and love. Harold started with the recommended dietary allowance (RDA) of 60 mg of vitamin C and increased the dosage by 100 mg per week until he felt no further increase in energy. His energy leveled off at a daily intake of 4300 mg. At the rate of increase mentioned, this part of the experiment would have taken 37 weeks (4300 − 600 = 3700 and 3700/100 = 37). He called this amount his dynamic daily allowance (DDA). Similar experiments were conducted with 13 other vitamins. Mrs. Prince likewise determined her DDA for these vitamins. She emphasizes the personal nature of the DDA and that each individual will probably terminate the experiment with a different quantitative mixture of vitamins. This statement is not surprising.

There are two aspects of the experiment that I find astounding. The first concerns its length. I estimate that it would require 2 to 3 years to determine the DDA for all 14 vitamins. During this lengthy period, the Princes measured their energy on a day-to-day, week-to-week basis and found a gradual, regular increase. Although I have not carried out such an experiment myself, I find it hard to believe that my energy level would consistently increase over a 2-year period independently of moods, illnesses, and the usual vicissitudes of life.

The other astounding aspect of the experiment is the Princes' use of energy as their estimate of a vitamin's effectiveness. With vitamin C, for example, despite the tremendous number of experiments that have been reported using large doses for the control of the common cold, none have mentioned an increase in energy as an effect. Pauling (1974) referred to increases in well-being and mental alertness that have been reported in some studies. In their large-scale, double-blind study of subjects receiving 1 g per day of ascorbic acid, Anderson, Reid, and Beaton (1972) found no difference in well-being between the controls and the experimental groups. Although well-being and increased energy may not be synonymous, I would expect some correlation between the two subjective feelings.

Is it possible that the Princes have discovered a new effect of vitamin C? It is unlikely, in my opinion. I suspect that Francine Prince provided the motivation for her husband's increased energy and that he just happened to be engaging in the vitamin experiment at the same time. In other words, she described a unique situation in which many different activities were going on, including a vigorous walking program. Possibly, because he was consciously varying his vitamin intake, Harold Prince attributed his increased energy to that variable rather than the half dozen others that were also changing in that 3-year period.

It is practically impossible for humans to regulate their lives to such an extent that they can carry out a one-variable experiment. This means that people can never be very sure of the cause of a result, even for themselves. When one decides on a cause, it is like picking a name out of a hat. A friend who accepts a recommendation based on private observations has about as much chance of benefiting as of winning the Irish Sweepstakes. Personal experiments are usually interesting and occasionally fascinating, but the conclusions are not generally applicable to others.

The qualifications I have mentioned above may give the impression that I believe that personal experiments have no value. That is not correct. I think that people who are aware of the variables in their lives can learn a great deal about themselves and, in general, gain considerable valuable information by performing personal experiments.

A Personal Experiment of the Author

As an example, I'll mention a personal experiment of my own. For many years I have consumed alcoholic beverages at parties where they were served. I have never been a heavy drinker but I occasionally would feel hung over the day after a party. In addition to the lassitude, my major symptom was diarrhea. Because my total consumption didn't vary a great deal, I began to wonder why the hangover occurred so capriciously and irregularly.

The first group of factors that I considered was psychological. Had I been depressed? Did I have a good time at the party? Had I become angry, anxious, or disappointed? I found no correlation between these factors and my symptoms. The next idea concerned food. Had I overeaten the hors d'oeuvres, seafood, or dessert? I like them all. But again I could find no correlation.

I finally considered the kinds of drinks I had consumed. I enjoy most kinds of alcoholic concoctions and am quite nonselective in my tastes. If the host offered martinis, I drank those; if it was punch, I drank it. I especially like Tom Collins or gin and tonic in the summer. Margaritas, Bloody Marys, whiskey sours, rum and cola, champagne, liqueurs, wine, and so on—I drank them all. If it was guest's choice, I took Scotch and water.

I soon discovered a correlation between gin drinks and my symptoms. If I had a hangover after a party hosted by a friend who had served drinks of unknown composition—at least to me—I would make a point of complimenting him later on his excellent bar and casually inquire what was in the drinks. It was invariably gin.

About this time the New Yorker ran a fascinating article on the history of gin. It was invented by a Dutch physician who had discovered that juniper berries contained a laxative. The water extract spoiled on storage, so he added alcohol as a preservative. The distilled product still contained sufficient juniper berry extract to flavor it—and to cause diarrhea in sensitive people like me. That cinched it. I had made the correlation, and the article provided the mechanism. I have not knowingly consumed any gin drink for over 20 years and my digestive system has been working just fine, thank you.

In retrospect I realize that I was very lucky in my little self-experiment. If there were more than one laxative in the drinks I had been consuming, or if other flavoring agents resulted in similar types of digestive upsets, I might be trying to sort them out even yet. I'll discuss other aspects of personal experiments in chapter 6.

The Role of Assumptions in Nutrition Research

Assumptions are as essential to mankind as breathing or eating. They are as necessary in science as they are in theology. One of the basic assumptions of science is that nature is regular. Einstein expressed this view when he said, "God does not play dice with the universe."

I consider being conscious of assumptions so very important—in daily living as well as in judging the validity of scientific generalizations—that I will italicize the words *assume* and *assumption(s)* in the remainder of this book so that you will become aware of how often they are employed in scientific discussions.

Nutrition research is based on many general *assumptions*. A few examples are that all the races of mankind have similar nutritional requirements; that calories from fat, protein, and carbohydrates are equivalent; and that the American RDAs cover the needs of 97.5% of healthy Americans. This last assertion, incidentally, is based on still another *assumption*: that the variation in nutrient requirements of Americans follows a symmetrical distribution. (This *assumption* is examined in more detail in chapter 5.) A few other widely held, but controversial, *assumptions* are that a carcinogen in one species is likely to act as a carcinogen in another (e.g., rats and humans) but the site of the tumor may vary; that "natural is better"; and that many food additives are carcinogens.

One of the by-products of research is to make *assumptions* explicit. Once exposed, they can be checked by experiments and, in some cases, removed. An interesting example is the *assumption* quoted above, *Natural is better*. This broad statement only has meaning when it is applied to something specific. Let's examine a few applications.

"Natural is better" is often applied to vitamins. I interpret it to mean that vitamins isolated from natural sources are nutritionally superior to synthetic ones. I am aware of extensive experiments on two vitamins in which the two sources have been compared. These are vitamins A and C. No significant differences were found (Irwin, 1980). Now we come to an interesting and important distinction between the scientific way of thinking and that of many self-styled experts and authors on nutrition.

The scientific generalizations are limited by the data at hand. In this instance, the generalization is restricted to the statement: purified samples of the synthetic vitamins A and C are equal to the natural forms with respect to the experimental comparisons of their vitamin functions that were made. Notice the possibility that differences may be found if additional tests were carried out on these two vitamins. Also notice that it leaves open the possibility that differences may be found in all the other vitamins.

Now, I'll quote—and comment on—statements by two popular authors. The first is from the book *From Eden to Aquarius* by Greg Brodsky (1974).

As for the controversy regarding natural vs. synthetic vitamins, there is more and more evidence that both natural and synthetic vitamins or food supplements contain highly beneficial elements which have not yet been isolated by science. The difference lies, however, in the fact that the unisolated substances now being found in the synthetics are proving to be of questionable benefit to the human organism. Whole natural foods and the vitamins they provide are complete, balanced, and in a state readily assimilable by the human organism. For this reason they are far more desirable than synthetic vitamins. (p. 100)

What does Brodsky mean by the phrase "highly beneficial elements which have not yet been isolated"? There is no hint here as to what kinds of experiments were carried out, what criteria were used in judging the beneficial effects, and how the unisolated elements were separated and distinguished from the known nutrients.

The last statement shifts the subject away from vitamins as supplements to that of whole natural foods. Is Brodsky implying that all natural foods contain a balanced mixture of vitamins? With regard to assimilability, has he not heard of the people with pellagra in the South who could not utilize the niacin in the corn they ate? I also wish to point out that in all these supposed statements of fact, Brodsky does not list a single reference. We have no way of knowing his source of information. If we accept his conclusions, it is because we *assume* that they are correct. I, for one, prefer not to make such *assumptions* on important questions like these.

Another example is taken from a chapter entitled "Bioflavonoids: The 'Useless' Vitamin We Need" in *The Complete Book of Vitamins* (Gerras, 1977). The chapter states,

Vitamin P . . . is a substance that occurs along with vitamin C in foods. So, when you take vitamin C made in a laboratory, you don't get any vitamin P, of course. And researchers have discovered that in many situations where vitamin C alone is not effective, the combination of the two will work wonders. (p. 363)

Note that the argument has been shifted away from whether natural vitamin C—a specific substance—is superior to synthetic vitamin C—a specific substance—to the possible advantages of eating bioflavonoids—substances that occur in many foods that contain vitamin C but are absent from synthetic vitamin C.

Vitamin P was first postulated by Rusznyak and Szent-Györgyi (1936). They observed that "under certain pathological conditions characterized by an increased permeability or fragility of the capillary wall, ascorbic acid is ineffective but the condition can be cured by the administration of extracts of Hungarian red pepper" (p. 27). The extracts were purified and found to consist of a practically pure flavonol derivative. This report stimulated considerable research on the new vitamin. Flavonols are a well-known family of plant pigments consisting of hundreds of chemicals. Other investigators subsequently tested many flavonols for vitamin P activity, but none were found active. As a result of these negative results, the Joint Committee on Nomenclature of the American Society of Biological Chemists and the American Institute of Nutrition (1950) recommended the discontinuance of the term, vitamin P.

Hughes and Wilson (1977) reviewed the work done with bioflavonoids since 1950 and concluded that the evidence was insufficient to include them in the group of essential nutrients (i.e., as a vitamin). They did leave open the possibility that flavonoids might act as growth factors under certain conditions. Thus, as often happens in nutrition research, an original claim may turn out to be invalid, but useful information may be found in the effort to reproduce it.

The lack of effect of bioflavonoids was published in many articles mentioned above, but the author chose to ignore it. Instead of accepting the conclusions from the facts available at present, the author chose to *assume* that a difference will be found in the future. Thus, the recommendation that natural vitamin C is preferable to synthetic because of the presence of bioflavonoids or other compounds in the former rests on an *assumption* that is unlikely to be realized. People who choose to pay extra for natural vitamin C because they agree with the *assumption* are, of course, free to do so. But we should be aware that unwarranted *assumptions* can be expensive luxuries.

The bioflavonoid myth goes on and on. In the *Vitamin Bible*, a best-seller by Earl Mindell (1979), he states that bioflavonoids are "necessary for the proper function and absorption of vitamin C. No daily allowance has been established, but most nutritionists agree that for every 500 mg of vitamin C you should have at least 100 mg of bioflavonoids" (p. 87). One wonders how extensive Mindell's readings were in the nutrition literature on this subject. Like Brodsky, he does not list a single reference. These claims have not been accepted by respected nutritionists for over 30 years (Committee on Dietary Allowances–Food and Nutrition Board [CDA], 1980).

Your Assumptions Can Affect
Your Diet and Your Health

One characteristic that Brodsky (1974), Mindell (1979), and the *Prevention* editors have in common is their authoritarian style of writing. The reader is soon convinced that they are experts who are giving the public the benefits of their long experience in presenting the "truth" about nutrition.

In contrast, scientists have learned to be skeptical of authoritarian writing. They do not assume that anyone, even a Nobel prize winner like Linus Pauling, should be believed, based on his or her word alone. As I have said previously, scientists can go to the original literature, search out the data, and form their own conclusions. Unfortunately, this route, which is the soundest that has yet been developed, is not feasible for most of the public.

My best recommendation for the public is to practice the scientist's policy of skepticism. Do not *assume* that authors—including me—are publicizing widely accepted generalizations just because they say they are. Be wary of any author who does not list references to the original literature to support his or her statements. In addition, note that trustworthy authors discuss both sides of a controversial topic.

Henry Ford was well aware of the importance of *assumptions*. An anecdote about him states that before hiring a new executive, Ford would take him to lunch. Besides the usual shoptalk, Ford observed if the man salted his food before eating it. If he did, Ford would not hire him. The man *assumed* too much.

To me, three characteristics of intelligent living are first, becoming aware of the *assumptions* that one makes; second, keeping the number of *assumptions* to a minimum; and third, becoming aware of other people's *assumptions*. If you follow this policy in nutritional matters for a year or so, I predict it will have a beneficial effect on your diet and your pocketbook. It did on mine! If you accepted this recommendation readily, I suggest that you reread the section on generalizing from anecdotal experiences.

Limitations of Epidemiological Research

The conclusions of epidemiological experiments apply to whole populations, not to individuals. The results may demonstrate that 10 or 100 subjects in a specific population may die of a disease each year, but the results do not identify which ones. Although this conclusion may be interesting scientifically, it has little practical value. Physicians and other people are interested in more detailed predictions than that. The idea of risk factors was developed to aid physicians and people alike in identifying those who are at the most risk of acquiring a disease before they actually develop symptoms. A *risk factor* is usually defined as a personal or cultural habit, a dietary constituent, a hereditary condition or tendency, or any other long-term factor that tends to increase a person's chances for acquiring a specific disease. *Risk factors do not predict which individuals will acquire a particular disease.* They are very useful in calculating the probability that a person with three risk factors, for example, will acquire the disease compared to the probability that a similar person with none, one, two, or eight risk factors will acquire the disease. People who have had their risk factors identified are then able, if they choose, to modify or eliminate them. People who modify or eliminate a risk factor are lowering the probability that they will acquire the disease. Risk factors for hypertension and heart disease are discussed in some detail in chapters 9 and 10.

A 40-year-old American male has heard that he is a prime target for a heart attack. If his doctor told him, "Change your habits or you will have a heart attack in the next 10 years," he would probably do so without question. But if his doctor said something like this: "With your present habits, your chances of having a heart attack in the next 10 years are one out of four, but if you change your habits according to these directions, your chances will decrease to one out of eight," he may wonder if the sacrifice is worth it. After all, he says he "never felt more fit in his life."

Unfortunately, our education has made us more comfortable with certainty than with probabilities. Besides, we have not been trained to take full responsibility for our own health. As promoters of wellness have discovered, the average American thinks he can overeat, overdrink, oversmoke, and overindulge in every way he can afford, and that it is the function of medicine to cure him so that he can be go back and do it some more.

The example above illustrates two of the most important points in this book. The first is that the doctor—representing medical science—cannot predict what will happen to the man with certainty. A physician should state predictions as probabilities. The second point is that only an individual can put scientific-medical advice into practice. Is there a contradiction here?

The first point was recognized by the Greek philosopher Aristotle (384-322 BC). His view can be summarized as:

> Medicine, for instance, does not theorize about what will help Socrates or Callias, but only about what will help to cure any or all of a given class of patients: this alone is its business. Individual cases are so infinitely various that no general knowledge of them is possible. (p. 981a)

Does this provocative statement still hold today? The sciences of medicine and nutrition have progressed a long way in the past 2,000 years. How are general conclusions applied to individuals?

The uniqueness of the individual is still recognized, but as members of the genus *Homo sapiens*, each of us shares in, or exhibits, a great many general characteristics. We are enough alike so that predictions based on averages work on a high enough percentage of people to be useful. Predictions and therapies on avoiding and treating illness are based on statistical averages. This realization, this advance in knowledge since Aristotle's time allows a physician to go from the general to the particular. The science of medicine deals with the general; the art of medicine deals with the individual. The science of medicine is taught in medical schools; the art of medicine is learned by a physician by seeing patients. I'll cite an example.

A middle-aged woman comes into a doctor's office not feeling well. On examination, the physician finds a number of symptoms such as chronic tiredness, depression, tenseness, and anxiety. She had seen a TV ad for an iron supplement some months ago and had been taking those pills, but they hadn't helped. Then a friend had mentioned how much better she had felt after taking vitamin pills; so the woman had been taking some of those also, but they hadn't helped either.

The physician confirmed that she had a severe anemia. From the type and number of cells that he could see under the microscope, the doctor diagnosed her condition as pernicious anemia. This disease is not usually caused by a nutritional deficiency but by a genetic defect in the synthesis of a carrier that is essential for the absorption of vitamin B_{12}. The symptoms of our patient were very general. They could have been due to a variety of deficiencies or other causes. The woman had tried two of the most obvious remedies but with no effect.

This example illustrates the similarity between diagnosis in medical practice and scientific research. A patient's symptoms suggest one or more hypotheses (diagnoses) to explain the cause or causes of the disease or condition. Additional tests provide facts that confirm or disconfirm the diagnosis—in this case, anemia. Now, there are many causes of anemia. Some are nutritional, some are not. The diagnosis cannot be made from the symptoms. To decide on the type of anemia, additional tests must be carried out. In medical terms, this process is called *differential diagnosis*. With most patients, it serves to limit the disease to a single cause. This hypothesis is checked by therapy. If the patient recovers, or is cured, the results are interpreted as confirming the diagnosis. If the patient improves but is not cured, the results suggest other factors are involved. The process is continued until a diagnosis is secured.

Sometimes the diagnosis is original: The patient has a disease not previously described. Sometimes there is no known therapy for the disease. Medical science is young, and there is much left to be learned. The point to this discussion is that progress in medical science, basic and applied, has disproved Aristotle. Medical science has learned to go from the general (the vast body of information about diseases and therapies) to the particular (application to an individual patient) and back to the general (diagnosis and therapy that links the individual to the general pool of information).

Nutritional science, however, in its application to a population of well individuals, has taken a different approach from medical science, which deals with sick people. It is obviously impossible to determine the nutritional requirements of each person in a large population. Nutritional research about quantitative requirements of essential nutrients studies relatively few people. The results are averaged and treated statistically, and a daily intake is calculated that will cover 97.5% of the population. This amount is called the recommended dietary allowance (RDA) for that population. Details of this calculation are included in chapter 5.

The Application of Animal Nutritional Experiments to Humans

The second limitation of nutritional research results from ethical considerations. Humans cannot be kept in cages like animals. The conclusions from animal experiments provide many insights into the human situation, but we can always expect differences in going from mice to men.

For example, a bioflavonoid user told me recently, "The fact that bioflavonoids have no effects in guinea pigs does not prove that they are ineffectual in man." In this she was quite correct. Nutritionists can only respond to statements of this type by saying, "There are no data that suggest that humans are different from guinea pigs in this respect." Users of bioflavonoids and some other pseudovitamins are *assuming* that differences exist.

A similar situation on species susceptibility to carcinogens occurs in cancer research. Most chemicals that have been demonstrated to be active carcinogens in humans have been found to be carcinogenic in one or more animal species. With a specific carcinogen, the sites of the tumors may vary from one species to another. What about the reverse situation in which a chemical has been shown to be carcinogenic in an animal species but has not been tested in man? Most cancer researchers make the reasonable *assumption* that the substance will likely act as a carcinogen in humans. This *assumption* lies at the heart of the controversy concerning whether formaldehyde should be banned in house insulation materials (Hanson, 1982; Perera & Petito, 1982).

Personal Responsibility for One's Health Is a Necessity

In a free society, it is expected (*assumed*) that each individual is responsible for his or her own care and safety—within limits. For some centuries the state has provided certain essential central services like police and fire protection, water and sewage services, utilities, and so on. Recently, the government has begun to regulate pollution of air, water, and foods to "safe" concentrations. How far the state should proceed in these endeavors raises very difficult questions with which Congress has been wrestling for many years. But in my view, government should not, because it cannot, monitor or control the health practices of each citizen. The responsibility of taking care of oneself, as an individual right in a free society, should be taught from kindergarten on. I've possibly stated another personal value judgment here. On the other hand, how does one protect oneself from the pollutants (poisons) of a technological society? In my view, protection requires education, awareness, and citizen participation in the political process.

The Intrusion of Politics and Business in Nutritional Decisions

Many people think that questions like, "Is saccharin a carcinogen in humans?" or "Does a diet high in saturated fat increase the risk of heart disease?" are straightforward, scientific questions to which there should be straightforward, scientific answers and therefore straightforward, scientifically based laws or recommendations to deal with them. Out in the real world things are not so simple.

Briefly stated, the data on saccharin as a carcinogen are equivocal. It is a weak carcinogen at worst. Besides, the data were obtained on rats. Are humans more or less susceptible? No matter what conclusion is considered, it involves an *assumption* of some type in the extrapolation from rodents to humans. Under these conditions, what can we expect from the politicians?

With regard to saturated fat in the diet, there are human as well as animal data. In applying animal data to humans, an *assumption* similar to that mentioned for saccharin is necessary. The great bulk of the human data was obtained in studies that fall in Categories 3 and 4 of Table 3.1. Nutritionists are not agreed as to whether conclusions from experiments at this level of credibility (40%–80%) should serve as a basis for a national nutritional policy. Under these conditions, what can we expect from the politicians?

The American Institute of Nutrition (1979) sponsored a symposium entitled *Translation of Scientific and Nutritional Findings to Social Policy*. J.P. Habicht, Chairman. A number of the speakers had worked with Congressional Committees on these questions. They were knowledgeable, and their answers shed considerable light on the problems on the incorporation of nutritional information into public policy.

Orlans (1979) said, "Knowledge of the nation's health and nutritional status is dated, uncertain, incomplete, and complex, whereas politicians demand simplicity and administrators practicability; and everyone wants more and better information" (p. 2553). He mentioned the changes in the wording of the goals of the Senate Select Committee on Nutrition and Human Needs (1977a, 1977b), *Dietary Goals for the U.S.*, between February and December 1977 (1st and 2nd editions, respectively). The basic facts had not changed in this 9-month period. The first edition recommended a "decrease in the consumption of meat" (p. 2554). The Chairman of the Committee was Senator McGovern of South Dakota, a state with a flourishing cattle-raising industry. It would be interesting to know what political pressures were brought to bear on the Senator between February and December and if such pressures were responsible for the deletion of this phrase from the second edition.

Senator Percy of Illinois, a rich agricultural state, also had a change of mind. In the February edition, he wrote, "Our national health depends on how well and how quickly Government and industry respond" (p. 2554) to the Committee's goals. In the December edition he noted "the lack of consensus among nutrition scientists about a general reduction in cholesterol intake" and went on to say that because "the value of dietary change remains controversial . . . science cannot at this time *insure* [italics added] that an altered diet will provide improved protection from certain killer diseases such as heart disease and cancer" (p. 2554).

The controversy to which Senator Percy referred surfaced after the February edition was published. Two respected American nutritionists, A.E. Harper, Chairman of the Food and Nutrition Board, and D.M. Hegsted, Director, Human Nutrition Center, U.S. Department of Agriculture, expressed sharply divergent views on dietary alteration. Harper (1979) maintained that the evidence relating nutrition to heart disease and cancer is relatively weak and insufficient to support a large publicity campaign to alter the American diet. Hegsted (1979) stated that diet is a well-recognized risk factor in both heart disease and cancer. As such, dietary alteration may be expected to help prevent, or postpone, death from these diseases.

I'll discuss this controversy in more detail in chapter 10. My reason for referring to it here is that, in my view, the difference in opinion as to what the government policy should be flows from the different *assumptions* of various experts. Harper, for example, *assumes* that the degree of certainty of the available data is too low to warrant a recommendation of diet change. To Hegsted, it isn't. I interpret the Harper position as being based on the *assumption* that some day there will be harder data and that a recommendation should be postponed until then. Hegsted, in contrast, may be *assuming* that many years may elapse, if ever, before more conclusive data become available. In the meantime, why not recommend on the data that we have? Many years ago, Bertrand Russell (1948) cleverly summarized this type of situation: "All knowledge is in some degree doubtful, and we cannot say what degree of doubtfulness makes it cease to be knowledge, any more than we can say how much loss of hair makes a man bald" (p. 516).

We elect members of Congress to make decisions, not to philosophize. As professional politicians, they are wary of controversy, especially when influential constituents favor the status quo. The insertion of the word *insure* in the revised recommendations by Senator Percy may be an illustration of political astuteness on his part. It seems like a reasonable request—to wait for more data before going overboard on a recommendation—but it could also be a dodge. It will be many years, if ever, before nutritional research can insure that diet will protect against the killer diseases.

In the chapters on these diseases I will point out numerous instances in which the call for more data is used as the reason for inaction. I can understand why the producer of a product or the owner of a factory whose products may be banned for health reasons would demand conclusive data before acceding to a law that he or she considers unfairly discriminatory. It is a long step from scientific conclusion to government recommendation or regulation; and in the process, *assumptions*, values, and motivations may overshadow or modify or cancel the original generalization.

R. Brandon (1979), in a provocative article entitled "Science, Senators, and Uncertainty," suggests three major factors that affect Congressional decision making. The first he calls the adversary nature of truth. This *assumption* arises from the competing views on a given subject a politician obtains from scientists, bureaucrats, friends, constituents, staff, and so forth. In this mélange, scientific truth is but one—and often not the most important factor—in the Senator's final decision to vote "yes" or "no" on a particular bill.

Secondly, Brandon mentions the new generation of Congresspersons who utilize models of decision making involving costs, benefits, and risks. These factors include values and assumptions that often are more important than scientific facts in influencing their votes.

Finally, Brandon has perceived that members of Congress somehow become aware of the degree of credibility in the scientific data pertaining to certain questions. Congresspersons utilize scientific recommendations as but one input into decision making, rather than as the sole basis for it.

I *assume* that many readers of this book are concerned about the relationship of their diet to their health and are expecting to find sufficient facts presented to enable them to make intelligent decisions on these questions independently of government recommendations. In arriving at these personal decisions, each of us is in a similar position to a Congressperson. We have many sources of information of varying degrees of uncertainty. We should become aware that our *assumptions* play an important role in decisions as to which facts and conclusions we accept and which we reject. In taking responsibility for our own wellness, we should recognize what degree of credibility seems reasonable as a basis for our own dietary modifications.

Summary

A major goal of scientific research is to increase knowledge. Knowledge consists of a compendium of assumptions, value judgments, definitions, observations, facts, conclusions, hypotheses, theories, and laws. Knowledge is increased by stating hypotheses and checking them by experiments. A publicly confirmed hypothesis often becomes a new fact which, in turn, is used to propose a new hypothesis, and so forth.

Conclusions of research experiments in the health sciences vary in applicability to other groups from quite high to very low relative certainty. Suggestions for judging credibility of conclusions are offered. The conclusions of large-scale, highly credible experiments, however, involve statistical calculations and thus apply to populations and not to individuals. The risk factor concept has been devised to help physicians aid healthy people in avoiding diseases by applying epidemiological results to individuals. While very useful in this objective, risk factors do not predict which individuals in a population will acquire a disease. Some risk factors are not under an individual's control. In these situations, it is suggested that health-wellness is best served by citizens' political action.

In Table 3.1, I have presented an estimate of relative certainties that certain types of experiments provide. You may be surprised at how low my estimates are. Most of us, I believe, are convinced that our friends and associates furnish more certainty than many of these experimental situations. When we make a date for lunch or tennis with a friend a week or a month in advance, we would be amazed if he or she didn't appear. If we drop a hot potato, we would be more than shocked if it didn't fall.

Planning our lives on a day-to-day or long-term basis requires *assumptions* of fairly high certainties. Even so, living contains surprises, many of them unpleasant. The divorce rate offers statistical evidence of shattered hopes and dreams. Risks abound, from being hit by a drunken driver, to slipping in the bathtub. We cannot anticipate all contingencies. *Assumptions* are essential. Awareness of *assumptions* allows us to vary them consciously, depending on our past experiences, and aids in evaluating fresh situations. Whether we allow unanticipated events to become stressful is often up to us and our attitudes toward certainty. These topics are discussed in the next chapter.

Chapter
4
Wellness and Stress Management

Handled well, stress is a friend that strengthens us for the next encounter.
Bernard R. Tresnowski

This chapter will help you

- recognize that the word *stress* has been so misused that it has become practically meaningless unless an author or speaker defines it;
- identify sources of psychological stressors;
- realize that stress management requires conscious coping;
- learn techniques that are helpful in combating stress;
- identify Type A characteristics in yourself and others and learn how to deal with them; and
- live with the uncertainties over which you have no control.

The American public has been deluged with articles on stress—as a situation to avoid, as a problem to overcome, as a cause of many diseases—since the publication of *The Stress of Life* by Hans Selye (1956). The subject of stress, however, really mushroomed after *Type A Behavior and Your*

Heart was published in 1974 (Friedman & Rosenman, 1974). In this book, Doctors Friedman and Rosenman describe a certain type of stressful behavior, which they term Type A, in great detail and identify it as a causative factor for heart disease. Stress has become a dirty word in these 14 years. It has become closely linked to Type A behavior, and many people think of them as synonymous. This view expresses an unfortunate oversimplification.

Another misleading oversimplification is that stress is often described as a condition that is always bad—a quagmire that traps the unwary—and that the stepping stones to happiness are composed of equal parts of tranquilizers and stress vitamins.

Stress has been part of human existence since prehistory. Think of the stress engendered in killing a woolly mammoth or tiger with Stone Age weapons, or the tensions built up when armies fought hand to hand. These topics were discussed by Cannon (1939) in *The Wisdom of the Body*. During millions of years of evolution, mammals developed characteristic behaviors of fight or flight on finding themselves in dangerous (stressful) situations. Carnivores obtain their food by fighting and killing. In contrast, many herbivores survive by running away. The human species, as it evolved, developed both types of behavior—sometimes fighting, sometimes fleeing—depending on the situation. There has been plenty of stress throughout history and prehistory. Yet, if we look at the pressures on people a bit more closely, we can conjecture significant differences between the types of stressors and their duration prevalent in preindustrial society versus industrial society.

What is new and different is not so much stress per se, but the rules that modern civilization has prescribed that limit one's responses to stressors. In modern society aggression is more frequently expressed verbally than physically. The fight-or-flight response is usually out of the question, but the sympathetic nervous system has not been civilized. Sensing the danger, it stimulates the secretion of hormones and the other physiological mechanisms that would be involved in the fight-or-flight response. These responses include an increase in concentrations of blood sugar and lipid as readily available sources of energy, a redistribution of the blood away from the digestive organs and towards the muscles, and a decrease in the blood's clotting time. It is obvious that all of these changes have survival value in fight-or-flight situations. Physical activity utilizes the energy liberated by these mechanisms, and when the danger has passed the person returns to a normal state of tension. The rates of hormone secretion slow down, the pulse rate and respiratory rate decrease, and by means of the processes of homeostasis (to be explained below), the body returns to its normal state.

As Freud realized, civilized humans are not permitted a physical outlet. They seethe in their own juices. They can sense their increased heart rates, rapid breathing, and pounding pulses, which signify an increased blood pressure, as well as their churning stomachs, and sweaty palms, but they are usually allowed only two alternatives: to respond civilly or to remain silent.

To study this question Hokanson and Burgess (1962) placed 80 college students under conditions of frustration. Their systolic blood pressures and heart rates were elevated compared with controls that were not frustrated. The frustrated group was subsequently allowed one of four types of aggression: physical, verbal, fantasy, or none. The blood pressures and heart rates of frustrated students allowed physical or verbal aggression against the frustrator soon returned to the levels of the nonfrustrated controls, whereas the blood pressures and heart rates of those restricted to fantasy or nonaggression remained elevated.

The Hokanson and Burgess study emphasizes the limitations in response to stressors that modern humans are forced to endure. Another difference, probably just as important as the first, originates from the major types of stressors that a person encounters. The major stressors in preindustrial societies were warfare, malnutrition, bacterial infections, exhausting labor with few if any protective devices, and lack of effective therapy after accidents. War, of course, was a very physical activity and may serve as a prototype of fight or flight. Malnutrition and infections have been and can be strong stressors; I classify them as physiological stressors. Hard physical labor can often be relieved by supper and a night's rest. This will allow sufficient recovery from the rigors of the day to enable the laborer to rise up and go out again the next morning, year after year. In the old days if one was born into the peasant class, one accepted that lifestyle as part of one's fate and died in peace and dignity at an average age of 40. Thomas Hobbes (1588-1679) a seventeenth-century English philosopher, succinctly described the condition of early humans: "In a state of nature, no arts, no letters, no society; and which is worst of all, continual fear and danger of violent death; and the life of man, solitary, poor, nasty, brutish, and short " (p. 65). Little wonder that the appearance of cheap distilled liquors in the sixteenth century was seized upon by many as an easy way to forget their troubles. Alcohol became the laborer's escape.

Sedentary work, which entailed very little physical activity, began to increase with the bookkeepers of Charles Dickens' day, but sedentary workers did not constitute a significant portion of the work force until the early years of the twentieth century. In the U.S. this fraction accelerated after World War I and has continued to increase ever since. In 1985, it was estimated that over 70% of the work force was engaged in sedentary work. This change in type of work, besides depriving a person of the automatic benefit of physical activity, has resulted in a great increase in the ratio of psychological to physiological stressors. It should be obvious that learning how to manage stressors so that they do not result in stress is a very important part of promoting wellness.

Defining the Word Stress

Stress has been used in engineering research and practice for many years. In this usage it means any external force directed at some physical object. The result of this force—a temporary or permanent alteration in the structure of the object—is called *strain*. This usage of stress and strain has been adopted by some writers in psychology and physiology, but not by all. The word stress was introduced into the psychological literature in 1945 by Grinker and Spiegel (1945) in their book, *War Neuroses*, which described the psychological effects of battle fatigue in airmen during World War II. As I understand the Grinker-Spiegel usage, the stressful conditions under which the fliers lived and fought for months at a time caused both physical and mental reactions in the men. This usage of stress as describing both the environment and a person's response to it is still common. An example follows.

"Don't Bring Stress Home" reads a headline in the *Salt Lake Tribune* summarizing an article about the health records of workers in 130 occupations (Smith, 1978). According to Dr. Michael Smith, Chief of Motivation and Research at the National Institute for Occupational Safety and Health (NIOSHO), the top six stress jobs were unskilled laborers, secretaries, assembly-line inspectors, clinical laboratory technicians, midlevel office managers, and foremen. Boredom, fatigue, and fast pace are the main problems of unskilled workers. Smith mentioned that deadlines add to the stress of secretaries and typists, and that the work is often boring. Deadlines by themselves are not necessarily stressful, Smith continued, if the work is interesting, as in newspaper reporting, practicing a profession such as medicine or law, or being a college professor. According to Smith, people who enjoy their work aren't stressed, merely strained.

Smith concluded that the six job categories mentioned above, as well as many others, include stresses that are as much a part of the job as the job description itself. These stresses are passed on automatically, inexorably, to the worker. Can you see that this use of the word stress demeans workers? It treats people as though they were inanimate objects that must carry the burden of stress that goes along with a job. In Smith's usage, stress means two things: an unpleasant component of a job, and a person's reaction to it. This usage leads to fuzzy thinking because one word is used with two quite different meanings. The ambiguity, in turn, leads to an absurdity, which Time magazine (1981) published: Stress, in addition to being itself and the result of itself, is also the cause of itself.

A third usage of stress places it solely inside an individual as a response to a stressor that may be either impersonal or personal. I favor this last usage for a number of reasons. It avoids the error of attributing stress to a job, per se. Stress is seen as closely related to the stimulus-response process—a well-studied phenomenon in physiology and psychology.

Stress responses are regarded as part of the process of homeostasis, the means by which the body maintains itself in a condition of constant composition and functioning. This view also allows for individual differences in responding to stimuli, for which there is abundant evidence. A minor annoyance for some people may result in other people's blowing their tops; some people enjoy working diligently and conscientiously, whereas others become angry and resentful if they are expected to work at a steady pace. The aphorism "One person's meat is another person's poison" applies to much more than food.

Frequent deadlines, overtime with no extra pay, boredom, or an office with blue walls, a pink carpet, or fluorescent lighting—any or all can be stressors or nonstressors. Whether they cause stress is based on a personal reaction. Many years ago I had a friend who worked as an analytical chemist. She analyzed organic compounds for their hydrogen and carbon content. This work was very precise, and she did it day after day. I thought it the most boring kind of work and wondered how an intelligent person could stand it. One day I said to her, "Thea, how do you put up with your boring job?" She replied, "Oh, it isn't boring. Every compound is different!" I learned something that day. It isn't what one does, it's how one looks at it.

For example, a welder may be expected to walk a narrow beam hundreds of feet in the air; a policewoman raps on a door, her answer may be a shot from inside; an auto racer cannot predict when the car ahead of him may blow a tire and cause a smashup. These occupations are known to be dangerous and are thus assumed to be stressful because a misstep, a deranged person, or a weak tire can set off a chain of events that may result in death or lifelong injury. In general, people who work at dangerous occupations learn to be careful, to concentrate on what they are doing, and to control their nervousness. Some people actually enjoy subjecting themselves to danger when they have been trained to meet it. Others, who do not learn to control their stress, change to a less hazardous job. It is really an individual matter. A stressor may be perceived as a threat or danger by one person, but as just another stimulus by another person.

Perceptions and judgment are involved in distinguishing a stressor from a stimulus. Lazarus (1966) and Lazarus and Folkman (1984) define a stressor as a troubled transaction between an individual and some aspect of the environment. This definition definitely places a stressor as a perceived threat or noxious, possibly dangerous, condition or substance with which one should be prepared to deal. In contrast, a stimulus may be negative, but it can also be neutral or positive. Ultimately, the distinction between a stimulus and a stressor becomes a matter of judgment.

The exercise of judgment presupposes that people are aware of what is happening in the environment—outside their skins. Many accidents occur, many stimuli and stressors are missed completely or are misjudged because of lack of attention. Persons engaged in work that bores them may get sleepy when they're not really tired and miss important stimuli because of inattention. A sizable number of auto accidents are caused each year by people falling asleep at the wheel.

In addition, individuals vary widely in their sensitivity to external stimuli and stressors. These differences have been studied in different people under similar conditions and in the same person under different conditions. Variations in sensitivity represent a continuum in both directions. For example, some people seem to have noses as sensitive as a dog's, whereas others are as insensitive as if they had a continuously stuffy nose. Similarly, sensitivity to stimuli varies with activity.

The sensation of pain functions to cut through, or overcome, distractions or inattention to stimuli or stressors and brings the injured area to a high priority for the conscious brain to deal with. Pain serves as a messenger to the brain that something serious is happening or has happened to us (i.e., wake up and do something about it!). The degree of pain also helps us to distinguish between stimuli of growing intensity and stressors.

The caricature of the absent minded professor becomes relevant here. Some professors, and many other people as well, engage in the unpopular habit of thinking at other places than their desks. Concentrating on a subject, problem solving, thinking of what to serve at one's next party, and so on shuts out the environment, and a person so engaged can carry an umbrella rather than put it up during a rainstorm, drive through a stop sign, or even be unaware of what another person has said. Some of these incidents may have humorous consequences and others serious. Concentration is essential in sports. The tennis players at the U.S. Open at Flushing Meadow have to learn to shut out the noise of the airplanes from nearby Kennedy airport or their concentration would be broken and they could not play well.

The recent emphasis on being aware of your body can be carried too far. If you have a pain, you should become aware of it; but to attempt to bring all of your sense organ signals into consciousness on a minute-to-minute basis—like a radar screen sweeping the sky—might make you incapable of doing anything else. Your mind should function as more than a wind sock or a thermometer—unless the wind begins to blow very hard or the mercury plunges precipitously. However, people who are engaged in any regular aerobic activity (e.g., jogging, running, cross-country skiing, backpacking, weight lifting, etc.), in which even slight injuries or metabolic aberrations such as dehydration or overheating may rapidly become serious if they are not noticed and attended to, need to follow the rule of listening to their bodies.

Five senses—taste, touch, sight, hearing, and smell—keep us aware of our environment. Each sense organ contains a type of receptor that is sensitive to a particular stimulus, and it sends nervous impulses to the brain on a continuous basis. The brain integrates all of the signals so that when we are conscious we know what is going on out there.

It should be mentioned that some stressors are not detected by our sense organ receptors. Carbon monoxide, for example, is a colorless, odorless gas that can kill before the person is even aware that something is wrong. Methane, another such gas, is the reason coal miners carry canaries into the tunnels with them. Birds have a higher rate of metabolism than humans and thus are more sensitive to lack of oxygen. Our visual receptors are sensitive to visible light but are damaged by ultraviolet light, which we cannot see. Sun blindness can result from unprotected eyes being exposed to reflections of sunlight on water or snow over a period of days or weeks.

Physiological Mechanisms of Stressor Responses

During the millions of years of evolution, animals, including humans, have been exposed to dangerous situations that could result in serious injuries. Survival of individuals has depended on two capabilities: quick action to avoid or outmaneuver a foe and the development of defense mechanisms if injured. At present, we think of threatening situations as being composed of one or more stressors. In a crisis, people have run faster and longer, jumped higher and farther, and lifted more weight than would have seemed humanly possible. In this section I'll discuss the mechanisms by which these feats are accomplished.

Figure 4.1 outlines the major pathways by which the body reacts to a stressor such as the cuts and bruises suffered in a car accident. Following an injury, the receptors in the skin stimulate nerves that carry signals up the spinal cord to the thalamus portion of the brain. Arrows in the diagram from the thalamus to the cerebral cortex indicate overall pathways in which stressors are identified and brought to the level of consciousness. The arrows from the cortex back to the thalamus represent some of the pathways of the response signals, which are part of the body's defense mechanisms toward stressors.

Response signals from the thalamus, as well as from other brain centers, feed into the hypothalamus—a complex nerve-*endocrine* organ. The endocrine portion of the hypothalamus synthesizes and secretes a number of hormone-releasing factors. These enter blood vessels that lead to the anterior pituitary gland and regulate the secretion of hormones from this gland. The major hormone involved in stressor responses is called adrenocorticotrophic hormone (ACTH). This hormone enters the blood and stimulates the adrenal cortex to secrete cortisol.

Three hormones—cortisol, epinephrine, and norepinephrine—are known as stress hormones. The secretion of epinephrine and norepinephrine increases almost instantly in response to a stimulus or a stressor that affects a receptor. The secretion of cortisol is somewhat slower. If the stressor acts for a long time, as from a broken bone, an extensive burn,

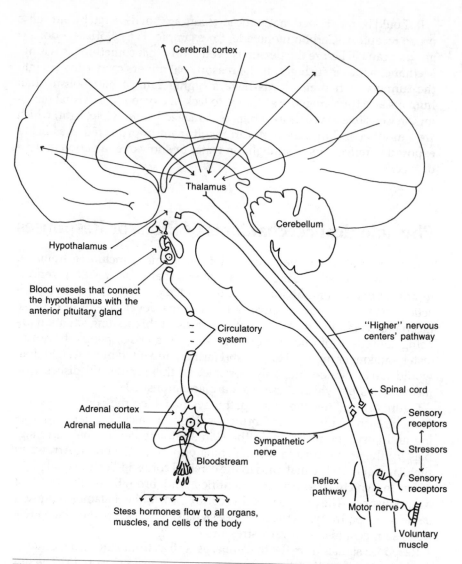

Figure 4.1　Pathways of stimulus-stressor responses.

or a major operation, secretion of these hormones is also prolonged. Cortisol and epinephrine affect the energy supplies so that the energy reserves become available for nerve and muscle action.

Now we come to an important distinction in the duration of action of stressors. Many physiological stressors are of short duration—from seconds to a few months. In contrast, malnutrition, infectious diseases, and serious trauma can result in long-term stresses. But there is another type of stressor, however, that may persist for years. This type includes psychological stressors that originate in the cerebral cortex and are shown in Figure 4.1 as arrows going from the cortex to the thalamic-hypothalamic area. These signals are handled by the nervous-endocrine systems in the same manner as physiological stressors. Thus psychological stressors also stimulate the secretion of stress hormones. We know that anger, fear, or anxiety can last from a few seconds to many years. In contrast to a short-term secretion that may save a person's life in an emergency, the chronic secretion of these same hormones may result in disease, disability, and even death.

It is useful to think of stress as a process or series of ongoing reactions whose original function is to aid the body in adapting to stressors, rather than as a static condition or situation.

A cold stimulus, for example, may cause a person to put on a sweater. If this action is insufficient to keep warm, and the person becomes aware that he or she may freeze if warmer clothes are not put on or movement away from the cold is not accomplished soon, then it becomes a stressor. In this example, it is clear that awareness and anticipation of harm are involved in evaluating the situation as stressful. Similarly, living in a smoggy area may be unpleasant to many people, but stressful to someone who has had a previous asthmatic attack because of it. Thus the appraisal of situations as possibly threatening or harmful is involved in distinguishing a stressor from a stimulus. If something or some situation is perceived as a stressor, people take steps to protect themselves before any stress occurs. It is obvious that perceptions of possible environmental threats followed by appropriate behavior play an important role in survival.

Another advantage of thinking in terms of stress reactions rather than stress per se is that most people know that reactions can vary in strength. For example, in an accident, a car hitting a person at 5 mph can cause injury, but at 50 mph, the injuries would be much greater. The person would be stressed, however, at either speed. We can take high blood pressure as another example. Hypertension is a well-known stressor of the circulatory system. A systolic/diastolic reading of 120/95, however, is in quite a different degree of seriousness from one of 180/120. Both people have the stress of high blood pressure, but the therapy would be quite different for the two. Likewise, two people may be stressed by the same stressor, but the stress reactions of one may be far more severe than those of the other, and as above, the suggested treatments would be quite different.

Stress research has demonstrated that our metabolic machinery is much better prepared to deal with short-term than long-term stressors. Long-term stressors that are unmanaged or mismanaged can be considered as similar to a disease process that results in irreversible physiological changes. A demanding boss, a nagging spouse, or an unrealistic ambition can pressure a person into some or many of the symptoms listed above, or into alcoholism or chronic illness. It is this extension of pathology from psyche to soma that emphasizes the importance of each person's learning to handle long-term psychological stressors.

Both stimuli and stressors may originate internally or externally. The arrows from stimuli and stressors to sensory receptors indicate the external ones. We become aware of them through our senses. It is worth noting that a stimulus or stressor that originates in another person in a social situation may affect or restrict our responses from slightly to strongly. Social settings exert a great influence on our response to stressors and whether we become stressed.

Due to the pioneering work of Hans Selye (1956) and his recent successors, we now have an outline connecting long-term stress to disease that is approaching a cause-effect relationship. For you to understand these mechanisms, I'll need to explain what is meant by the dynamic steady state and how it is altered by stress reactions.

Stress Upsets the Normal Dynamic Steady State

In his classic book, *The Wisdom of the Body*, Cannon (1939) used the term *homeostasis* (*homeo*, Gr. = always the same, unchanging; *stasis*, Gr. = tendency towards stability), as the sum of the processes by which the body maintains itself at relatively constant composition. Research with a variety of isotopes has demonstrated, however, that constant composition is an oversimplification of the actual situation. Although a person's total fat or protein content may not vary much from day to day, the actual components of the fat and protein—glycerol, fatty acids and amino acids, respectively—can vary widely. The enzymes in a normal person are constantly synthesizing and breaking down fat and proteins. The sum of these reactions is called *turnover*, a dynamic process, and homeostasis itself is understood as representing the sum of all the turnover reactions. In other words, homeostasis is now considered as representing a dynamic condition, which is more accurately expressed as *the dynamic steady state*.

This important idea can be understood by use of the analogy of a parking lot. Imagine a parking lot outside of a large shopping mall with room for 1,000 cars. If the cars actually present were counted once each hour and the numbers averaged from 8:00 a.m. to 6:00 p.m., the result would be 532 cars. If counts were made every day, we could calculate the daily average number and the standard deviation as 531 ± 61 cars. This number represents the homeostatic condition of the parking lot. But if we look at the parking lot in more detail, we see that some cars are entering and other cars are leaving most of the time. In other words, the actual composition of the population of cars is changing even though the total number remains constant. This exchange amounts to turnover, and we can explain the constancy of the homeostatic condition as a result of the dynamic steady state.

As we shall see, stimuli, stressors, and especially stress form a series of activators that change the dynamic steady state. The change may be temporary or long-term. For example, the normal steady state concentration of glucose in the blood is 80 ± 10 mg/100 ml. The concentration rises after an acute stress (trauma, burns) and then slowly returns to the normal range. If it remains high in the absence of stress, it is taken as a sign of a disease (probably diabetes).

The dynamic steady state can be compared to a physiological gyroscope. Like a gyroscope, it has the capacity to right itself if given a quick push. The dynamic steady state is different from a toy gyroscope in that the toy runs down in time but the dynamic steady state is kept running by the energy derived from the food we eat. A stimulus or stressor actually increases the energy that is available for fight or flight so that the person is able to cope with an emergency on an instant's notice.

For example, I recall an incident while backpacking in southern Utah. We were walking down a gully, and I saw one of the members of our group suddenly jump sidewards about 3 feet; at about the same time I heard a rustling in the leaves. Catching up to them, I inquired what had happened and was told that she had heard the rattling of a rattlesnake. She estimated that it was probably never closer to her than about 5 feet. When things had quieted down a bit, I asked her what her very first sensations were on becoming aware of the snake. She said that a feeling of warmth had run up the leg that was closest to the snake.

To understand the speed of her responses as well as the warming of her leg, I'll need to explain what goes on inside us when confronted with a sudden stimulus or stressor. Figure 4.1 outlines the pathways of stressor responses, both fast and slow. I'll describe the fast ones first as they are simpler to understand than the slow ones.

Immediate Stressor Responses: Reflex Pathways

Accidents sometimes happen so suddenly that, if we had to think about the response to make, it would take too long for signals to ascend the spinal cord, be processed in the cortex, descend the spinal cord, and activate a voluntary muscle to move an arm or a leg to avoid the stressor. A person might be killed or seriously injured in the second it would take for this response. To speed things up, reflex pathways have been developed, one of which is outlined towards the bottom of the spinal cord in Figure 4.1. If you have ever cut yourself while using a sharp knife, you may have noticed that your arm moved immediately—before you felt any pain. The sensory receptors at the place of injury signaled a peripheral nerve in the spinal cord. This nerve stimulated another nerve that led directly to a muscle in the arm, and—almost before you knew it—the arm had moved. Very fast reactions like this one, where the signal does not go to the brain first, are called reflex actions. They play an essential role in surviving unexpected bumps and injuries.

There was no physical contact in my friend's encounter with a rattlesnake, yet her visual and/or auditory systems were stimulated, the signals were processed in the cerebral cortex as coming from a snake, and immediately a long neurone in the spinal cord activated a peripheral nerve to stimulate her leg muscles to contract so that she could jump away. These responses are almost as fast as reflex actions.

The nerve-muscle junctions in the leg, when stimulated, are known to release the nerve-transmitter substance acetylcholine, which, in turn, stimulated the muscles to contract by hydrolyzing the energy-providing chemical adenosine triphosphate (ATP). Other reactions follow very rapidly, and heat is released in the process. The incident illustrates that, in a split second, a sudden shift in the dynamic steady state provided the energy for her jump.

At the outset of an emergency it is impossible to predict whether the stimulus will remain a stimulus or become a stressor. The body's defenses adapt to a dangerous situation much as a fire department sends in more equipment if a conflagration increases despite attempts to control it. In the incident I've described everything returned to normal in a few minutes. If, however, the woman had been bitten, she would have gone into stress almost immediately, and the dynamic steady state would have been altered to a greater extent and for a longer time while the body's defenses against rattlesnake toxin were being marshaled. In an emergency the dynamic steady state can change much faster than the cars in a parking lot. Emergencies demonstrate the value of maintaining normal muscle cell tension. The engine is always running and fuel—glucose—is always circulating; a quick response can be obtained by facilitating the entrance of the fuel into the muscle cells that use the energy for movement.

Longer Term Stressor Responses

Suppose my friend had severely sprained her ankle in jumping away from the snake? How else would her defense mechanisms have responded to the new stressor? She would have felt pain, which would result in emotional responses such as anxiety and fear. Behavioral responses such as crying or feeling cold might also have occurred. In addition, physiological changes would follow the activation of the sympathetic nervous system as well as stimulation of certain hormonal secretions that were described earlier.

The effects of these neurohormonal changes would be to increase the blood sugar concentration, increase the heart rate and blood pressure, and decrease blood flow to the viscera and skin. A feeling of being cold would result and it would be intensified by increased sweating. These symptoms are included in what Selye (1956) has called the *alarm reaction*. Depending on the severity of the injury, these changes might last from an hour to one or more days.

The Role of the
Three Stressor-Response Hormones

The actual functions of epinephrine, norepinephrine, and cortisol are quite different, and detailing them illustrates beautifully how the body responds to and protects itself in an emergency. The two hormones, epinephrine and norepinephrine, have similar chemical actions. Because they are released in different locations in the body, they stimulate different tissues. Norepinephrine is released by the sympathetic nerves in close proximity to the smooth, involuntary muscles. Once inside the muscle cell, it stimulates the hydrolysis of glycogen to glucose and fats to fatty acids—both sources of energy for the muscles. This response is backed up by the similar effects of epinephrine on the liver and fat depots. Epinephrine stimulates these two organs to release glucose and fatty acids into the blood, which in a few seconds bathes the voluntary muscles and provides these energy-utilizing tissues to burn the sugar and fatty acids for movement.

Cortisol acts as a backup to epinephrine and norepinephrine. Extra secretion of cortisol begins after a few minutes and may continue for hours, days, or as long as a stressor is acting. Cortisol stimulates the breakdown of proteins into amino acids. This effect accomplishes two purposes: first, most amino acids can be converted to glucose by the liver, which serves as an energy reservoir; second, because eating may be impossible during a stressful situation, the released amino acids can be used to synthesize new protein in case of injury. Cortisol raises the blood glucose concentration during a stressful period. Cortisol also redistributes fats from the fat depots to peripheral tissues, including the coronary arteries. This effect explains in part how long-term stress may increase the likelihood of strokes and heart attacks. A discussion of the role of fat deposition in the development of coronary artery disease is included in chapter 10.

The mechanisms by which psychological stressors increase blood pressure are also being gradually worked out. Light, Koepke, Obrist, and

Willis (1983) stressed young men who had either a family history of hypertension or borderline hypertension by having them compete in mental tasks. Under these conditions this group retained more sodium than a normal group. Sodium retention has long been considered a major factor in the development of hypertension (as I shall discuss in chapter 9), but this is the first report demonstrating its retention during stress in a high-risk group.

Figure 4.2 may help in clarifying the differences in effects between stimuli and stressors, and also between acute and chronic stress. The diagram omits the nerves, the portions of the central nervous system, and the stress hormone secretion system that were shown in Figure 4.1.

Stimuli are sensed by the sensory receptors, and their signals to the central nervous system aid in maintaining normal muscle cell tension. These processes are largely automatic, and we are hardly conscious of them. As stimuli become stronger, the sensory receptors send more signals to the nervous system, which results in excess muscle cell tension. At this point, a person should become conscious of the change in the environment and begin adapting to it. This process is called stressor management, and its objective is to reduce excess muscle tension back to normal muscle tension.

Figure 4.2 also summarizes a number of important differences and similarities between stimuli and stressors. The double arrow between stimuli and stressors indicates that the two form a continuum—if stimuli become stronger, they merge into stressors; if stressors weaken they may be judged as stimuli. A short stimulus may become a stressor if prolonged.

It is important to remember that what may be a stimulus for one person may be a stressor for another. The distinction between the two is based on individual judgment. As I have emphasized previously, judgment is always involved in the interpretation of an event. One person who has just flunked a test may be stimulated to try harder the next time, while another person may conclude that he is a failure and decide to commit suicide.

External stimuli may be either positive, neutral, or negative, whereas external stressors are by definition negative. Decisions about stimuli and stressors, however, are often uniquely individual. We tend to think of an external stimulus such as the smell of bread baking as desirable. But for a person on a reducing diet, such an aroma may act as a stressor.

External stimuli and stressors both act by stimulation of the sensory receptors. The intensity of the signals from the receptors allows the central nervous system to decide whether the stimulus is benign or a stressor. A strong stressor may bring a person to a condition of temporary stress very quickly. If the stressor is short-lived or if it is handled well, the person may return to a condition of excess or normal psycho-physiological responses quite rapidly. On the other hand, if the stressor is mismanaged or results in serious physiological damage, chronic stress may result.

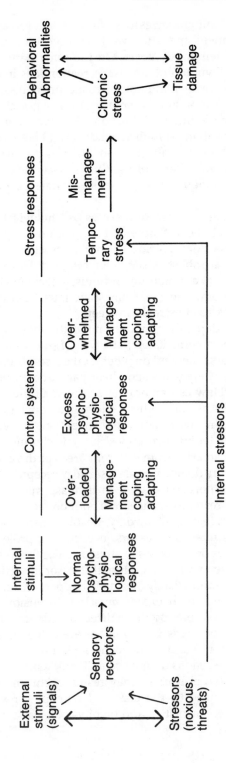

*The pathways of signals between the nerve-hormonal systems and the psycho-physiological system are omitted. These pathways are outlined in Figure 4.1.

Figure 4.2 Stimulus and stressor responses.

Many external stimuli and stressors affect us involuntarily. They are part of the environment and often we have no choice but to adapt to them—at least on a temporary basis. On the other hand we may seek out enjoyable stimuli voluntarily. Most recreation falls in this category. Occasionally a pleasurable stimulating situation may become stressing, such as being caught in a sudden snowstorm in light clothing.

In a remarkable article titled "Reflections: Experiencing Places" Tony Hiss (1987) describes varying stimuli in buildings and places in and around New York City and how they affect mood. He uses the term *simultaneous perception* to describe the effects of multiple sensations in creating feelings of wonder and tranquillity and a sense of shared experience in the midst of urban life.

Continued stimulation may lead to excess psychological-physiological responses. As we shall see in chapter 7, fatigue is one way of preventing excess muscle tension from developing into a stressful situation. Under most conditions, we are able to sleep when fatigued. During sleep external stimuli tend to be at a minimum and muscle tension also decreases. Fatigue due to boredom, however, may sometimes be circumvented by a change in activities as preferable to sleep.

External stressors, depending on their intensity, may rapidly result in temporary stress almost immediately. The type of stress management that is suitable will, of course, depend on whether the stress is primarily physical or psychological. Many years ago I heard an Arab proverb put in the form of a question: How can an animal be given all the food it can eat and yet remain thin? Answer: Tether a sheep in an open space and place a caged lion nearby. In this situation the sheep's usual type of stressor management, flight or hiding, was impossible, and chronic stress resulted.

Internal stressors can arise from different areas of the central nervous system. These stressors do not stimulate sensory receptors but do stimulate the sympathetic nervous system to increase muscle cell tension, psycho-physiological responses, and stress hormone secretions. Disturbed affects, such as anger, fear, guilt, anxiety, hostility, depression, love, and hate can function as internal stressors, especially if prolonged.

There are three types of responses to stressors. The first is excess muscle cell tension. If intense enough, an internal stressor like grief may result in temporary stress immediately, as may happen when a loved one dies suddenly. Second, both excess muscle cell tension and psycho-physiological responses may be normalized by adaptive behavior and coping. These types of stress management are achieved by a rational analysis of the stressor(s) and by devising a plan to deal with them so that long-term stress reactions do not occur. Third, temporary stress from either internal or external sources may result in chronic stress if mismanaged or unrecognized by the person. Non-coping responses often result in behavioral eccentricities and/or physiological abnormalities.

Behavioral eccentricities include alcoholism or other types of drug abuse, eating disorders, extreme shyness or loudness, hypochondria, Type A behavior, migraine headaches, and misanthropy. Stuttering, stammering, and other speech disorders can also occur. Some of the most serious effects of mismanaged psychological stress are on cognitive functioning. Thought processes, problem solving, perceptions, judgment, and perceptual motor skills are all decreased.

Tissue damage as an end product of mismanaged stress was studied extensively by Selye, who identified the following pathological changes: enlargement of the adrenal cortex, atrophy of lymphatic tissue, and ulceration of the stomach, to name a few.

He defined a class of diseases that he called diseases of adaptation to chronic stress. This class includes cardiovascular disease, high blood pressure, allergic reactions, connective tissue disease, kidney disease, and others. The connections between chronic stress and hypertension are discussed in chapter 9, and cardiovascular disease in chapter 10. It should be clear that managing stress is essential in two important ways concerning health: in the prevention of disease, as discussed above, and as a key group of techniques in the pursuit of wellness.

Short-Term Psychological Stresses Have Survival Value

I have the impression from reading the popular literature that stress is often described as an extreme condition, a quagmire in which you are caught, unless you take stress vitamins, tranquilizers, or some other medicine from which someone is making a profit. The harmful effects of stress are so overemphasized that people believe that all stress is to be avoided. This conclusion in inaccurate. Psychological stressors, like physiological ones, serve an important function.

A person who is not fearful when crossing a busy street is foolish. A man who does not become anxious and see a doctor when he has a pain in his chest is acting suicidally. Worry that leads to planning ahead is often valuable. The difference between a normal stimulus or signal and a stressor is not a difference in kind but in amount. Just as a short exposure to cold may be invigorating and a long exposure dangerous, a short anger may key up a person in a dangerous situation, but long-term hostility towards fellow workers is not only pointless, it may also become debilitating.

Psychological Stresses
and the "Diseases of Civilization"

Although the term stress had not entered the medical vocabulary at the time Freud was writing *Civilization and Its Discontents* in the 1920s, there is little doubt that he was describing what are now called psychological stressors. We can now understand the reason for Freud's emphasis. In civilized societies a person may expect to encounter many more psychological stressors per year than physiological ones.

For example, a person may imply or state that you have been dishonest or incompetent when you know that the statement is unfair and inaccurate. If a friend or acquaintance makes such a remark, you may become angry and tell him or her off either physically or verbally. Under these conditions, the stress that has been generated may be relieved. But if your boss or supervisor makes a derogatory remark about you, these outlets are not permissible—unless you don't mind losing your job. Often in modern society when such an incident happens, your only recourse is to suffer in silence, to hide your anger and anguish, and to attempt to answer civilly and politely, if any answer is allowed. Under these conditions, the stress reactions are unrelieved, and it is this lack of opportunity to react naturally that distinguishes the major stresses of modern times from those of previous times.

Complaining to a friendly third party about one's problems at work or home is often nonproductive for a number of reasons. The direct antagonist or source of threat is usually absent. A gripe-session serves mainly to bolster the ego of the threatened person and neither probes into the reasons behind the perceived threat nor considers possible resolutions of conflict. Unloading your troubles on a friend is only a verbal exercise. The session may increase your stress, not lower it. A tense, stressed person would probably feel better if he or she learned to relax, engaged in some form of active exercise, or took out his or her frustrations in a game or sport.

Stress represents the end response to a stressor that has not been managed; that is, the stressor has overcome the person's defenses against it. Stress responses to a single psychological stressor may proceed in a regular series. First, brief emotional reactions like hate, hostility, impatience, worry, and anxiety occur; these are accompanied by a hypernormal secretion of the stress hormones. If the stress becomes chronic, the so-called stress hormones continue to be secreted in larger amounts than normal. These hormones, especially cortisol, affect a wide variety of tissues, including the nervous system, and the continued hypernormal secretion leads to tissue damage by altering the metabolism of the person in significant ways.

Because the shift from normal feelings and healthy emotions to pathological ones is a continuum, many people are unable to realize when they have slipped over the line. Who is to say how much anxiety is healthy and how much is sick? There are too many variables to allow a general answer. I have written above as though there were quantitative scales for measuring the emotions and feelings. In all honesty, there aren't any, although psychologists are attempting to develop them. We have no devices to measure anxiety as we have for blood pressure. The usual measures of anxiety come from what a person tells us about it or else is inferred from his or her behavior. Neither is quantitative. We are a long way from the hypothetical situation in which a physician tells a patient,

> Your anxiety index is 7.9 on a scale of 10. Unless you bring the index down to at least 5.5 in the next 6 months by employing the psychic exercises that the anxiety specialists will train you in, you will probably develop high blood pressure, because you have a familial tendency in that direction. Good luck, and don't forget to have your anxiety index checked regularly.

Pathological Effects of Stress: Soma Directed

Examples of the effects of stress on the cardiovascular, digestive, and muscular systems are included in Table 4.1. The behavioral and cognitive aspects of stress responses are presented in Table 4.2, and stress-related diseases and conditions are listed in Table 4.3.

The wide variety of conditions and diseases listed in these tables raise an interesting question: How can stress reactions possibly result in all of them? Medical scientists are now tracing the pathways between types of stressors, neurohormonal responses, and pathological effects. The results suggest that there are common routes—common denominators—by which stress reactions produce such widespread damage.

Long-term stress has been shown to decrease the functioning of the immune system. This system makes the antibodies that help protect us against a wide variety of infectious agents and allergens. If the immune system loses effectiveness, a person becomes more susceptible to more infections and diseases than otherwise. The immune system provides an example of a common denominator that helps explain how long-term stress acts as a disease-enhancing process.

Jemmott et al. (1983) measured the amounts of immunoglobulin A in the saliva of dental students during the course of a school year. This protein helps protect against a variety of viruses, including those of colds. While the amounts of the immunoprotein dropped in all the students at

Table 4.1   Examples of the Effects of Stress on the Cardiovascular, Digestive, and Muscular Systems

Cardiovascular	Elevated heart rate
	Increased blood pressure
	Increased heart rate variability
	Coronary heart disease
Digestive	Burning sensation in stomach, chest, and throat areas (due to increased stomach acidity)
	Nausea
	Loss of appetite
	Reduction in the flow of saliva
	Ulcers
	Disruption of rhythmic peristalis (making swallowing difficult, causing diarrhea, etc.)
Muscular	Tense muscles
	Tension headaches
	Tightness of chest cavity
	Spasms of the esophagus/colon (Diarrhea/constipation)
	Backache
	Tension at back of neck
	Tension around the stomach

Note. From *A Behavioral Approach to the Management of Stress* (p. 9) by H.R. Beech, L.E. Burns, and B.F. Sheffield, 1982, New York: Wiley. Copyright 1982 by Wiley. Adapted by permission.

Table 4.2   Stress Responses: Behavioral and Cognitive Aspects

Behavioral	Decreased performance level
	Overcompetitiveness
	Attempt to control situations and people
	Egotism
	Impatience with others
	Generalized hostility
	Passivity/inertia
Cognitive	Distortions of thinking
	Lowered intellectual functioning
	Unproductive, ruminative, anxiety-generating patterns of thinking
	Indecisiveness

Note. From *A Behavioral Approach to the Management of Stress* (p. 11) by H. R. Beech, L.E. Burns, and B.F. Sheffield, 1982, New York: Wiley. Copyright 1982 by Wiley. Adapted by permission.

Table 4.3   Examples of Stress-Related Diseases and Conditions

Cardiovascular system	Coronary artery distress Hypertension Strokes Rhythm disturbances of the heart
Muscular system	Tension headaches Muscle contraction backache
Locomotor system	Rheumatoid arthritis Related inflammatory diseases of connective tissue
Respiratory and allergic disorders	Asthma Hay fever
Immunological disorders	Lowered resistance Autoimmune diseases
Gastrointestinal disturbances	Ulcer Irritable bowel syndrome Diarrhea Nausea and vomiting Ulcerative colitis
Genitourinary disturbances	Diuresis Impotence Frigidity
Dermatological diseases	Eczema Neurodermatitis Acne
Other problems	Fatigue and lethargy Type A behavior Overeating Depression Insomnia Diabetes

Note. From *A Behavioral Approach to the Management of Stress* (p. 13) by H.R. Beech, L.E. Burns, and B.F. Sheffield, 1982, New York: Wiley. Copyright 1982 by Wiley. Adapted by permission.

the time of a particularly difficult exam, it decreased less in the more relaxed students. It also rose faster in the relaxed group after the stress of the exam was over.

Suls and Fletcher (1985) checked the hypothesis that stress resistance is related to a predisposition to focus on internal aspects of the self. This type of introspection is termed *private self-consciousness*. A private self-consciousness inventory was filled out by 120 adult subjects as well as a list of recent life events and a symptom checklist. The incidence of stress-ful life events predicted subsequent illness in subjects low in private self-consciousness but not in subjects high in private self-consciousness. These results confirm those of other experiments that support the conclusion that so-called stressful events and their effects are not determined by what happens to you, but by how you react to them—by what happens *in* you.

We thus have clear indications that chronic stress can result in debilitat-ing diseases and shortened lives. Recently, publicity has coupled psy-chological stress to susceptibility to cancer. I'll discuss this possibility next.

Stress and Cancer

During the past few years there have been a number of articles in the media that postulated that susceptibility to cancer was related to chronic stress. My first reaction was that these claims were pretty farfetched, and I didn't pay much attention to them. Since, as has been mentioned, stress can impair the immune system and the immune system is involved in controlling the spread of cancer in an individual, the possibility of a con-nection between stress and cancer is worth investigating.

An eminent American physician, Willard Parker (1885), noted that strong grief often preceded the onset of breast cancer. Recent work tends to confirm these observations, but the evidence to support the connection between chronic stress and cancer is still tenuous. In this sec-tion I'll present the pros and cons of these interesting and important controversies.

During the 1950s, LeShan (1959) and colleagues studied the link be-tween catastrophic events and cancer. They examined mortality data of widows and widowers and determined whether the survivor subse-quently died of cancer more frequently than would be expected by chance. They concluded that cancer was more frequent following the loss of a partner. Greene (1966) obtained similar results in patients with leukemia and lymphoma. On the other hand, Muslin, Gyarfas, and Pieper (1966) compared breast cancer patients to those having benign tumors with regard to a loss of someone to whom the patient was deeply and emotion-ally attached. They found that the emotional loss did not correlate with the subsequent incidence of benign and malignant tumors.

Schmale and Iker (1966) investigated a possible relationship between cancer of the cervix and feelings of hopelessness in 51 women who were essentially healthy, had no gross evidence of disease, and were under age 50. Predictions of cancer were made on the basis of reported responses of hopelessness to a life event during the preceding 6 months. They cor-rectly identified 11 out of 19 women with cancer and 25 out of 32 without cancer.

Graham, Snell, Graham, and Ford (1971) studied the relation of social trauma to cancer of the cervix and breast in a large number of women. Social trauma was defined as death, divorce, unemployment, economic want, or prolonged illness in the family for the previous 5 years. Social trauma was not correlated with the incidence of cancer in this population. These conflicting results do not permit firm conclusions to be drawn concerning the relationship of stress to subsequent incidence of cancer.

Is There a Cancer Personality?

An English physician, Sir Richard Guy (1759), suggested that cancer of the breast was more common in women who were nervous and given to hysteria and depression. The hypothesis that a certain kind of person is more likely to develop cancer than someone with a different personality is now being evaluated carefully by a number of psychologists. A person with a cancer personality is passive and goes through life expressing little or no emotions. The pent-up emotions of such people are thought to weaken the immune system. This effect may make a person more susceptible to cancer as well as other diseases. Besides being relatively apathetic, these people do not struggle in the face of hardship, but just give up.

As we saw in chapter 3, prospective studies in general lead to firmer conclusions than retrospective ones. This caution is especially relevant to investigations of the cancer-personality hypothesis because the disease has such a long induction period, and the patient's personality may be affected before overt symptoms occur. In addition, significant components of lifestyle may have been forgotten or misemphasized by the patient. These limitations become even stronger in investigations of emotional trauma due to death of a family member and the attempt to relate the loss to the subsequent development of cancer. For these reasons, the conclusions of the retrospective studies mentioned below are to be considered more as suggestions of possible relationships than as established generalizations. Another reason for caution in accepting the conclusions of retrospective studies of the cancer-personality hypothesis is the large number of publications that do not confirm it.

Studies at Kings College Hospital in London found a positive correlation between suppressed anger and incidence of breast cancer in women. The more passive women also died sooner after they developed the disease than the more feisty ones who expressed their emotions. Claude and Marjorie Bahnson (1969) and Claude Bahnson alone in a later project (1980, 1981) studied patients with and without malignant disease and found significant differences in personality. Cancer patients, and those who were cancer-prone, repressed emotions related to deaths in the family.

In addition, they found that cancer patients denied that they experienced feelings of defeat, failure, frustration, and lack of acceptance or love.

Greer and Morris (1975, 1978) interviewed and administered personality tests to 160 women admitted for breast tumor biopsy. Breast cancer was significantly related to extreme suppression of anger. Patients over 40 also suppressed other feelings. No significant differences were found between patients and controls in a variety of other characteristics such as psychiatric disorders, marital relations, interpersonal relations, work and leisure activities, verbal intelligence, hostility, extroversion, or neuroticism.

Morrison and Paffenbarger (1981) summarize all these studies as proving nothing. They criticize the retrospective studies for ignoring the long latent period of cancer that might affect the personalities of the subjects. Known risk factors for cancer, such as smoking, have not been controlled, and many inconsistent results have been reported indicating that other important variables have not been controlled.

There are relatively few prospective studies that have investigated the cancer-personality hypothesis. Hagnell (1966) reported the results of one of the few prospective studies that attempted to relate personality types and cancer. In 1947 he classified 2,550 people in Sweden on a 5-point personality test. In males, he found cancer incidence over the next 10 years to be independent of personality. Women with cancer, however, were more socially oriented, warm, hearty, and more interested in people than those without the disease. On the other hand, Shekelle et al. (1981) gave a personality test to over 2,000 men, and checked death certificates 17 years later on how many had died from cancer. Those who had been depressed were twice as likely to have died from cancer than the others ($p < .001$). There was no significant difference in non-cancer death rates ($p = .131$).

Thomas and colleagues (1974, 1976, 1977, 1979) had been administering psychological tests and questionnaires to over 1,300 Johns Hopkins medical students since 1948. By 1979, 48 had developed cancer. Examination of the questionnaires of the cancer group when in medical school revealed a lack of closeness to parents compared to those who did not acquire the disease. This study, however, has been faulted in two aspects. First, Thomas did not consider the role of smoking as a cancer-causative agent that would act independently of the psychological factors she was evaluating. Second, the differences that she found were not statistically significant. On the other hand, the Thomas research was designed more as a pilot study to examine possibilities than as a study that would prove or disprove a hypothesis. It is possible that the early cancers in the Thomas study may be more closely related to personality factors than later cancers—where long-term carcinogens may be expected to become more important. Unfortunately, despite Thomas' cautions about the limitations of the study, it has been widely publicized as demonstrating the effects of personality on susceptibility to cancer.

Sources of Psychological Stressors

Most of the popular literature on stress, and some textbooks as well (Zimbardo, 1979), assume that a person's major stressors are out there in the environment. This category contains life crises (Holmes & Masuda, 1974; Sarason & Johnson, 1976). The list includes bad events like death of a partner or other loved one, divorce, loss of a job, and the like. By and large, many of these are unavoidable, and the stress they induce is dependent on the person's ability to adapt or otherwise adjust to them. Job-induced stress is the other major source. This category includes work overload—too much pressure to produce, either products per se, or sales—and work underload—frustrations, boredom, lack of a feeling of accomplishment, and so forth. In the environmental model, stressors are like chuckholes in the street: one tries either to avoid them or, failing that, to drive slowly enough so that running into a hole doesn't cause stress.

A second category of psychological stressors is that imposed on the young by their parents, relatives, older friends, or acquaintances. These may include the usual moral imperatives against lying, cheating, stealing, hurting other people either physically or psychologically except in self-defense, and destroying or damaging other people's property maliciously. I suspect that much of the meaning of the verb to mature lies in the gradual realization of the discrepancy between the morality taught in Sunday school and the morality that is practiced downtown. Yet most of us learn to rationalize the hypocrisy we observe, with certain reservations for exceptional circumstances, without a great deal of stress. We also learn that personal freedom stops at the end of another person's nose.

An exception to this group of constraints are those dealing with various aspects of sex. Too many children are brought up to believe that the sex act is dirty and immoral, except by married couples who desire children. This bias has resulted in a refusal to allow sex education in the public schools with the excuse that it is the responsibility of the parents to impart this knowledge as well as the accompanying morality. This procedure might work out satisfactorily if it were carried out by a majority of parents. My perception is that in home presentations morality takes precedence over the facts of reproduction, with a consequent large number of unwanted pregnancies resulting.

The reproductive urge is strong in all species—including the human—otherwise they would not have survived. The phrase, "The human race is part of nature," is popular in some circles, but in matters of sexual activity, many cultures have forbidden doing what is natural. I recall my teenage urges and the stresses that resulted. Perhaps, if I hadn't obtained my sex information in the gutter, I could have handled the situation with less stress than I endured.

Masturbation, especially, is surrounded by a mythology that predicts everything from criminality to insanity for those who practice it. Perhaps it would be a more satisfactory substitute for the sex act by teenagers if the guilt could be removed from it. Adolescent, middle-class Americans are placed in a catch-22 situation. They are prohibited from doing what their hormones are urging; they are told it is sinful to even think such thoughts. I suspect that society has burdened the young with enough stress on sex matters alone to insure a large number of lifelong maladjusted people.

To help avoid sex guilt or to help overcome it, I am pleased to recommend two excellent books on human sexuality: *The Facts of Love* by Comfort and Comfort (1979) and *Sex Without Guilt* by Ellis (1966). The Comforts' book is addressed to young people and their parents. Ellis discusses touchy subjects like "Adultery, Pros and Cons," "Why Americans Are So Fearful of Sex," and "How American Women Are Driving American Males Into Homosexuality."

A third category of psychological stressors includes those that originate in people and are communicated to their friends and associates. Whether a person is conscious of stressing others or does it unconsciously, the effects are negative, and interpersonal relations suffer.

Psychologically aggressive people can be divided into two groups. The first is the Type A category (Friedman & Rosenman, 1974) whose manner of coping leads them to stress others. Psychologists consider Type A behavior as an example of defective coping and stress mismanagement, and it will be discussed in that section of this chapter. The second group of aggressive people is composed of those who habitually stress others due to faulty use of language, who have not learned to distinguish opinion—their opinions—from fact.

The problem I am describing can be considered as a semantic one—a question of meaning. People who make a statement about something or about other people know what they mean or think they do. Whether their words express their ideas clearly is another matter. How often do you hear a person exclaim in the middle of a heated discussion, "But what I meant was . . ." And often what was meant is quite different from what was being argued. Many people express personal opinions about the world and about other people as generalizations. For example, how often do you hear someone speak of another person's actions in terms of *good* and *bad*? This manner of expressing a judgment pins a highly inflammatory label on a person, and if the judgment is expressed directly to the person or if he or she hears it from a third party, he or she can be sorely stressed by it. To make matters worse, sometimes in the heat of an argument a person slips from calling an action bad to implying that another person is bad. Then watch the stress hormones flow! My point is that these judgments flow directly from one's value system and have no validity as generalizations beyond it. The use of ambiguous, ultimate terms like good and bad, right and wrong, polarize situations and relationships. They often leave little room for discussion and decrease chances for a less emotional, rational analysis of the subject.

If we can but remember that there are two sides to every argument, that there may be alternate yet reasonable viewpoints to our own, that few conclusions are all right or all wrong, we won't get slapped down so often. To discuss prickly questions with other people and still retain them as friends requires two attributes, one of which is dependent on the other. The first is learning not to put the person on the defensive. Unless you are discussing hard science, don't try to prove anything—it generally can't be done. It isn't a sensible objective. Most arguments revolve around judgments—and who is infallible? Becoming adept at general conversation is aided considerably by becoming aware of your own value judgments and your own basic assumptions. The other attribute is the one mentioned above: Do not express opinions as facts and avoid absolute terms, which are the verbal equivalent of poison.

The solution to not stressing others is really quite simple, that is, simple to write about. It amounts to stating an opinion as an opinion and only as an opinion yet avoiding the criticism of being considered opinionated! To avoid being considered as opinionated, you need to become aware of both verbal and nonverbal responses to your own statements. A verbal response that tells you that you have overstated a position is, ''What is there to say?'' You are being told very politely that your remark has left no room for discussion. If you want feedback, you need to give people adequate psychological space. If your remarks are perceived as a threat by others, they may threaten you right back. If you often feel stressed in social situations where you didn't anticipate any, it may be advisable to consider that you are the source of the original stressor. Telling people off may give you a sense of power, but it will lose you friends faster than cheating at golf.

Some people deal with the difficulties of expressing themselves by saying very little. They simply will not express an opinion. That may be a safe way to avoid stressful experiences, but it also results in a very dull life. Speaking for myself, I have found it much more satisfactory to express an opinion without driving other people up the wall than to sit silent for fear of offending. I think of it as practicing a game.

The Verbal Expression of Human Perceptions Often Results in Interpersonal Stressors and Needless International Antagonisms

As mentioned previously, our sense organs are responding to stimuli of various types, 24 hours a day as long as we live. Many of these stimuli give rise to nerve impulses that are carried to the central nervous system, including the higher centers, where they are interpreted and we become conscious of them. The interpretation includes our past experiences so that, in addition to our sensations of what is out there, we also form perceptions about the environment. These judgments include the distinctions between ordinary stimuli and stressors, between beauty and ugliness, and so forth. Because these perceptions are dependent on an individual's sense organs, and past experiences as well as his or her assumptions and value judgments, they are unique and therefore subjective, not objective.

It appears that most animals possess these types of sense organ receptors and responses. But animals can communicate only a few of their perceptions, as in cries of warning of danger or the use of scents to mark territories; only humans talk. This ability of humans has inestimable survival value, but the widespread, worldwide failure to recognize the subjective factors in our verbal expressions has made for serious errors in communication that have destroyed countless personal relationships as well as played an important role in inciting war.

It seems obvious to me that the verbal expression of our perceptions should overtly recognize their subjectivity. The subjective aspect of our generalizations, however, is often ignored. People assume that they are being objective when they are not, or a second party will assume that he or she is being given objective information when he or she is not.

A common error is that of stating personal perceptions as facts. Instead of expressing our perceptions as personal opinions, we say, "That is a beautiful building" or "Isn't she homely?" We assume that our perception is the correct one and state it as such. This habit places someone else with a different perception with the difficult task of disagreeing without questioning our judgment and/or intelligence. In my opinion we should state our perceptions as personal judgments; for example, "I think that the building is beautiful" or "She strikes me as homely." If you start listening to how many people express their opinions about objects, other people, ideas, and so on you will find that you usually learn more about the person than about the object.

First, an example dealing with an object. A couple built a log house in our neighborhood—the only one in this part of town. It is distinctive but doesn't fit the style of the other houses. Still, as long as people don't violate the zoning laws of a given community, they can build the kind of house they desire where they choose. Imagine then, the new couple cleaning up their front yard when a longtime resident passed by and asked them why they had built such an ugly house! A fine welcome for a new neighbor! What a way to commence a friendship! Suppose she had said, "In my opinion your house is ugly." Would the situation have been less tense? What is the possibility that, in phrasing her remark as an opinion, she may not have said it at all?

Recognizing the subjectivity of our generalizations and judgments also has another important consequence. It weakens the connections between our conclusions and our egos. In other words, a criticism is deflected from our easily hurt ego—as solely responsible for an error—to include our sense organs, which most of us learn to recognize as fallible. Recall the errors in perception that have been studied by Loftus (see chapter 3, "The Validity of Eyewitness Testimony").

Another complication resulting from our manner of verbal expression, and one with enormous potential for interpersonal and international antagonism and conflict, is that humans treat abstractions similar to how they discuss concrete objects and processes.

Consider another example with international overtones. During his first term, President Reagan remarked publicly that the U.S. represented the forces of good in the world whereas the Russian government represented the forces of evil. The use of these terms includes the assumption that everyone agrees on their meaning—which to me seems highly improbable. I interpret the use of the terms *good* and *evil* in this manner as a gratuitous insult that hardly befits the office of President. Recall, however, that Secretary Khrushchev's remark some years ago that "We will bury you" is in the same genre. Does this manner of speaking promote peace?

This type of misuse of language by rulers and rabble-rousers has been used repeatedly over the centuries to stir up passions against "the enemy." In a democracy we have the privilege of electing our leaders. Fortunately or unfortunately, we elect our leaders in our own image. The fact that President Reagan was re-elected with a solid majority *after* he made the above statement indicates that this manner of thinking and talking is typical of how the American people think. I suggest that public education on the use and misuse of language—starting in the first grade and continuing through high school—would help reduce both interpersonal and international tensions (stressors).

Echo Stressors and Silent Echoes

People receiving psychological stressors from others may respond aggressively—verbally or physically. If the stressor-initiating persons were unconscious of the stressors they were broadcasting, they may be surprised and astounded at the response. Their own stress can be increased considerably and rapidly. I call this type of response the *echo effect*. If the original persons are astute and realize what has happened, they can often defuse the situation by a neutral remark or an apology. If they are not aware of what has happened, or have become stressed themselves, they may respond in kind and fight until exhausted—physically or emotionally. People who encounter echo stressors in social situations without recognizing themselves as the source need practice in sharpening their insights and in controlling their stressor output.

Many people are polite by either training or necessity; their response to a verbal stressor is silence. Depending on how threatened they feel as a result of being the object of a verbal stressor, they will leave stressing persons as soon as politeness allows and will avoid them in the future.

These *silent echoes* give rise to questions like "Why didn't I get promoted?" "Why doesn't Roger call me any more?" "Why does May avoid me?" Direct answers to questions of this type are difficult to come by. They comprise some of the major, long-lasting uncertainties of living. Stressing persons don't know whether they may have insulted someone inadvertently, received a higher grade on a test, or beat them out for a promotion. To add to the uncertainty, if they ask, they probably won't get an honest answer; and if they did get a response they might become stressed because those who were silent have now pointed out a fault.

Don't Let Continuing Uncertainty Become Stressful

In chapter 3, I mentioned that scientists have become used to living with uncertainty and that, insofar as the general public is aware of and dependent on scientific advances, it is being forced to accept the uncertainties that go along with them. The uncertainty of the role of cholesterol in heart disease, however, is insignificant compared to the uncertainties encountered in daily living.

In fact, living is closer to a free-floating crap game than it is to science. Personal relations probably provide far more uncertainty than any other source. We think we know our friends and depend on them for solace and support—and suddenly they are less sympathetic, and we don't hear from them as often as we used to.

We look at ourselves in the mirror, recognize our friends day after day, year after year, and conclude that we—and they—change very little. Appearances are deceiving. As I mentioned earlier, the dynamic steady state keeps functioning, and we keep changing as long as we live. The major changes are internal. Our bodies and faces are like masks that hide the changing people inside.

If we repress our thoughts and emotions we become strangers to ourselves. To me, this is the real meaning of the expression *hollow people*. In these people, the connections between their rational thoughts and their extrarational impulses seem broken. Unpleasant things just happen to them, and they become stressed by events that they don't understand. Over 2,000 years ago Socrates wrote, "The unexamined life is not worth living." I will be brash enough to paraphrase it as, "The unexamined life is often damned stressful." How do we manage to avoid stress in the midst of the shocks and uncertainties of everyday living? By learning to cope.

Symptoms of Chronic Stress

For the past 20 years or so I have seen estimates that 60% to 80% of the people who make appointments with physicians are not objectively sick.

Articles in the press, as well as TV ads, have publicized the symptoms of these people. For completeness, I'll list them again: Depressed, anxious, feel unloved, neglected, lonely, and no longer enjoying life; always tired; often bored, at work and at home; frequent colds and other respiratory infections; frequent headaches, usually termed migraine; loose bowel, chronic insomnia; a feeling of cold, even in a warm room; excessive use of alcohol or other drugs; allergies.

These people obviously aren't well, but if they visit a doctor and no evidence of physical disease is found, neither are they classified as sick. They are not cheered if the doctor says, "Congratulations, there is nothing wrong with you." They know better. They know they aren't enjoying their lives as much as they feel they should. On one hand, they want to recover the pep and energy they had years ago. On the other hand, they don't want to be told, "It's all in your head." They also know that they are not mentally ill with all that implies. Many physicians try to soothe the patient by talking of the stressful time we are living in and acknowledging that everyone's nerves are on edge.

At this point, I want to say a few words about how our medical system works. For various reasons, many physicians engaged in family practice or internal medicine—those who see the majority of the general public—do not choose to get involved in the psychological problems of their patients. Most physicians have been trained to treat and cure diseases with known causative factors. Therapy usually involves prescribing a medication. They have not been trained to treat psychological conditions or diseases. Prescribing Valium® or some other tranquilizer for what physicians recognize as a psychological disease fits in with their usual practice of drug therapy. As they give patients the prescription, physicians may smile and say, "These pills will help to calm your nerves." The habit of prescribing drugs for just about every medical ailment is so deeply ingrained in American medical practice that if a physician does not prescribe one, a patient may judge him or her as unsatisfactory and go to another doctor. Apparently what people are looking for is a pill that will pep them up and make life seem worth living.

The Medical Approach to Stress Management

There are sound reasons why Valium® is a very widely prescribed drug in America. It makes people feel better. Do you remember the story of Ponce de Leon's search for the Fountain of Youth? He died an old man, never having found it. In my view, looking for a health pill is just as futile. Our brains are so complicated that if a chemical like Valium® is found that promotes certain desirable feelings, it is probably also going to result in some undesirable side effects. If the pharmaceutical industry ever develops peace of mind in a bottle, it will be at the cost of being human, of being aware of and responding to stressors, and, ultimately, of being aware of and responding to the needs of others.

Tranquilizers (antianxiety drugs) are recognized as depressant drugs. They sedate people and produce drowsiness. Most people do adjust to this side effect after a short time. To me, the most serious drawback in taking tranquilizers is that they don't help people cope with their problems. The person is just less disturbed by them. Over a period of months or years the unmanaged stressors may become more serious or new ones may develop, and the person on a tranquilizer may respond by taking larger and larger doses. A person on chronically large doses of a tranquilizer is subject to more serious side effects than drowsiness. Alcohol intake has to be markedly restricted or even prohibited or psychotic episodes may occur. Large amounts of these drugs are addictive. What started out as an easy solution to a person's problems may end in his or her being hooked. I suggest that people think of these common long-term effects before they choose that route to happiness. They may have bought happiness at the price of becoming less human.

A Personal Approach to Stress Management

If you are chronically bothered by one or more of the symptoms listed above, you may suspect that stress is at the bottom of them. It is not wise, however, to assume this. Don't diagnose a disease from its symptoms. It is advisable as a first step to visit a physician and request a thorough physical examination. If you are told that there is nothing wrong, you are lucky. The doctor may prescribe Valium® or some other tranquilizer for the control of your symptoms. The prescription is your physician's way of telling you that he or she thinks that your symptoms are due to unrecognized or unmanaged stress. It is at this point that the personal approach branches off from the medical. If you are smart, you can interpret the prescription as a signal for you to start taking your life into your own hands. Your first act in this endeavor will be to drop the prescription into the first wastebasket you pass. Take the money you have saved on pills and have a good time that evening. Consider it as your first night in your fight for personal freedom—your first step on a path toward wellness. If this recommendation seems too brash, you may find a physician/counselor or stress management expert who will supervise non-drug therapy.

But let's face it. You have accepted a difficult challenge with no assurance or guarantee that you will succeed. You may be encouraged, however, to learn that millions of people have taken this same path and have emerged as more capable, healthier human beings. There is nothing magical in their achievement. I'll outline below a step-by-step procedure that you can use as a guide to set up your own program.

Step one amounts to a decision on your part whether to accept the doctor's diagnosis that your symptoms are due to stress. If you have any question about it, you may wish to obtain additional evidence. Fortunately, this evidence is easy to get. For starters, you can answer the questionnaires in the appendix at the end of this chapter. These tests not only give an indication of how stressed you are, but also help identify the types of psychological stress that are bothering you the most.

Many people have been helped by counselors who specialize in working with stressed clients. A number of state health departments support ongoing programs in stress management. You can obtain expert counseling at reasonable group rates from this source. Or you may prefer a private psychological counselor. Counselors can administer still other questionnaires and tests that will help identify your stressors. This information helps you to focus on major areas of concern. Joining a class in stress management early on is an easy way to get going without the delay of wondering what to do first. In addition to having the benefit of the professional expertise, you will find that you are not alone and that the mutual interaction with your classmates serves as an immediate support group. Sooner or later, however, you will need to break free and become an independent coper.

Stress Management Requires Conscious Coping

Do you remember when you were 15 1/2 years old and were taking driving lessons? Many students, especially those who had never driven a car before, became quite nervous the first few times they sat behind the wheel. The world suddenly looked different from that position. We suddenly became aware that the force under the hood was the greatest we had ever controlled. If we didn't maintain control it could inflict awesome damage on ourselves and others. Most of us soon learned the knack of driving, and it wasn't long before we began to enjoy it and the new degree of freedom that we had earned.

After learning the essentials of manipulating the car in traffic, we began to learn about defensive driving. These sessions emphasized the necessity of conscious, continuous awareness of factors along the road in the environment we were traversing. We learned not only to adjust our speed to the road conditions, but also to anticipate dangerous situations created by others before they happened. With practice, defensive driving became second nature. In short, we learned that a good driver copes well on the road.

As with driving, coping in various aspects of living can be learned by almost anyone who wants to make the effort. Unfortunately, there are few after-school classes for beginning copers as there are for beginning drivers. Most of us have to learn the hard way by making mistakes and then wondering what went wrong. If you are involved in an auto accident, the police come and review the events leading up to it in great detail. If you are found at fault, you are given a ticket, told what mistake you had made, and advised to attend traffic school so that your driving will improve. Living itself can be looked at as a school with yourself as both teacher and pupil. If you become too aggressive and subsequently realize that you are offending others, pretend you have sent yourself to a private coping school and let the teacher in you instruct you as pupil in how and why you aggressed. In the long run it is up to you to decide how well you are doing.

Successful coping requires decision making based on the exercise of judgment. "Should I look for another job? Should I marry Solomon? Should I tell my roommate I can't stand her anymore?" One's value system and assumptions are deeply involved in personal questions of this type and in the answers that a person will find satisfactory. I'm not attempting to compete with Ann Landers here, but I am suggesting that, if people are aware of their value systems and accompanying assumptions, they may become more able to solve their personal problems.

In some situations even well-trained, competent people can be overwhelmed, drowned in work. John Curley (1983) describes the plight of a number of public utility workers in Texas and other states following the breakup of the American Telephone and Telegraph Co. Alan Erwin,[1] the 38-year-old chairman of the Texas Public Utility Commission, works 65 hours a week, lunches on peanuts and diet Coke, and still has to work at home nights and on weekends. He rarely plays soccer with his sons anymore or has time to attend Boy Scout meetings. He and his wife rarely entertain friends and he no longer has time to work on his novel—his real passion. He may have to give up before the end of his 6-year term as a regulator at $55,000. "I doubt if I'll make it to 1989," he says.

Peggy Rossen, another Texas commissioner, works 16 hours a day, has no social life, and has made no friends since moving to Austin. She meditates daily and also reads the Bhagavad-Gita regularly.

How can you cope when work takes over your life on a long-term basis? Curley mentions that in Texas 5 out of 11 attorneys, and 5 out of 12 economists have quit in the last 4 months. In my opinion there is no general answer to the question of forced overwork. People in this type of situation need to solve it in terms of their own value systems.

Developing Your Own Style of Coping

As I've mentioned previously, stressors are very personal. Your own list will be as different from anyone else's as your fingerprint. Similarly, your

---

[1]I called the Texas Public Utility Commission in May 1987 and was informed that Mr. Erwin was no longer an employee and that Ms. Rossen was still employed.

particular style of coping will also be individualistic. I suggest that you follow your intuitions and do what comes naturally for you. Pounding on the desk and shouting may work for a friend or your boss, but if you are not comfortable with it, don't behave in that fashion; it won't work for you. On tough stressors you may seek advice on coping tactics. Your friends will tell you what worked for them on similar problems and will assume that it will also work for you. It probably won't unless you feel that it's right for you.

One advantage of conscious coping is that it leads to thinking of alternatives. You will soon realize that there is usually more than one way of dealing with a particular stressor. For example, suppose you live in an apartment house and the people on the floor above play loud music until 2:00 a.m. every morning. It disturbs your sleep. You ask the landlord if there isn't a quiet time after which loud music is prohibited. He replies that they pay their rent on time, and he doesn't want to lose them as tenants. He doesn't seem concerned about you.

What is your next step in coping? You can make a list of possibilities:

- Move out yourself.
- Buy earplugs.
- Play loud music yourself.
- Pound on the ceiling at midnight and shout for quiet.
- Call on them and discuss it.
- Start working the graveyard shift.
- Grit your teeth and decide you are not going to let it bother you any more.

In this example, the list divides into two types of coping: adapting to the stressor, or attempting to lessen, remove, or eliminate the stressor. In many other situations, however, your list may include far more adaptations on your part than ways to eliminate the stressor.

Constructing a Successful Coping Foundation

Probably all of us know some people who seem to manage their lives well; no matter what complications, problems, or disasters they have had to live through, they have survived without bitterness. Fate may have been unkind, but it has not struck them out. In contrast, other people become upset and thrown off the track by what seems to us a little thing or by trivial complications. In my observations on these two kinds of people, I find that there are significant differences in how they handle their problems. The effective copers tend to accept their problems as a personal responsibility. They may seek advice from friends and experts, but they realize that final decisions must be made by themselves. Another characteristic of effective copers is their rational approach to problem solving. They identify their chronic stressors and then work out strategies that result in unstressful responses, similar to playing a game or doing an exercise.

Many readers of this book may agree with my analysis and description of successful copers and realize that they don't possess those characteristics. My position is that people can ascend the disease/health-ease continuum and become well *if they truly desire to do so*. It won't be easy, and it may not be quick, but it can be done if the desire is strong enough.

The discussion of coping so far has emphasized it as a means of dealing with stressors, or events and experiences that threaten us. This emphasis is probably justified, but it has ignored one essential aspect of coping: the psychological base from which we operate. By this term I mean that if you cope with a negative attitude by going through the motions but not really expecting to accomplish anything, chances are you won't accomplish anything. The first steps along the psychological path to wellness require a certain minimum of self-confidence to be effective. I suspect that half the battle in coping is in feeling that it has a good chance of working. The first objective then in coping is getting yourself in a positive frame of mind. There are a number of ways of accomplishing this objective. The first two are private; the others involve other people.

Chronic physiological stressors may contribute to a negative attitude. For example, some people have low amounts of the enzymes that are necessary for lactose utilization. Other people do not metabolize alcohol effectively. Still others have allergies to certain foods. For these people, consuming milk, alcohol, or seafood upsets the digestive system and may lead to serious illness if ingested regularly. If you suspect or know that any foodstuff or type of alcoholic drink can act as a stressor for you, avoid it, even though it may mean giving up a long-standing habit like drinking with friends. Don't give up the association, but choose some drink that does not stress you.

There are few people who are not competent in at least one activity, hobby, or skill. It may be having a green thumb, cooking a special dish, knowing a great deal about a particular spectator sport, helping others, and the like. Whatever it is, harvest the maximum satisfaction that you can from it. Use the activity as a springboard to try something else that you would enjoy. Whatever it is, cherish it. It can be your first stepping-stone towards wellness.

I am suggesting activities that are totally apart from responsibilities at work or at home. I am talking about your secret desires: those things that you would like to do for yourself, for your own satisfaction, rather than for applause, recognition, approbation, advancement, or pleasing others. Whatever it is, make it yours—not something you bought, saw, heard, were given, found, or stole. Also, whatever it is, don't be competitive about it. If you have done your best, be satisfied with the result. You will improve with practice, but there will probably always be someone who is better at it than you. Be grateful for these people; you can learn from them.

Are good copers born that way or is it something they have learned? As with most nature-nurture questions, there is no simple answer. My impression, based on the experts I have read, is that nurture, what one has experienced in early life, outweighs nature, the role of heredity in coping. Due to varied backgrounds, large differences in coping ability are already present by adolescence. To make things even more complicated, the stressors we face as we mature and become independent vary widely in number and severity. In dealing with stressors, people establish a pattern of coping, which is their own particular style. This style may range from being very effective to being very ineffective, as a continuum. Fortunately, if people realize at age 20, 30, 50, or 75 that they are not coping very effectively, they can improve if they so desire. This statement is not a pie-in-the-sky example or a claim that everyone can become millionaires if they give themselves pep talks. Further, it is not based on anecdotal experiences of the man down the street but on measured improvements in millions of people who have attended stress management classes over the past 20 years. The strategy practiced in these classes is based on the principle of accepting yourself where you are and going on from there. In many of these classes, people are given the opportunity to describe how they solved or dealt with a difficult stressor. These descriptions, in turn, help others to realize that they are not alone, and to give them confidence that they, too, can learn to deal with stressors.

There is no reason, however, why people cannot probe into their past on their own and attempt to understand what they have done and why they have done it. The goal, as I see it, is to go beyond the vapid rationalizations of justifying one's mistakes and errors and to become more objective in self-evaluation. For this goal, reviewing one's past as though it were a historical autobiography becomes a fascinating and useful pastime.

Who Am I?

Unless you are a very unusual person, you will never answer this question with finality. My own answers keep changing as I grow older, but I find it fun to mull over the question from time to time. It is like painting a picture of yourself to which you add new brush strokes every day. In more technical language, Antonovsky (1979) calls this very personal activity the *search for ego identity*.

If you persevere in these ruminations, you will begin to see yourself not just as a struggling person but as an individual composed of a myriad of capabilities, talents, and weaknesses. You will come to recognize that intelligence, for example, is not a single attribute but is composed of many subsidiary qualities like logical thinking, memory, imagination, keenness of observation, resourcefulness, and so forth. You will see that you are weak in some of these and strong in others, as are your friends. If you enjoy this first journey of self-exploration, you may want to take other inward journeys and include speculations about yourself and your friends (in an objective way, of course), which may include character, motivation, intuitions, and awareness of the environment. After some years of these forays into the unknown, you may journey to a strange land and recognize one of the inhabitants as yourself. If this being smiles at you in a friendly fashion, congratulations; self-knowledge is a most valuable resource in coping.

Meet Wayne Cook

I take the view that we are all limited to some degree (e.g., Einstein was just a mediocre violinist). What impresses me are those people who are so limited that we consider them physically and/or mentally handicapped. Many of them don't mope, they cope. They engage in wheelchair Olympics, tennis, and basketball; learn to read foreign languages in braille; dictate books; become self-employed; and help others. They are indomitable. They are marvelous! And so can you be. The unfettered human spirit knows no boundaries, recognizes no limits, and does not admit defeat. The story of such a person is reprinted here (Mooney, 1983).

The Twin Resources of Knowledge and Intelligence

Coping ability is definitely related to what is called knowledge-intelligence and these in turn are affected by education. For example, a person whose education was terminated early and who can barely read and write is far more likely to score low on an intelligence test compared with someone who graduated from high school. Does this correlation have any significance? I do not accept the definition of *intelligence* as what intelligence tests measure. It may be years, if ever, before we can measure intelligence adequately, by which I mean functionally. In the meantime, I think intelligence profiles, which attempt to measure some of the attributes mentioned above as separate components, furnish more accurate estimations of a person's capabilities than the standardized tests that are now so widely used. General education reveals how the world works, and this knowledge is very useful in coping. If your education was terminated before obtaining a bachelor's degree, I would recommend taking correspondence courses or classes in continuing education in nonvocational subjects that interest you. However, many intelligent people who were somehow deprived of a college education have managed to educate themselves superbly by devising a reading program for themselves.

Meet Wayne Cook

by John Mooney

Maybe you read the story under the headline "Judge Won't Let Quadriplegic Starve Herself to Death" in Saturday's *Salt Lake Tribune*. Elizabeth Bouvia, 26, a cerebral palsy victim, had decided life was not worth living and wanted to end it all by starvation.

But does a crippling disease mean the end of a person's usefulness?

Consider Wayne Cook of Denver, who will play an exhibition racquetball match against Jeff Congdon Tuesday at 7 p.m. at the Racqueteer, 615 East 9800 South.

Born with the crippling birth defect, cerebral palsy, Cook, 32, is technically considered a triplegic as both legs and his right arm are affected by the disease.

But Wayne miraculously has overcome his handicap to become a physical education teacher, professional public speaker, real estate agent, and athlete.

Because he refused to recognize his handicaps as unsurmountable, Wayne has become proficient at tennis, snow skiing, basketball, golf and racquetball.

Starting last Wednesday, Wayne launched a 16-city racquetball exhibition with all the proceeds from voluntary admission contributions and those from the corporate sponsors of the tour going directly to United Cerebral Palsy.

Cook anticipates raising between $50,000 and $100,000 through the tour and if you know someone who needs inspiration, Wayne Cook's exhibition Tuesday night could be just what the doctor ordered.

Wayne's slogan is "inspiration through action" and he argues, "When I was young, I used to think, 'Why me? Why has this happened to me?' But I realized thinking about it wouldn't change anything, that this attitude was self-defeating, that I had to make the most of what I am."

Since Wayne's western tour will take him into that area, wouldn't it be wonderful if he could see that young cripple who hopes to die in Riverside and convince her life can be worthwhile, if she will work for a goal?

Reprinted with permission.

Knowledge of health data is also useful in coping. If you are a one-pack-a-day smoker and don't know the odds of your developing lung cancer compared to a nonsmoker, you should. If you refuse to get the information, that fact tells you something about yourself. If you are a woman who doesn't want to get pregnant, you should know about methods of birth control along with their relative effectiveness and side effects. Good copers know what community services are offered by their local health department. They also know how to distinguish a quack, faker, or fraud from a legitimate physician or businessman. What questions should you ask before investing your life's savings with a stranger who offers you a 50% annual return on your money?

Other personal factors that can help you to maintain a decent quality of life and also aid in survival are included under adaptability. In this rapidly changing world, each of us needs to learn how to adapt to changes at physiological, psychological, cultural, and social levels. Many of these adaptations have been discussed previously in relation to tension management.

It seems like good common sense to avoid stressors that may lead to disease if unrecognized. The following preventive measures are now taken for granted by millions of Americans: vaccinations, Pap smears, regular checkups (physical examinations), breast examinations, not smoking, general and aerobic exercise, and a healthy diet.

Finally, we come to money and what it will buy in coping with stressors. This resource is so obvious that I will need to treat it only briefly. Suffice it to say that it is not coincidental that people below the poverty level have a lower quality of life as well as a shorter life span due to inadequate shelter, food, and clothing.

Cognitive Appraisals

It is interesting that Plato placed reason above all the other virtues. His perfect man was above emotion. In the computer age, we recognize that Plato was describing a fully programmed robot rather than a human being. Even so, those people who do not use whatever reasoning abilities they possess to the maximum are penalizing themselves needlessly. Some people apparently see reason and emotion as in opposition to each other. I consider this view an error of the greatest magnitude. Reason and emotion are words that separate physiological processes that are not separable in actuality. Our nervous systems are wired in such a way that our emotions enter into everything that we do, even solving a problem in mathematics. Thus, to cope well, which basically means to overcome the threats that we meet daily, calls for the maximum use of rationality. We need to assess threats as accurately and objectively as possible.

Once we have made an analysis of a threat, we should devise flexible tactics in dealing with it. As we perceive a change in the situation, as we obtain new information about the threat, we will need to change our tactics. Farsightedness is another factor that helps in dealing with serious stressors. If we can anticipate a change in a probable long-term stressor before it happens, we are in a position of a basketball player with an extra free throw in a tight game.

A general characteristic of effective copers is that they act! After the analysis and planning, they don't fret and worry; they do something.

Appropriate action is the crucial final phase of coping. Action often requires courage, especially if it means bringing up an emotional, touchy subject with a friend, spouse, or employer. In these situations, the words used, the tone of voice, and the attitudes expressed may spell the difference between a satisfactory solution (often a compromise) and a shattered relationship.

Interpersonal Relations as a General Resource

"Misery loves company" is a folksaying that I have long interpreted as meaning that people who are out of luck share their misfortunes as a means of verbal touching—an emotional massage that eases the pain. The phrase, however, can be looked at positively: "Two heads are better than one." People who feel that they are not facing a hostile world all alone but have friends and acquaintances they can call on possess a most valuable resource in dealing with stressors.

Similarly, a cultural background does more than give us a place in the world. The fact that a culture has survived over many generations demonstrates that it has developed a set of responses to stressors, which is available to every individual in the group. Antonovsky (1979) calls this resource *ties to the community.* By getting involved in community projects and activities, you will meet dozens of other people like yourself. Fortunately, the world is full of people with vision who can see beyond their own problems and are busily engaged in trying to make this world better. Engaging in these activities helps place one's own problems in a perspective that makes them more bearable and more easily solvable. The beauty of this approach is that you can start with your present friends and broaden your interests and activities at your own pace. The first few steps may be the hardest because it may be new to you. But remember, there is nothing to lose but your stress.

Norman Cousins, in his books *Anatomy of an Illness* (1979) and *The Healing Heart* (1983), has provided us with two outstanding anecdotal examples of the value of interpersonal relations in overcoming the stressors of serious illness. This approach is a long way from being scientifically validated, but in a life-or-death struggle, what is there to lose by trying it?

Coherence—A Possibly New and Valuable Viewpoint

For years I have thought that the one most valuable personality characteristic that parents could inculcate in their children was that of self-confidence. Although I still think it is a sound idea, the means of achieving it have remained elusive. Nowhere have I run across a recipe for instilling self-confidence, and discussing it with friends and psychologists has provided no definite suggestions. For these reasons, I was pleased that Antonovky (1979) suggested a different, and perhaps even broader, organizing principle that could serve as a foundation to help a person maintain wellness. He calls it the *sense of coherence* and defines it as follows: ''A global orientation that expresses the extent to which one has a pervasive, enduring though dynamic feeling of confidence that one's internal and external environments are predictable and that there is a high probability that things will work out as well as can reasonably be expected'' (p. 123).

The similarity between Antonovsky's description of coherence and my description of the attitudes of scientists in chapter 3 is striking. Both groups of people assume that nature is regular, that predictability in experimental situations and in daily life is worth testing, and that what actually happens is assessed on the basis of available facts and logical reasoning.

Antonovsky emphasizes the important distinction between a sense of coherence and a sense of control. People with a sense of coherence recognize the laws of nature, the laws of the country they are living in, the reasons for the regulations in their place of work, and the rules that one should follow in creating a happy home. Well people accept the view that they are not in control of most situations that influence their own wellbeing. This acceptance does not imply passivity or fatalism. It means that one struggles to achieve what one can in all areas of one's life but does not throw a tantrum, create a scene, or have a nervous breakdown when one's desires have not been achieved. I'll return to a sense of control in discussing Type A behavior as an example of miscoping.

Sources of Coherence

Because coherence represents a global viewpoint, it is not surprising that various psychologists attribute its origins to childhood experiences. If a child is reared in an environment in which things happen to it willy-nilly and its own actions seem to play no part in whether it is punished or praised, it is likely that the child may give up trying to figure things out after a few years and withdraw, act helpless, and adopt an attitude of hopelessness. Similarly, if a child is raised with no rules, it may find itself in situations and faced with problems that are beyond its means to solve. Under these conditions a child may conclude that there are no rules in the world and that there is no way to figure things out, and thus not develop a feeling of coherence. A third, and often ignored, impediment to developing a sense of coherence is that of poverty. People living on welfare for long periods of time are forced to learn to cope with a system that is often impersonal, cruel, arbitrary, demeaning, and seemingly irrational in its rules and the way they are applied. I think that it would be difficult to maintain a sense of coherence under these conditions, especially if a person experienced them as a child.

These childhood experiences are similar to those mentioned as contributing to Type A behavior, which can be considered as one means of handling stress. I consider that these people are struggling against a severe handicap. The first step toward wellness lies in recognizing the problem. The second is admitting you have it. These people are similar to alcoholics. They are trapped until they can admit to themselves that they have a disease. The symptoms of what might be called *global stress* are more subtle than those of alcoholism, but for starters, here are a few that may be useful in self-diagnosis: the feeling that chance governs your life, that luck is more important than competence, that whom you know is more important than what you know, and that only suckers believe in the hard-work myth. Many of these people are also susceptible to various conspiracy theories; for example, the AMA is in league with the pharmaceutical companies for their mutual profit; a small group of International Bankers is controlling the business of the world to their own advantage; and the little guy never has a chance. Admittedly, there are anecdotes that support these stories and hypotheses. The fatal step is generalizing from them and then using the false generalization as an explanation of what is going on in the world. These are some of the consequences of early stressful experiences.

Positively speaking, if a child is encouraged to figure things out and is rewarded when it does, and if its failures are analyzed in terms it can understand, it will in time develop self-confidence in problem solving and approach problems as puzzles that can be solved by the application of general rules. Such a child-maturing-into-adult will gradually learn that dealing with people as persons includes a certain range of problems, whereas dealing with people as representatives of institutions or organizations, in which rules and regulations are sometimes interpreted in what seems an arbitrary and capricious way, includes quite a different set of problems. To me, the term *coping* means learning to deal with both types.

If, on reading this description of what a sense of coherence entails, you feel that you do not possess it and you also feel that your coping abilities need strengthening and that your stressors are getting out of hand, what do I suggest? For people in this situation, but otherwise in good health, I would suggest joining a class in stress management and, if you like the instructor, paying for a number of private sessions until you feel you have constructed a firm enough foundation to build it up further on your own.

A Perspective on Stress Management

Humans have lived under stressful conditions from time immemorial. Most people seek happiness, and chronic stress is incompatible with that elusive goal. Although the contemporary usage of *stress* is of relatively recent origin, its control and management have been sought after for thousands of years. All the great leaders of human history have been concerned with living the good life and thus with stress management. Imagine what the world would be like if we could behave according to the golden rule of Confucius and love our neighbor as Jesus suggested. What prevents these behaviors?

It is my impression that the present emphasis on stress and its control is based on the assumption that modern society is more stressful than those societies of the past. Because stress surveys, like the ones at the end of this chapter, hadn't been invented 50 or 500 years ago, any such comparisons are guesstimates at best. Another impression of mine is that people are puzzled by the amount of stress they observe in others as well as in their own lives. Stress is a cloud that covers the whole country. The sought-after attributes of affluence, power, and position not only are incapable of blowing stress away, but strangely, when achieved, often seem to increase it.

In a recent TV program on housewives and stress, experts on stress management mentioned some causative factors in stress: the fast pace of modern society—one has to hurry just to keep up, the lack of personal control in decision making, and the desire to be perfect in all aspects of living. They spoke of the *superwoman syndrome*. Many young working mothers have kept as many goals for themselves as they had before the children were born or before they began to work. It is virtually impossible for a mother of young children to work and yet spend as much time with them as they need and in addition function as an excellent homemaker, shopper, lover, and interesting conversationalist! No wonder burnout now refers to people rather than to candles. The experts suggested that working mothers identify their goals and reduce them to a reasonable number, slow down and relax more, and especially take time during the day for activities that are personally satisfying.

The interdependence of the muscular and nervous systems is illustrated very clearly in the analysis of stressor origins and controls. A majority of stressors originate from unpleasant and/or threatening interpersonal relations (i.e., psychological phenomena), which, if not managed competently, results in muscle tenseness. Conversely, if the mind is cleared (by whatever means), muscles relax, at least temporarily.

Direct Approaches to Stress Management

Broadly speaking, stressors can be managed directly or indirectly. The direct approach uses cognition as its tool. The person analyzes his or her problems and devises a plan of action to solve them.

By direct management, I mean that a person realizes consciously which conditions, problems, and people act as stressors and takes direct action to control them. This approach is the one first suggested by Buddha. The philosophy of Buddha was directly concerned with how to attain happiness. The goal cannot be achieved as stated but can be approached by mastering a series of less ambitious objectives. The first is learning to avoid frustration. Frustration (i.e., internal stresses) can be circumvented by controlling desires, which, in turn, are controlled by desiring only those things that can be attained. The analysis and control of these psychological constructs is developed in detail, but no universal solution is proposed. It is left to the individual to work out what seems most satisfactory (Bahm, 1962). In this analysis, Buddha's use of opposites is, to me, positively brilliant. His description of Nirvana is ''when one enjoys one's tenseness untensely'' (Bahm, 1962, p. 74). He obviously had an excellent sense of humor.

The indirect approach on the other hand, utilizes diversions. The person escapes from the stressors, mentally, physically or both. These escapes can vary from those who have a special room or place to be alone, to those whose lives are spent traveling the world in search of themselves. Diversions include religious, philosophical, and psychological beliefs and activities. A person seeks privacy, calmness, and clarity; and frequently, things sort themselves out. Another type of escape involves more active pursuits: work, one or more hobbies, participant and spectator sports, travel, and so forth.

Recently, Friedman and Rosenman (1974) and Friedman and Ulmer (1984) have advised Type A personality people to analyze their behaviors and change them. I suspect that this approach will require expert counseling for most Type As to effect significant, long-term behavioral changes.

Indirect Approaches to Stress Management

By far the greater number of procedures for stress management utilize indirect approaches. These include relaxation techniques, autogenic training, sensory awareness, imagery, altered states of consciousness, physical exercise and sports, active hobbies, and moderate use of alcohol.

Relaxation Techniques

One of the most widely practiced conscious relaxation techniques is *meditation*. It was invented about 4,000 years ago by the yogic sages as an adjunct to study of the Upanishads, the Bhagavad Gita, the Veda, and the Yoga Sutras of the Hindu religion. The objective is to develop self-knowledge and thus the ability to manage stressors.

Just as stress is a nonspecific response to an unmanaged stressor, there is also its opposite: an antistress response to relaxation. The major objective of meditating is to become totally relaxed. Benson (1975) describes the characteristics of the relaxation-response as decreases in muscle tension, heart rate, blood pressure, and rate of breathing (Benson, 1975). The conditions necessary to bring about the relaxation response are simple: a quiet environment for 10 to 20 minutes, twice a day; a comfortable sitting position; closed eyes; and a repetitive word or symbol which, in the Orient, is called a mantra.

Muscle relaxation is somehow dependent on getting one's mind off one's problems. A meditator can choose from a wide variety of nonpersonal subjects to think about. They may be pleasant thoughts or none at all. Relating oneself to a greater power, as in many types of prayer, has helped millions of people relax.

In a more recent work, *Beyond the Relaxation Response*, Benson (1984) advocates the use of a "Faith Factor" as an adjunct to meditation. The term Faith Factor refers to a faith-rooted focus word that is based on one's personal belief system. The word used should have a positive significance so that each day the meditator will obtain positive psychological reinforcement in employing it. The word may or may not refer to religious symbols. In this book, Benson includes many anecdotal accounts of the value of meditation in controlling a variety of medical conditions and, in general, of promoting wellness.

Ainslie Meares, in *A Way of Doctoring* (1985), has written a profound and moving book that describes his experience in introducing "still-mind" meditation to a wide variety of patients. I highly recommend that readers of *Pathways to Wellness* read Meares.

A recently discovered fact that now seems well established is that *anxiety cannot exist in a completely relaxed person* (Gaarder & Montgomery, 1981). Thus, if you can learn to relax, you can banish anxiety and its counterpart, tenseness. Although the mechanism is not understood scientifically, a person who can relax at will is somehow better able to deal with stressors that occur at other times. Meditation supplies you with a rudder and keel so that you have some command of the direction of your life. The most widely publicized type in the U.S. is transcendental meditation, in which instruction is available for a fee.

Yoga meditation, as practiced in India and now in many parts of the world, emphasizes concentration on respiration, that is, becoming aware of one's inhalations and exhalations in concert with pronouncing a mantra. The yogis use the sacred syllable, *om* (pronounced slowly, "ooohm"), but any suitable sound or word can be used. For example, one can say "re-lax," the first syllable when inhaling and the second when exhaling. Meares (1985) suggests that quiet meditation, a stillness of the mind in which one thinks of nothing, is the most relaxing.

Autogenic Training

Autogenic training was developed by Schultz (1932) and was updated and translated into English by Schultz & Luthe (1959). It employs sensory awareness of physiological processes such as muscle relaxation, feelings of warmth, and rhythms of heartbeat and respiration. According to Jencks (1979), autogenic training is especially effective in calming upsets in the autonomic nervous system, that which is involved in the regulation of the internal processes of the body. The method includes six exercises by which an altered state of consciousness is produced that allows a person to control heartbeat, rate of breathing, and body warmth.

Sensory Awareness

Sensory awareness training originated in Europe in the nineteenth century, primarily for training in the performing arts. Elsa Gindler recognized its value in muscle relaxation, correction of shallow breathing, and improvement in circulatory disturbances. Jencks (1979) credits Charlotte Selver (1957) for coining the term *sensory awareness* for this series of exercises. Jencks describes sensory awareness as emphasizing primary sensations instead of thoughts and emotions, active instead of passive participation, and relating to present reality instead of that of the past or an anticipated future. Sensory awareness depends completely on conscious sensory perceptions, and if an altered state of consciousness occurs, such as feelings of floating or changes in body image, the person must immediately stretch or inhale deeply before continuing. In distinction to meditation, the subject should keep the eyes open. It is advisable for anyone considering sensory awareness training to begin under the supervision of a trained person. I also suggest that Jencks' (1979) book, *Your Body, Biofeedback at Its Best*, be consulted before deciding on a particular form of psychological training or relaxation exercise. Massages of various types may also include sensory awareness. Although I have seen no studies on the psychological benefits of massages, I suspect there must be some or the practice would not have survived as long as it has.

Imagery and Altered States of Consciousness

Both imagery and altered states of consciousness are admirable techniques for inducing relaxation by individuals. They have not been as widely utilized in the West as in the Orient. Imagery includes the formation of images in the mind's eye, in the back of the head, or out there in perception, thought, feeling, memory, and fantasy (Jencks, 1979).

Individuals differ greatly in their ability to call forth images. Small children often experience imagery but usually are not encouraged to continue the practice. Wide variation also occurs in the type of imagery one person may engage in. For those who desire them, the ability to invoke images and to keep their memory may be increased by practice. An outstanding example of the use of images in tennis, as well as other aspects of living, is found in Tim Gallwey's (1974) book, *The Inner Game of Tennis*. In this book, Gallwey explains how relaxed concentration can be achieved, on or off the court. The principle involves bringing harmony between Self 1 (the judgmental ego, mind) and Self 2 (the body). The goal is realized by letting things happen, not making them happen. These ideas are reminiscent of Buddha's.

An altered state of consciousness occurs in all people when they go to sleep. Additional examples are dreams, daydreams, and hallucinations not induced by drugs. In other words, altered states of consciousness are not to be feared. Spontaneous hallucinations have frequently been described by people doing repetitive or boring work, as by truck drivers (especially at night) and by jet pilots flying straight and level at high altitudes. These are the conditions under which unidentified flying objects (UFOs) have been observed.

Self-induced hypnosis is another example of an altered state of consciousness. The state may last from seconds to hours and vary from pleasant to most unpleasant. Altered states can also occur during a period of attention, as at a lecture or religious service, or during a period of inattention in the same situations. What is not widely realized is that altered states can be utilized to promote relaxation; induce sleep; decrease pain, fears, and anxieties; and utilize the subconscious in problem solving. It is interesting that altered states are desirable and valuable in meditation but are prohibited in sensory awareness sessions.

Physical Exercises and Sports

A list of widely practiced exercises includes hatha-yoga, tai chi chuan, kung fu, and karate. Notice that all of these originated in Asia. In addition to requiring active physical movement, proficiency in each involves acquiring a mental attitude of relaxed concentration. Once acquired, this attitude can be applied in daily living, including stress management.

In this connection, jogging, running, swimming, cross-country skiing, walking, and many other noncompetitive physical activities that are engaged in over a period of years result in psychological benefits that are relatively unappreciated by nonparticipants. Mind–body harmony is probably more readily accomplished in noncompetitive activities than in competitive ones. The benefits of these activities are discussed in more detail in chapter 7.

Active Hobbies Are Great for Relaxing

Hobbies are probably the most popular group of relaxing activities. There is little need for me to list any. There are, however, two points about hobbies that I think are worthy of emphasis. The first concerns selection. Do not take up a hobby because it is popular or because your friends are doing it. As with the other types of relaxing activities, if there is no particular hobby that attracts you, shop around a bit and try different ones before selecting one. The most important thing about choosing a hobby is that it appeals to you as an activity.

Here we come to the second major point. The hobby should be an active one, in which you do something. Whether it involves making something as in sewing/quilting; producing something as in cooking/gardening; creating something as in any form of art, engaging in active sports, or playing a musical instrument; observing nature as in bird watching or rock collecting; helping others as in tutoring or volunteering at a social agency; or taking risks as in white-water kayaking, sky diving, or gliding, the person acts as a participant not as a spectator. Thus I exclude most TV watching as a beneficial hobby as well as spectator sports and listening to background music. These passive activities provide entertainment and temporary relaxation and relief from problems, but in my opinion, they have little or no carryover after the activity.

Moderate Use of Alcohol Aids in Stress Management

There is evidence that humans have drunk alcoholic beverages throughout history and its use probably extends well into prehistoric times. Alcohol has been used as an adjunct to feasts and celebrations, in religious rites, as a medication, and as a food. Most of these practices are still in use today. In many ancient civilizations its use was proscribed except under special circumstances. I interpret these taboos as indicating that mankind has been aware of the dangers of overindulgence for a very long time.

As with many other practices, the conditions under which people are allowed to drink alcohol has got off the track in Western cultures compared to those of the past. One possible explanation for this difference has to do with technology. Ancient peoples drank wine, ale, and beer, which are all products of fermentation, but with a relatively low alcohol content.

The significant technological development was that of distillation. In the twelfth century alchemists discovered that distilling wine yielded a product that was almost pure alcohol. Whereas wine contains about one part alcohol to nine parts water, the distilled product, first known as *aquae vitae* (water of life), contains about nine parts alcohol to one part water.

The introduction of distilled spirits into Northern Europe opened a new chapter in people's love affair with alcohol. Fermented beverages had long been used in Europe on a daily basis as a substitute for water because water supplies were generally contaminated. In addition, drinking a pint of wine or beer with meals tasted good, seemed to help digestion, and was relaxing. Distilled spirits, however, could not be consumed in these quantities without resulting in drunkenness. The liver, the organ where alcohol is metabolized, was overwhelmed by the amount of alcohol in an 8-oz glass of gin or whisky, and in time, the brain itself was affected. Hogarth's realistic drawings, "The Rake's Progress," vividly portray the effects of excess alcohol consumption shortly after the importation of gin into England.

There seems to be no question that a moderate amount of alcohol is relaxing. One or two drinks containing a maximum of 4 oz of 80-proof alcohol consumed over 2 hours produces a carefree sensation, releases tensions, and makes life seem more pleasant. For these reasons, many physicians suggest one or two drinks before or during dinner. Wine has recently become popular in the U.S. as an aperitif. One should remember that it, too, contains alcohol and that 12 oz of wine is equivalent to 4 oz of whiskey. For most people, a third drink produces noticeable effects in speech and walking, and if consumption has been at the rate of 8 or 10 oz in 2 hours, a person appears to be very drunk, staggers, is incoherent, and becomes a severe threat behind a steering wheel. The safety factor for alcohol—the ratio between unsafe and safe quantities, as discussed in chapter 5—is less than two, one of the smallest of any known substance. Moderate amounts of alcohol aid in stress management, but in slightly larger amounts it changes into one of the most vicious stressors known.

Temporary Stressors Can Be Fun

Although some people abhor risks, especially voluntary ones, other people find living without risks dull as dishwater. Risk taking can be primarily physiological, as mentioned above, or primarily psychological, as in card playing for high stakes. By definition, risk-taking hobbies involve stressors. The first has to do with duration. Many people enjoy severe stressors that may last from minutes to hours. As I've mentioned previously, most people can handle short-term voluntary stressors well.

My view of living dangerously is, if you enjoy it, do it, but be prepared to take the consequences of an accident. A friend of mine broke his leg after 7 years of skiing. "If a broken leg every 7 years is the price of skiing, it's worth it," he replied, when I expressed sympathy about his tough luck. A participant should think through the entire experience including the seriousness and length of confinement of a possible accident. Is the attraction of skydiving in the thrill of the drop or in not thinking about the consequences of a malfunction, or both? Is playing poker for high stakes exciting because it combines skill and daring, or because you can't afford to lose as much as you have bet, or both?

Taking Unnecessary Risks Is Stupid

Risk taking for thrills is a very private decision, and only the person involved can equate the enjoyment with the danger. However, many people take risks from which they receive no thrills. Driving without a seat belt, driving while under the influence (DUI), or operating a piece of equipment improperly so that what should not be a dangerous job in actuality becomes one are examples of what I call stupid behavior.

Type A Behavior:
An Example of Stress Mismanagement

In previous sections I have discussed the consequences of stress mismanagement primarily from a physiological point of view, that is, how stress mismanagement acts as a risk factor for many diseases. The psychological effects of stress mismanagement are perhaps even more common than the physiological effects. *Type A Behavior and Your Heart* by Friedman and Rosenman (1974) covered both aspects of stress mismanagement but emphasized its role as a causative factor in heart attacks. This aspect of stress will be taken up in chapter 10, "Risk Factors and Heart Disease." In the following section, Type A behavior is discussed as a kind of unconscious coping with stress that often leads to aberrant, unproductive, and self-defeating behavior.

How to Recognize Type A Behavior

In their early research on identifying Type A behavior, Friedman and Rosenman discovered that it was composed of a number of specific behaviors. Few individuals exhibited all of them; to be classified as a Type A required typical behavior in at least two or three of them. The main characteristics of Type A behavior are

1. a chronic sense of time urgency,
2. a highly competitive drive,
3. a free-floating, easily aroused hostility,
4. a strong drive to achieve self-selected but poorly defined goals,
5. a persistent desire for recognition and advancement,
6. a strong feeling of insecurity unrelieved by recognition and success,
7. a necessity to prove superiority even in noncompetitive situations,
8. feelings of guilt when not working or thinking about work, and
9. a necessity to control the environment, including other people.

To identify Type A individuals, Friedman and Rosenman devised an interview in which the interviewer purposely attempted to provoke the subject. Their term for this unique form of verbal harassment was the *structured interview*. For example, a very simple question might be put to the subject very slowly as though it were a question that was difficult to understand. Type A people generally answered the question before the interviewer had finished stating it, or they would answer it angrily as though the interviewer had insulted their intelligence, or they would interrupt and ask the interviewer to talk faster; Type B people would answer calmly (see below). Obviously, the interviewers had to be carefully trained in asking the questions and evaluating the responses, because the content of the answers was less important than the manner in which they were answered. The results of this test admittedly contain a large subjective component. To decrease subjectivity, Friedman and Rosenman had the subjects read a very emotional appeal by a military commander to his troops before a battle and recorded the voiceprints electronically. Oscillations on the graph when certain key words were pronounced were much larger for Type As than for Type Bs. This addition increased the objectivity of the interview somewhat.

In an important section Friedman and Rosenman point out that Type A behavior has no relation to kind of work, degree of success, or economic status. In other words, they find this type of individual in unskilled, manual laborers, in clerks and bookkeepers, and on higher rungs of the corporate ladder. They also find it in women. Type A behavior is independent of age in the range from 30 to 60 years.

In contrast to Type A, Friedman and Rosenman also postulate its opposite, Type B. These people never (or almost never) suffer from a sense of time urgency, are not hostile to others, can relax and engage in sports for the fun of it rather than to prove their superiority, and do not feel guilty when they are not working or thinking about their work. Types A and B represent extremes; most people fall somewhere in between. Friedman and Rosenman postulate that it is the extreme Type A person who is most at risk of heart disease, and accordingly, they have focused on procedures to identify Type A.

Is Type A Behavior a Form of Stress Or Is It a Stress Response?

In my view, Type A people are chronically stressing themselves. They compete when there is no need to, they hurry when they have plenty of time, and they become angry at the drop of a hat. Furthermore, they become uptight in situations where they are not in control. There are some events, however, where it is recognized that a person is not in control, such as death of a member of the family, divorce, loss of a job, or retirement. These events can act as strong stressors and many people are stressed by them. Recent studies suggest that Type A individuals respond to these events with more sickness than Type B individuals.

According to Glass (1977), Type A subjects are engaged in a perpetual struggle to retain control. They attempt to avoid anxiety in coping with situations and people by gaining mastery over them. If these attempts to control their environment are unsuccessful, Type As give up and act helpless. Glass proposes that the cycle of active coping and controlling followed by giving up when their efforts are unsuccessful is correlated with large fluctuations in the secretion of catecholamines by the sympathetic nervous system.

Self-Assessment of Behavior Type

In *Type A Behavior and Your Heart*, Friedman and Rosenman (1974) devote a number of pages to self-assessment techniques. How many of us go through life acting a part, playing a role, with neither understanding of why we do the things we do, nor insight into the reasons behind people's reactions to us? The objectives of self-assessment questionnaires are to increase self-awareness, to give us insight into the motivations of our own actions, and to help us seek other bases for ego-justification than the shaky rationalizations that we have relied on heretofore. Obviously, these objectives are a very large order.

In summary, it appears that Type A people cope very inexpertly. They create more stress in themselves and in others by their efforts to control situations. The first step in getting well is admitting to yourself the possibility that you are a Type A person. The second step includes answering some personal questions, such as those in the appendix at the end of this chapter. If the results indicate that your behavior falls into the Type A category, I suggest taking those further steps that lead to more effective coping tactics.

Reversibility of Type A Behavior

In talking about Type A behavior to many friends and acquaintances, I have found that most of us can recognize one or more Type A behaviors in ourselves at least some of the time. These characteristics are obviously quite common in a culture where over half of the male population has been classified as Type A. Percentages of this magnitude raise a number of questions. Is Type A behavior a prevalent human characteristic? Might the kind of society or social system in which a person is raised bring out, or even demand, Type A behavior for survival? Does Type A behavior have a hereditary basis? How early can it be recognized? Is Type A behavior reversible? Answers to some of these questions are known, and others are being researched at the present time.

There are a sufficient number of Type B people around to indicate definitely that Type A behavior is unnecessary for survival or for success in the business world—the area in which competitive striving is most pronounced. In fact, Friedman and Rosenman suggest that the Type A people are frequently their own worst enemies. Their overbearing attitudes, frequent outbursts of anger, and other demonstrations of hostility often outweigh their hard work, loyalty, and occasional brilliance.

I suspect that Type A behavior people may be similar to alcoholics: They refuse therapy until they admit to themselves that they have a problem. This recognition may come only after years of hardship, blows, and damaged human relations. The cure for alcoholics is to stop drinking. What is the cure for Type A behavior? How reversible is it? How does one go about changing one's behavior?

Friedman and Rosenman discuss these important questions in the last quarter of *Type A Behavior and Your Heart*. They take the optimistic view that behavior can be changed. They state in large letters, "YOU CAN CHANGE YOUR BEHAVIOR PATTERN," but they admit that it isn't easy. Because I believe that a Type A person is unwell, I'll briefly summarize some of their suggestions for reducing Type A behavior. I consider these suggestions as steps on the path to wellness.

Friedman and Rosenman relate the experience of a Type A New York physician who scheduled himself to work long hours—frequently until midnight. In addition to a large practice, he lectured at a medical school and was at the beck and call of his patients. He was not overweight, hypertensive, or hypercholesteremic, but he had a heart attack at age 49. While he was recuperating, he decided that his Type A behavior must have been responsible for the attack, and he resolved to change it. He stopped scheduling patients after 5:30 p.m., cut down on his teaching and phone calls, and moved from Manhattan to Long Island where he could spend more time with his wife and family. He consciously tries to keep his hostility asleep, and says he never enjoyed life more than during this recent period. His experience raises the questions, "Why wait for a heart attack before modifying your Type A behavior?" If you start now before a myocardial infarction, you not only may live longer, but will begin to enjoy your life in ways that you can hardly imagine.

The first step in accomplishing this objective is an honest self-appraisal—an admittedly difficult undertaking. Friedman and Rosenman present a list of ten suggestions that a person should probe as honestly as possible. This list is not an assessment of whether you are Type A. Rather it asks you to examine your psyche as deeply as you can so that you can find out what kind of person you actually are, what your ambitions and goals are, what enjoyment you are getting out of life outside of your work, and what activities you engage in from which you derive no income. I'll discuss some items from this list and add some comments of my own.

Consider your sense of humor. Is it largely made up of anecdotes and jokes or does it serve to give you a long-term view of what's going on in the world, and an insight into your own activities? Do you ever find your own actions amusing, if not ludicrous? Do you ever think of human activities as a game?

Examine your interests. How many of your activities, outside of your work, have to do with art, music, literature, drama, philosophy, science, and protecting the environment? Do you enjoy talking to persons of the opposite sex of your own social class or to anyone not in your social class on a person-to-person basis? If not, why?

You need to become aware of the basis of your hostile feelings. What nurtures them? What satisfactions are you getting from them? How are they related to your feelings of insecurity?

"You must dare to examine critically your ethical and moral principles. How honest have I been in my life, how often and under what circumstances have I cheated, lied, and borne false witness against my neighbor?" (p. 219).

Persist in asking yourself over and over until you have answered the question, **"What, apart from the eternal clutter of my everyday living, should be the essence of my life?"** (p. 219).

In other chapters, Friedman and Rosenman discuss altering specific Type A characteristics head on. **Do you suffer from hurry sickness?** They consider the hurry sickness as one of the major contributors to Type A behavior. They are quite incisive and definite in what should be cut down or cut out. Schedule only really important appointments, and cut out as many meetings as you can. Refuse all but the most urgent telephone calls. Get up 15 minutes earlier in the morning so that you can have a relaxed breakfast, a chat with your wife and children, and a look at the garden before rushing off to work. Use the extra time so gained by these changes to muse, daydream, or even think about your life and yourself as a person.

Begin the search for aloneness. When you stop the common urge to acquire things worth having, with your new free time you can work to achieve becoming a being worth knowing. In other words, become a person of substance and of some intrinsic worth who does more than mouth the headlines that the media presents; a reader for whom this book is written—a thinking person!

The distinction between aloneness and loneliness is an important one. In my visits to large cities where I may know few, if any, people, I am lonely though surrounded by thousands of persons, each rushing on some individual business. How many people acknowledge that others are even present unless they are shoved into the gutter? How many people look like they are enjoying themselves? I have heard of cities being rated by their pace, with plaudits being given to the fastest. Excitement of this type may appeal to a spectator or tourist but is expensive in human costs and damaging if one is caught up and contributing to the race.

Learn to slow down. In addition to detailing why the hurry sickness is so damaging, Friedman and Rosenman list some drills that can help a person slow down. I'll mention a few of them. Try to find the cause of your own hurry sickness. This objective may take considerable probing over a period of time. The rationale here is that, if a person understands the cause, he or she can treat it directly rather than treating its symptoms.

The authors suggest reminding yourself at least three times a day that life is always unfinished. You can't accomplish all your objectives. Learn to accept what you can accomplish on a day-to-day basis. Quit trying to think of more than one thing at a time. Friedman and Rosenman call this habit *polyphasic thinking*. It often occurs in talking to another person. You can become so busy thinking of what you are going to say next that you lose track or become disinterested in what the other person is saying. From time to time stop using music as background to whatever you are doing. Put down your book or your dustrag, sit down, and concentrate on the music. Try to hear every note of a piece that you like. It can be a rewarding experience as well as an excellent drill in concentration, or *monophasic thinking*.

Go with a friend to a restaurant or theater at which you know you will have to wait in line. Instead of fuming at the delay as you usually do, make a point of engaging in interesting conversation during the interim. The next drill is one that I am working on myself. It concerns increasing speed in a car in order to get through a yellow light at an intersection. When you find yourself doing this, penalize yourself by going around the block, returning to the intersection, and waiting for the light if necessary. They also suggest following a slow car on a street or highway even though you could pass it. If you get stuck in a freeway jam, smile at the other drivers who are alongside you. If you are engaged in some job that you know will be stressful, interrupt the work at intervals before you become stressed and relax by doing something pleasant.

Incorporate relaxation periods into your routine activities. Many people have found that short periods of meditation interspersed throughout the day will prevent stress for hours afterwards. Participating in a yoga class or aerobic exercise on a regular basis also has long-term relaxing effects for many people.

Reduce hostility. With regard to hostility, I'll suggest a change in the aphorism, "Forewarned is forearmed" to "Forewarned is unarmed." By this I mean that if you know that you are going to meet someone with whom you have been hostile, resolve in advance not to react in a hostile manner. Be pleasant, even though it hurts. Occasionally, you may be surprised that the other person will act with less hostility than you had imagined he or she would. Friedman and Rosenman offer some sage advice for situations like these. Keep your mouth buttoned tight. Say the minimum. If these tactics don't work, they suggest seeing the other person(s) as little as possible.

Shift your objectives. As a final drill, Friedman and Rosenman suggest that you become aware of how much of your efforts, interests, and income are used in acquiring things. Have you become a caretaker of the creative efforts of others at the cost of losing your own because of disuse?

These authors refer to a point concerning opinions mentioned in chapter 3 of this book. Consider most of your conclusions and opinions as provisionally correct, especially in the areas of race, religion, and politics. Handling these controversial subjects diplomatically is much more of a feat than juggling seven sharp swords. Expressing certainty or being dogmatic when there is no basis for such a position can be more dangerous than catching a sword by the blade instead of the handle. If you don't know something, admit it. This tactic is preferable to making a fool of yourself and being placed in the position of defending a statement that is doubtful or very controversial. Finally, they suggest that you enrich your life with intellectual activities. Become familiar with arts, humanities, and sciences, or any other area that turns you on.

On the Origin of Type A Behavior

For some Type A people, understanding how they got that way may be helpful to them in changing their behavior. Matthews and Siegel (1983) suggest that Type A behavior may originate from an environment that strongly encourages productivity but includes ambiguous standards for evaluating that productivity. This combination may give rise to the impression in a child that time is insufficient to accomplish all of his or her goals. One has to hurry continually because there is never enough time.

According to Festinger (1954), comparing one's performance with that of peers often starts in childhood. The tendency is to compare oneself with someone who is superior in ability and/or productivity. This type of comparison amounts to adopting an ambiguous standard that is unrealistically high. It often leads to the self-perpetuating hurry sickness. These studies suggest that one way to encourage high productivity in people without the side effect of Type A behavior would be to include objective standards of evaluation as frequently as possible.

Frequently, comparisons of one child to another are made by parents. These comparisons can cover any activity or type of behavior: getting good or bad grades in school, picking up one's room, helping with the dishes, minding one or both parents, and so forth. Generally, such comparisons bring out the deficiencies of the child being addressed or scolded. If positive comparisons are never or seldom made, over a period of years children may acquire strong feelings of inferiority, insecurity, and hostility, especially if they feel that the comparisons are unfair. Without standards, the comparisons tend to be viewed as always unfair. Later on, when children compare themselves with their peers, it is usually with those who are superior to them in some sport, game, or grade on a report card. Unfair comparisons tend to deepen feelings of insecurity, and, in time, these children come to view the whole world as hostile. Such people demand to get even by whatever means they can muster.

If the psychological basis of the various Type A behaviors includes an underlying insecurity and a general lack of self-confidence, then the value of objective standards of comparison becomes clear for both child and parents. Realistic standards can serve as a reminder to parents to not always compare their child's performance to the best in the class or to that of older children. In my view, if a child gets the feeling of competence in one or more areas of school/play and learns early that overall he or she is better than some and worse than some, overambition, arrogance, and overcompetitiveness will take care of themselves.

In reviewing my own life, that of my children, and what I have learned from friends and acquaintances, I have come to the view that feelings of self-worth can be nourished in the home environment by parental encouragement of some activity either physical or mental in which there are objective standards of comparison. Self-esteem, self-confidence, or self-worth—call it what you will—serves as the anchor which helps prevent one's frail craft from being swept into the unknown seas of overpowering uncertainty and competition with hostile strangers. If parents are patient with their children and teach them to be patient with themselves, all normal children can learn to be proficient in some activity in which they are interested. Bright adolescents may require extra-curricular challenges and, if the child is well coordinated, physical as well as mental activities.

An anecdotal account of two generations in one family neatly illustrates some of these points. I have a friend, a physician whose specialty concerns the effect of heredity on heart disease. I have not sensed any hostility in him, even when he showed me a manuscript that had been refused by a prestigious medical journal. He classes himself as Type A based on the following behavioral characteristics: He is a very fast eater, extremely time conscious, extremely competitive even when playing games, and overly devoted to his work. A work day of 14 to 16 hours is not uncommon and 10 to 12 hours is routine.

His parents gave him a set of golf clubs when he was 12, and he enjoyed the game even though he lost his temper on making poor shots to the extent of throwing or breaking the clubs. No one enjoyed playing with him. His parents insisted that he continue golf as a way of learning to be patient, and as a lesson in self-control. His parents punished him when he lost his temper. In retrospect, he considers that he did learn some valuable things from golf and from his parents discipline. He also learned to play the piano at an early age, and later shifted to the clarinet. He now thinks that the hours of practice on musical instruments were also valuable in his learning patience, self-control, and concentration.

He first recognized Type A behavior in one of his sons at age four. The boy ate rapidly and was very impatient when waiting in line to attend a movie. Now at age eleven, these behaviors have changed very little, and the boy's competitiveness has become stronger. He does well at school, but his grades are no higher than his Type B sister. He spends hours practicing video games so that he can beat his father. (Two Type As competing at Pac-Man must be something to watch!) The son is not generally hostile, but if one of his siblings disturbs something in his garden, he becomes very angry. His parents punish him when his anger becomes too uncontrolled. It will be interesting to see if he, like his father, will remain unhostile.

Does this boy's behavior resemble his father's so closely because of hereditary influences? Or were similar factors present in both their early environments to bring out Type A behavior? As with most nature–nuture questions, we shall probably never come to a final conclusion. Rahe, Herrig, and Rosenman (1978) measured the heritability of Type A behavior by a variety of procedures. Data obtained from the Structured Interview, Jenkins Activity Survey, and the Thurstone Temperament Schedule showed significant correlations with both Type A behavior and heritability. On the other hand, a list of adjectives, which people could check in describing their behavior correlated with Type A but not with heritability. It appears from these preliminary results that some components of Type A behavior may be heritable and others not. The nonheritable ones were: Self-confidence, change, dominance, autonomy, achievement, and acceptance of counseling suggestions.

From the anecdotal example we can speculate that, if a child knows that he or she is being punished for a certain type of behavior and that his or her parents still love him or her and are not reacting angrily, the child's hostility can be kept to a minimum. As a parent, I know that these maxims are easier written than done!

Insecurity, the Necessity for Control, and Living With Uncertainty

You may recall from chapter 3 that I discussed the necessity of scientists learning to live with uncertainty, and suggested that the lay public should also. In that discussion I didn't specify to which type of uncertainty I was referring. It is the uncertainty that comes from realizing the difficulty of drawing correct inferences from events and experiences. It is the uncertainty that develops when a person learns to distinguish facts from hypotheses and realizes how many decisions are based on hypotheses because the facts are not available. It is the uncertainty that grows as we become aware that most of our generalizations are overgeneralizations; that a single incident is not sufficient basis for any generalization. Finally, if we are challenged over a weak, or faulty, generalization, we should admit error at once. Remember: Unwarranted certainty often leads to stressful situations.

Another type of certainty concerns people. We expect our friends and acquaintances to act in a regular, predictable manner. Examples of behavioral uncertainty like Dr. Jekyll and Mr. Hyde are rare enough to be publicized by the media. In our culture, time plays an important part in the certainty of both people and events. Suppose a man arrives home from work at 6:00 p.m. every day. His wife regularly serves dinner at 6:15. On one occasion, he doesn't arrive at 6:00, 6:05, or 6:15. He had not phoned to inform his wife that he would be late. Such a tardy arrival had not occurred for 20 years. At what time might his wife start to get nervous? At 6:05, 6:15, 6:30, or 7:00? At what time should she call the police, her mother, her husband's best friend? What other factors might affect her decision as to when to call someone: How much she loved him, her degree of dependency on him, her plans for the evening? Other things being equal, would a Type A woman call sooner than a Type B?

I ask all these hypothetical questions because degree of certainty and degree of control are closely related. A person who is basically insecure (Type A) and seeks to control situations to achieve a feeling of greater security, might be expected to be threatened earlier by the situation described above because the uncertainty was beyond her control. It is possible that if the husband arrived home at 11:00 p.m., sober and uninjured, the woman's first reaction might be one of anger because she had been deprived of 5 hours of certainty. The man had better have an impeccable reason for his lateness. Seen in this light, the control or dominance that Type A persons seek in a situation is not because they enjoy controlling or dominating for its own sake, but as a means of achieving security.

In real life there are few situations in which one has such complete control as a scientist conducting an experiment. Real-life situations contain uncertainties of both events and people. In addition, real-life situations are usually unique—they are not repeatable as an experiment. If it is an important event like a murder trial in a courtroom, the two leading lawyers prepare for it meticulously: They coach their witnesses, have all the facts at their fingertips, and have prepared explanations of their client's actions to place them in as favorable a light as possible. Each side wants to affect the outcome by exerting maximum possible control over the jury.

This example sheds some light on how extreme Type A people approach many everyday events. They are competitive, achievement oriented, compelled to win, and insecure. They attempt to decrease their insecurity by controlling as many events and people in the situation as they are able. In this way they hope to influence the outcome to suit their own objectives. But unlike the scientist described above, whose security increases with repeated accurate predictions, Type As remain insecure no matter how many times they win. Their behavior seems independent of their success.

Internally Produced Stressors: Premenstrual Syndrome

While many stressors arise in the environment and are perceived by means of our nervous systems, others may be generated internally and affect soma, psyche, and behavior. These internally produced stressors at present can be grouped into two types. The first group includes those acting as neurotransmitters in the brain, an unbalance of which is thought to be involved in psychoses such as manic-depressive psychosis, depression, and schizophrenia. These diseases present complicated medical problems and will not be discussed here. The other, which affects almost half of the human race to varying degrees, has a hormonal origin. I am referring to premenstrual syndrome (PMS). It is estimated that up to 10% of adult women are subject to spontaneous, recurrent stress of considerable magnitude and discomfort.

If you are an adult male, try to imagine what it must be like to lose control of your behavior from a few days to 2 weeks every month! Imagine having little control over your emotions, going from tears to anger in a few minutes, acting irresponsibly, being irritable and depressed for half your days, and not being able to stop the irrational behavior, not understanding why or how it happens, and not finding anyone in the medical or allied professions who could provide any real help.

PMS received worldwide attention in 1982 when the defense in the murder trial of two women in England claimed that they should not be held accountable for their actions because they were suffering from untreated PMS. The women were acquitted on probation with the proviso that they receive therapy as long as required. What physician was responsible for this novel defense? She was Dr. Katharina Dalton, who had experienced many of the symptoms mentioned above while still a medical student. Because of her lack of control, she was in the process of seeing her dreams and aspirations go down the drain, when fortunately she was treated by a physician who prescribed the hormone progesterone as therapy. In the past few years PMS has become an openly discussed disease. Women from all walks of life are requesting, even demanding, that the medical profession help them to live normal lives. Many young professional women are no longer willing or able to suffer in silence. Is it a fad, like hypoglycemia—an excuse for nonproductivity—or has another barrier at last been broken in women's demands for fairness and understanding in medical diagnosis and therapy? In my opinion, PMS presents a serious, recurrent, legitimate problem to many women. Estimates of the prevalence of PMS range from 40% to over 90%. Keye (1983) thinks it likely that only 5% to 10% of women have premenstrual distress that causes serious problems.

What Is PMS?

PMS does not include every menstrual disorder or discomfort. The diagnosis of PMS is based on the occurrence of certain physical, mental, and behavioral symptoms during the week preceding menstruation. Over 150 symptoms have been reported. Some of the most common symptoms of all three types are listed in Table 4.4. The symptoms highlight one of the difficulties of classifying or evaluating PMS as a disease; most of the symptoms are quite subjective. In my opinion women are as suggestible as men. If one woman tells a friend that she had a ringing in her ears before her last period, the second is likely to experience it too.

Thus, placing PMS on a sound diagnostic basis requires the prospective charting of symptoms throughout the entire menstrual cycle. A diagnosis of PMS based on memory and recall alone may be incorrect. This diary needs to be constructed in conjunction with a woman's physician. PMS is no longer considered as a single syndrome with a single cause. As with so many other medical conditions, increased knowledge has led to an understanding of its complexity. As of 1985, the major causative factors in PMS were thought to be physical, psychological, and social. Evaluation of the importance of these three factors should precede a therapeutic regime.

PMS Therapies

The list of treatments for PMS is a long one. Some of them are exercise, special diets, diuretics, oral contraceptives, progestins, progesterone, tranquilizers, lithium, and psychotherapy. None has stood the test of a controlled double-blind study. None are effective as a general therapy. Katharina Dalton and the two murderers were lucky. Progesterone worked for them.

Research by Endicott, Halbreich, Schacht and Nee (1981) and Halbreich, Endicott, and Nee (1983) suggests that PMS is not a homogeneous entity

Table 4.4   A First Step in the Diagnosis of PMS

1. Do you suffer regularly from many of the following symptoms?
   -Depression
   -The need to be alone
   -Anger
   -Incoordination
   -Headache
   -Anxiety
   -Fatigue
   -Bloating
   -Irritability
   -Breast tenderness and swelling
   -Cravings for sweets or salty foods
   -Confusion or forgetfulness
   -Other persistent physical or emotional afflictions
2. With the above symptoms do you suffer
   -cyclically, in conjunction with menstruation?
   -to the extent that it interferes with the quality of your life?
   -in a way that you feel out-of-control?
   -for reasons that can't be identified?
3. Are you an otherwise competent, accomplished, happy, and responsible person for at least a portion of every month?

If you answered a frantic yes to all or most of these questions, there's a good chance you are suffering from premenstrual syndrome.

Note. From "Pre-Menstrual Syndrome: The Phantom Disease Millions of Women Have Denied" by M. Dickson, 1983, *Network,* **6**(3), p. 13. Copyright 1983 by *Network.* Adapted by permission.

that can be treated as a single disease. Some of the specific subtypes of depressive premenstrual symptoms resemble those of depressive affective disorders. A high percentage of women who have premenstrual depression have had a major depressive episode in their past. These women are also at increased risk for future episodes of major depressive disorders. As diagnoses become individualized, therapies will follow.

Seeking Help

I suspect that people realize when their coping is inadequate. Responsibilities pile up, mistakes occur more frequently, feelings of inferiority deepen, periods of despondency or depression lengthen, and the world grows blacker day by day. Even under these conditions, many people will not seek aid on their own. Often, a family member, close friend or confidant, physician, minister, or priest is necessary to provide the initiative.

However the decision is arrived at, the first question to be answered is, what next? There are two major routes in seeking professional help. Often the counselor knows a psychiatrist or clinical psychologist to whom you can be referred. This type of therapy is called *one-on-one* because it is private. The other route is some form of group therapy: a class in stress management, assertiveness, or relaxation techniques. In general, classes are cheaper than private therapy. In addition, finding many other people in similar circumstances may provide encouragement and friendship, and maintain ties to the human race at a crucial period in a person's life.

With either type of therapy it is important that people not feel obligated to continue if, after a few weeks, they do not feel that they are making progress. People who have become aware of their own assumptions may recognize similarities or differences in the assumptions of the therapist-leader. If a person feels strange, uncomfortable, or embarrassed, it is likely that assumptions don't fit, and help should be sought elsewhere.

Objectives of programs are just as important as assumptions in assessing whether a class or a therapist is right for you. A person whose appraisal of problems is deficient may feel out of place in a class whose main objective is teaching techniques for coping with identified problems. To be effective, any stress management program must teach a person new techniques of appraisal and coping with stressors.

A less clinical approach towards problem recognition and solving is provided by EST training (now called The Forum) or by Lifespring. Both of these groups offer a free, noncommittal, get-acquainted session for people who want to understand themselves better and desire more satisfactory personal relationships than they are experiencing.

After Stress Management, What?

The condition known as stress is very common in industrialized countries. It is estimated that three-quarters of visits to physicians are the result of stress-related symptoms and feelings of disease. Many of these symptoms might be handled without medications if people learned the techniques of recognizing and managing their stressors.

Is successful stress management equivalent to wellness? Not in my book. To me, stress management contributes importantly to survival, but wellness suggests a positive factor in living that survival does not. Successful stress management should provide a foundation of self-confidence that will lead to a person's taking the next step toward wellness—that of enjoying an active life. In my opinion, well people have earned the freedom of doing what they want to do in their spare time. I call this type of behavior responsible hedonism. The behavior is earned. Whatever turns you on, do it and enjoy!

Summary

This chapter has emphasized the distinctions between stressors and stress. Stressors were defined as perceived threats to a person, either physiological or psychological. If stressors are recognized and managed, they need not necessarily result in stress. Stress results when the normal psycho-physiological responses to stressors are overwhelmed for a long enough time to allow behavioral abnormalities and/or tissue damage to develop. A wide variety of diseases are known to be stress related. Similarly, chronic stress can result in behavioral changes in which Type A behavior is a well-known example.

The chapter deals with three major themes: first, managing stressors so that they do not cause stress; second, if stress reactions have already occurred, recognizing the symptoms and mobilizing resources to prevent stress reactions from becoming chronic; third, realizing that stress management provides a springboard in the pursuit of wellness.

Appendix 4A
Stress Awareness and Management Self-Questionnaire

You may be dissatisfied with one or more areas of your life but don't know where or how to begin to change them. The following self-evaluations may help you identify and become aware of those areas where stress arises. You are probably already aware of them, but filling out the questionnaire may place them in a perspective and increase your consciousness of them. The main objective of scoring is to help you to identify the areas of problems and permit you to focus on specific objectives.

Your problem areas may vary in number from 1 to 10 or more. It is suggested that you not tackle too many at once—perhaps not over 3. You may have identified a group of areas that are linked together and are making you most uncomfortable. Try to devise a strategy on a step-by-step basis that will solve the problem(s) and reduce your stress. If you cannot think of a plan by yourself, confide in a trustworthy friend, clergyman, or counselor whose judgment you respect. Answering this questionnaire will not solve anything. But it can serve as the first step in stressor management.

Stress Test Part One

Choose the most appropriate answer for each of the 10 questions as it actually pertains to you.

1. When I can't do something my way, I simply adjust to do it the easiest way.
   a) **Almost always**   b) **Usually**
   c) **Usually not**   d) **Almost always not**

2. I get upset when someone in front of me drives slowly.
   a) **Almost always**   b) **Usually**
   c) **Usually not**   d) **Almost always not**

3. It bothers me when my plans are dependent upon others.
   a) **Almost always**   b) **Usually**
   c) **Usually not**   d) **Almost always not**

4. Whenever possible, I tend to avoid large crowds.
   a) **Almost always**   b) **Usually**
   c) **Usually not**   d) **Almost always not**

5. I am uncomfortable having to stand in long lines.
   a) **Almost always**   b) **Usually**
   c) **Usually not**   d) **Almost always not**

6. Arguments upset me.
   a) **Almost always**   b) **Usually**
   c) **Usually not**   d) **Almost always not**

7. When my plans don't flow smoothly, I become anxious.
   a) **Almost always**   b) **Usually**
   c) **Usually not**   d) **Almost always not**

8. I require a lot of room (space) in which to live and work.
   a) **Almost always**   b) **Usually**
   c) **Usually not**   d) **Almost always not**

9. When I am busy at some task, I hate to be disturbed.
   a) **Almost always**   b) **Usually**
   c) **Usually not**   d) **Almost always not**

10. I believe that all good things are worth waiting for.
    a) Almost always   **b) Usually**
    c) Usually not   **d) Almost always not**

To score: Questions 1 and 10   a = 1, b = 2, c = 3, d = 4
                        2-9   a = 4, b = 3, c = 2, d = 1

This test measures your vulnerability to stress from being frustrated (i.e., inhibited). Scores in excess of 25 suggest some vulnerability to this source of stress.

Stress Test Part Two

Circle the letter of the response option that best answers the following 10 questions.

How often do you

1. find yourself with insufficient time to complete your work?
   a) Very often b) Fairly often c) Seldom d) Never

2. find yourself becoming confused and unable to think clearly because too many things are happening at once?
   a) Very often b) Fairly often c) Seldom d) Never

3. wish you had help to get everything done?
   a) Very often b) Fairly often c) Seldom d) Never

4. feel your boss/spouse simply expects too much from you?
   a) Very often b) Fairly often c) Seldom d) Never

5. feel your family/friends expect too much from you?
   a) Very often b) Fairly often c) Seldom d) Never

6. find your work infringing upon your leisure hours?
   a) Very often b) Fairly often c) Seldom d) Never

7. find yourself doing extra work to set an example to those around you?
   a) Very often b) Fairly often c) Seldom d) Never

8. find yourself doing extra work to impress your superiors?
   a) Very often b) Fairly often c) Seldom d) Never

9. have to skip a meal so that you can get work completed?
   a) Very often b) Fairly often c) Seldom d) Never

(Cont.)

10. feel that you have too much responsibility?

a) Very often b) Fairly often c) Seldom d) Never

To Score: a = 4, b = 3, c = 2, d = 1

Total up your score for this exercise.

This test measures your vulnerability to overload (i.e., having too much to do).

Scores in excess of 25 indicate vulnerability to this source of stress.

Stress Test Part Three

Answer all questions according to how true they are for you in general.

1. I hate to wait in lines.
   a) Almost always   b) Usually
   c) Seldom   d) Never

2. I often find myself racing against the clock to save time.
   a) Almost always   b) Usually
   c) Seldom   d) Never

3. I become upset if I think something is taking too long.
   a) Almost always   b) Usually
   c) Seldom   d) Never

4. When under pressure, I tend to lose my temper.
   a) Almost always   b) Usually
   c) Seldom   d) Never

5. My friends tell me that I tend to get irritated easily.
   a) Almost always   b) Usually
   c) Seldom   d) Never

6. I seldom like to do anything unless I can make it competitive.
   a) Almost always   b) Usually
   c) Seldom   d) Never

7. When something needs to be done, I'm first to begin, even though the details may still need to be worked out.
   a) Almost always   b) Usually
   c) Seldom   d) Never

8. When I make a mistake, it is usually because I've rushed into something without giving it enough thought and planning.
   a) Almost always   b) Usually
   c) Seldom   d) Never

9. Whenever possible, I will try to do two things at once, like eating while working or planning while driving or bathing.
a) **Almost always**   b) **Usually**
c) **Seldom**   d) **Never**

10. When I go on a vacation, I usually take some work along, just in case I get a chance.
a) **Almost always**   b) **Usually**
c) **Seldom**   d) **Never**

Score: a = 4, b = 3, c = 2, d = 1

This test measures the presence of compulsive time-urgent and excessively aggressive behavioral traits.

Scores in excess of 25 suggest the presence of one or more of these traits.

Stress Test Part Four

How do you cope with the stress in your life? There are numerous ways, some of which are more effective than others. Yet some coping strategies may actually be as harmful as the stress they are used to alleviate. This scale was created largely on the basis of results compiled by clinicians and researchers who sought to identify how individuals effectively cope with stress. This scale is an educational tool, not a clinical instrument. Its purpose is to inform you of ways in which you can effectively and healthfully cope with the stress in your life. A point system will give you an indication of the relative desirability of the coping strategies you are currently using.

Simply follow the instructions given for each of the 14 items listed below. When you have completed all of the items, total your points and place that score in the box provided.

___ 1. Give yourself 10 points if you feel that you have a supportive family around you.

___ 2. Give yourself 10 points if you actively pursue a hobby.

___ 3. Give yourself 10 points if you belong to some social or activity group that meets at least once a month (other than your family).

___ 4. Give yourself 15 points if you are within 5 lb of your ideal body weight, considering your height and bone structure.

___ 5. Give yourself 15 points if you practice some form of deep relaxation at least three times a week. Deep relaxation exercises include meditation, imagery, and yoga.

___ 6. Give yourself 5 points for each time you exercise 30 min or longer during the course of an average week.

___ 7. Give yourself 5 points for each nutritionally balanced and wholesome meal you consume during the course of an average day.

___ 8. Give yourself 5 points if you do something that you really enjoy which is just for you during the course of an average week.

___ 9. Give yourself 10 points if you have some place in your home that you can go in order to relax and/or be by yourself.

___ 10. Give yourself 10 points if you practice time management techniques in your daily life.

___ 11. Subtract 10 points for each pack of cigarettes you smoke during the course of an average day.

___ 12. Subtract 5 points for each evening, during the course of an average week, that you take any form of medication or chemical substance (including alcohol) to help you sleep.

___ 13. Subtract 10 points for each day, during the course of an average week, that you consume any form of medication or chemical substance (including alcohol) to reduce your anxiety or just calm you down.

___ 14. Subtract 5 points for each evening, during the course of an average week, that you bring work home that was meant to be done at your place of employment.

Now calculate your total score and place it in the box on the left. A perfect score would be 115 points. If you scored in the 50-60 range, you probably have an adequate collection of coping strategies for most common sources of stress. However, you should keep in mind that the higher your score, the greater your ability to cope with stress in an effective and healthful manner.

Note. Adapted from *What Do You Know About Stress?* (DHEW Publication No. PHS 79-50097; pp. 1-4) by G.S. Everly, 1979, Washington, DC: Department of Health and Human Services, U.S. Government Printing Office. Copyright 1979 by Department of Health and Human Services. Adapted by permission.

Reduce Stress—
Any Place, Any Time
(Breckenridge, 1987)

People under stress tend to breathe in short, shallow breaths. Deep breathing provides you with maximum oxygen and allows you to relax.

Concentrate on inhaling through the nose and exhaling slowly through the mouth. Slowly breathe in until you can't take in any more air, and slowly exhale until you've squeezed every last bit of air from your lungs.

Practice 5 breaths a time at least once a day so that you will feel comfortable doing it under stressful situations. Notice your body relaxing as you continue to breathe in this manner.

Chapter

5

Nutrients and Wellness

Serenely full, the epicure would say,
Fate cannot harm me, I have dined today.
Sydney Smith

This chapter will help you

- recognize the differences between proteins, carbohydrates, and fats as calorific essential nutrients;
- understand that, while ethyl alcohol furnishes calories, it is classified as a drug and not a food;
- recognize the roles of vitamins, inorganic elements, water, and possible dietary fiber, as essential noncalorific nutrients;
- comprehend the experimental basis and meaning of the Recommended Dietary Allowances (RDAs) and how to use this information in reading labels while shopping for food; and
- utilize nutrient density in planning your meals and snacks.

We eat food, not nutrients. And yet an adequate diet must contain all the essential nutrients in certain amounts or deficiencies will develop and wellness will be impossible. A knowledge of nutrients is thus essential in making food choices that will ensure an adequate diet. For this reason, I will introduce the large topic of nutrition with a discussion of nutrients. This type of information will not insure that the dietary strand of wellness will be strong, but without this information, dietary wellness is difficult to achieve. You might ask, How did people manage before scientific knowledge on diet became available? As Tannahill (1973) describes in *Food in History*, things were chancy in the old days. Obtaining enough to eat was a recurring problem, and what we recognize now as vitamin-deficiency diseases were endemic in many parts of the world.

Essential Nutrients

Dietary essential nutrients are of two types: those that supply energy (calories)—proteins, fats, and carbohydrates—and those that are noncalorific but necessary for the utilization of energy. This latter group contains the vitamins (13 substances), the essential elements (22), water, and dietary fiber, which I consider to be a group of six essential nonnutrients. In addition, there are nine essential amino acids and essential fatty acids. These latter 11 substances not only participate in noncalorific essential functions but also are ultimately used for energy.

By definition, essential nutrients cannot be synthesized by humans. They are necessary for three vital functions: maintenance of health, growth, and reproduction. A chronic lack of any one essential nutrient will result in a gradual diminution of wellness, and eventually death will ensue.

A number of living organisms do not require organic nutrients. They can synthesize them. For example, certain bacteria will grow and reproduce if they are supplied only with a source of energy, a source of nitrogen, water, carbon, and a few elements—inorganic nutrients. Their needs are few. As we ascend the evolutionary ladder to more complicated organisms, however, nutrient needs increase. We probably know more about the nutrient requirements of rats than of any other species. They require 46 nutrients in addition to energy. Humans require 47—the 46 of the rat plus ascorbic acid (vitamin C).

Human nutrition would certainly be simpler if our dietary requirements were as few as the bacteria mentioned above. There is a price to pay, however, for being self-sufficient. In bacteria, genes are required for the synthesis of the enzymes that produce the small organic molecules called coenzymes that are necessary for still other enzymes to function. In contrast, humans have lost these genes, and we now rely on our diet to furnish us with these essential nutrients. We call them vitamins. If we could synthesize all 13 vitamins, our gene pool (genome) would have to be much larger than it is. Geneticists have speculated that, if we retained the genes for synthesizing vitamins, we might not have been able to develop those that are responsible for our unique and complicated nervous system. Better to talk than to make our own vitamin C!

Sources and Expenditure of Calories

The potential energy from proteins, carbohydrates, and fats is released by a series of reactions that are called oxidations and phosphorylations. Although all of these reactions do not involve oxygen directly, oxygen gas in the air is essential for them to continue. In the process, the carbon atoms these substances contain are oxidized to carbon dioxide (CO_2), which we exhale when we breathe out. The overall process is similar to burning gasoline in our automobiles, but the biological process is much more complicated and subject to many more controls than an engine.

In an engine the CO_2 that is produced by the oxidation occupies a much larger volume than the original volume of gasoline. The CO_2 gas exerts pressure on the cylinders, they move, and by a series of connections, the power is transferred to the wheels. In an animal, the synthesis of adenosine triphosphate (ATP) is coupled to the oxidations, and this energy-rich substance is utilized to provide energy for muscle movement and other vital functions.

Energy is used in two broad categories: first, to keep alive, or to furnish energy to, our organs such as the brain, liver, and kidneys to carry out their functions; and second, for muscle movement. Organ usage of energy, called basal metabolism, remains relatively constant from day to day, but muscle movement can vary widely from minute to minute. A table of Daily Energy Expenditures is included at the end of this chapter (see Table 5A.1). These estimates are handy in calculating one's dietary energy requirements.

It is important to realize that the amount of energy that we obtain from a unit of weight of food varies quite widely. Fats furnish the most—9 kcal per gram, whereas proteins and carbohydrates furnish equal amounts of 4 kcal per gram. It is obvious from these numbers that it is easier to keep one's weight in line on a low-fat diet than on a high-fat diet.

The Proportion of the Three Energy-Supplying Foods May Affect Health

Apart from total energy intake, does the proportion of the three foodstuffs matter? Are there specific effects of a high-protein, a high-fat, or a high-carbohydrate diet? The answer is a resounding yes.

Excess protein (over 15%) places an extra burden on the liver and on the kidneys. The liver is forced to synthesize more urea, the chemical by which most of the body's nitrogen is excreted. The kidneys are required to excrete the excess urea. In this connection, a high-protein diet requires a high-liquid intake to prevent toxic concentrations of excretory products from building up (Chopra, Forbes, & Habicht, 1978). Also, high-protein diets result in a higher excretion of calcium. This effect is thought to be a factor in the high incidence of osteoporosis in the U.S.

High-fat diets (40% and above) tend to result in high blood cholesterol levels and the building up of *atheromas* in sedentary people. High-fat diets are also correlated with the occurrence of certain types of cancers. In general, nutritionists and many diet-conscious physicians suggest that total fat intake be restricted to about 30% of total calories. In my opinion this hypothesis is not proved—as was discussed in chapter 3—but it seems reasonable, especially for sedentary people.

If these suggestions are followed, they result in carbohydrates contributing 60%-65% of the total calories. It is interesting that these proportions are similar to those calculated for human diets over past millennia when the human race was largely engaged in agriculture and other types of manual labor.

It is important to keep in mind that, when you see a reference to fat contributing to 30% or 49% of a diet, it is referring to percentage of calories, not to percent by weight. For example, a 2%-fat milk carton label contains the following:

NUTRITION INFORMATION
Per serving
Serving size   1 cup
Calories   121
Protein   8 g
Carbohydrate   11 g
Fat   5 g

The total weight, ignoring that from water and salts, is 24 g, of which fat contributes 5 g = 21% on a dry weight basis. In calculating percentage as calories, however, fat percentage comes out much higher.

Protein: 8 g × 4 kcal/g = 32 kcal
Carbohydrate: 11 g × 4 kcal/g = 44 kcal
Fat: 5 g × 9 kcal/g = 45 kcal

The total calories equals 121, of which fat contributes 45 = 37%. From this calculation, you can see that even 2% milk is high fat. Two percent milk furnishes more calories as fat than that from either protein or carbohydrate. To emphasize this important distinction, I shall specifically indicate in subsequent chapters which type of percentage I am referring to (i.e., % [cal] as calories, or % [wt] as weight). In case you are wondering where the 2% fat calculation fits in, it refers to the weight of fat in 100 g of milk wet weight.

Essential Carbohydrate

The third energy source, carbohydrate, is required in the diet in some form, but in distinction to proteins and fats, there is no essential, specific carbohydrate. This statement means that the major sources of dietary carbohydrate—starch and sugars—can be converted to all the different sugars found in our bodies.

Yet, there is a requirement for some minimum amount of carbohydrate in the diet. How can this be? If the carbohydrate content of a person's diet is reduced to 20% of calories or below, the person will develop a condition known as ketosis. In this condition, fats are incompletely oxidized, and a percentage of them is excreted in the urine and breath as three chemicals: acetoacetic acid, β-hydroxybutyric acid, and acetone. The three collectively are known as the ketone bodies.

There are two conditions under which the ketone bodies are formed in large amounts. The first occurs when a person is consuming a high-fat, low-carbohydrate diet, such as the Atkins diet. This diet is effective in weight loss because, for some reason not yet understood, the ketone bodies depress appetite. A complication, however, is that the long-term excretion of these acidic substances results in a depletion of the body's supply of cations such as sodium and potassium. The excretion of these ions in excess amounts may unbalance the person's electrolyte system with serious consequences. The other condition in which ketone bodies are excreted is in uncontrolled diabetes. This similarity in the effects of a low-carbohydrate diet and diabetes makes the point that the diabetic who excretes sugar in the urine because it cannot be utilized is in a similar metabolic condition to the person on a very low carbohydrate diet. A function of insulin is to allow the sugar to be metabolized.

Sources of Carbohydrates

The human digestive tract has developed to handle diets that are high in polymers like starch and fairly low in sugars. This distribution is found in the traditional diets of mankind in various parts of the world. For example, sweeteners like honey and sugar were quite rare in the diet of Europeans until cane sugar began to be imported in the sixteenth century.

Although the consumption of cane sugar was originally restricted to the nobility and the wealthy, as production increased its price was lowered until almost everyone could afford it. Consumption in England was about 10 kg per person per year in 1850, 30 kg in 1930, and 50 kg in 1960. The average American eats about 50 kg of sugar per year. This amount calculates to about 600 kcal per day of sweeteners, most of them in the form of refined and processed sugars and sweetening agents. Is this large consumption of refined carbohydrates harmful?

Sweet and Dangerous?

Sweet and Dangerous (with no question mark) is the title of a book by an English physician, Dr. John Yudkin (1972). His thesis was that refined sugars were responsible for the huge increases in heart disease, diabetes, and obesity that have occurred in developed countries. Actually, many of these ideas were first publicized by another English physician, T.L. Cleave, in a series of papers that were summarized in a book for physicians entitled *Diabetes, Coronary Thrombosis and the Saccharine Disease* (Cleave, Campbell, & Painter, 1969). Unfortunately, most of the epidemiological studies on which these ideas were based were flawed in that the fat and fiber contents of the diets were not controlled. In addition, differences in physical activity between members of underdeveloped and developed cultures were overlooked by almost everyone.

Despite these serious flaws, the notion that refined carbohydrates are poison was accepted and widely publicized by popular writers like Adelle Davis (1965), H. L. Newbold (1978), Robert Atkins (1977), and Carlton Fredericks (1965). Are we dealing here with a legitimate controversy or with a pseudo-one in which a storm has been stirred up by popular writers searching for simplistic solutions to complicated questions? First I'll summarize the known effects of diets high in refined carbohydrates and sugars and then discuss the evidence that these dietary components are causative agents in a wide variety of diseases.

Most nutritionists agree that a meal high in sugar results in the prompt secretion of insulin. This hormone facilitates the absorption of glucose into cells where it is oxidized, stored as glycogen, and/or converted to fat. In some way, as yet unknown, blood glucose concentration is involved in appetite control. The appetite regulator, sometimes referred to as the *appestat*, is located in the brain, in or near the hypothalamus. A low blood glucose stimulates the regulator, and the person feels hungry. Eating food is followed by digestion and absorption, and in about 20 minutes the blood sugar concentration begins to rise, the appestat is turned off, and hunger subsides. These facts and hypotheses help us understand an important effect of how the composition of the food affects the rate at which the blood sugar level rises, which in turn affects the rate at which insulin is secreted, and finally the frequency of the desire to eat.

If a meal or snack contains mostly refined carbohydrates and sugars, digestion and absorption are relatively fast, blood sugar tends to rise rapidly, and large amounts of insulin may be secreted. Blood glucose drops promptly to the fasting level or below, and the person may feel hungry just 30 minutes after eating. It is easy to understand how this type of diet can lead to obesity. The person is hungry most of the time.

If a meal or a snack contains appreciable amounts of proteins and fats in addition to carbohydrates, digestion and absorption take longer, and it also takes time for the liver to convert the excess amino acids derived from protein into sugar. A mixed meal of this type will maintain the blood glucose level above the fasting level for a long time, and the person may not become hungry for hours, even though the caloric intake may not be higher than it was from the refined carbohydrate meal. Some of the thinnest people I know eat heartily at meal time but, due to their selection of foods, do not get hungry until the next meal. They seldom snack between meals because they do not have the urge.

This hypothesis of appetite control also helps us to understand why a slow eating rate makes it easier to avoid overeating. A hungry person who eats rapidly may finish the meal in less than 20 minutes. An excess of calories may have been consumed before the appetite control mechanism had a chance to work. A slow eater who takes a minimum of 30–40 minutes to finish a meal becomes aware of the satiety signal and cuts down or stops eating before consuming an excess of calories. With this in mind, the European custom of leisurely dining appears as more healthful than the American one of rapid eating of fast foods.

Now we come to a fascinating and important relationship between obesity and insulin receptors on cells. Before insulin can act to facilitate the entrance of glucose into cells, it must first react with a receptor on a cell. In obese people there are fewer insulin receptors per cell. Consequently, to prevent blood glucose from remaining high, the pancreas secretes more insulin. It is now a confirmed fact that the concentration of blood insulin is higher in obese than in nonobese people. Although the detailed explanation has not yet been worked out, this fact serves as the cornerstone of the hypotheses linking chronic obesity to the development of diabetes in middle-aged, obese people.

Diets high in refined carbohydrates and sugars have also been linked to a condition known as hypoglycemia. Due to wide publicity in the popular press, hypoglycemia became the fad disease of the mid-1970s. Newbold (1978) estimated that 20-40 million Americans have it. Its so-called symptoms reflected most of the common ailments of the human race. Some of the usual symptoms are: depression, dizziness, drowsiness, headaches, faintness, cold hands and feet, lack of concentration, insomnia, confusion, aggressiveness, and hostility. Here, we encounter the serious mistake of defining a disease by its symptoms. People with these symptoms—and who of us doesn't have some of them from time to time?—would go to their physicians and ask to be treated for hypo-glycemia! Americans had reached the apogee in self-diagnosis. The predictable happened. A subspecialty, which became known as the hypoglycemia doctors, appeared that treated the patients for a handsome fee. Often the so-called therapy went on for years.

In the meantime, legitimate physicians wrung their hands. The term *hypoglycemia* means low blood sugar. As I've mentioned, blood glucose increases after a meal and then declines. Its concentration after an over-night fast is taken as a standard condition. The medical diagnosis of hypoglycemia is based on the results of a glucose tolerance test in which a large amount of glucose is administered to a fasting person and the blood glucose concentration measured at intervals for 5 to 6 hours. It is the same test that is used in the diagnosis of diabetes. If the blood glucose rises well above the average after an hour and tends to remain high for 3 to 4 hours, the glucose tolerance curve strongly suggests diabetes. In con-trast, if, at some time, the blood glucose concentration decreases to a sig-nificant amount below the fasting level, the data suggest hypoglycemia. A valid diagnosis requires that a number of psychological symptoms oc-cur concomitantly with the low point of blood glucose.

Many of the physicians who carried out both a glucose tolerance test and psychological tests on their patients obtained very confusing results. Some patients were definitely hypoglycemic but showed none of the psy-chological symptoms mentioned above. Others were not hypoglycemic but did exhibit one or more of the symptoms. A small percentage of patients (about 10%) had both. Many in this last group did respond favor-ably to a dietary change that decreased refined carbohydrates and sugar in meals and snacks and increased protein and fat (Gray & Gray, 1983).

Ethyl Alcohol: A Calorific Drug

The fourth widely used source of energy in many parts of the world is alcohol. The use and misuse of alcohol by the human race has a long and infamous history. Some societies have been wise enough to proscribe its use to ceremonial functions, but in many civilized countries alcohol can be purchased by almost anyone old enough to hold a dollar up to the counter.

Ethyl alcohol—commonly referred to as alcohol—is usually formed by fermentation of carbohydrates. Alcohol is classified as a drug and not as a food. To my knowledge it is the only widely used drug that furnishes energy. We obtain 7 kcal per gram from alcohol. Its energy yield is a bit lower than fats and higher than that of protein and carbohydrates. I think that the energy content of alcoholic drinks should be emphasized because many people will have a drink or two before a hearty dinner with wine and not be aware that they have consumed 300 or more kcal over and above their food intake. At this rate of overconsumption, a person can gain an extra pound every 12 days. Table 5.1 below lists the calorie content of the three most widely used types of alcoholic beverages.

Table 5.1   Energy Content of Alcoholic Beverages

Beverage	Amount oz	Energy kcal
Beer (12-proof)	12	140
Whiskey, gin, vodka, rum (80-proof)	1.5	105
Table wine (27-proof)	3.5	90

Consumption of alcoholic drinks faster than about one per hour affects the behavior of most people. Alcohol is widely thought to act as a stimulant because people act more lively after a few drinks. Actually, alcohol acts as a sedative, and people feel livelier because it sedates their inhibitory nerves sooner than their excitatory ones. Long-term consumption of excess alcohol can definitely shorten life because it damages many organs such as liver, kidneys, brain, and muscles. For these reasons, alcohol is classified as a drug and not as a food.

Alcohol is a generic term that includes thousands of chemical substances. To my knowledge ethyl alcohol (ethanol) is the only one that is not a strong poison. Have you ever wondered why it is that we can imbibe fairly large quantities of ethanol (e.g., 6 oz. of whiskey) in a short time, become intoxicated, and yet recover from it with no obvious ill effects if the practice is not repeated too frequently? Many people who have consumed comparable quantities of wood alcohol (methanol) just once, in contrast, have become permanently blind for their indiscretion. What about rubbing alcohol? Its technical name is isopropanol. What about the alcohol in mouthwashes? It contains specially denatured ethanol so that its taste is not pleasant. Table 5.2 shows the comparative toxicity of a few alcohols commonly found around the home. The LD_{50} (lethal dose) gives the dosage at which 50% of the rats died.

To return to my question above: A possible reason that ethyl alcohol is so much less toxic than the other alcohols is that it is produced in very small amounts in normal metabolism. As a result, the liver contains enzymes that oxidize it to *acetic acid*, the main constituent of vinegar, and then to carbon dioxide and water. These reactions furnish energy. What is important to understand is that the capacity of these enzymes is limited, and if a person drinks the equivalent of over two drinks a day for an extended time, the alcohol itself, as well as other chemicals produced from

Table 5.2 Relative Toxicities of Some Common Alcohols

Alcohol Common Name	Technical Name	LD_{50} (oral)[1] g/kg
Wood alcohol	Methanol	12.9
Alcohol	Ethanol	13.4
—————	n-Propanol	1.9
Rubbing alcohol	Isopropanol	5.8

[1]The numbers in the column show that the LD_{50} of methanol, the lethal dose to kill 50% of the rats, is not much lower than that of ethyl alcohol. The LD_{50}, however, does not take into account the side effect of methyl alcohol on vision loss.

it, can affect the function of the liver, muscles, and brain. One of the long-term, irreversible effects of chronic overdrinking is called *cirrhosis of the liver*. This disease is possibly the oldest known lifestyle disease.

Effects of Alcohol on Absorption and Excretion of Nutrients

According to Iber (1971), large amounts of alcohol interfere with the absorption of vitamins A and B_{12}, thiamin, and folacin, as well as fat and amino acids. On the other hand, McDonald (1979) refers to one of the few metabolic studies on wine, carried out at the Human Nutrition Laboratory in Berkeley, California, in which it was found that consumption of 22% to 25% of total calories as wine or as United States Pharmacopeia (U.S.P.) ethanol had quite different effects. The consumption of wine resulted in considerably higher absorption of calcium, phosphorus, magnesium, zinc, and iron than did the consumption of ethanol or water. Dealcoholized wine was even more effective in increasing the absorption of these elements than regular wine. The authors conclude that it is the *congeners* in the wine and not the alcohol that are responsible for the increased absorption.

Alcoholics exhibit numerous nutrient deficiencies, because of both a decreased consumption of food and an increased excretion of nutrients (Halsted, 1976). The two elements most affected seem to be zinc and magnesium. Zinc deficiency, in turn, is associated with decreased release of vitamin A from the liver. Magnesium deficiency has also been related to increased excretion of this element due to alcohol. Solomon (1976) describes a patient who was depressed, anxious, and irritable. She had been on a reducing diet in which alcohol was not restricted and had been drinking heavily for some time. Blood analysis showed low magnesium. This deficiency was responsible for most of her problems, as her mood improved and she lost weight after being treated with magnesium and placed on a nutritious, alcohol-free diet.

Specific Calorific Dietary Essential Nutrients

The liver has the ability to convert every six-carbon sugar found in foods to glucose. For this reason, even though glucose is the carbohydrate fuel used for energy production by the cells, glucose is not essential in the diet. The same condition does not hold for fats and proteins. There are two fatty acids and nine amino acids that the body cannot synthesize. They are required in the diet and are called *dietary essential fatty acids* and *dietary essential amino acids*.

Essential Fatty Acid and Linoleic Acid

There are three types of fatty acids: saturated (SFA), monounsaturated (MFA), and polyunsaturated (PUFA). Of the dozens of fatty acids found in foods, linoleic acid, a PUFA that contains 18 carbon atoms and two unsaturated bonds, is one of two that cannot be synthesized in the body. It must be present in the diet or deficiency symptoms, such as skin irritations, occur. Linoleic acid serves as a precursor molecule for another PUFA called arachidonic acid. This acid, in turn, is the starting point for the synthesis of *prostaglandins, prostacyclins, thromboxanes,* and *leukotrienes*. These four types of chemicals are widely distributed in the body and are involved in a variety of inflammatory and allergic reactions. Aspirin, for example, reduces fever because it interferes with the synthesis of the prostaglandin family of molecules.

In general, red meat contains much more SFA than linoleic acid. For example, ground beef (3 oz), 21% (wt) fat, contains 7.0 g SFA and 0.4 g of linoleic acid, a ratio of 0.4/7.0 = 0.37. Chicken breast (2.8 oz) contains 1.4 g SFA and 1.1 g of linoleic acid, a ratio of 1.1/1.4 = 0.79; and ocean perch (3 oz), 2.7 g SFA and 2.3 g of linoleic acid, a ratio of 2.3/2.7 = 0.85 (Adams & Richardson, 1981). Vegetable oils from corn, safflower, and soybeans are excellent sources of linoleic acid.

The other dietary essential fatty acid is called linolenic acid. It contains 18 carbon atoms like linoleic acid but has three unsaturated bonds. For many years after it was discovered, its role as an essential fatty acid was in doubt. In 1982 Holman, Johnson, and Hatch presented a case history of a girl who had been shot in the abdomen and had to be nourished by intravenous solutions. After months of this type of feeding, she developed a number of symptoms that were very unusual, including numbness, weakness, inability to walk, leg pain, and blurred vision. Analysis of the solution showed that it was quite deficient in linolenic acid. Addition of this acid to the solution was followed by remission of symptoms. Since then, additional research has established linolenic acid as an essential fatty acid for humans.

Another fatty acid that is very similar in structure to linolenic acid has the long name of eicosapentaenoic acid (EPA). This fatty acid contains 20 carbon atoms and five double bonds. Although it is not established as an essential fatty acid, it has become of considerable interest in that its high concentration in fish and fish-eating animals is postulated as a reason that Eskimos do not develop heart disease even though their diets are high in fat. The role of EPA in avoiding heart attacks is discussed in chapter 10.

Dietary Essential Amino Acids

Of the 20 natural amino acids found in proteins, the 9 dietary essential amino acids are treated no differently from the other 11 by the energy-producing system. As proteins are *turned over*, all 20 amino acids are utilized for energy. Their names are glycine, alanine, valine[1], leucine[1], isoleucine[1], serine, threonine[1], aspartic acid, asparagine, glutamic acid, glutamine, lysine[1], arginine, cysteine, methionine[1], tyrosine, phenylalanine[1], tryptophan[1], proline, and histidine[2].

Proteins are essential in the diet not because they are a source of energy. There are other sources of energy that are just as adequate as proteins. Proteins are essential in the diet because of their content of nine amino acids that we cannot synthesize in our own cells. Without these nine, we could not synthesize new proteins, and our lives would be rapidly terminated. These amino acids occur in different proportions in different proteins, and for continued health, it is necessary to know something about their distribution in foods and how to assure obtaining them with a maximum of gustatory pleasure and a minimum of fuss and bother.

---

[1]Indicates dietary essential amino acids.

[2]Indicates dietary essentiality under some conditions.

Comparison of Animal and Vegetable Sources of Protein

To understand why there are differences in the nutritional value of animal and plant proteins for humans, you need first to learn how proteins are synthesized. Proteins are *polymers* that are composed of amino acids linked together in long chains. The amino acids are present in a protein in a definite sequence like the letters in a word. If the letters in a word are transposed, it may change meaning or it may lose meaning. For example, the word *action* loses sense in four out of five transpositions, and the meaning is changed in the fifth.

The sequence of amino acids in a protein is directed by the structure of the DNA in our genes. If a mutation changes the structure of DNA, the sequence of amino acids in a protein may be altered, and if the protein acts as an enzyme, the enzyme may lose all or some of its activity. If the DNA calls for the insertion of a particular amino acid in a protein but that amino acid is missing, the cell protein synthesis will stop. I'll explain how this happens by a letter-word example.

Let the word *antianthropocentric*, which contains 19 letters, stand for a protein. The word contains 10 different letters, each of which represents a particular amino acid. Now suppose that the amino acid *i* is missing from the amino acid mixture in the cell where protein synthesis is taking place. What happens? A partial protein with the structure *ant* would be synthesized, and then the synthesizing mechanism would stop. The protein fragment would soon be destroyed. Because, as far as we know, all proteins have functions, the organism would lose that function and would be less likely to survive. Now, let's return to the topic of animal and plant sources of proteins as food sources.

Plants have the ability to synthesize the 20 amino acids from simpler molecules like carbon dioxide (CO_2) and ammonia (NH_3). These amino acids are then incorporated into proteins under the direction of the plant DNA. The plant kingdom contains thousands of proteins, but humans utilize a relatively few of them as sources of energy and amino acids. The most common plant proteins that we consume come from cereal grains such as wheat, rice, and corn and from legumes such as soybeans, other beans, and peas.

Many plant proteins do not contain even approximately equal quantities of each of the 20 natural amino acids. We speak of such proteins as unbalanced. Kidney-bean proteins, for example, are relatively low in the amino acid methionine and relatively high in the amino acid lysine. Wheat proteins are relatively low in lysine and relatively high in methionine. If animal herbivores or human *vegan* vegetarians ate only beans or wheat as a source of protein, they would have to consume very large quantities indeed to permit their own growth to proceed at a normal rate because of the limiting amount of methionine or lysine.

On the other hand, what would result if a human vegan vegetarian ate both beans and wheat pasta at one meal? Once the protein is digested and its amino acids are present in the blood, their source is of no significance, and it is as though the person had eaten a balanced protein. This matching of proteins so that the weakness of one is matched by the strength of another is known as protein complementarity (see Table 5.3). It is not a modern discovery but has been known for centuries in different parts of the world where meat has been absent or in irregular supply. I have outlined the principle of complementarity in the table below. *Diet for a Small Planet*, Frances Moore Lappé (1971), has worked out complementarity for a large number of plant proteins, and in this book and a companion volume called *Recipes for a Small Planet* by Ellen Buchman Ewald (1975), there are hundreds of recipes containing delicious combinations for hungry vegetarians and others who want to expand their protein sources.

You might wonder how herbivores like wild horses or field mice manage. They have to eat a lot. They spend most of their waking hours searching for food. Farmers and producers of pet foods know about complementarity, and tame animals are fed a variety of grains. Ruminants like cows, sheep, and goats with their multistomachs comprise a special class. The digestive systems of these herbivores contain billions of bacteria that synthesize complete proteins. When the bacteria are themselves digested, the amino acids of their proteins enter the bloodstream of the

Table 5.3   Protein Complementarity

Plant Protein	Weakness	Strength
Beans	Methionine	Lysine
Wheat	Lysine	Methionine
Beans and wheat mixture	None	Lysine plus methionine

Other excellent traditional complementary protein combinations and area of origin are

Soybeans + Rice   (China)
Beans   + Corn   (Native Americans)
Peas   + Wheat (Middle East)

ruminant and are used for its protein synthesis. Cows have been raised with urea as the sole source of carbon and nitrogen!

To continue, most of the proteins of all animals are complete: they contain 20 amino acids. The same 20 amino acids are required for the synthesis of human proteins. Thus nonvegetarians don't have to worry about complementarity. We can synthesize 11 amino acids in our own cells, and the 9 that we cannot synthesize are the dietary essential amino acids. In this sense the dietary essential amino acids are comparable to vitamins and the 11 dietary nonessential amino acids to other substances that we synthesize in our cells like ATP or *acetylcholine*, which are also essential for growth and metabolism.

Protein synthesis and turnover are going on in our bodies all the time, in adults as well as in growing infants and children. An adult who is not regularly consuming all nine of the dietary essential amino acids will gradually become weaker due to loss of muscle tissue and become increasingly anemic due to loss of hemoglobin. A baby or child will soon cease to grow. It is for this reason that an adequate diet is so important for children. Eventually, however, the carbon chains of all the amino acids will be oxidized and utilized for energy.

Calorie Sources in Natural Food Mixtures

Natural foods very seldom are composed of just one type of energy source. Vegetables, meats, grains, dairy products, eggs, and fruit are all mixtures of various proportions of proteins, fats, and carbohydrates. For example, many people will pay more for choice beef because it has more flavor than standard grade. The difference in flavor is due not to a difference in the protein of the meat, but to the fact that choice meat contains more fat. Besides providing more flavor, the fat also provides more calories— lots of them. Choice cuts of meat furnish more calories as fat than as protein. In this connection, with the present emphasis on cutting down on fat, it is noteworthy that meat markets are now offering low-fat meats, both fresh and cold cuts.

In contrast to meats, protein in plant products such as wheat bread, pasta, rice, and corn is surrounded by carbohydrates. For this reason, vegetarian diets tend to contain less fat than carnivorous ones. In addition, diets high in minimally processed plant foods contain dietary fiber which adds bulk to the diet and is also low in calories. Animal foods contain no dietary fiber. These facts favor a predominantly vegetarian diet. It is recommended that omnivorous people adopt the Chinese custom of using meats mainly as a condiment.

Effects of Other Factors on Calorific Nutrient Needs

Growth is an expensive process in terms of calories. Babies eat far more per pound of weight than adults. Also, have you ever tried to fill up a healthy adolescent male? Protein requirement, however, is no higher for a 16-year-old than for an adult man.

Pregnancy and Lactation

These two conditions obviously require more calories to support the growth of the fetus and the production of milk. The advice of the woman's obstetrician and pediatrician should be followed with regard to desirable weight gain during pregnancy and how many extra calories are required for milk production. Some general figures are included in Table 5A.2 at the end of this chapter.

Age

With many people a discrepancy develops between appetite and activity. Many young bachelors gain weight shortly after marriage. Many young mothers retain the weight they gained during pregnancy and lactation. At some point in time—often in the early thirties—people will realize that their appetite is as large as it was 10 years previously but that their physical activity has decreased significantly. This situation amounts to a prescription for weight gain.

It is at this point that lifelong, conscious control of appetite should begin. Along with this restriction on intake, an increase in aerobic activity becomes very valuable, both for its own sake as well as for weight control. A moderate aerobic program that utilizes an average of 200 kcal per day, multiplied by 200 days equals 40,000 kcal per year. A pound of fat represents 3,500 kcal, so that this extra activity will result in a yearly weight loss of slightly over 11 lb without dieting! The question of weight control will be discussed in more detail in chapter 8.

Metabolic Factors

Weight gain represents energy storage, and it seems that some people are more efficient than others in storing energy as fat rather than radiating it as heat. Aerobic exercise has been found effective in increasing heat production, not only during the activity but also for hours afterwards. Metabolically speaking, fatty tissue uses fewer calories per pound for maintenance than muscle tissue at rest. This difference helps explain why fat people have a harder time losing weight than their more muscular counterparts.

Noncaloric Essential Nutrients

Food should provide us with more than energy. To convert food into a form that we can utilize requires a whole host of enzymes and accessory factors organized in a wonderful and marvelous fashion.

The following experiment furnishes some idea of the importance of noncalorific essential nutrients in the diet. Rats are divided into three groups, and two groups are provided with diets that are equal in calories but one of these is deficient in one or more noncalorific essential nutrients. The third group is starved. The rats receiving the deficient diet will die faster than the one receiving the complete diet. This result is not surprising. What is surprising is that the deficient rats will die faster than those of the third group that received no food at all. The starved rats reduce their activity as they use up their stored energy supplies. In addition, turnover of their proteins, coenzymes, and essential elements slows down, and they become much more efficient in utilizing what they possess. The fed animals metabolize and excrete their stores at the usual rate, and they die shortly after essential substances are exhausted.

Experiments of this type demonstrate why it is so important to eat foods that contain all the essential nutrients. It has been demonstrated repeatedly that deprivation of an essential nutrient over a long time, either willfully, through ignorance, or because of the unavailability of foods containing it, will result in sickness and finally death.

Vitamins

Vitamins are *organic* compounds and are divided into two groups based on their solubility. Nine are soluble in water. Their scientific names (common names given in parentheses) are thiamin (vitamin B_1), riboflavin (vitamin B_2), pyridoxine (vitamin B_6), cobalamin (vitamin B_{12}), biotin, folacin, niacin, pantothenic acid, and ascorbic acid (vitamin C). Four vitamins are insoluble in water and are called fat-soluble because they are fatty substances and are soluble in fat solvents like acetone. Their names are retinol (vitamin A), 1,25-dihydroxycholecalciferol (dihydroxy vitamin D), alpha-tocopherol (vitamin E), and phyloquinone (vitamin K).

Vitamins were discovered as a result of deficiencies in human populations. Beriberi, for example, affected millions of Asiatic people because they discarded the rice bran, a source of thiamin. Another widespread deficiency disease was known as pellagra, which is Italian for rough skin.

Corn was brought back to Europe by Columbus, and it soon supplanted rye as the major grain in southern Europe. Pellagra was first recognized in Spain and Italy in the eighteenth century and was thought to be an infectious disease.

Pellagra was endemic in many southern states of the U.S. early in the twentieth century. Its incidence was highest among the economically disadvantaged. Sebrell (1981) noted an interesting correlation between the increase in the price of cotton and the disappearance of pellagra during World War I. After the war, the price of cotton fell and pellagra reappeared. With benefit of hindsight, we can now recognize that, as the price of cotton increased, people's income also rose and they could afford higher quality diets. The brilliant researches of Joseph Goldberger from 1910 to 1922 solved the problem of pellagra by showing that it was definitely a nutritional-deficiency disease and that people who had to rely on corn as their major source of energy and protein were not receiving a sufficient amount of some essential factor. This factor has since been identified as niacin (Sebrell, 1981).

Many low-income Mexican Indians also use corn products as their major energy source, but they do not get pellagra. Why should these people be resistant when the disease was so common north of the border? Carpenter (1981) examined the cooking habits of the Mexicans in detail and found that they treated their corn flour with lime, which increases the available niacin content. Nutrition science has confirmed the value of many folk practices such as this one. We shall probably never know, however, how or when the lime treatment originated. A list of the common vitamin-deficiency diseases is presented in Table 5.4.

Inorganic Essential Nutrients

The second type of essential noncalorific nutrients is the inorganic elements. These are often called minerals, but I prefer the term elements

Table 5.4 Some Essential Nutrient-Deficiency Diseases

Deficient Essential Nutrient	Disease
Vitamin A	Xerophthalmia
Vitamin D	Rickets
Vitamin C	Scurvy
Vitamin B_1	Beriberi
Vitamin B_{12}	Pernicious anemia
Niacin	Pellagra
Iodine	Goiter
Iron	Anemia
Zinc	Dwarfism

because it is more accurate. The essential elements are divided into two groups based on the amounts found in the body. The seven major elements—called macronutrient elements—are present in amounts larger than 5 g. I'll list them in decreasing order: calcium, phosphorus, potassium, sulfur, sodium, chlorine, and magnesium. The allowances of these elements in the diet roughly follow the same order.

The 15 trace elements—also called micronutrient elements—are present in the body in amounts of less than 5 g. Because the allowance of only 9 of these has been worked out, I'll list all 15 in alphabetical order: arsenic, chromium, cobalt, copper, fluorine, iodine, iron, manganese, molybdenum, nickel, selenium, silicon, tin, vanadium, and zinc. The amounts required for some of these are so small that, to produce a deficiency, the food must be especially purified, the air of the animals being used in the experiment must be filtered, and the water that they drink must also be especially purified. As might be expected, human deficiencies of the trace elements are rare.

I have listed all the elements by their proper names. Few occur in foods as the free, unreacted element. Most occur in the *ionic* form, and it is in this form that they are taken up and metabolized by most animals, including humans. This distinction is important, because fluorine, for example, is extremely toxic as the free element and is required as the ion (F^-), which has the chemical name fluoride. Carbon occurs as the free element in charcoal, graphite, and diamonds, none of which are very nutritious. But when carbon combines with other elements, such as hydrogen, oxygen, and nitrogen, it forms all the organic compounds found in nature.

Some of the essential elements (e.g., magnesium and zinc) function as direct cofactors for a variety of enzymes. Others (e.g., cobalt and chromium) function only when associated with an organic molecule. For example, cobalt is not utilized by mammals when ingested in the ionic form, Co^+ or Co^{++}, but only when combined as part of the vitamin, vitamin B_{12}. This situation raises the question whether ionic cobalt should be listed as an essential element.

Although not of nutritional concern, certain bacteria in the human colon can synthesize vitamin B_{12} if provided with ionic cobalt. The vitamin cannot be absorbed, however, because these bacteria occur below the absorbing area of the intestine. The vitamin is excreted in the feces. It is thus possible that people who are not consuming sufficient vitamin B_{12}, and are exhibiting deficiency symptoms, may be excreting a quantity that would protect them if they could but absorb it. These facts may explain why many herbivores engage in *coprophagy*. Such are the marvels of nutrition research. Table 5.4 also lists some of the well-known deficiency diseases that have been identified as due to a trace-element shortage in the diet.

The increased knowledge that nutritional research has contributed during this century has made possible the great decrease in diseases due to lack of essential nutrients that has occurred in developed countries. Occasional cases of vitamin-deficiency diseases are found in the U.S. in impoverished areas and among alcoholics. Unfortunately, nutrient-deficiency diseases, as well as starvation, are still too common in many parts of the world.

Dietary Fiber

The last group of possible essential substances I'll mention is called dietary fiber, which is a very complex mixture containing dozens of different chemicals. It contains six major groups called cellulose, hemicelluloses, lignins, pectins, cutins, and gums. These materials are largely indigestible and add bulk to our feces.

A few words about the meaning of the term *fiber* may be in order here. In the first place, nutritionists state that fiber occurs *only* in plant material. There is none in animal foods. Yet everyone has heard of muscle fibers, and tendons and ligaments certainly seem fibrous when encountered in a drumstick or hock. Why aren't they included as fiber? To complicate the question even further many plant fibers are gelatinous rather than fibrous. What is the basis for the distinction? The distinction goes back to the early years of this century when methods of analysis of plant materials were being developed. After many extractions, including fat solvents, acid, and alkali, some plant material had not dissolved (i.e., it was still insoluble). The dried residue looked fibrous, so it was called *crude fiber*. This method is still used, and when you see the word "fiber" or "crude fiber" on a box, it refers to this material.

With the recent interest in plant fibrous substances, it was realized that the crude fiber methods were too drastic. Human stool, by definition, contains the insoluble material of the diet plus a goodly number of bacteria. It became obvious that crude fiber was not the same as the excreted material. Crude fiber was too small in weight, and it did not contain a number of plant insoluble materials. This realization has resulted in two advances. First, the new methods of analysis have permitted the identification of six chemical classes in the fiber fraction mentioned above. These are listed in Tables 5A.3 and 5A.4 along with examples of foods in which they occur and their functions. Second, the sum of the weights of the six fiber fractions exceeds that obtained by the old method by two to six times. To distinguish the material obtained by the new method from the old, the new is called *dietary fiber*.

In my opinion, present knowledge of dietary fiber and its uses is about as advanced as knowledge of vitamins 60 years ago. Dietary fiber has not yet been proved to act as an essential nonnutrient, but considerable data have been obtained to strongly suggest this conclusion.

In addition to helping avoid constipation and straining at stool, which leads to hemorrhoids, fiber has been suggested as aiding in the prevention of colon cancer, diabetes, and cardiovascular diseases. Please note that I have said *suggested*, not *demonstrated*. These questions are being researched at the present time and are still quite controversial. Bran, especially wheat bran, has received the most publicity, as in Reuben's *Save Your Life Diet* (1976), which mentions hardly any other type of fiber. His claims for the numerous beneficial effects of wheat bran have not been substantiated.

As shown in Table 5A.3, other types of fiber may have special effects. Pectins (Kay & Truswell, 1977) and hemicelluloses (Kies & Fox, 1977) in the diet have been reported to reduce serum cholesterol levels. Guar gum and gum tragacanth are more effective than most types of fiber in flattening the rise of blood glucose after a meal. If a person consumes a diet high in plant products, eight servings per day of fresh fruits and vegetables, and whole-grain products, it is probably not necessary to supplement with bran or other forms of dietary fiber.

Our need for liquid is so obvious that some authors have not even included it as an essential dietary constituent. The old dictum of eight glasses of water a day or their equivalent still holds, and its importance cannot be overemphasized. To mention an extreme situation: most people deprived of food but allowed water will live for at least a month and some have gone for a year. But a person allowed food but no water will be dead within 2 weeks. Water requirement is probably more closely related to climate and activity than any other nutrient, because physical exertion in hot weather may increase water needs many times. Thirst generally serves as an adequate guide of water need, and it is important that an active person satisfy it.

Have All the Human Nutrients Been Identified?

The first 52 years of the twentieth century were the heyday of vitamin research. During that period all the known vitamins for humans were isolated, and their structures were determined. Despite the continued search for additional vitamins, none has been identified in the last 35 years. There have been claims, such as those for the so-called vitamins B_{15} and B_{17}, but they have not stood up to critical scrutiny. Yet we are not justified in saying that all the vitamins have been discovered. A valid claim might be made at any time.

It is another matter, however, with the essential elements. Mertz (1981) states that the list of essential elements has been increased by seven in the past 30 years. It is likely that more will be added in the future. In contrast to the organic nutrients, which are members of an almost infinite class of compounds, the essential elements are limited in number by the size of the periodic table. Thus, at some point in time it should be possible to say that all of the essential elements have been discovered.

So far I have mentioned six groups of essential nutrients, which include 46 specific substances and 6 types of fiber. I expect that most experts would agree with this list, except for the fiber. The disagreements and controversies begin when we shift from qualitative to quantitative requirements. The cutting edge of nutrition research is honed by quantitative experiment, and hypotheses rise and fall as our quantitative knowledge increases. These topics will be discussed next.

Determining Human Requirements for Essential Nutrients

After a particular vitamin was discovered and it became possible to measure it quantitatively, answers to questions like "How much vitamin C is necessary to prevent scurvy?" and "How much vitamin A is needed to prevent night blindness?" were forthcoming. These studies led to the idea that the requirement for a nutrient was the minimum amount that would just prevent deficiency signs or symptoms (Harper, 1974).

In actual experiments that determine human nutrient requirements, the conditions are very carefully controlled and resemble those with guinea pigs or rats. Human subjects (formerly students or prisoners, nowadays paid volunteers) live in a restricted environment and have no direct contact with the outside world. Their food is adequate except for the nutrient being studied. They eat the same fare day after day. During this period their blood and excreta are frequently sampled and analyzed. They are not allowed to smoke or drink alcoholic beverages. They exercise on stationary bicycles, and their recreation is limited to reading or watching TV.

It often takes months for deficiency symptoms to develop. This phase of the experiment is necessary to drain the stored reserve of the nutrient from the subject. The onset of symptoms serves as an objective baseline for the rest of the experiment. When a deficiency has been established, the minimum amount of the nutrient that will remove it is determined. This part of the experiment may take as long or longer than the first part. Some symptoms may disappear faster than others. Even when the subject is symptom free, the blood levels of the nutrient may still be lower than is considered normal, and the amount necessary for achieving normal blood concentrations may take additional time to determine.

Suppose a person wanted to know his or her individual requirements for only 10 nutrients. The experiment might take 5 or 10 years! In the meantime, the person would be a voluntary prisoner on a monotonous diet. Unless the subject had an independent income or could work under these conditions, the experiment would be economically impossible. In addition, the costs of the special diet, chemicals, and technicians add to the expense. For these and other reasons, I have come to the conclusion that it is practically impossible for a person to know his or her requirement for even a single nutrient. The price in time and expense far exceeds the value of the information.

Individual Variability in Nutrient Requirements

Our genes are responsible for individual uniqueness. The differences extend from the size of our noses to the shape of our stomachs. Just as our looks and temperaments vary, so do our nutrient requirements. Roger Williams, the discoverer of pantothenic acid, and his colleagues have emphasized these differences in a provocative series of researches (Williams, Heffley, Yew, & Bode, 1972). They showed that the needs for eight amino acids varied from 2-fold for valine to 7-fold for lysine. This group also measured a 4.6-fold variation in the requirement for calcium and a 3.9-fold variation for thiamin. The number of subjects in these investigations was small; the largest was 50 people. Williams et al. correctly pointed out that the variations probably would be greater if 1,000 or 10,000 people were studied. This study reveals a practical question: Because it is not possible to measure the nutrient requirements of individuals *en masse*, on what basis should nutrition recommendations be made?

Recommended Dietary Allowances

Realizing these difficulties, and yet recognizing the need for some type of dietary recommendations, the Committee on Dietary Allowances, Food and Nutrition Board, National Research Council, in 1943 devised a statistical approach to the problem. As mentioned above, all healthy individuals do not require the same amount of any selected nutrient. The purpose of the RDAs is to select an amount for each nutrient that will be satisfactory for most people in a given population. It is assumed that nutrient requirements, like most biological variables, follow the statistical distribution known as the *normal distribution*, the familiar bell-shaped curve, which is drawn in Figure 5.1.

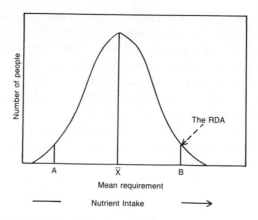

Figure 5.1   The statistical basis for the RDAs.

The mean for a certain nutrient requirement ($\overline{X}$) is determined for a random sample of healthy individuals, and the standard deviation is calculated. The standard deviation is a statistical measurement of how much variation from the mean is present. It is a property of the normal distribution that 95% of the population will lie within 2 standard deviations of the mean. These are indicated as A and B of Figure 5.1. The remaining 5% of the population are equally divided between the two tails; that is, 2.5% of the values are less than A, and 2.5% of the values are larger than B. Thus, by selecting the RDA at the amount designated by B, the allowance will cover 97.5% of the population. It is assumed that the 2.5% of normal, healthy individuals not covered by the RDA will not be seriously deficient in any nutrient if they ingest the RDA.

It is necessary to point out that, while the *Gaussian curve* of Figure 5.1 provides an admirable theoretical basis for the RDAs, the experimental basis is weak. To my knowledge, there is not a single RDA for which the data on which it is based are sufficient in number and distribution to justify the application of the bell-shaped curve. It is most unfortunate that, at this centerpiece of human nutrition, the RDAs, we encounter assumptions instead of facts.

The objective of the RDAs (National Research Council, 1980) is to "provide standards to serve as a goal for good nutrition" (p. v). The ninth revision of these allowances is reproduced in Table 5A.5. The RDAs are widely used by many health professionals: nutritionists, dieticians, nurses, physicians, and public health workers. Persons who are attempting to work out their own dietary needs and who want to understand the information on food labels will find an understanding of the RDA concept most helpful. Because there are many misconceptions and misstatements about RDAs, I'll review the highlights in the next few paragraphs.

First, a definition: The RDAs suggest a daily intake of essential nutrients judged to be adequate to meet the nutritional needs of almost all healthy people. It should be emphasized that the RDA for a specific nutrient, for example vitamin A, is an average figure that applies to millions of people but does not apply to any particular individual. *RDA should not be confused with individual requirements.* There are also gaps in our knowledge about the RDAs. Essential nutrients are still being discovered so that the list is probably incomplete. The human requirements of a number of essential nutrients are unknown at present so that an RDA cannot be calculated. As stated above, the RDAs list a satisfactory intake of nutrients for healthy people and are not meant to cover therapeutic needs, which occur during infections, or for chronic diseases, metabolic disorders, effects of medication on nutritional requirements, or particular foods that may affect absorption of nutrients. These restrictions should be recognized by anyone who is using the RDAs either professionally or personally.

Even if 2.5% of the population have needs above the RDA, they still are at little risk of nutritional deficiencies, because the allowances for most nutrients are set well above the level at which deficiency symptoms might occur. Some people have extra high requirements—tens or hundreds of times above the RDA—due to hereditary changes in protein structure that may result in malfunctioning of enzymes and other proteins. These people should be receiving medical care. Because the available data are so incomplete, many of the individual RDAs are admittedly the best judgment or "guesstimates" of the committee. We can expect some of the RDAs to change as more data are secured.

In addition to these limitations, there are complications that also must be taken into account in dealing with a large population. The needs of infants and children for essential nutrients are generally considerably higher than those for adults per unit of body weight. Women, in general, have lower requirements than men. Other factors such as pregnancy, lactation, old age, physical activity, and climate can affect needs of some nutrients and not of others. A number of these special allowances are included in Table 5A.5. Specific habits like alcohol consumption, smoking, and use of oral contraceptives also affect allowances. The effects of specific habits on allowances will be discussed in the section on nutrient supplements.

How RDAs Are Calculated

In this section I'll describe some of the general procedures that have been used in calculating RDAs for nutrients. Anyone desiring to know how the RDA for a specific nutrient was arrived at can find it in the RDA booklet (National Research Council, 1980).

Energy

An adult's energy requirement is the sum of that which is necessary for maintenance, the basal metabolism, and that which is utilized for physical activity, both for work and for recreation. It is interesting that the brain's requirement for energy is independent of what it thinks about or how much it is utilized.

The RDA booklet recommends an intake of 2,700 ± 400 kcal for a 70-kg (154 lb) male, and 2,000 ± 400 kcal for a 55-kg (120 lb) female in the age range 23–50 years. The variation is due to physical activity. Younger people require slightly more calories and older people slightly less calories than those in their midyears. The RDA for energy is the same as the energy requirement. If this were not so, the energy RDAs would be encouraging obesity!

Vitamins and Elements

A variety of procedures and techniques has been utilized in securing the data on which the RDAs are based. I'll briefly summarize them here.

The two most common methods are balance studies and analysis of blood concentration of the nutrient in question. Balance studies involve measurements of intake and excretion. When the two amounts are equal for a specific nutrient over a sufficient period of time, the person is said to be in balance. Excretion of more of the substance or its metabolic products than is being ingested is called negative balance because the body's stores are being decreased. The condition of positive balance is just the opposite. The person is ingesting more than is being excreted. Positive balance is normal and desirable in growing children and pregnant women.

The average blood concentration of a nutrient in a healthy population is a convenient, and therefore widely used, method for calculating nutrient needs. The amount of a nutrient required in the diet to maintain the normal blood concentration defines its RDA. Another method, not as widely utilized recently as in former times, is the measurement of the amount of a nutrient that will just prevent deficiency symptoms and doubling it for the RDA.

Four vitamins are synthesized by bacteria in the digestive tract. They are vitamin K, biotin, folacin, and cobalamin (B_{12}). Dietary sources of the first three substances would not be required by many people. However, it would be expensive, time consuming, and inconvenient to identify those people who required them and those who did not. In addition, the use of oral antibiotics may deplete the numbers of digestive tract bacteria to such an extent that food sources of these vitamins are necessary, at least temporarily. For these reasons, an RDA for folacin is included in the RDA table, and tentative values for biotin, pantothenic acid, and vitamin K are included in Table 5A.5. Cobalamin is synthesized in a section of the large intestine where absorption does not occur.

Limitations of the RDAs

The function of the digestive tract is to transform the food we eat into soluble substances that can be absorbed and subsequently distributed by the blood and utilized in all parts of the body. The part which is not solubilized is called dietary fiber. To be absorbed, the products of digestion must be not only soluble but also small. In the digestive process, large molecules are converted into small ones. For example, a single protein of molecular weight 100,000 or larger may be *hydrolyzed* into 20 amino acids of average molecular weight of 110; a complex carbohydrate may form six or eight simple sugar derivatives.

Nutrient Interactions

The digestive tract can be compared to a gigantic test tube filled with dozens, if not hundreds, of reactive substances. The composition of the mix keeps changing due to enzyme activity, absorption of some substances, and the addition of new ones from the most recent meal or snack. Chemical reactions can be expected to occur on a random basis in this melange. Some of the products may be beneficial to the person who is their unwitting host, and others may be harmful. Types of interaction among these products that tend to form insoluble precipitates or complexes will decrease their absorption. Diet-conscious people should be aware of these interactions because they may lead to shortages of essential nutrients, and alterations in the diet or supplements may be necessary.

In a sense, adequate nutrition is as much dependent on how much of a nutrient gets absorbed as it is on how much is present in the food eaten. A person may be eating an adequate diet but may still exhibit deficiency symptoms due to poor absorption of one or more nutrients. The RDAs take these reactions into account for all nutrients on which there are data. The RDA value assumes that the percentage of absorption of a particular nutrient is similar to that found with an experimental diet. Efficiency of absorption is calculated as the ratio of the amount of a nutrient that is absorbed to that present in the diet. Absorption from average diets varies from a low of 10% for iron to over 90% for water-soluble vitamins. To make the points definite, I'll discuss interactions that affect the absorption of calcium and iron in some detail.

Calcium absorption is affected by many factors. Some increase it; some decrease it. The RDA figure of 800 mg for adults assumes an average absorption in the range of 30% to 50% of dietary calcium. Calcium absorption is facilitated by vitamin D (this action is one of this vitamin's chief functions), proteins, lactose (the major sugar of milk), and a calcium/phosphorus ratio near 1:1. Calcium absorption is decreased by the formation of insoluble salts such as with long-chain fatty acids, oxalates, and phytates, and by excess dietary phosphate. These chemicals are found in fatty foods, rhubarb, spinach, and cereal grains, respectively.

The American RDA for calcium is much higher than that for most of the rest of the world. The reason is not that Americans are less efficient in absorbing calcium than other peoples, but is due to two components of the American diet. It is unusually high in phosphate and in protein.

The attempt to measure calcium retention in humans under multivariable dietary conditions of calcium intake, phosphate intake, protein intake, type of protein, time of ingestion of the three nutrients, and hormonal levels as a function of age and gender is obviously a very complicated one. The variety of results and lack of confirmation of hypotheses could be predicted from Barry Commoner's phrase, "Everything affects everything else." The specific situation is stated succinctly by Schuette and Linkswiler (1984):

Because of the interrelationships among calcium, phosphorus, and protein it is difficult, if not impossible, to select a single calcium requirement for any age group. It is clear that an increase in protein intake affects [increases] urinary calcium and calcium retention opposite to the effect of an increase in phosphate intake. (p. 408)

The authors hypothesize further that the low protein intake of people in developing countries may explain why they can remain in calcium balance with calcium intakes in the range 400-500 mg/day.

An impasse such as this one on an important topic is not neglected but stimulates more research. Up to this point I have written of protein intake as a factor in calcium excretion. But all proteins are not alike in composition. Some contain more sulfur-containing amino acids than others, and the sulfur is oxidized to sulfuric acid in the body, which is excreted and makes the urine more acidic. This situation, in turn, lowers the reabsorption of calcium in the kidney and thus more is excreted in the urine. I should add that this hypothesis is offering new insights into the relationships of calcium absorption, protein composition, and calcium excretion ("High Protein Diets," 1981).

I mention these details because they reveal how puzzling problems are approached in research. In addition, the results will probably have some bearing on dietary advice (i.e., aid) to Third World countries. It suggests that perhaps they should not follow our *luxus* consumption of animal protein with its attendant complications on requirements of other nutrients.

Milk and milk products are excellent sources of calcium and phosphate, and they also have desirable calcium/phosphorus ratios of close to 1/1.

For people who do not consume the equivalent of two 8-oz glasses of milk per day, obtaining the RDA for calcium is difficult.

Because milk and milk products are our major source of calcium, I suggest that those people who have cut down or cut out these items from their diets should return to milk. For those who are concerned about the saturated fat content of milk, I suggest 1%-fat milk, skim milk, buttermilk, nonfat dried milk, or very low-fat cheeses or yogurt as excellent sources of calcium that are low in fat. Other alternatives are to seek out on a regular basis such foods as sardines or other small fish with bones, tofu, or broccoli. Many elderly women are using calcium supplements to assure themselves of an adequate intake, which should be in the range of 1,000-1,200 mg per day. Some years ago, bone meal and dolomite, both natural sources of calcium, were found to be contaminated with toxic quantities of lead. It is dangerous to use these products unless their lead content has been analyzed and found to be absent or below toxic levels.

Osteoporosis: A Multifactorial Disease

Osteoporosis is a disease of weakened bones. The weakening occurs in the inorganic portion, which is composed of calcium phosphate and contributes about two-thirds the mass of bone. The other major component is the protein collagen. Both of these components turn over; that is, they are continuously formed and dissolved throughout life. Calcium has many essential functions in the body in addition to its role in bone structure. Bone, however, acts as a calcium reservoir, and if people chronically consume too little calcium, it is withdrawn from bone and the bones become weaker. These relationships explain why osteoporosis is often considered a calcium-deficiency disease. However, osteoporosis is far more complicated than a simple nutritional deficiency.

Why do a higher proportion of elderly women develop osteoporosis than elderly men? There are two reasons: A common one affects both sexes and the other affects mostly women. The common reason is based on the turnover mentioned above. With age, resorption (dissolution) of bone tends to exceed formation, and weakening occurs. The smaller bones of women weaken faster than the larger bones of men. When the small, weakened bones can no longer support the weight of the body, they break. This chain of events furnishes a very good reason for elderly people to keep their weight in line. Many overweight osteoporosis patients with broken hips or vertebrae are confined to wheel chairs for the last years of their lives.

A variety of drugs, including alcohol, can contribute to an early onset of osteoporosis. The use of aluminum-containing antacids, which can be bought over the counter and used in unregulated dosages for long periods, has been found to result in extensive bone demineralization and ultimate osteoporosis (Spencer, Kramer, Norris, & Osis, 1982).

Dietary Factors in the Prevention of Osteoporosis

From this analysis, we can understand the necessity of consuming adequate amounts of calcium throughout life and why women are being encouraged to ingest 50% more than the RDA shortly before and after menopause. This recommendation, however, does not have a firm experimental basis. Numerous studies in normal Western populations show no significant correlation between calcium intake and postmenopausal bone density (Gordon & Vaughn, 1986).

Phosphate and vitamin D are other dietary factors that are known to affect calcium absorption in the intestinal tract. Vitamin D deficiency is quite rare in developed countries, and while phosphate imbalance has been shown to decrease calcium absorption in experimental studies, this condition does not appear significant in the free-living population (Spencer, Kramer, & Osis, 1982). In summary, diet does not appear as either the major preventive factor or the cure for osteoporosis.

The role of fluoride in strengthening bones as well as teeth has been known for many years. Madans, Kleinman, and Coroni-Huntley (1983) have carried out an interesting ecological study of the correlation between the fluoride concentration of water supplies and the incidence of osteoporosis in people over age 45. Although the data are inconclusive, they found some indications that concentrations of fluoride higher than 0.7 ppm in the water might have a protective effect for women. This study illustrates the point made in chapter 3 that even inconclusive correlations of this type can suggest large-scale studies to test the hypothesis that fluoride may help prevent osteoporosis.

Physical activity is acknowledged as a major factor in the prevention of osteoporosis for both sexes. This conclusion is supported by the well-known loss of bone on immobilization of a limb either in a cast or in space. Special exercises are now being developed for astronauts. Ordinary people can obtain sufficient exercise to help prevent osteoporosis by engaging in the graded walking program that is presented in Table 7.7.

Estrogen in the Prevention of Osteoporosis

The sex-specific reason is based on one of the actions of the female sex hormone, estradiol. The hormone aids calcium absorption in the intestine, which in turn helps keep the bone resorption/formation ratio in balance. The decrease in the rate of the secretion of estradiol after menopause allows resorption to exceed formation, and women's bones also grow weaker for this reason.

An encouraging therapy for postmenopausal osteoporosis has been described in a small-scale study by Gordon and Genant (1985). These researchers found that a calcium intake of 1,500 mg per day did not prevent bone loss in women subjects, but the combination of this amount of calcium with 0.3 mg of estrogen actually increased vertebral bone mass. This amount of estrogen is too small to affect the endometrium. Consequently, side effects are less likely than with larger doses.

Anemia

Anemia is the name of a condition in which the blood hemoglobin is low. Other symptoms are a chronic tired feeling, lack of energy, and chronic fatigue. There are many other causes for anemia than a deficiency of dietary iron. As I have said before, to leap from a symptom to a diagnosis of a disease is not only unjustified, but also foolhardy and dangerous. Thus, to take a commercial iron preparation with or without added vitamins for "that tired feeling" is dangerous and foolhardy. Feeling tired is a symptom of a disease or a condition that is seldom related to iron intake. Popping an extra pill or so a day, besides being ineffective, will delay finding the actual cause. In medicine, delays in accurate diagnosis often have serious consequences.

As evidenced by the prevalence of anemia, especially among women, iron is also deficient in American diets. The reason for this sex difference in iron need stems from the fact that males have no mechanism for excreting it. Outside of accidents in which blood is lost or by donating blood, men add to their store of iron over the course of their entire lives. This capacity for storage leads to few complications unless iron ingestion is especially high. Alcohol increases iron absorption, and because wine also contains iron, chronic, heavy consumption of wine may result in *hemochromotosis*—an excess of stored iron in the liver. A more localized and exotic form of this disease occurs among the Bantu of South Africa who consume large amounts of Kafir beer. This beer has been traditionally brewed in iron pots, and in the process, the liquid dissolves considerable iron from the pot. Long-term ingestion of Kafir beer results in a serious form of iron-storage disease.

Between the ages of approximately 15 and 45, women lose iron by menstruation. Although the average male loses 1 mg of iron per day via skin, nails, and hair, the average woman loses 1.5 mg. Consequently, a fertile woman's requirement is 50% higher than a man's. Numerous surveys have reported a higher incidence of anemia among women than among men.

Some interesting and significant differences occur in the efficiency of iron absorption, depending on its chemical form in different foods. Iron occurs in plant sources in the ionic form, Fe^{++} (ferrous), or Fe^{+++} (ferric). In these forms, efficiency of absorption is only about 10%. In animal sources, however, considerable iron occurs associated with heme in the proteins hemoglobin and myoglobin, and absorption jumps to 35%. Consequently, women who are able to secure sufficient meat run less risk of iron-deficiency anemia than those restricted to a vegetable diet.

Of the two forms of ionic iron, the Fe^{++} is absorbed more efficiently than the Fe^{+++}. Ascorbic acid (vitamin C) is able to reduce Fe^{+++} to Fe^{++}. Cook and Monsen (1977) showed that including ascorbic acid in a meal doubled iron absorption from vegetable sources. This observation suggests a way of increasing iron absorption without increasing the iron content of the diet. It suggests that women eat an orange or another good source of vitamin C with their meals.

The Effects of Dietary Fiber on Absorption of Nutrients

I have listed dietary fiber as an essential nonnutrient, and a good case can be made for this conclusion even though the effects of a completely fiber-free diet have not been studied in humans. The ingestion of large amounts of bran (16 g per day for 3 weeks) resulted in higher excretion in the stool of sodium, potassium, and magnesium than control subjects (Eastwood & Mowbray, 1976). People who consume a high-fiber diet— for example, vegans and those who supplement with bran—need to eat diets especially high in potassium and magnesium. A list of high-fiber foods and a discussion of whether fiber should be used as a supplement are included in chapter 6.

I have described these examples of interactions of nutrients to give you some idea of the complex interrelationships among energy sources and nutrients once they enter the digestive tract. As I mentioned, the RDAs are designed to furnish sufficient absorbable amounts of the nutrients in average diets so that most people need not be concerned with detailed calculations on the nutrient composition of their diets. The objective of eating a nutritionally adequate diet can be achieved by consuming a varied assortment of foods selected from the four food groups.

The RDAs Do Not Distinguish Between Energy Sources

The RDA for energy is based on age, sex, and physical activity. The sources of energy are protein, carbohydrates, and fats. Does the proportion of the three foodstuffs in the diet matter? Probably. The RDA book (National Research Council, 1980) (see Table 5A.1) lists recommended energy intakes but says nothing about the sources of the calories. Many nutritionists and public health specialists believe that the fat/carbohydrate ratio influences tendencies toward a number of diseases as cancer and heart disease. These topics are discussed in chapters 8 and 10. The effects of a high-animal protein diet have been discussed above. This omission can be considered a serious oversight in a publication "designed for the maintenance of good nutrition of practically all healthy people in the U.S.A." (p. 1).

The RDA Table Should Footnote the Importance and Sources of the Essential Amino Acids and of Vitamin B_{12}

The RDA table lists the protein allowances for various age groups, for the two sexes, and for pregnant and lactating women. The topics of amino acid requirements and nutritive value of proteins are briefly but adequately discussed (National Research Council, 1980, pp. 42-46), but some vegetarians may not be aware of the essential amino acid deficiencies of most vegetable proteins and of the lack of vitamin B_{12} in vegan diets. Footnotes would correct these oversights.

The Bases for Setting the Mean Requirements Are Not Specified

The RDA book does not explicitly state the value of the mean requirement for a nutrient or the basis on which it was selected. It has been stated by Harper (1974) as the amount at which no deficiency symptoms appear. This vagueness allowed Pauling (1974) to write with regard to vitamin C, "The principal consideration in setting these values has been the prevention of scurvy" (p. 4445). Because the amount of vitamin C that will prevent scurvy has been known for many years to be approximately 10 mg per day, Pauling's statement reflects his strong bias in favor of larger amounts. At the time of his article the RDA for vitamin C was set at 45 mg/day.

Pauling (1974) continues, "It is, I believe, misleading to call these intakes the Recommended Dietary Allowances, permitting them to be interpreted, as is often done, as the intakes that lead to the best of health. . . . I suggest that instead they be called the Minimum Dietary Allowances" (p. 4445). In this remark, Pauling's enthusiasm for larger amounts of vitamin C takes him well beyond the evidence that was available in 1974 to support such a position. The RDA for vitamin C has received the most publicity of any vitamin in recent years, not because its basis is more suspect than the others, but because of Pauling's writings on the subject.

Pauling's criticism of the RDA for vitamin C brings out the dilemma of the Food and Nutrition Board. On the one hand, they are attempting to recommend an amount that will maintain health for which there are no long-term data; and on the other hand, they need to recognize the economic constraints of their recommendations. If all the governmental and commercial kitchens in the country, as well as school lunch programs, were to increase the vitamin C content of their meals by a factor of 10 to 450 mg/day, the extra expenses would be considerable. The Food and Nutrition Board would be subject to justified criticism if they recommended such an increase without considerably more evidence than is now available. In the meantime, the vitamin C enthusiasts, and there are millions of them in the U.S., are at liberty to consume as much extra vitamin C as their pocketbooks and opinions will allow.

In *Nutritional Requirements of Man*, Irwin (1960) has presented the world data on requirements of three vitamins, four elements, and protein and amino acids. The mass of data included in this book highlights the problems of the Food and Nutrition Board. It is perhaps surprising and certainly disappointing that such a small percentage of the research bears on the stated objective of the RDA table: "the maintenance of good nutrition of practically all healthy people in the U.S." This objective, although laudable, is well beyond present or foreseeable evidence to support it. In concluding this discussion of the RDA table, I consider it, at best, a guideline or "guesstimate" of suggested human intakes of nutrients. Even though it contains deficiencies, it is still the best guideline available for Americans. Additional guidelines have been published by the Canadian Government (Department of National Health and Welfare, 1977) and the World Health Organization (WHO) as cited by Pike and Brown (1984, pp. 824 & 826, respectively). These guidelines differ only slightly from the 1980 RDA values.

Summary

One of the objectives of this chapter has been to discuss the three sources of calories and how their variations in the diet can affect health. The energy content per gram of proteins, carbohydrates, and fats is 4, 4, and 9 kcal, respectively. Due to the high energy content of fats, it is especially important to monitor their intake in controlling weight. Ethyl alcohol also provides energy, 7 kcal per gram, even though it is not a food, but a drug. The roles of the dietary essential amino acids and fatty acids have been mentioned. I have also explained the importance and use in diet planning of protein complementarity.

The classes and number of the noncaloric essential nutrients are vitamins (13), elements (21), fiber (6) (not yet proved essential), and aqueous liquids (1). I have explained the relation between the human requirement for each of these and the recommended dietary allowance (RDA). The requirement is very difficult to measure.

The RDAs avoid the difficulty of measuring individual requirements for a large number of people by employing a statistical approach to calculate a daily intake that is sufficient to maintain health but avoid excess. I have concluded the chapter with a discussion of some limitations of the RDAs.

Table 5A.1   Examples of Daily Energy Expenditures of Mature Women and Men in Light Occupations

Activity Category[a]	Time (hr)	Man, 70 kg Rate (kcal/ min)	Man, 70 kg Total (kcal)	Woman, 58 kg Rate (kcal/ min)	Woman, 58 kg Total (kcal)
Sleeping, reclining	8	1.0–1.2	540	0.9–1.1	440
Very light Sitting and standing activities, painting trades, auto and truck driving, doing laboratory work, typing, playing musical instruments, sewing, ironing	12	up to 2.5	1,300	up to 2.0	900
Light Walking on level at 2.5–3 mph, tailoring, pressing, doing garage work, working in the restaurant or electrical trades, doing carpentry work, working in a cannery, washing clothes, shopping with light load, golfing, sailing, playing table tennis or volleyball	3	2.5–4.9	600	2.0–3.9	450
Moderate Walking 3.5–4 mph, plastering, weeding and hoeing, loading and stacking bales, scrubbing floors, shopping with heavy load, cycling, skiing, playing tennis, dancing	1	5.0–7.4	300	4.0–5.9	240
Heavy Walking with load uphill, tree felling, working with a pick and shovel, swimming, climbing, playing football or basketball	0	7.5–12.0		6.0–10.0	
Total average intake	24		2,740		2,030

[a]*Recommended Dietary Allowances* (National Academy of Sciences, 1980). *Note.* Adapted from *Energy, Work and Leisure* by J.V.G.A. Durnin and R. Passmore, 1967, London: Heinemann Educational Books. Copyright 1967 by Heinemann Educational Books. Adapted by permission.

Table 5A.2 Recommended Daily Dietary Allowances[a] Designed for the Maintenance of Good Nutrition of Practically All Healthy People in the U.S.A.

	Age (years)	Weight (kg)	Weight (lb)	Height (cm)	Height (in.)	Protein (g)	Vitamin A (μg RE)[b]	Fat-Soluble Vitamins Vitamin D (μg)[c]	Vitamin E (mg α-TE)[d]
Infants	0.0-0.5	6	13	60	24	kg × 2.2	420	10	3
	0.5-1.0	9	20	71	28	kg × 1.0	400	10	4
Children	1-3	13	29	90	35	23	400	10	5
	4-6	20	44	112	44	30	500	10	6
	7-10	28	62	132	52	34	700	10	7
Males	11-14	45	99	157	62	45	1,000	10	8
	15-18	66	145	176	69	56	1,000	10	10
	19-22	70	154	177	70	56	1,000	7.5	10
	23-50	70	154	178	70	56	1,000	5	10
	51+	70	154	178	70	56	1,000	5	10

Females							
11-14	46	101	157	62	46	800	10	8
15-18	55	120	163	64	46	800	10	8
19-22	55	120	163	64	44	800	7.5	8
23-50	55	120	163	64	44	800	5	8
51+	55	120	163	64	44	800	5	8
Pregnant					+30	+200	+5	+2
Lactating					+20	+400	+5	+3

Note. Adapted from *Recommended Dietary Allowances* by the National Research Council, 1980, Washington, DC: National Academy of Sciences. Copyright 1980 by National Academy of Sciences. Adapted by permission.

[a] The allowances are intended to provide for individual variations among most normal persons as they live in the United States under usual environmental stresses. Diets should be based on a variety of common foods in order to provide other nutrients for which human requirements have been less well defined. See text for detailed discussion of allowances and of nutrients not tabulated. See Table A5.1 for suggested average energy intakes.

[b] Retinol equivalents. 1 retinol equivalent = 1 μg retinol or 6 μg β carotene. See text for calculation of vitamin A activity of diets as retinol equivalents.

[c] As cholecalciferol. 10 μg = 400 IU of vitamin D.

[d] α-Tocopherol equivalents. 1 mg d-α tocopherol = 1 α-TE. See text for variation in allowances and calculation of vitamin E activity of the diet as α-tocopherol equivalents.

(Cont.)

Table 5A.2 (Cont.)

Age (years)	Weight (kg)	Weight (lb)	Height (cm)	Height (in.)		Vitamin C (mg)	Thiamin (mg)	Riboflavin (mg)	Niacin (mg NE)[e]	Vitamin B6 (mg)	Folacin[f] (µg)	Vitamin B12[g] (µg)
					Water-Soluble Vitamins							
Infants												
0.0-0.5	6	13	60	24		35	0.3	0.4	6	0.3	30	0.5[g]
0.5-1.0	9	20	71	28		35	0.5	0.6	8	0.6	45	1.5
Children												
1-3	13	29	90	35		45	0.7	0.8	9	0.9	100	2.0
4-6	20	44	112	44		45	0.9	1.0	11	1.3	200	2.5
7-10	28	62	132	52		45	1.2	1.4	16	1.6	300	3.0
Males												
11-14	45	99	157	62		50	1.4	1.6	18	1.8	400	3.0
15-18	66	145	176	69		60	1.4	1.7	18	2.0	400	3.0
19-22	70	154	177	70		60	1.5	1.7	19	2.2	400	3.0
23-50	70	154	178	70		60	1.4	1.6	18	2.2	400	3.0
51+	70	154	178	70		60	1.2	1.4	16	2.2	400	3.0

Females										
11-14	46	101	157	62	50	1.1	1.3	15	1.8	400	3.0
15-18	55	120	163	64	60	1.1	1.3	14	2.0	400	3.0
19-22	55	120	163	64	60	1.1	1.3	14	2.0	400	3.0
23-50	55	120	163	64	60	1.0	1.2	13	2.0	400	3.0
51+	55	120	163	64	60	1.0	1.2	13	1.0	400	3.0
Pregnant					+20	+0.4	+0.3	+2	+0.6	+400	+1.0
Lactating					+40	+0.5	+0.5	+5	+1.5	+100	+1.0

[e]1 NE (niacin equivalent) is equal to 1 mg of niacin or 60 mg of dietary tryptophan.

[f]The folacin allowances refer to dietary sources as determined by Lactobacillus casei assay after treatment with enzymes (conjugases) to make polyglutamyl forms of the vitamin available to the test organism.

[g]The recommended dietary allowance for vitamin B$_{12}$ in infants is based on average concentration of the vitamin in human milk. The allowances after weaning are based on energy intake (as recommended by the American Academy of Pediatrics) and consideration of other factors, such as intestinal absorption; see text.

(Cont.)

Table 5A.2 (Cont.)

	Age (years)	Weight (kg)	Weight (lb)	Height (cm)	Height (in.)	Calcium (mg)	Phosphorus (mg)	Minerals Magnesium (mg)	Iron (mg)	Zinc (mg)	Iodine (µg)
Infants	0.0-0.5	6	13	60	24	360	240	50	10	3	40
	0.5-1.0	9	20	71	28	540	360	70	15	5	50
Children	1-3	13	29	90	35	800	800	150	15	10	70
	4-6	20	44	112	44	800	800	200	10	10	90
	7-10	28	62	132	52	800	800	250	10	10	120
Males	11-14	45	99	157	62	1,200	1,200	350	18	15	250
	15-18	66	145	176	69	1,200	1,200	400	18	15	150
	19-22	70	154	177	70	800	800	350	10	15	150
	23-50	70	154	178	70	800	800	350	10	15	150
	51+	70	154	178	70	800	800	350	10	15	150

Females										
11-14	46	101	157	62	1,200	1,200	300	18	15	150
15-18	55	120	163	64	1,200	1,200	300	18	15	150
19-22	55	120	163	64	800	800	300	18	15	150
12-50	55	120	163	64	800	800	300	18	15	150
51+	55	120	163	64	800	800	300	10	15	150
Pregnant					+400	+400	+150	[h]	+5	+25
Lactating					+400	+400	+150	[h]	+10	+50

[h]The increased requirement during pregnancy cannot be met by the iron content of habitual American diets nor by the existing iron stores of many women; therefore the use of 30-60 mg of supplemental iron is recommended. Iron needs during lactation are not substantially different from those of nonpregnant women, but continued supplementation of the mother for 2-3 months after parturition is advisable in order to replenish stores depleted by pregnancy.

Table 5A.3   Sources and Functions of Fiber Types

Celluloses
  Natural sources
  Soy bran (soybean hulls)
  Fruit juice sacs (e.g., from citrus
    fruits)
  Legumes (e.g., beans, peas)
  Carrots
  Artificial sources
  Solkafloc^R powdered cellulose,
    from wood, highly purified and
    standardized
  Avicel^R microcrystalline cellulose,
    from wood highly purified and
    standardized
  Methylcellulose, a polymer derived
    from cellulose by alkali and
    other treatments
  Carboxymethylcellulose (CMC), a
    synthetic, water-soluble polymer
    derived from cellulose
  Functions
  Aids regularity. Adds bulk.

Hemicelluloses
  Natural sources
  Corn hulls (maize)
  Barley hulls
  Oat hulls
  Corn bran
  Wheat bran
  Brewer's grains, residues from
    malting, mainly barley; mixture
    usually contains rice and some-
    times other grains as well
  Soy fiber concentrate, residue after
    soy protein has been extracted
  Artificial sources
  Masonex^R extract of wood fibers
    by acid hydrolysis
  Xylan, the polysaccharide polymer
    of D-xylose units extracted from
    various plant sources
  Functions
  Adds bulk

Pectins
  Citrus pulp
  Apple pulp
  Cabbages and other brassicas
  Sugarbeet pulp
  Legumes (e.g., peas and beans)
  Alfalfa leaves
  Sunflower heads
  Functions
  Reduces blood cholesterol

Cutins
  Apple peels
  Tomato peels
  Berries (seeds of)
  Peanut skins
  Almond skins
  Onion skins
  Functions
  Slows gastric emptying
  Binds bile acids

Gums
  Guar gum, from ground endo-
    sperms of the legume, *Cyamopsi
    tetragonolobus* (L) Taub
  Gum arabic, from locust beans
  Oat gums, from oat flour
  Agar, a phyllocolloid, polysaccha-
    ride mixture of agarose and
    agaropectin derived from red
    algae
  Gum tragacanth, a mixture of
    polysaccharides of galactose,
    fructose, xylose, arabinose, and
    glucuronic acid from *Astragalus
    spp.*, legumes
  Alginate, from kelp (seaweed),
    mixtures of hydrophilic colloids
  Xanthan, a polysaccharide from
    prickly ash trees
  Psyllium or fleaseed, from plan-
    tains (*Plantago spp.*)
  Glycan, from yeast
  Functions
  Slows gastric emptying
  Binds bile acids

Table 5A.3 (Cont.)

Lignins
  Wheat straw
  Cottonseed hulls
  Alfalfa stems
  Bagasse, the sugarcane residue
    after sugar has been extracted
  Tannins, e.g., $C_{75}H_{52}O_{48}$ or penta-
    (m-digalloyo)-glucose; gallic acid
    derivatives found widely in
    plants
Functions
  Reduces blood cholesterol
  Binds bile acids and metals

Note. Adapted from "Fiber—Standardized Sources" by L. Crosby, 1980, *Nutrition and Cancer, 1*, pp. 15-26. Copyright 1980 by *Nutrition and Cancer.* Adapted by permission.

Table 5A.4   Foods to Provide 25 g Dietary Fiber per Day

Fruit group: About 2 g fiber per serving; use four or more per day

Apple, 140 g; 5 oz   Peach, 87 g; 3 oz
Banana, 56 g; 2 oz   Pear, 82 g; 3 oz
Strawberries (raw), 100 g; 4 oz   Plums, 133 g; 5 oz
Cherries (20 large), 130 g; 5 oz

Bread and cereal group: About 1 g fiber per serving; use four or more per day

Whole wheat bread (1 slice), 14 g;   All Bran (1 tbsp), 3 1/2 g; 1/8 oz
  1/2 oz   Corn Flakes (2 cups), 56 g; 2 oz
Shredded Wheat (1/2 biscuit), 24 g;   Oatmeal (cooked, 1/2 cup), 110 g;
  1/2 oz   4 oz
Grape-Nuts (1/4 cup), 28 g; 1 oz   Puffed Wheat (2 cups), 28 g; 1 oz
White bread, 42 g; 1 1/2 oz

Vegetable group: About 2 g fiber per serving; use four or more per day (these values are for cooked portions)

Broccoli (1/2 stalk), 50 g; 2 oz   Green beans (1/2 cup), 60 g; 2 oz
Brussels sprouts, 70 g; 2.5 oz   Potato, 58 g; 2 oz
Carrots (1/3 cup), 54 g; 2 oz   Tomato (raw, 1 medium), 142 g; 5 oz
Corn on the cob, 42 g; 1 1/2 oz   Baked beans (canned, 1 tbsp), 27g;
Lettuce (raw, 2 cups), 133 g; 5 oz   1 oz

Miscellaneous group: About 1 g fiber per serving

Peanut butter (1 tbsp), 25 g; 1 oz   Pickle (1 large), 66 g; 2.5 oz
Peanuts, 14 g; 0.5 oz   Strawberry jam (5 tbsp), 85 g; 3 oz

Note.   Adapted from "A Guide to Calculating Intakes of Dietary Fiber" by D.A.T. Southgate, B. Bailey, E. Collinson, and A. Walker, 1976, *Journal of Human Nutrition*, *30*, pp. 309-311. Copyright 1976 by *Journal of Human Nutrition*. Also adapted from *Food Values of Portions Commonly Used* (pp. 226-227) by J.A.T. Pennington and H.N. Church, 1985, Philadelphia: J.B. Lippincott. Copyright 1985 by J.B. Lippincott. Adapted by permission.

Table 5A.5   Estimations of Nutrient Adult RDAs[1]

Nutrient	Tentative RDA
Vitamins	Vitamin K 70-140 µg Biotin 100-200 µg Pantothenic acid 4-7 µg
Microelements	Copper (Cu) 2.0-3.0 mg Manganese (Mn) 2.5-5.0 mg Fluoride (F) 1.5-4.0 mg Chromium (Cr) 0.05-0.2 mg Selenium (Se) 0.05-0.2 mg Molybdenum (Mg) 0.15-0.5 mg
Macroelements	Sodium (Na) 1.1-3.3 g Potassium (K) 1.9-5.6 g Chloride (Cl) 1.7-5.1 g

[1]Adapted from *Recommended Dietary Allowances* (p. 178) by the National Research Council, 1980, Washington, DC: National Academy of Sciences. Copyright 1980 by National Academy of Sciences. Adapted by permission.

Chapter

6

Food and Wellness

From a conversation between Dr. David
Livingston and the Bayeiye Chief Palani:
"I gave him a piece of bread and
preserved apricots; and as he seemed to
relish it, asked if he had food equal to that
in his country. 'Ah,' he said, 'Did you
ever taste white ants?' "

Source unknown, possibly apocryphal

This chapter will help you

- eat a nutritious, delicious diet by applying the idea of nutrient density to the foods you commonly eat;
- distinguish between nutritious foods and junk foods objectively;
- understand the role of food additives;
- realize that any and all nutrients or other substances found in foods can be toxic if ingested in excess amounts (it follows that dietary supplements should be monitored with care); and
- work out a procedure for conducting nutrition experiments on yourself that will be useful to you in obtaining a healthy diet.

The *adequacy* of food quantity can be judged by the number of calories per day it furnishes. Food *quality*, however, is not so readily defined. In general, food quality in previous societies and in industrialized countries up through the 1940s has meant a sufficiency of appetizing, well-prepared foods in accordance with the traditions of the culture.

In some societies food quality is related to scarcity, as with caviar, or to time required in preparation, as with sauces. In America, quality is often related to a swell taste, as with Mom's apple pie or home-baked bread. A sweet taste is prized in most cultures and humans are said to possess a sweet tooth. In my experience, fatty foods are also frequently prized. Consider the popularity of whipped cream, high-fat cheeses, and dips. Most desserts and candies contain both sugar and fats.

According to Tannahill (1973), Middle East peoples for centuries have prized meat fried in the fat (alya) of the fat-tailed sheep. Figure 6.1 gives some idea of the value these people place on the tails of these animals.

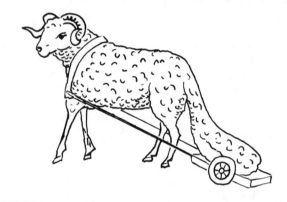

Figure 6.1   The main asset of the fat-tailed sheep had to be protected from wear and tear. *Note.*   From *Food in History* (p. 176) by R. Tannahill, 1973, London: Eyre and Spottiswoode. Copyright 1973 by Eyre and Spottiswoode. Reprinted by permission.

Recent research has established that the appetite of rats for vegetarian foods is similar to that of humans. A rat provided with a standard chow diet *ad libitum* will average between 10% and 20% body fat. If the fat content of the diet is raised 30% to 60% above the usual chow content of 2% to 6%, rats will become obese. Even though rats eat less high-fat food than low-fat food, they do not compensate for the extra calories per gram of the fat, and consequently gain weight faster (Carlisle & Stellar, 1969; Hamilton, 1964). Mice and dogs also become obese when provided with high-fat diets. Both of these research groups found that rats, when given a choice between foods differing in fat content, strongly preferred the foods containing the most fat. We now have a reason for baiting mouse and rat traps with cheese.

When victuals are scarce, food quality is often considered identical to food quantity. On the other hand, Walter Kerr (1962) quoted Eric Gill as saying that it is sinful to eat inferior ice cream (p. 277). I interpret this remark to mean that if one is treating oneself or one's family to a luxury food, primarily for its taste, other factors should not count. There are times when there is no substitute for quality.

In recent years the definition of food quality has been broadened to include the content of essential nutrients. These substances were discussed in the previous chapter, and I won't repeat their names or functions here. A nutrient-dense food is defined as containing a high content of essential nutrients per calorie as found in milk, whole wheat bread, and broccoli. Examples of low-nutrient-density foods are soft drinks containing sugar, doughnuts, and potato chips.

Foods to which large amounts of sugar or fat are commonly added during preparation or processing may receive poor marks when graded by nutritive quality standards, even though these foods may be delicious to eat. Michael Jacobson (1975), in *Nutrition Scoreboard*, has worked out a grading system for foods in which points are given for nutrient content and points are subtracted based on sugar, fat, or white flour content. This viewpoint illustrates an extreme definition of food quality. The word *taste* does not appear in the index.

This dual definition of food quality neatly illustrates the difference between scientific definitions and classical ones based on perceptions. The classical definition is overtly sensual and qualitative. The scientific one explicitly emphasizes the quantitative idea of nutrient density—and that is all. These two different approaches are not necessarily incompatible. Attractive, delicious dishes and meals can be prepared that are also nutritious. The first chapter of that widely used cookbook, *The Joy of Cooking* (Rombauer & Becker, 1974), presents a clear summary of nutrition information. Perhaps an even more impressive example is found in *Cuisine Minceur* (Guerard, 1976). In this book, the famous French chef Michael Guerard describes a cuisine for slimness and demonstrates that taste need not be sacrificed on the guillotine of calories.

The idea of nutrient density allows a simple statement of the main objectives of satisfactory, healthy nutrition. It is to eat appetizing foods under pleasant conditions, which furnish sufficient, but not excess, energy and supply the essential noncalorific nutrients in adequate amounts. As with some other natural functions, civilized peoples seem to have made a very complicated business out of fulfilling their gustatory desires. One of the main objectives of this chapter is to provide readers with sufficient information on foods and nutrition so that they can make informed choices when they go to market or order a meal. Knowledge of nutrient density and how it is estimated from information on labels is crucial to this objective.

Nutrient Density

Nutritive wellness is based on two factors. The first is that of essential nutrient adequacy. As mentioned previously, each person must ingest sufficient amounts of each of the 50 essential nutrients on a regular basis. Illness and even death may result if a chronic deficiency is not corrected. The second factor is that of calories. Each person requires a certain number of calories in order to live and engage in activities. If excess calories are ingested over an extended period of time, overweight/obesity will result. This condition is not considered to be healthy.

The term *nutrient density* relates nutrient content to calories in a quantitative manner. Theoretically, each and every food has approximately 50 nutrient densities—one for each nutrient—per serving or per unit weight of food or per 1,000 kcal. One common definition of nutrient density is obtained from the equation:

$$\text{Nutrient density} = \frac{\% \text{ of RDA of an essential nutrient in a food (wt., serving or kcal)}}{\% \text{ of RDA for kcal in a food for a person (wt., serving or kcal)}}$$

Because the RDAs for essential nutrients vary with a person's age, sex, and condition (i.e., pregnancy or lactation), and for calories depending on physical activity, these must be specified for the calculation to be useful. The RDA book suggests the following estimated caloric intake for average U.S. adults:

Reference man: Energy expenditure = 2,700 kcal/day
Reference woman: Energy expenditure = 2,000 kcal/day

Fortunately, it is not necessary to remember a list of RDAs when you're shopping. Present-day labels furnish considerable information, as shown in Table 6.1, which reproduces the label on Campbell's Old Fashioned Beans. All you need remember is your RDA energy expenditure—say 2,700 kcal/day. One serving of these beans contains 270 kcal, or 10% of your daily needs. In the list of essential nutrients, protein, vitamin C, calcium, and iron are present in concentrations of 10% or more of the RDAs. Thus this food contains four essential nutrients with a nutrient density of 1.0 or more.

This calculation of nutrient density has been termed the *index of nutritional quality* (INQ) by Hansen (1973). If the ratio is 1 or above, the food is considered nutritious for that nutrient. For example, 3.2 oz of frozen, diluted orange juice contains 45 kcal and 45 mg of vitamin C. For an adult female whose recommended energy intake is 2,000 kcal, 45 kcal represents $45/2,000 = 0.0225$ (2.25%) of the daily energy. For vitamin C, 45 mg represents $45/60 = 0.75$ (75%) of the RDA. Dividing the percentage of the RDA for vitamin C furnished by this volume of orange juice by the percentage of the daily energy it furnishes, we obtain the following: nutrient density = 75%/2.25% = 33.3. This high number tells us that

Table 6.1   Campbell's Old Fashioned Beans

Nutrition information per serving

Serving size . . . . .8 oz (227 g)
Servings per container 2
Calories 270
Protein (grams) 11
Total carbohydrates (grams) 49
   Simple sugar (grams) 20
   Complex carbohydrates (grams) 29
Fat (grams) 3
Sodium . . . . .1,100 mg/serving

Percentage of U.S. Recommended Daily Allowances (U.S. RDA)

Protein 15		Riboflavin 2
Vitamin A . . . .*		Niacin 2
Vitamin C 10		Calcium 10
Thiamin . . . .*		Iron 20

*Contains less than 2% of the U.S. RDA of these nutrients.

Ingredients: Prepared pea beans, water, tomatoes, invert sugar, pork fat, brown sugar, molasses, salt, corn syrup, sugar, dehydrated onions, spice, apple concentrate, and natural flavoring.

Note: The fat content can be calculated in your head.

3 g × 9 kcal/g = 27 total kcal from fat
27 kcal/270 total kcal = 10% fat as calories

Also note the high sodium content (1,100 mg/serving).

orange juice is an excellent source of vitamin C. It is nutrient dense with regard to this vitamin.

Let's calculate the nutrient density of orange juice with regard to another nutrient—protein. The same volume of orange juice mentioned above contains 0.7 g of protein, which is 0.7/44 = 0.015 (1.5% of the protein RDA for a 55-kg woman). Again, dividing the nutrient RDA percentage by that of the daily energy percentage for the reference female, we find the following: nutrient density = 1.5%/2.25% = 0.66, a number less than one. This number tells us that orange juice is a poor source of protein compared to milk, which has a nutrient density for protein of 2.4.

Another way of comparing orange juice with milk as sources of protein is to calculate the volume of each that would be necessary to obtain the daily allowance for protein. Orange juice would require 44 g/0.7 g = 63 portions of 3.2 oz each, or a total of 201 oz, which amounts to 6.3

qt! A similar calculation for whole milk shows 44 g protein/8.5 g per cup, or 5.2 cups. If the woman obtained all her protein from milk, she would be ingesting 827 kcal. If the woman attempted to obtain all her protein from orange juice, she would find that the 6.3 qt per day was providing her with 2,835 kcal! However, someone who attempted to obtain the RDA for vitamin C from milk would be required to drink 5.5 qt daily. This volume of milk would furnish them with 3,487 kcal.

These calculations demonstrate the absurdity of attempting to meet the RDA for a nutrient from a food in which its nutrient density is low. It is theoretically possible to obtain many of the essential nutrients from candy bars or ice cream, but in the process, one would be consuming so many calories that one would resemble a balloon rather than a person. For those people who are trying to consume a diet that is adequate in all the essential nutrients as well as within the range of their energy requirements—and this should include everyone who is responsible for his or her own or others' diets—a working knowledge of nutrient densities of common foods is essential.

I need to emphasize that there are as many nutrient densities per foodstuff as there are nutrients. However, this large number—about 50—is never used. One reason is that it is neither convenient nor necessary. Another reason is that there is probably no food that has been analyzed for all the essential nutrients. To make up for these lacks, labels on processed foods must list a minimum of eight essential nutrients. The eight nutrients are protein, niacin, calcium, iron, and vitamins A, C, B_1, and B_2. Recent surveys in the U.S. have found that many of these nutrients are deficient in the food of 20% of the population.

To simplify the problem of obtaining a nutritious diet, Guthrie (1977) and colleagues have examined the interrelationships among the noncalorific essential nutrients. From the results of a recent nutritional survey, Jenkins and Guthrie (1984) identified four index nutrients: calcium, iron, and vitamins A and B_6, which, if adequate, assured comparable intakes of six additional nutrients: magnesium, phosphorus, and the vitamins riboflavin (B_2), thiamin (B_1), cobalamin (B_{12}), and ascorbic acid (C).

Three out of the four index nutrients are now listed on the labels of n ¬y processed foods. As shown in Table 6.1, these three are vitamin A, calcium, and iron.

The Importance of Reading Nutrition Labels and the Small Print of Ads

In these days of self-service supermarkets, most people recognize the food products they are looking for by brand names or generic names. Many printed cartons contain both. In addition, the name of the manufacturer and the net weight of the contents must always appear on the front of the package. The list of ingredients on the front or side panel gives the ingredients in order of amount present. Lables of products with standards of identity need not include an ingredient list.

Nutrition-wise consumers also look for the nutrition information panel. This panel, if present, must contain the following information:

- Serving or portion size
- Servings or portions per container
- Calorie content per serving
- Protein, carbohydrate, and fat content per serving
- A minimum of eight constituents
- Protein, vitamins, and elements as percentages of the U.S. RDA

It may surprise you to learn that the terms *U.S. RDA* and *RDA* are not synonymous. The U.S. RDA values that appear on labels are the RDA values for adults that were current in 1968. The RDA values are revised approximately every 5 years so that there are small differences between the current (1980) RDA values and those of 1968. If a nutrition claim for a product appears on the label, information of the nutritional value, as described above, must also appear.

Some other labeling laws that also are valuable to consumers are listed below:

- Any food labeled "low in calories" must state the number of calories per serving and must contain no more than 40 calories per serving as a maximum.
- Any food labeled a "reduced-calorie food" must contain at least a third less calories than the food it most closely resembles.
- Additives listed on labels must state their functions.

Another helpful aid to nutrition-wise Americans occurred on July 1, 1986 (Lecos, 1986). On that date the FDA ruled that all FDA-regulated processed foods that carry nutrition labels must list the sodium content. For the first time, hypertensives and others who wish to monitor their sodium intake are able to obtain the sodium content per serving of a wide variety of processed foods. This important step by the FDA can be interpreted as another example that government, as well as industry, responds to the desires of nutrition-conscious consumers.

It is also valuable to know the definitions of a few terms that commonly appear on labels. An *enriched* food contains nutrients in about the same amounts found in the whole food. Thus, white bread or flour is enriched (with iron, riboflavin, thiamin, and niacin) to bring these four nutrients to about the same concentration found in whole-wheat flour or bread. A *fortified* food, on the other hand, may contain added nutrients in higher amounts than were present originally, or that were not even present in the original food. For example, iodized salt; milk and margarine to which vitamins A and D have been added; and fruit drinks to which large amounts of vitamin C have been added are all examples of fortified foods.

Now that the importance of polyunsaturated/saturated fatty acid ratios (P/S) has been recognized, many more people have begun to look at margarine labels. Most margarines state their P/S ratio on the label. Unfortunately, some consumers assume that all margarines have high P/S ratios. They do not. Some margarines may contain as low a P/S ratio as butter; others may possess ratios in the range of 2–3. Corn or safflower oils are commonly used to increase the polyunsaturated fatty content of margarines.

All margarines are hydrogenated to some degree so that they remain solid at room temperature and yet spread more easily than butter. Soft margarines have had air blown through them to expand their volume. They contain about three-quarters as many calories per tablespoon as ordinary margarine.

Idaho russet potatoes have a wide reputation as a very high-quality product and sell at a premium price. Many people think that all russet potatoes are Idaho grown. Some growers buy their seed potatoes from Idaho sources and label the bags as Idaho russet potatoes, even though they were not grown in Idaho. For example, the Idaho Public Service Commission is ordering the Idaho Potato Co. to state in larger letters on their potato bags that their product is grown in Canada. Consumers who are used to reading labels, of course, would not be taken in by such a ruse. Do you know where your potatoes are grown?

Consumers can save money by buying beef or pork by the quarter or half directly from a butcher and placing the meat in freezers. Besides the usual grades of meat, there is one known in the trade as the *cutting yield*. This term refers to the pounds of meat actually obtained per 100 lb of original total carcass. The highest cutting yield is given a grade of 1 and the lowest 5. The difference is due to unusable fat content. A side of beef with a cutting yield of 1 will contain about 30% (wt) of fat that will be discarded. In comparison, a cutting yield of 5 will contain about 60% (wt) of discardable fat. Thus, in a 1,000-lb carcass, the number 1 will yield 700 lb of meat and bones, whereas the number 5 will yield 400 lb.

It is not uncommon for cut-rate meat processors to advertise a very low price in large letters and, near the bottom, state the cutting yield of 4 or 5 in small letters. Often, one can obtain more tasty meat per dollar by paying a few cents more per pound for meat with a cutting yield of 2 or 3. Knowledge and observation pay off.

Uses of Nutrient Density

Nutrient density calculations provide a basis for defining a nutritious food. In discussing this question, Guthrie (1977) introduces the term *nutrient calorie benefit ratio* (NCBR), which corresponds to the nutrient density as defined above. She defines a nutritious food as one that has a nutrient density of one (1.0) for at least four nutrients, or a nutrient density of two (2.0) for at least two nutrients. Notice that this definition represents a value judgment. Guthrie applied this definition to 112 common foods that are found in the four food groups and to a miscellaneous group of 23 items. Using the criterion of a nutrient density of at least one for four nutrients, she found that 65% of the foods qualified as nutritious. On this basis, the foods in the miscellaneous group, which were high in fat and sugar, failed to qualify. Her calculations are summarized in Table 6.2.

In *Nutrition Scoreboard*, Jacobson (1975) has given plus scores for foods high in five vitamins, two elements, protein, and natural carbohydrate and has assigned negative scores for saturated fat, excessively high total fat, and the addition of sugar to a food. Snack foods such as peanuts, raisins, apples, and pretzels rate positive scores while cookies, candies, and soft drinks rate negative scores. This system has the advantage of simplicity. One positive or negative number sums it all. But does it?

These procedures can be very useful for consumers in evaluating foods. As with any type of simplifying scheme, however, persons using them should be aware of their limitations. The conclusions are based on value judgments, and the attempt to make them quantitative is tricky. Jacobson's point score, for example, reflects his biases on the consumption of refined sugar and saturated fat. If you think his scoreboard is useful, look at his numbers and decide if his assumptions about the numerical value of each item and yours agree. Feel free to modify it if you choose.

Another area in which consumer judgment is necessary concerns the nutritive value of highly processed foods. A manufacturer could add a few nutrients to almost any food to improve its score even though most of the natural nutrients might be missing.

As mentioned above, the present emphasis on nutrient content of foods has resulted in a variety of terms to express the relation between nutrients and calories. This relation is important, but I think that nutrient density, or similar term, should not be used synonymously with food quality. I refuse to throw the taste of foods to the winds of scientism. It is on this basis that I suggest the term *index of nutritional adequacy* (INA) as less loaded than the term *index of nutritional quality* (see Table 6A.1).

A definition of a junk food might be one in which no calorific essential nutrient has an INA as high as 1.0. Table sugar or cooking fat that has not been fortified both qualify as junk under this definition. Because both of these foods contain calories, and because the enzymes that produce utilizable energy (ATP) require a steady input of cofactors that contain organic or inorganic essential nutrients, it means that junk foods actually deprive the metabolic system of necessary cofactors. In this way we can understand how a steady diet that is high in junk foods can result in nutrient deficiency symptoms. Nature insists that we either eat right or else!

Table 6.2   135 Foods Used to Evaluate Concept of a Nutritious Food

Food Group	Number of Items	Examples	Number Qualifying as Nutritious NCBR Criterion 1*	2+
Milk and milk products	16	Milk, cheese (Swiss, Cheddar, and cottage), ice cream, yogurt	13	13
Meat and meat substitutes	22	Bacon, beef liver, pork chops, perch, eggs	16	17
Fruits and vegetables	45	Green beans, peas, potatoes, corn, broccoli, prunes, tomatoes	35	37
Breads and cereals	19	Bread (enriched, whole wheat), crackers, waffles, rice	15	6
Mixed dishes	10	Macaroni and cheese, chili con carne, pizza, tacos	8	9
Miscellaneous	23	Butter, cakes, cookies, pies, gelatin, potato chips, popcorn	0	1
Total	135		87	83

*A nutrient: calorie benefit ratio of one for four nutrients.
+A nutrient: calorie benefit ratio of two for two nutrients.
Note.   From "Concept of a Nutritious Food" by H. Guthrie, 1977, *Journal of the American Dietetic Association, 71*, pp. 16-17. Copyright 1977 by the American Dietetic Association. Adapted by permission.

Junk foods have received tremendous publicity in recent years and have been declared the culprits in many cases of behavioral problems in children. Here we have a fascinating example of cause and effect thinking being applied in complex family situations such as hyperactive children.

A very widely publicized cause of hyperactivity during the 1970s was the Feingold hypothesis (1975), which stated that the behavioral problem was due to artificial flavors and colors in foods. He suggested that the child's diet be changed to one that contained only natural foods with no additives or artificial colors. Many parents changed their hyperactive child's diet in this way and were delighted to find that more normal behavior followed. Did the results prove the Feingold hypothesis? Not by any means. Why is my conclusion so negative?

In the first place, the behavior of the parents changed markedly. They paid more attention to the child and were probably more supportive and less critical than they had been. In the second place, a natural food diet not only contains fewer additives, it was probably richer in nutrients than the previous diet. The child may have been suffering from a number of partial nutrient deficiencies. Behavioral changes such as irritability, aggressiveness, depression, and emotional instability have been linked to deficiencies of thiamin, riboflavin, niacin, pyridoxine, folacin, cobalamin, ascorbic acid, iron, copper, magnesium, and zinc. I suggest that the diets of people with psychological problems be examined as carefully as the other aspects of their environment. To conclude: a junk food diet may result in behavioral problems, not from its high content of sugar or fat, but due to a lack of essential nutrients.

Now that we have discussed the questions of what is meant by nutritious food, we are ready to tackle the larger problems of selecting, preparing, and eating a nutritious diet. Fortunately, there are some guidelines that make a detailed knowledge of the RDAs unnecessary.

The Four Food Groups (Plus One)

In planning a week's menu for a family of four, a person would be faced with a tiresome and time-consuming task of going from the RDA table to a list of food compositions to be assured that he or she was preparing nutritious meals that were adequate in all the essential nutrients. To make nutritious meal planning easier, many years ago the U.S. Department of Agriculture (USDA) began to publicize the four food groups: (a) milk and milk products, (b) meat and meat products, (c) fruits and vegetables, and (d) bread and cereals.

The idea was that, if people ate a specified number of servings each day from each of the four food groups, they would be ingesting an adequate diet. The four food groups plus one, sample foods from each group, and the main nutrients they contain are shown in Table 6.3.

As I've mentioned before, the goal of nutritious eating is to obtain all the essential nutrients without getting fat (i.e., without ingesting too many calories). It may surprise you to learn that by careful selection it is possible to include the essential nutrients in a diet that contains no more than 1,000 cal per day (Hamilton, Whitney, & Sizer, 1985). In this plan,

Table 6.3 The Four Food Groups (Plus One)

Food Group	Sample Foods	Main Nutrient Contributions*	Servings/ Day (Adult)	Serving Size
(1) Meat and meat substitutes	Lean beef, pork, lamb, fish, poultry, eggs, nuts, legumes	Protein, fat, iron, riboflavin, niacin, microelements	2	2-3 oz cooked meat, fish, or chicken; 1 cup cooked legumes
(2) Milk and milk products	Low-fat or skim milk, yogurt, cheese, cottage cheese, buttermilk, soy milk, ice milk	Calcium, protein, fat, carbohydrates, riboflavin, vitamins A and D	2**	1 cup (8 oz) milk, 1-2 oz cheese
(3) Fruits and vegetables	Dark green or yellow vegetables	Vitamin A, vitamin C, iron, riboflavin, fiber, PUFA	4+	1/2 cup fruit, vegetable, or juice
(4) Grains (bread and cereal)	All whole wheat flours and products	Riboflavin, niacin, iron, fiber, carbohydrates, microelements	4++	1 slice bread, 1/2 cup cooked cereal, 1 cup ready-to-eat cereal

(5) Low-nutrient density	Most desserts, canned fruits in heavy syrup, Jell-O, pancake syrup, presweetened cereals	Sugar	O C C A S I O N A L L Y
	Butter, margarine, potato chips, hard cheeses	Fat	
	Pickles, other highly salted foods	Salt	

*Thiamin is equally distributed in all four groups.

**For children up to 9, 2-3 cups; for children 9-12, 3-4 cups; for teenagers and pregnant women, 3-4 cups; for nursing mothers, 4 cups or more.

+One should be rich in vitamin C; at least one every other day should be rich in vitamin A.

++Whole grain products only.

Note. From Nutrition, Concepts and Controversies (p. 19) by E.M.N. Hamilton, E.N. Whitney, and F.S. Sizer, 1985, St. Paul, MN: West. Copyright 1985 by West. Adapted by permission.

high-nutrient-density, low-fat, low-sugar foods are emphasized. For example, skim milk, lean meat, and low-fat cheeses rather than their higher fat counterparts; whole-grain products rather than enriched; and fresh fruits with minimum sugar rather than canned in heavy syrup are routinely consumed. Even for people on a moderate diet, selection of high-nutrient-density foods as the major constituents allows extra calories to be chosen from favorite foods, desserts, or alcoholic beverages.

Needless to say, like any other simplifying recommendation, the four food groups have been criticized. Some nutritionists have claimed that people following this regime tend to overeat and gain weight. Others have pointed out that it is possible to follow the four food groups and still consume a diet that is deficient in one or more essential nutrients. Eating according to the four food groups, like any other human activity, does require judgment and knowledge. Selections can be made from each group that are nutrient rich (a high-nutrient density) or nutrient poor (a low-nutrient density). Selections high in the former type will result in a satisfactory diet, and those from the latter in an inadequate diet. Similarly, if the same foods are eaten repeatedly for long periods, it is possible to miss some essential nutrients. It is important to choose a varied selection in each group.

The Berkeley Co-Op (Black, 1980) has modified the four food groups by separating the vegetable-fruit group into three sections: vitamin-C rich, dark green vegetable, and potato or other vegetable or fruit. The Co-Op nutritionists have also added one modest serving of fat or oil to insure adequate intake of linoleic acid. This food guide, which provides between 1,100 and 2,200 kcal per day, is presented in the appendix for chapter 6 (Table 6A.2).

I cannot emphasize too strongly that a nutritious diet and a tasty, attractive diet are not incompatible! Become aware of all the information that your taste buds furnish. You can readily learn to sense those foods high in fat and/or sugar. Don't think of cutting them out of your diet—that is the road to dietary failure—but enjoy them on an occasional basis.

Food Additives in Highly Processed Foods

Additives have been used in food preservation for millenia. With the rapid growth of urbanization in industrialized countries, the demand for processed foods has markedly increased. Table 6.4 lists the major functions of food additives and a few examples of the chemicals used in each category.

Table 6.4   Functions of Food Additives

Function	Chemicals Added
Flavoring agents:	
Sweeteners	Aspartame, sugars, corn syrup
Salt	Salt
Texturizers:	
Emulsifiers	Lecithin, mono- and diglycerides of fatty acids
Stabilizers	Gums, alginates
Thickeners	Modified starch, pectin
Preservatives:	
Anti-microbial	Sugar, salt, benzoic acid
Anti-oxidants	BHA (butylated hydroxyanisole), vitamins C and E
Sequestrants	EDTA (ethylene diamine tetraacetic acid and its salts)
Appearance enhancers:	
Colors	Tartrazine, dyes
Bleaches	Benzoyl peroxide
Flavor enhancers:	MSG (monosodium glutamate)
Nutrients:	
Fortifiers	Vitamins A, C, and D, iron
Enrichers	Thiamin, riboflavin, niacin, iron

Sweeteners

In terms of quantity, sweeteners are by far the number one food additive in the U.S. The average American adult consumes 128 lb of sugars of various types as additives in processed foods every year. Although the amount of sugar added to breakfast cereals has scandalized many people, you might be surprised to see how much sugar is being added to a variety of other common foods (see Table 6.5).

According to the present regulations on labels, it is impossible to esti-mate the sugar content of most processed foods. Additives are listed in decreasing order of concentration. If one sees sucrose listed first, it is a good indication that a high percentage of the total calories will be pro-vided by this substance. But how many people recognize that in addi-tion to sucrose, fructose, glucose (dextrose), corn syrup, corn sugar, honey, invert sugar, and molasses are all commonly used as sweeteners? When two or more of these additives are included in a food, it is im-possible to calculate the amounts of *simple sugars* that are present.

Table 6.5 Sugar Content of Some Foods and Beverages

Foods and beverages	% (wt/wt)	kcal/fl oz	Cereals	% (wt/wt)	kcal/oz
Beverages, carbonated			Cheerios	3.6	4.
Cola soda	11.	13.6	Corn Flakes	7.	8.
Ginger ale	8.	9.7	Froot Loops	46.	52.
Orange soda	12.	15.3	Fruit & Fibre, Apples & Cinnamon	26.	30.
Tonic water	8.5	10.4	Granola, Nature Valley	25.	28.
			Nutri-grain, Wheat	7.	8.
Beverages, noncarbonated			Nutri-grain, Raisins	25.	28.
Kool-aid, from mix	10.	12.	Puffed Wheat	0	0
Tang, orange	22.		Puffed Rice	0	0
			Raisin Bran	32.	36.
Salad dressings			Shredded Wheat	0	0
Buttermilk, Good Seasons	5.6	7.2	Sugar Smacks	57.	64.
French Old Fashioned, Good Seasons	3.1	2.0	Wheaties	11.	12.
Italian	2.5	3.2			
Italian, Low cal.	7.8	4.2			

Soups

Beef, mushroom, chunky	1.	1.1
Chicken, noodles, chunky	1.	1.1
Tomato	7.4	8.

Syrup

Log Cabin	65.	101.

Candy

		kcal/oz
Chocolate chips, semi-sweet	61.	68.
Crunch bar, Nestle	50.	57.
Krackel	51.	58.
Milk chocolate	57.	64.
Mr. Goodbar	41.	48.
Reese's Pieces	57.	64.

Frozen Entrees

Beef Oriental, Stouffers Lean Cuisine	0.8	0.9
Chicken Glazed, Stouffers Lean Cuisine	1.6	2.
Meatball Stew, Stouffers Lean Cuisine	2.8	3.2
Fish Fillet, Divan, Stouffers Lean Cuisine	1.7	2.

Fruits

Apple, raw	9.9	11.
Banana, raw	14.	16.
Dates, dried	66.	76.
Orange, raw	8.	10.
Raspberries, raw	5.	6.
Raspberries, frozen, sweet	22.	25.
Strawberries, raw	5.	6.
Strawberries, frozen, sweet	19.	21.
Mixed fruit, frozen, sweet	22.	24.

Note. From *Food Values of Portions Commonly Used* (pp. 236-239) by J.A. Pennington and H.N. Church, 1985, Philadelphia: Lippincott. Copyright 1985 by Lippincott. Reprinted by permission.

The other major source of sugar consumed by Americans is in soft drinks. According to Brewster and Jacobson (1978), Americans consumed over 500 8-oz servings of soft drinks per person in 1976. One-fourth of the U.S. sucrose consumption was in the form of soft drinks, and of these, cola drinks made up over half. Eighteen percent of the total calories consumed in the U.S. in 1976 consisted of sweeteners. Does this statistic reveal a serious flaw in the American diet? Some people think so.

I am not one of those who consider sugar and sweeteners as poisons or as contributing directly to heart disease, cancer, and diabetes. My concern about these additives is that they may easily become a major source of calories even though they are devoid of noncaloric nutrients. Sugar sweeteners lower nutrient density. They may be consumed if desired, but in moderation.

Sugar has been cursed with the epithet "empty calories." Its purity is its Achilles heel. If we eat much sugar, we will need to eat more of other foods to satisfy our requirements for the noncalorific essential nutrients. These other foods also furnish calories, so that, unless we pick them very carefully, we run the risk of becoming obese.

For me, it is simpler to keep my sugar consumption to a minimum and to eat a variety of other foods, than to consume a lot of sugar and have to worry about sources of essential nutrients that are low in calories so that I won't get fat. Nutrient density is one of the most important ideas discussed in this book.

Salt

Common salt is the second most widely used food additive. It is composed of sodium and chloride ions, which are both essential elements. The estimated safe and adequate daily dietary intake for sodium is 1.1–3.3 g/day. This amount calculates to 3–8 g/day of sodium chloride. The average intake for adult Americans is estimated at 10–20 g/day of salt. In contrast to these amounts, the actual requirement for salt is about 0.5 g/day. Salt occurs in practically all foods to some extent, but approximately two-thirds of the salt Americans consume is present in processed foods as an additive. Because of its close association with hypertension, the salt content of many foods will be presented and discussed in chapter 9.

In contrast to sugar, salt contains no calories. As I've mentioned, our actual requirement is quite modest and can be attained solely from animal and plant foods without our adding any salt to the food we eat. Although there are other risk factors for hypertension than excessive salt intake, there is a dose-response relationship between salt consumption in the world and the incidence of high blood pressure. Mark Hegsted (1978), former head of the Human Nutrition Center of the USDA, has commented: "The current level of salt intake by Americans is about half the toxic dose. If salt were a new food additive, it is doubtful if it would be classified as safe, and certainly not at the level that most of us consume" (p. 1507).

Fat

Fat occurs naturally in many foods, but it can be considered an additive in many others. Fried foods, for example, contain much more fat than those that are broiled or baked. Frying in deep fat is fast and produces a tasty product, hence its popularity in fast-food establishments. Many of these products are listed in Table 6.6. In the last column I have calculated the percentage of calories derived from fat. Pizzas and shakes are among the lowest in fat, with the fried foods falling in the 50%-60% range.

In my opinion, excess fat in the diet is comparable to excess sugar. They both add extra calories (fat, 2 1/4 times as much as sugar per gram) without contributing any other essential nutrients, with the possible exception of linoleic acid in some vegetable fats.

The conversion of the nutritious baked potato into less nutritious french fries and even less nutritious potato chips is illustrated in Table 6.7. As the fat content increases, the nutrient density decreases for protein, iron, thiamin, niacin, and vitamin C. In other words, the calories in potato chips are over 6 times more concentrated on a weight basis than those in a baked potato. It should be obvious that overeating can occur much more readily on calorie-concentrated foods than with calorie-diluted foods.

The Nutritional Adequacy of Fast Foods

It is estimated that in recent years about 40% of North American meals are eaten in restaurants, especially in fast-food establishments. It is, therefore, important to consider the nutritional adequacy of the products available at the Double Arches and similar eateries.

The first point I want to make about the fast-food chains is that their products cannot fairly be called junk foods. The composition of many fast food items is shown in Table 6.6. The nutrients present in a hamburger, french fries, and shake add up to an impressive contribution to a day's nutritional needs. According to Finberg, Landis, and Harlan (1976), a hamburger provides 42% of the RDA for protein and contains all the essential amino acids and many of the noncalorific essential nutrients. They reported that it is low in vitamins A and C, and folacin. The fries contain 42% fat calories—a bit high—especially when coupled with 66% fat calories in a hamburger. People who add much ketchup to their hamburger and fries should remember that it contains 29% sucrose on a weight basis— the fat floats on a high-calorie tomato puree.

Table 6.6 Calorie Content and Energy Sources of "Fast" Foods

Item	Calories	Protein (g)	Carbohydrates (g)	Fats (g)	Kcal From Fat %
McDonald's Big Mac	541	26	39	31	52
Burger King Whopper	606	29	51	32	48
Burger Chief Hamburger	258	11	24	13	45
Arthur Treacher's Fish Sandwich	440	16	39	24	49
McDonald's Filet-O-Fish	402	15	34	23	64
Kentucky Fried Chicken Original Recipe Dinner—drumstick & thigh	830	52	56	46	50
Kentucky Fried Chicken Extra Crispy Dinner—drumstick & thigh	950	52	63	54	51
McDonald's Egg McMuffin	352	18	26	20	51
Burger King French Fries (reg.)	214	3	28	10	41
Arthur Treacher's Coleslaw	123	1	11	8	59
McDonald's Apple Pie	300	2	31	19	57
Burger King Vanilla Shake	332	11	50	11	30
McDonald's Chocolate Shake	364	11	60	9	22

Note. From *Food Values of Portions Commonly Used* (pp. 54-60) by J.A.T. Pennington and H.N. Church, 1985, Philadelphia: J.B. Lippincott. Copyright 1985 by J.B. Lippincott. Reprinted by permission.

Table 6.7 Nutrient Dilution of Potatoes by Fats (Isocaloric Comparison of Baked Potato, French Fries, and Potato Chips)

Potatoes, Baked in Skin
161 g, which supply 150 kcal of energy

Nutrient	Amount	INA	% RDA
Energy	150.000 kcal	1.00	7
Protein	4.194 g	1.22	9
Calcium	14.516 mg	0.17	1
Iron	1.129 mg	0.88	6
Vitamin A	0.000 IU	0.00	0
Thiamin	0.161 mg	2.05	15
Riboflavin	0.065 mg	0.65	5
Niacin	1.742 mg	2.74	20
Vitamin C	32.258 mg	10.04	72
Pantothenic acid	0.613 mg	1.72	12
Vitamin B_6	0.165 mg	1.15	8
Vitamin B_{12}	0.000 g	0.00	0
Fat	0.000 g	0.02	0
Saturated fatty acid	0.000 g	0.00	0
Unsaturated oleic	0.000 g	0.00	0
Unsaturated linoleic	0.000 g	0.00	0
Cholesterol	0.000 mg	0.00	0
Carbohydrate, total	34.032 g	1.76	13
Fiber	0.968 g	2.51	18
Phosphorus	104.839 mg	1.22	9
Sodium	6.452 mg	0.02	0
Potassium	811.290 mg	2.84	20

Nutrients as proportion of energy

(Cont.)

Table 6.7 Cont.

Potatoes, French Fried
55 g, which supply 150 kcal of energy

Nutrient	Amount	INA	% RDA
Energy	150.000 kcal	1.00	7
Protein	2.354 g	0.69	5
Calcium	8.212 mg	0.10	1
Iron	0.712 mg	0.55	4
Vitamin A	0.000 IU	0.00	0
Thiamin	0.071 mg	0.91	6
Riboflavin	0.044 mg	0.44	3
Niacin	1.697 mg	1.70	12
Vitamin C	11.496 mg	3.58	28
Pantothenic acid	0.208 mg	0.58	4
Vitamin B$_6$	0.056 mg	0.39	3
Vitamin B$_{12}$	0.000 g	0.00	3
Fat	7.226 g	1.10	8
Saturated fatty acid	1.642 g	0.92	7
Unsaturated oleic	1.642 g	0.70	5
Unsaturated linoleic	3.832 g	2.15	15
Cholesterol	0.000 mg	0.00	0
Carbohydrate, total	19.708 g	1.02	7
Fiber	0.547 g	1.42	10
Phosphorus	60.766 mg	0.71	5
Sodium	3.285 mg	0.01	0
Potassium	466.971 mg	1.63	12

Nutrients as proportion of energy

Potato Chips
26 g, which supply 150 kcal of energy

Nutrient	Amount	INA	% RDA
Energy	150.000 kcal	1.00	7
Protein	1.400 g	0.41	3
Calcium	10.563 mg	0.12	1
Iron	0.475 mg	0.37	3
Vitamin A	0.000 IU	0.00	0
Thiamin	0.055 mg	0.71	5
Riboflavin	0.018 mg	0.18	1
Niacin	1.268 mg	1.27	9
Vitamin C	4.225 mg	1.31	3
Pantothenic acid	0.100 mg	0.28	2
Vitamin B_6	0.048 mg	0.33	2
Vitamin B_{12}	0.000 mg	0.00	0
Fat	10.511 g	1.60	11
Saturated fatty acid	2.641 g	1.48	11
Unsaturated oleic	2.113 g	0.90	6
Unsaturated linoleic	5.282 g	2.96	21
Cholesterol	0.000 mg	0.00	0
Carbohydrate, total	13.204 g	0.68	5
Fiber	0.423 g	1.10	8
Phosphorus	36.708 mg	0.43	3
Sodium	89.789 mg	0.31	2
Potassium	298.415 mg	1.04	7

Nutrients as proportion of energy

Note. From "Nutritional Quality Index Identifies Consumer Needs" by B.W. Wyse, A.W. Sorenson, A.J. Wittwer, and R.G. Hansen, 1976, *Food Technology,* **30,** p. 33. Copyright 1976 by *Food Technology.* Adapted by permission.

The original shakes were made with milk and were called *milk shakes*. USDA regulations require that a milk shake be made with milk, although whether it contains whole, 2%, or skim milk need not be stated. The word *shake* by itself indicates that the beverage does not contain liquid milk although it does contain nonfat milk solids, vegetable oils, and coloring and flavoring agents. Shakes contain significant quantities of protein, fat, calcium, riboflavin, and niacin. The largest difference between a shake and an equal volume of whole milk is in the carbohydrate content. A shake contains 50-60 g of carbohydrate (most of it as sucrose), whereas milk contains 12 g of carbohydrate per cup (as lactose). This difference explains both the greater sweetness of a shake compared to milk as well as the large difference in calories (325-360 kcal vs. 160 kcal).

What then is missing? Have the fast-food chains discovered the ideal diet? The major attractions at fast-food chains (hamburgers, french fries, and milkshakes) certainly provide essential nutrients. My main concern is that these three popular foods have low-nutrient densities for a number of essential nutrients. The nutrient densities of a shake and burger and of a pizza have been graphed by Wyse, Sorenson, Wittwer, and Hansen (1976) as shown in Tables 6.8a and 6.8b. To show the ease of using these graphs, I have included the nutrient density of 7 nutrients in 23 representative foods in Table 6A.1. On this list of eight nutrients, the duo stacks up moderately well. However, iron, vitamin C, niacin, and thiamin show INQs of 0.66 or less. A glance reveals that the pizza is richer in the listed nutrients than the burger-shake combination. Dietary fiber is probably low in both.

The sensible action for a person whose diet is unbalanced in this fashion is to make up for the deficiencies by eating other foods that are rich in vitamins and dietary fiber such as yellow and green vegetables (asparagus, fresh beets, broccoli, brussels sprouts, corn), legumes (black-eyed peas, lima beans), and liver. Table 6.9 contains sources of foods rich in vitamin E, vitamin B_6, magnesium, zinc, and iron.

In *Food for Nought*, Hall (1974) intones against the advertisements and blandishments of the food industry, and implies that consumers have lost control of their diets and are but pawns in the machinations of agribusiness. Personally, I am not so pessimistic. Consumers are undoubtedly strongly influenced by advertising and prices; but the success of the health food stores, for which neither advertising nor price is the main attraction, demonstrates the economic power of knowledgeable consumers. It is also significant that the supermarkets have added more and more health food items to their shelves, such as high-P/S margarines, low-salt soups, canned fruit in light syrup, and low-fat dairy products. I wonder what it would take for McDonald's to offer a choice of whole wheat or white rolls? I am confident that they would do it if enough people wrote to the management: McDonald's Corp., McDonald's Plaza, Oak Brook, IL 60521. Some fast-food outlets already provide this choice.

Table 6.8a Nutrient Profile of a Hamburger and Milk Shake

Nutrient	Amount	INA	% RDA	0%	25%	50%
Energy	637.38 kcal	1.00	32			
Protein	24.43 g	1.18	38			
Vitamin A	1218.30 IU	0.76	24			
Vitamin C	10.08 mg	0.53	17			
Thiamin	0.31 mg	0.66	21			
Riboflavin	0.71 mg	1.31	42			
Niacin	0.60 mg	0.60	19			
Calcium	408.49 mg	1.28	41			
Iron	2.59 mg	0.45	14			

Hamburger with lettuce, tomato, and catsup
Milk shake (12 oz)

Table 6.8b Nutrient Profile of a Pizza—Pepperoni, Sausage, Vegetables (1/4 of 14″ pie)

Nutrient	Amount	INA	% RDA	0%	25%	50%
Energy	599.05 kcal	1.00	30			
Protein	37.13 g	1.91	57			57%
Vitamin A	1235.10 IU	0.82	25			
Vitamin C	14.49 mg	0.81	24			
Thiamin	0.37 mg	0.83	25			
Riboflavin	0.53 mg	1.03	31			
Niacin	7.06 mg	1.18	35			
Calcium	337.66 mg	1.13	34			
Iron	5.34 mg	0.99	30			

Note. From "Planning for the Inevitable: Snack Foods in the Diet" by R.G. Hansen and B.W. Wyse, 1979, *Family and Community Health,* 1, pp. 31-39. Copyright 1979 by *Family and Community Health.* Reprinted by permission.

Table 6.9 Good Sources of Vitamin E, Vitamin B₆, Magnesium, Zinc, and Iron

Vitamin E (> 2.0 IU/svg[1])	Vitamin B₆ (> 200 g/svg)	Magnesium (> 20 mg/svg)	Zinc (> 1.0 mg/svg)	Iron (> 2.0 mg/svg)
Nuts	Meat, poultry, fish	Nuts	Milk	Leafy greens
Vegetables	Legumes	Legumes	Meat, poultry, fish	Legumes
Leafy greens	Wheat germ	Leafy greens	Legumes	Beef, lamb, pork
Wheat germ		Milk	Whole grain cereals	Shellfish
		Meat, fish	Wheat germ	Eggs
		Wheat germ		
		Wheat cereal		

Note. From "Evaluation and Modification of the Basic Four Food Guide" by J.C. King, S.H. Cohenoni, C.G. Coruccini, and P. Schneeman, 1978, *Journal of Nutrition Education*, **10**, p. 28. Copyright 1978 by *Journal of Nutrition Education*. Reprinted by permission.

[1]A serving (svg) equals 3 oz meat, poultry, fish; 2 eggs; 3/4 cup cooked legumes; 1 oz nuts; 3/4 cup cooked leafy greens or 1 cup raw; 1 cup milk; 1 tbsp wheat germ; 1 oz dry cereal; 3/4 cup cooked cereal or pasta; 1 slice bread; 1 tbsp vegetable oil.

Effects of Processing on Nutrient Content of Foods

Processing of foods is an all-inclusive term that covers everything that happens to a food after it is harvested or slaughtered. Before the twentieth century, the major aim of food processing, preparatory for storage, was to keep it edible and prevent spoilage. For most foods, this objective was accomplished by two procedures: the removal of fats, which become rancid when kept at room temperature; and the removal of moisture to prevent microbial growth. Alternative procedures relied on high concentrations of salt or sugar in solution to inhibit bacterial or mold growth. Classical processing procedures almost invariably resulted in a loss of nutrients.

Different types of processing are important and sometimes essential in making a food safe to eat, either when fresh or after storage. An outstanding example concerns the treatment of the cycad nut. The palm-like cycad tree grows in tropical and semitropical regions and has been used by natives as a staple food and medicine for generations. When first harvested, however, it is very toxic; acute jaundice, hemorrhage, and partial paralysis result from eating it. It is necessary to repeatedly wash the sliced nuts and fruit to remove the toxin, which has recently been isolated and identified (Miller, 1973). One wonders how many people died before this procedure was perfected.

Fresh fruits and vegetables are usually washed in water to remove contaminants like dirt, bird droppings, insecticides, and the like. With modern refrigeration techniques by the wholesaler, retailer, and consumer, fresh produce retains attractiveness and nutrient content much longer than it used to.

Food preservation is another major objective of processing. The phrase "feast or famine" may sound poetic, but learning to preserve food when it was available for times when it was not could mean the difference between survival and extinction for a tribe. Washing food, pickling, salting, smoking, drying, heating, and cooling have all been tried at one time or another, and many of these procedures are still used today.

Canning was introduced in the eighteenth century as an industrial process and is also widely practiced by thrifty householders. The history of canning can serve as a thumbnail sketch of how the application of technology improves a process. The original objective was merely to exclude air from the foodstuff. After Pasteur demonstrated that many bacteria could reproduce under these conditions, but could be destroyed by heat, the widescale heating of canned foods and milk was introduced. Using taste as the criterion, the industry has changed the appearance and flavor of canned peas from hard, leather-like nodules to green spheres with a definite pea-like flavor. With the discovery of vitamins in the early twentieth century, analyses of these nutrients have been included in the evaluation of nutritional adequacy.

After washing, the food to be canned is blanched briefly in steam or longer in boiling water. The heat treatment destroys antidigestive factors in grains and legumes and also inactivates enzymes that destroy vitamins. In general, the shorter and hotter the blanching, the less the nutrient loss. Steam blanching of spinach results in 90%-100% retention of vitamins B_1, B_2, and C, and niacin, while boiling water blanching lowers retention of the same vitamins to 65%-90%.

These results are typical. The vitamins that are the most heat-unstable are thiamin, pantothenic acid, and ascorbic acid (vitamin C) (Nesheim, 1974). Most of the vitamin losses in industrial processing occur during blanching. The same principles apply during home blanching or cooking; steaming for as short a time as possible is preferable to a lower temperature for a longer time.

A guide to the storage of many processed foods in the home is presented in the Appendix (Table 6A.3). Storage at room temperature (70 °F) reduces shelf life considerably compared to storage at 40 °F. It is advisable when buying foods at case-lot sales or in warehouses to determine the age of the products if you can. Sales items may be near the end of their designated shelf life.

In terms of taste, I think most people would agree to a descending order: fresh, frozen, canned. In this connection, with the state of California providing about half the total fruit and vegetables for the U.S., it is possible that something that appears on your supermarket shelf as fresh produce was picked anywhere from 7 to 14 days ago. Fortunately, the same conditions that will preserve freshness and attractiveness are those that will maintain vitamin content.

In my opinion, a frozen vegetable that was probably picked at the peak of freshness, blanched at the optimum conditions of time and temperature, quick frozen, and kept at the optimum freezing temperature (0 °F or lower) is likely to retain more nutrients than a fresh vegetable that is wilted because it was not kept cold and moist.

To summarize: Harris and Karmas (1975) state that frozen vegetables lose about 25% more of the water-soluble vitamins on cooking than fresh vegetables. Canned vegetables lose more water-soluble vitamins than frozen vegetables. Similar losses are found when frozen are compared with fresh fruits.

The Problem of Milk Storage

From the very earliest times milk has been recognized as a superb food for adults as well as for babies. Without refrigeration in mild climates, however, keeping it sweet for over a day is next to impossible. Because most people don't like sour milk, one long-used ploy has been to control the types of organisms, and thus were cheese and yogurt invented.

Marco Polo (with an assist from Tannahill, 1973) described how the Tartars dried mare's milk. They heated it to almost boiling, skimmed off the cream from the top, and let the remainder dry in the sun. The product was as stable as our modern dried milk, which is dried under high vacuum.

Pasteurization, Then and Now

As mentioned above, heat treatment of foods was discovered long before Louis Pasteur showed that microorganisms were present in foods, but could be killed by heat. One of the early applications of Pasteur's research was heating milk to sterilize it partially. The treatment was appropriately called *pasteurization*. The difference between Pasteur's use of heat and the Tartars' is significant. The Tartars' experiments were empirical since they had no conception of bacteria or fermentation. Pasteur established that heat killed the bacteria that not only were responsible for souring milk but also caused many human diseases. Further research has led to other advances that will be described below.

Due to additional applications of technology, pasteurized milk now has a much longer shelf life than previously. Two recent treatments have lengthened shelf life even more. The first is called ultrapasteurization, which involves heating milk to at least 100 °C (212 °F) for 0.01 second. This treatment has increased storage time over conventional pasteurization, but the product must be kept cold. The second is a method of sterilizing milk that does not result in an unpleasant taste.

Recently the FDA has approved the marketing of ultra-high temperature (UHT) processed milk. This milk can be stored unrefrigerated for at least 3 months. To achieve this stability, the milk is heated to 138 °C (280 °F) for at least 2 seconds, which sterilizes it. The fluid is then transferred *aseptically* to sterilized containers. Once it is opened, bacteria enter, and the milk should be kept cold like ordinary milk.

Food Irradiation

Another method of food sterilization that is waiting in the wings utilizes irradiation by *gamma rays*. This procedure can sterilize foods without loss of nutrients. Precooked meats can have a shelf life of up to 7 years. Irradiated bacon would be free of the botulism organism without adding nitrite as at present. The Japanese irradiate potatoes to prevent sprouting during storage. With ethylenedibromide (EDB) banned as a preservative for stored grain because it acts as a carcinogen, why is it that the procedure of irradiation is not being used?

The sad fact is that the American public is scared of the word *irradiation*. It reminds us of hydrogen bombs and fallout. Actually, controlled radiation of foods at low doses was shown to be safe over 30 years ago in research by the U.S. Army. The food of our astronauts is sterilized by radiation. The U.S. Congress will need to change the law that considers irradiation as a food additive rather than a process; this is a necessary first step in clearing the way for the widespread introduction of this valuable procedure (Sun, 1984). Food irradiation has become controversial, and its economic advantages are suspect. It may be years before widespread use of this technique will be common (Zurer, 1986).

A Comparison of White and Whole Wheat Breads

The outline of a wheat kernel (see Figure 6.2) illustrates at a glance the difference between white and whole wheat bread. The latter contains the three components endosperm, germ, and bran. The white bread of commerce contains only, or mostly, the endosperm. The color of the natural flour suggests its composition. The endosperm contains starch and protein, both white substances. Wheat germ is yellow, and the bran or husk is brown. Thus, whole wheat bread has a much darker appearance than bread from which the bran and germ have been removed.

Another example of the human attempt to preserve a valuable food source is provided by the repeated efforts to produce a white wheat flour. Since Roman times, and possibly even earlier, humans have preferred white flour to brown. The reason had nothing to do with color but with stability on storage. Wheat germ contains many polyunsaturated fatty acids and the natural antioxidant, vitamin E. On long-term storage, however, the fatty acids become oxidized and the flour becomes rancid and inedible. As not every farmer could own and operate his own flour mill, length of storage had important economic and military consequences. Because the husk enclosed the germ, it was also removed in the process. The whiteness of the flour was used as an index of the degree of removal

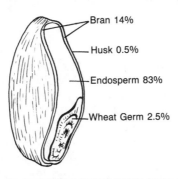

Figure 6.2 Anatomy of a wheat kernel.

of the husk and germ and thus of its quality, which in those times was equated with storability.

Crushing the wheat seeds between stones was the only method available until the industrial age. In the nineteenth century, steel roller mills were developed that, for the first time in history, cleanly allowed the separation of the endosperm from the other components. White bread was popularized in England by advertisements showing upper-class people eating it in preference to brown. To consume white bread became a status symbol. This factor outweighed nutritional considerations. Magendie reported in 1826 that dogs fed white bread did not survive beyond 50 days, while those fed brown bread survived indefinitely.

Long-term storage of flour had still another advantage. The baking qualities of flour stored for a few months improved. About 1900 it was found that this process could be sped up by treating the flour with either agene gas (NCl_3) or chlorine gas. In recent years bromates and iodates have been used as maturing agents.

The terms used to describe flours may be confusing to the uninitiated. Standard white flour is 70% extraction, and the term means that the flour contains 70% of the original wheat berry. Whole wheat flour is 100% extraction. Some whole wheat flours state that they are stone ground, in contrast to steel roller milled. Stone ground is preferable for two reasons. First, the wheat berries are not subjected to as high temperatures as with steel milling, and they retain more B-vitamins and vitamin E. Second, the oils from the germ are spread more evenly over the flour and are less subject to becoming rancid than in the high-speed methods.

Do not use the color of the bread as an index of whether it is made from whole wheat flour. If the label says *enriched*, it means that ordinary white flour was used and was colored brown with molasses, caramel, or a dye. The term enriched as applied to flours means that the vitamins thiamin, riboflavin, niacin, and the element iron have been replaced to the level in the original flour. As you can see from the comparison of nutrients in Table 6.10, whole-grain products contain significantly more B-vitamins, elements, and bran than refined/enriched.

A Rat Growth Experiment
Comparing White and Whole Wheat Breads

As mentioned above, whole wheat flour contains more essential elements and vitamins than white. Does it follow that whole wheat bread is more nutritious than white? Consumer's Union (1982) attempted to answer this question in a rat-feeding experiment. Ten samples of each type of bread were fed to young rats as the sole source of nutrients for 18 weeks. Weight gains were measured as the criterion of nutritive quality. Six of the white breads were ranked very good or excellent compared to only four of the

Table 6.10   Mean Energy and Nutrient Content of Whole Grain Cereals Versus Enriched/Refined Cereals

Item and Unit[1]	Whole Grain (n = 8) Mean ± SEM[2]		Enriched/Refined (n = 15) Mean ± SEM[2]		Whole Grain/ Refined
Energy, kcal	95	± 16	94	± 9	—
Protein, g	3.2	± 0.3	2.6	± 0.3	—
Vitamin A, IU	0		26	± 10	—
Vitamin E, IU	0.45	± 0.23	0.10	± 0.08	2
Vitamin C, mg	0		0		—
Thiamin, mg	0.13	± 0.03	0.08	± 0.01	1.6
Riboflavin, mg	0.04	± 0.01	0.05	± 0.01	—
Niacin, mg	0.91	± 0.26	0.67	± 0.11	1.3
Vitamin B_6, g	96	± 30	28	± 6	3.4
Vitamin B_{12}, g	0		0		—
Free folacin, g	15.1	± 4.7	1.7	± 0.3	8.9
Calcium, mg	17	± 2	20	± 5	—
Phosphorus, mg	92	± 17	43	± 6	2
Magnesium, mg	31	± 7	13	± 3	2.4
Iron, mg	0.9	± 0.1	0.7	+ 0.1	—
Zinc, mg	1.0	± 0.2	0.3	± 0.1	3.3
Iodine, g	2.7	± 0.5	2.5	± 0.3	—
Bran (% dry wt.)[3]	8.5		2.7		3.1

[1]Amount per 1 slice bread, 1 oz dry cereal, or 1/2 cup cooked cereal.

[2]Standard error of the mean.

[3]From "A Guide to Calculating Intakes of Dietary Fiber" by D. Southgate et al., 1976, *Journal of Human Nutrition*, **30**, p. 309. (bread only)

Note.   From "Evaluation and Modification of the Basic Four Food Guide" by J.C. King et al., 1978, *Journal of Nutrition Education*, **10**, p. 28. Copyright 1978 by *Journal of Nutrition Education*. Reprinted by permission.

whole wheat varieties. The results surprised many people. Most nutritionists, myself included, consider whole wheat bread as more nutritious than white. Are we misleading the public? Because *Consumer Reports* is read by millions of people, I will comment on the article as an illustration of the care that must be taken in the planning and interpretation of the results of two variable nutritional experiments.

The data are presented in two columns: sensory rating and nutritional rating. Weight gain was used as the criterion of nutritional rating. But weight gain is dependent on two independent factors: the amount consumed and the quality of the protein in the food. If the quality of the protein in different breads is being evaluated, then the amount consumed should be held constant, or measured, and the gain per unit of food consumed calculated. No indication of whether these two measurements were made separately in this experiment is given. The use of weight gain as a measure of protein quality is unwarranted if the amounts consumed varied.

The characteristics listed under sensory rating were based on human perceptions rather than rats. Breads that were supplemented with egg protein or milk protein were preferred over those that contained only wheat protein. These were the same brands that scored highest in nutritional quality. The supermarket diet experiments mentioned in chapter 5 demonstrated the similarities in rat and human food preferences. Thus it is probable that the rats ate more of the supplemented breads. The results suggest that, if you choose a bread of which you like the taste, it will probably rank high in nutritional quality.

Consumer's Union also discusses the difference in bran content between whole wheat and white bread and the effects of bran on possibly decreasing the absorption of a number of essential elements. Because no analyses of the absorption of elements were done, the experiment added no new knowledge on this question. The average American diet is low in dietary fiber, and whole wheat bread contains considerably more than white. Whole wheat bread seems preferable on this count alone.

To my knowledge, very few North Americans obtain all their protein from bread. Thus, the question of protein quality is not the paramount one in choosing a bread. If protein quality is important to you, then choose a bread that has been supplemented with egg or milk proteins. In summary, the results of this poorly designed experiment hardly justify its cost.

What Is Safe?
Toxic Concentrations of Nutrients, Contaminants, and Additives

Thousands of suicides are reported each year in which the person has taken an overdose of a drug. From these sad news items, the public has learned that even a common and valuable drug like aspirin can be lethal if taken in an excessive quantity. It is my impression, however, that the public has not yet grasped the generalization that literally anything, any substance, can be deadly if ingested in large enough amounts over a sufficient time period. The sixteenth-century physician, Paracelsus (1488-1541), expressed this idea well: "Poison is in everything, and nothing is without poison. The dosage makes it either a poison or a remedy." Pachter (p. 86). Scientists have learned that it is not possible to categorize substances as safe or toxic. The real concern is with the risk, hazard, or benefit associated with the amounts consumed.

The essential nutrients are included in this generalization. One person killed himself by drinking a gallon of water a day. Eventually his *electrolytes* became so unbalanced that his heart stopped. Another drank a quart of carrot juice each day. At the time of death he was as yellow as a ripe squash, and his liver had ceased to function. It may surprise you to learn that water and carotene can act as toxic chemicals. This statement is a half-truth because it omits any mention of concentration. The public has been led to believe that, if something is toxic, it is toxic at all concentrations and that if something is beneficial, it is harmless at all concentrations. Both of these viewpoints are dangerous oversimplifications.

The situation, as we understand it at present, is illustrated in Figure 6.3 (Mertz, 1981). The graph shows that a nutrient may be essential at one concentration and toxic at another. A person may become ill, or even die, from a deficiency of an essential nutrient or from an excess of it.

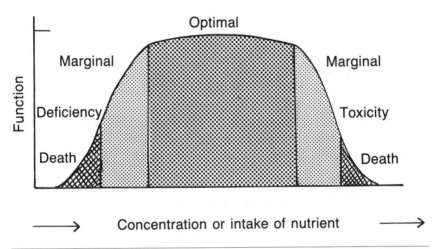

Figure 6.3 Dependence of biological function on tissue concentration or intake of a nutrient. *Note.* From "Essential Trace Elements" by W. Mertz, 1981, *Science,* **213**. Copyright 1981 by *Science.* Reprinted by permission.

Table 6A.4 in the appendix lists the RDAs and the toxic doses (if known) of the vitamins and the essential elements. The term *safety factor* is calculated as the ratio of the toxic daily dose to the RDA value. This number gives some idea of the length of the optimal portion of the curve in Figure 6.3. The smaller the number of the safety factor, the more cautious one should be in taking supplements containing these nutrients. There are cases on record where people have suffered serious illnesses, or have died, from chronic overdoses of vitamins A and D.

As a group, the water-soluble vitamins have larger safety factors than the fat-soluble ones. This difference is mainly due to the water-soluble vitamins being readily excreted, whereas the fat-soluble ones tend to be stored in the body. With the essential elements, however, water solubility has no predictive value on the size of the safety factor. Numerous substances accumulate in tissues or form insoluble products and thus tend to have small safety factors. Many of the essential microelements have small safety factors; it is more dangerous to take a supplement of them than one of water-soluble vitamins.

It is also important to recognize that, just as there are a number of deficiency symptoms for lack of nutrient, there are multitoxic symptoms when too much is ingested. These, of course, may differ from the trivial to the serious. Whichever particular toxic symptom one chooses to define, the safety factor is largely a matter of judgment. In the controversy over fluoridation of public water supplies for example, the opponents of fluoridation cite as toxic the concentration that produces a whitish area on the teeth that can only be seen by microscopic examination by a trained observer. This effect is considered trivial by knowledgeable dentists.

Yiamouyiannis and Burk (1977) of the National Health Federation, however, have called 1 part per million of fluoride poisonous in the campaign to defeat referenda on fluoridation in various cities of the U.S. Taves (1979) has discussed this controversy and pointed out the errors in Yiamouyiannis' and Burks' interpretations of the data. However, Taves also criticized the National Cancer Institute for its procrastination in addressing this issue. Unfortunately, this scare tactic has been successful. The public schools should educate students on the importance of quantification in evaluating claims about toxic symptoms of food additives and environmental pollutants.

To summarize: Any or all of the essential nutrients can be toxic if consumed in sufficient quantities for a long enough time. As you will see in the section on dietary supplements, I am not opposed to supplements, but the amounts taken should be carefully monitored.

The second source of toxic food components comes from naturally occurring substances, contaminants, or additives. There are a large number of naturally occurring toxicants in foods (Wilson, 1984). Research has recently demonstrated that plants produce a wide variety of substances that repel or harm insects. In other words, there are natural products that serve the same functions as man-made insecticides or pesticides. Many of these toxicants are carcinogens or mutagens. They are usually present in very small quantities, and the human race has built up defenses against them. It has been said that if potatoes were offered as a new food in 1986, the FDA would not approve them because of their content of a toxic chemical called solanine. In contrast, the flavoring matter of root beer is now a synthetic chemical because the natural flavoring agent, safrole, is too toxic in the amounts consumed by enthusiastic root beer drinkers. As another example, coffee contains many carcinogens, but epidemiologists have not yet demonstrated that any of the common forms of cancer result from coffee consumption. Because natural toxicants are present in different foods in different concentrations, we have here another reason for eating a wide variety of foods.

Toxic Substances in the Common Environment

In addition to toxic effects of the nutrients when ingested in amounts beyond their safety factors, we are also subject to pollutants of various types that may be present in the air we breathe, the food we eat, and the water we drink. They may be generated by industry and emitted from smokestacks, or chemical dumps that may contaminate groundwater supplies. Our everyday practices, such as driving automobiles, may also produce large amounts of toxic products such as the lead aerosols that come from the tetraethyl lead added to gasolines to improve performance.

A Trail of Lead:
Rome, U.S. Inner Cities, and Mountain Meadows

Every schoolchild has heard about the fall of the Roman Empire. From Gibbon on, historians have speculated on the reasons for the fall. A recent hypothesis that is gaining favor among nutritionally minded historians emphasizes the importance of lead contamination of wine and food of the Roman nobility and upper classes (Gilfillan, 1965; Nriagu, 1983).

Many Roman emperors who reigned between 30 BC and 220 AD— among them Claudius, Caligula, Nero, and Tiberius—as well as members of the Roman upper classes, were prodigious drinkers of wine. The color and bouquet of their wine was enhanced by adding a grape syrup that had been boiled in leaded containers. According to Jerome Nriagu (1983), one teaspoon of this syrup would have been sufficient to cause chronic lead poisoning. In addition, upper-class Roman kitchens cooked food in lead-containing utensils, and unscrupulous tradesmen regularly added red lead to pepper to increase its weight. The end result of these practices is now interpreted as a widespread epidemic of lead poisoning in Roman nobility and their friends.

Chronic lead poisoning results in numbness, insomnia, digestive problems, and malfunctions of the nervous system such as memory loss, headaches, drowsiness, convulsions, and stupor. Two other symptoms— decrease in fertility and gout—are also known to have occurred in the

Roman upper classes. Taken together, all of these effects, lasting over many generations, may have contributed greatly to the decline of the Roman Empire.

In modern America, a high percentage of inner-city black children have elevated blood levels of lead. The National Center for Health Statistics (1984) reported that 4% of all U.S. children have blood levels greater than 30 μg per deciliter—the cutoff point for referring children for medical follow-up. In contrast, 18.6% of inner-city black children have elevated levels compared to 4.5% for inner-city white children. The most common sources of lead in inner cities are paints, aerosols from gasoline, food, dust, soil, and drinking water.

Lead pollution, however, is not confined to inner cities or to urban areas. Hirao and Patterson (1974) found evidence of lead inputs in Thompson Canyon located in the crest of the High Sierras in California. They estimated that 1 kg of lead entered the watershed by dry deposition on foliage during the 4 summer months and 12 kg of lead coprecipitated with snow during the 8 winter months. They estimated that 97% of the aerosol lead entering the canyon came from smelter fumes and gasoline exhausts.

To counteract the growing lead pollution in the U.S., the Environmental Protection Agency (EPA) on March 4, 1985 ordered refiners to reduce the lead content of their gasolines by 90% by the end of the year. In a surprise move, the EPA ordered that lead be completely removed from gasoline by 1988 rather than the original date of 1995 (Sun, 1985). This step-up was prompted by two recent studies (Pirkle, Schwartz, Landis, & Harland, 1985) that found a strong statistical correlation between blood lead concentrations and high blood pressure in white males 40 to 59 years.

It should be mentioned that the Roman example is speculative. It is not proved, and it is unlikely that experiments can be devised to prove it. In contrast, the extent of U.S. lead pollution is based on analyses of children's and adults' blood, of dust, air, and vegetation. These examples provide a valuable contrast between reasonable scientific hypotheses that are without proof, and the dangers of U.S. lead pollution, that is backed up by analytical data.

Imitation Foods

Another dividend from our burgeoning technology is a new class of foods called *imitation foods*. This class includes synthetic foods or those that are nutritionally inferior to the food imitated. With the present emphasis on low-calorie foods, those that contain less than 90% of the U.S. RDA of a vitamin, element, protein, or calories of a food for which it is a substitute for must be labeled imitation. An amusing example of this practice concerns imitation margarine, which was originally developed as a butter substitute! Actually, the imitation margarine available in stores is regular margarine that has had air whipped into it so that a tablespoon now contains 70 kcal rather than the usual 100 kcal of regular margarine.

Essential Nutrients as Dietary Supplements

The use of pills, especially vitamin pills, as dietary supplements supports a huge industry in America. Surveys in which the percentage of people taking one or more supplemental nutrients show more than half of any given group consume extra vitamins. Perhaps this practice is part of Adelle Davis' legacy. In *Let's Get Well* (1965), she speaks of clients who placed their day's allotment of pills in a big bowl on the table and called it their "Davis Cup." *Prevention* magazine has touted supplementary nutrients for decades. Many of the popular nutrition books of the sixties and seventies contained glowing accounts of the effects of extra vitamins. Testimonies promoting supplements are common in *Preventive Organic Medicine* by Kurt Donsbach (1976), or *Secrets of Health and Beauty* by Linda Clark (1969). The so-called health food stores are replete with advertisements pounding the same drum.

In addition to these reasons, others contribute to the widespread use of dietary supplements. Agribusiness, supermarkets, and the foods they grow and sell have become suspect. It is as though the nutrients have been sucked out of supermarket products. Brodsky (1976) writes in *From Eden to Aquarius*, "The heating process used to pasteurize and homogenize milk kills harmful bacteria which it may contain, but it also kills the beneficial bacteria and necessary enzymes, leaving the product almost void of nutritional strength." I have seen similar statements in books by Paavo Airola and Jane Fonda. None of these authors support their statements with evidence. Additives have been castigated as somehow neutralizing the nutrients in foods. It seems to me that authors Davis, Donsbach, Brodsky, and Clark *assume* the following:

1. Processed foods purchased in supermarkets have lost their nutrients (vitamins and elements).
2. Unprocessed foods, such as fresh vegetables and fruits, are loaded with pesticides unless they were grown organically.
3. Natural vitamins are more effective than synthetic ones.
4. Many, if not most, diseases are caused by nutritional deficiencies and thus may be prevented and/or cured by a natural diet supplemented with megavitamins and minerals.

In my opinion these assumptions tend to overemphasize nutrition as a causative factor for disease. I submit that these assumptions are unrealistic at best and unwarranted at worst.

Another reason for taking supplements can be ascribed to the prevailing drug culture. We take pills for so many things, why not for nutrients too? Many people know that they aren't eating nutritiously. They are too busy to care and too busy to take the time to eat a proper breakfast, and to prepare an appetizing and nutritious dinner. They take a pill as insurance to supplement their known inadequate diet.

Who Needs Supplements?

For millions of years the human race survived, and often thrived, without the use of food supplements. Suddenly, in the past 40 years, supplements have been touted in many health food magazines as essential. What is behind this development? Does the greed of vitamin purveyors explain it all? There are a number of reasons that help explain what has happened.

Science-technology has provided the basis for supplements by creating the vitamin concept, determining the structure of vitamins and their mode of action, and finally synthesizing most of them in the laboratory. Products need markets, and in our type of society, advertising can create markets. All this has occurred. In addition, Americans have become acutely nutrition conscious since World War II. The existence of the RDAs, the federal surveys that have revealed nutrient deficiencies in various age groups and in all stratas of society, have made many people uneasy about their own diets.

The Results of Federal Dietary Surveys

Since 1965 the U.S. government has carried out five large surveys of the nutrient intake of Americans. The findings have been remarkably consistent. Nutrients whose intake was 70% or less of the RDA in 20% or more of the population surveyed were classified as *problem nutrients*. Vitamin A occurred in this group in four out of five surveys, vitamin C in all five, riboflavin in two, and pyridoxine and thiamin in one. In the group of essential elements, both calcium and iron occurred four times and magnesium once. Unfortunately, not all nutrients were surveyed. The status of zinc and folacin (folate) is not known. What should a person do about it? There are two obvious solutions: eat an adequate diet or take a supplement. Which is preferable?

I want to say at the outset that I am not opposed to supplements *in toto* for all people at all times. I cannot make a blanket statement on nutritive supplements for individuals. Nutrition-conscious people who know about nutrient density of foods and the four food groups can probably do well without supplements. It takes some work to acquire the knowledge to keep nutrients in mind while shopping or ordering a meal in a restaurant. If this rather boring activity can be avoided by popping a One-a-day vitamin, why not do it?

Pros and Cons of Dietary Supplements

Taking a daily multivitamin pill as insurance is easy, is relatively cheap, and gives one peace of mind so that even if one's diet isn't all that it should be, one believes one has a cushion to prevent a serious deficiency disease from developing. Then there is the *placebo* effect. If people think that a supplement will make them more attractive, grow hair, and improve not only their sex life but also their golf game, then the added confidence may actually improve their performance. Still another factor revolves around the idea of individual differences. Many people are aware that they do not know their nutritive requirements, have heard about individual differences, and assume that their requirements may be above the mean. The solution? Take a supplement. However, most professional nutritionists advocate obtaining one's nutrients from foods unless a person has special requirements. What are their reasons? I'll mention six.

First, eating should be an enjoyable experience whether one is eating alone, with friends and family, or at a banquet. To consider food as a kind of prescription or primarily as a source of nutrients is to miss the point. Eating a variety of foods makes life more interesting as well as providing us with energy and nutrients. Learning enough about the nutrient content of foods in relation to health fits into this viewpoint without becoming a fetish. To paraphrase a popular expression: Eating food is the natural way to obtain good nutrition.

Second, supplements contain only noncalorific nutrients, and a person taking them may fall into the habit of thinking they are more important than source of calories. Actually, the problems with food selection these days is not so much with the noncalorific nutrients as with the calorific ones. The major diseases of the developed world are more closely related to overeating and high-fat diets than to vitamin-element deficiencies.

Third, I consider fiber as a noncalorific nutrient. It would be difficult to obtain a fiber supplement that contained balanced amounts of the six types of dietary fiber.

Fourth, available supplements contain far more than the recognized essential nutrients, and their contents are subject to fads. A few of the supplements that can be purchased in health food stores contain kelp, lecithin, inositol, choline, chelated minerals, and vitamins B_{15} and B_{17}. If a person is taking supplements because he or she doesn't want to learn about nutrition, how is he or she going to handle this question? Have you ever met a vitamin salesperson who advised you not to buy one of their products? Ignorance makes a person a sucker for every quack that comes along. Also, don't expect to get sound nutrition information from the brochures in health food stores. Their function is to sell products, not educate.

Consumer Reports (1985) discusses the use of supplements in some detail. The publication lists 42 products that make unproven claims in violation of federal law and emphasizes five products considered especially dangerous because the claimed benefits concern various life-threatening diseases, such as diabetic cataracts, cancer-producing processes, coronary heart disease, angina pectoris, adrenal insufficiency, and osteoporosis. These five products are Bio-flavonoid complex, Padma 28, Meganephrine,

DMSO, and Rheumoid. A person with symptoms or suspicions of these diseases who ingests any of these products instead of seeing a physician is acting dangerously.

Fifth, uncareful use of supplements may lead to overdosages. This caution holds true especially for vitamins A and D but also for some of the water-soluble vitamins, as well as elements that are not readily excreted. Refer to Table 6A.4 for quantitative amounts.

In the past few years a new form of mineral supplement has been introduced called *chelated minerals*. The pitch here is that through *chelation* the inorganic essential nutrients like calcium, magnesium, zinc, and iron become more soluble and the percentage absorbed will be increased. Absorption may well be increased, and herein lies the danger. As indicated in Figure 6.3, all nutrients have an optimum maximum concentration in the body. If this amount is exceeded, the nutrient acts as a poison. Thus, if you purchase and use chelated mineral preparations, you should be very careful that you do not overdose yourself.

For example, the RDA for zinc is 15 mg/day. Up to 30 mg/day is considered safe. The zinc supplements that are available in stores include dosages of 10, 22, 30, 50, and 100 mg. What might happen to a person taking the larger amounts on a regular basis? Excess zinc decreases the absorption of copper, which in turn, may result in *hypercholesterolemia*, a risk factor for *atherosclerosis* and heart disease. How many people know of this relationship between zinc and copper? If more copper is taken as a supplement, still other complications set in. The answer? Obtain your copper and zinc from foods, not supplements. You are far less apt to run into serious complications.

Sixth, and finally, is the matter of expense. I have a rich friend who said that he could not afford to buy the amino acid tryptophan. When I asked him the reason, he said that he had calculated the cost of a pound of it compared to obtaining it in milk or meat. He said that at these prices for amino acids he would soon go broke if he bought them as supplements.

Tryptophan: 500 mg, 30 tablets $6.57 (before tax) K Mart = about $200/lb
Lysine: 500 mg, 100 tablets $5.69 (before tax) drugstore = about $50/lb

In recent years, I have seen protein supplements on sale at health food stores and weight-lifting studios. It may seem reasonable that people with big muscles, which are made up of proteins, should need more protein in their diets. Here, we have another example of how common sense can be misleading. An adequate diet that contains 12% protein provides enough to furnish all the amino acids for the synthesis of large muscles. Protein supplements, sold as muscle-building pills and powders, are a very expensive way to obtain energy. I consider them as completely unnecessary and possibly semitoxic on a long-term basis, for the reasons given in chapter 5, if a person is already eating an adequate amount of protein.

Now for an exception. Adults who dislike milk products may have an insufficient calcium intake. They may benefit from a daily calcium supplement to bring their total intake into the range of 800-1,500 mg/day. Some natural sources of calcium such as dolomite and bone meal have been found to be contaminated by relatively large amounts of lead. I would suggest that you purchase only those brands that have been analyzed and shown to be lead free.

There are two special groups of individuals whose needs for supplements require separate consideration. The first group are those people who do not control their food supply, such as those who eat in restaurants or boarding houses most of the time. Many elderly people are also in this category. Food that has been kept hot for an indefinite period of time may lose considerable amounts of heat-sensitive vitamins. If people have no choice but to eat overcooked vegetables, they may be subject to low intake of both vitamins and essential elements. If I were in this position, I would buy fresh fruits and eat at least two a day all year long.

The other group consists of smokers, heavy drinkers, and contraceptive pill users. Blood analyses have shown that smokers are low in vitamin C, and the others in a variety of B-vitamins. As mentioned earlier, heavy drinkers are often low in magnesium. Smokers might be advised to reach for an orange instead of a smoke. The others could just as easily correct their presumed deficiencies with foods rich in B-vitamins as to take a multivitamin pill.

The special requirements of infants and pregnant and lactating women are well recognized and are included in the RDA Table A5.2. Vegans who use no animal products need a supplementary source of vitamin B_{12}. Teens who drink a lot of soft drinks and little milk may require extra calcium. A modern myth that I hope is dying is that athletes, especially body builders, require extra protein. Physically active people require more calories, preferably in the form of plant starches, and that is all.

Public Supplements

There are two sources of nutrient supplements in the public food supply. The first is in enriched grains such as wheat and rice products. Actually the word *enriched* is something of a misnomer because what is added brings back the amounts of thiamin, riboflavin, niacin, and iron to the same concentration as was in the original flour. The other comes from the addition of vitamins A and D in dairy products and margarine. Fluoride is added to the drinking water in many cities in the eastern half of the U.S. This practice has been demonstrated as one of the most effective Public Health measures ever implemented. Antifluoridationists in various parts of the U.S. have raised fears that fluoridation will increase cancer incidence, cause chromosomal damage, and result in unsightly mottling of teeth. These claims are without scientific foundation (Taves, 1979). In areas where the water is not fluoridated, it is advisable, especially if children are involved, to obtain a physician's prescription for sodium fluoride or some other source of fluoride.

The Dual Nature of Vitamin D

Vitamin D has the distinction of becoming the first hormone to be classed as a vitamin. This statement may strike you as odd, inconsistent, or even wrong. Everyone knows that a vitamin is a chemical that we require in our food and a hormone is a chemical that we synthesize within our own bodies. Why should we require something that we can make ourselves? Working out the answer required years of research. Sunlight is necessary for us to synthesize the hormone. This result implies that humans evolved under conditions where they were exposed to sunlight the year around. Fair-skinned people can obtain their daily supply of the hormone in 30 minutes of exposure to sunlight; dark-skinned people may require up to 3 hours. This difference in exposure requirement has been used to explain why the peoples of Northern Europe are fairer skinned than those from Southern Europe.

A derivative of cholesterol is converted by sunlight in the skin to a chemical that is called previtamin D_3. This substance is changed by body heat to vitamin D_3 which enters the blood stream and, after undergoing enzymatic alteration in the liver and kidney, circulates as the active hormone. It functions to increase calcium absorption in the gut and and deposition in bones. In the absence of vitamin D hormone, the bones are weak and mis-shapen due to a lack of calcium. The disease is called rickets. Now, human exposure to sunlight is highly variable. Hunter-gatherers and later agricultural peoples labored outside from sunrise to sunset, on cloudy days and on clear. What was to prevent them from getting an overdose of the hormone on a succession of clear, sunny days? According to Holick, MacLaughlin and Doppelt (1981), extra sunlight converts previtamin D_3 to inactive products that remain in the skin and are sloughed off. These reactions regulate the amount of vitamin D_3 that can be formed in a day and prevents the synthesis of toxic amounts.

The vitamin D_3 that is present in foods or in vitamin supplements, however, is not subject to physiological regulation. All of it is converted to the active substance. This important difference in control mechanism may explain why vitamin D exhibits one of the narrowest windows of safety of any essential nutrient. The RDA for adults is set at 200 IU, but 100 IU is sufficient to prevent rickets. The RDA for children with growing bones is set at 400 IU. Milk is fortified with 400 IU of vitamin D per quart so that someone who drinks this much milk daily is already ingesting

2 times the RDA for an adult. Many cold breakfast cereals, butter, and margarine are also fortified with vitamin D.

Possible Dangers of Vitamin D Toxicity From Normal Diets

To my knowledge, no survey has been made that has attempted to measure the number of people who are sensitive to extra amounts of vitamin D in their diet. The amounts of vitamin D that are added to milk or allowed in vitamin supplements (400 IU) were set in 1968 and represent the information available at that time. I suggest that the safe amounts for some people are lower than what is now permitted. Until the regulations are changed, I further suggest that readers of this book examine labels of foods and vitamin supplements carefully to prevent ingesting toxic amounts of vitamin D. Remember that, if you are out-of-doors very much, you need little, if any, vitamin D in foods. Toxic side effects have been found on a daily intake as low as 1,000 IU. Thus, a milk drinker who also takes a vitamin supplement may be close to a toxic dose.

Miller and Hayes (1982) state that a daily intake in excess of 50,000 IU is needed to produce toxicity in most adults. Some of the symptoms are muscle weakness, nausea, vomiting, constipation, dehydration, *hypercalcemia*, and calcification of soft tissues such as arteries, kidneys, and lungs. Taylor (1972) reported that several years intake of modest amounts of vitamin D (1,000-2,000 IU per day) may result in the passing of stones in the urine. This condition is often painful and may also become serious medically.

On the other hand, smaller excesses may produce complications in sensitive individuals. The effects of moderately high intakes on hypercholesterolemia will be discussed in chapter 10. Table 6.11 lists the vitamin D content of some common foods. The first five are fortified.

Principles and Perils of Nutritional Self-Experimentation

Whether you cook for yourself or a family, or whether you eat out most of the time, you are making many decisions each day about what food you eat and how it is prepared. Practically speaking, you are acting as an amateur nutritionist, comparable to a professional who is in charge of a dining facility for a thousand people. The main difference between you and her is that she has been trained for her job and you have not. Fortunately, you can readily learn the principles.

Table 6.11   Vitamin D Content of Some Common Foods and Multivitamin Preparations

Food	Vitamin D Content, IU[1]
Milk, 1 qt	400
Special K, 1 oz	50
NutriGrain, 1 oz	50
100% Corn oil margarine Premium, Mazola, 3.5 oz	320
Butter, 3.5 oz	40
Egg yolk, 3.5 oz	25
Herring, fresh or canned, 3.5 oz	900
Liver, 3.5 oz Beef, pork	45
Chicken	50-70
Mackerel, fresh, 3.5 oz	700
Salmon, fresh or canned, 4 oz	150-550
Sardines, canned, 3.5 oz	300
Shrimp, 3.5 oz	105

Multivitamins and Elements	Suggested Dosage	Vitamin D Content IU[2]
Multicebrin	1 tablet/day	1,000
Theragran	1 tablet/day	400
Vi-Daylin, chewable	1 tablet/day	400
Calcium plus (GNC)	3 tablets/day	400
Nutriplus	1 tablet/day	400
Naturemade, Mega 1000	1 tablet/day	400
Myadec	1 tablet/day	400
Geritol complete	3 tablets/day	1,200
One-A-Day	1 tablet/day	400
Therapeutic M	1 tablet/day	400

[1]Vitamin D content of foods from *Food Values of Portions Commonly Used* (p. 215) by J.A. Pennington and H.N. Church, 1985, Philadelphia: Lippincott. Copyright 1985 by Lippincott. Adapted by permission.

[2]Vitamin D content of multivitamin preparations collected by S.R. Dickman, 1986, unpublished.

But on further reflection it becomes obvious that your situation is even more complicated than that of a professional nutritionist. She is not directly concerned with the health of her clients. She may not know them personally or be aware of their personal idiosyncracies about food. You have the double responsibility of selecting a diet as well as evaluating its effects.

In this dual role, you are literally acting like a scientist in the laboratory whose objective is that of discovering new facts about nature. You, like a scientist, utilize the knowledge at your disposal to help you make decisions on diet. If you try something different, like taking a vitamin supplement, you, like a researcher, are in a position to draw conclusions from the new facts at your disposal. Changing some aspect of your diet or lifestyle is easy. Drawing sound conclusions from the results of that change is difficult.

For example, on eating breakfast with a group of friends, a young man said, "I can't eat eggs." On being questioned, he didn't know if a portion of an egg would make him sick, if the manner of cooking would make a difference, or if eating eggs included in potato salad would have a similar effect. He was pressed for more details about his unusual inability to digest eggs. He said it all began after an all-night drinking party with friends. They went out to breakfast at a hash joint, and he had ordered two fried eggs. They were very greasy but he ate them anyway. Later, he became sick and threw up. Since then, eating eggs has made him feel so queasy that he has stopped ordering them. He wondered what had happened to his digestive system because he had always enjoyed eggs before this incident.

When it was pointed out to him that it was probably the combination of alcohol and fat that had upset his digestive system, and not the eggs, he immediately went to a cafe, ordered a three-egg omelette, and has been eating them happily ever since.

This example illustrates three common traps. The first is that of placing two events in a cause-effect relationship in the presence of many other variables. The next was not being aware of the importance of subjective factors (feelings) in his response to later incidents. As a result, he committed the third error of generalizing from a single incident.

I suggest that we all should become expert in the art of testing; that is, experimenting on ourselves to decide if a given effect is repeatable or is a onetime event. The facts that you discover and the conclusions you draw from them will apply to you alone. You should also be prepared for the tricks that your own psyche will play on you. Let me explain.

It is now recognized that humans respond to experiments in peculiarly human ways. If 100 people are given a pill that may contain vitamins or chalk, a majority of them will report some beneficial effect even though they didn't know which pill they took. This is called the *placebo effect* and is thought to be due to the positive effects of receiving attention (placebo, Latin, = I shall please). To overcome this effect in nutritional experiments, the actual material being tested is shifted back and forth with the placebo so that the subjects become used to being tested. These are called single-blind experiments.

But expectations of what the results should be are also present in the scientists in charge of the experiment, who are also human. In examining the subjects, if the scientists anticipate a positive effect, they are apt to find one, and vice versa. For this reason, in carefully controlled nutritional experiments where some of the results are based on human judgment, the examiners are unaware of what substance the subject has consumed. This is also a single-blind experiment but of a different type from the one mentioned above. In the most carefully controlled experiments, neither the subject nor the examiner knows what has been consumed. This is called a double-blind experiment and furnishes the most objective results.

Now let us contrast the double-blind situation with a typical one in which a person is taking a multivitamin supplement for the first time. His friends have assured him in advance that he will feel better, he will have more pep and energy, his golf game will improve, and he will feel 10 years younger. In addition, he believes that if something costs over a dollar a day, it has to do some good. With all this psychological buildup, the person does feel and perform better than he has for some time, and another person joins the list of suckers of health through pills.

If we examine this situation from a scientific standpoint, we can easily recognize that it was not an experiment at all. An x number of vitamins have been added to his usual consumption of food and drink. His daily life remained as variable as ever with the exception that his ego has received a big boost from his friends. The only data are his subjective feelings, which, as we have seen above, are unreliable. The net effect of his taking vitamins is as inconclusive as most events in a person's life.

Having introduced the subject of self-experimentation with a negative example, I now feel obliged to say that it is not an impossible situation. If it is to have any value, much more care in its planning and execution will be necessary than in the example cited above. I'll mention a few criteria that should be followed in personal experiments of this type and then illustrate the principles with positive examples.

The criteria used should be as objective as possible. By this I mean quantitative measurements of such things as blood pressure, pulse rate, weight, and angle that a limb can bend, should be included whenever possible. These measurements should be made at least once a week and should also be inexpensive and convenient.

The self-experimenter needs to be patient. It may take months to establish a single conclusion. Frankly speaking, it will require considerable motivation to keep at the experiment long enough to establish anything. Time is necessary to even out the variables and even then an emotional upset resulting from a divorce or separation, loss of a job, or other major disappointment can invalidate the whole enterprise.

This brings me to the subjective factors, which are the trickiest variables of all. Most of us rationalize our actions and reactions so that no matter what happens, we can justify what we did. The rational person has learned to poke holes through this screen. We must try to look at ourselves and to evaluate our actions as though they were carried out by someone else. It is for this reason that I emphasized that objective measurements above. They provide a little reality to which you can tie your experiment. Most people who attempt to judge the effects of an experiment by their feelings will either be disappointed or fall into the trap formed from their own illusions.

Before you start, you should realize the objective of the experiment very clearly. State it to yourself, or better, write it down. In addition to knowing what evidence you are looking for, you need to know how frequently you will obtain results to judge how the experiment is going. You should also have a definite idea as to how long the experiment is to last. Can you expect results in a week, a month, a year, 10 years?

You should choose what you are going to do very carefully and be aware of the limitations in the choice. Are you going to take extra vitamin A to see if your complexion will improve? How much will you take every day? Is it by itself or present in a capsule with other vitamins? Is anyone besides yourself going to judge your complexion? Is there anything else you should examine, like cold sores, skin condition on other parts of your body, or the lustre of your hair?

One of the main questions people need to answer before beginning a dietary modification is whether they just want results, or whether they want to know if the change in diet was responsible for the results in case there are any. What I have written in this chapter is directed to people in the second category.

Roger J. Williams (1975) has described a fairly common type of self-experimentation. A science professor was bothered by sores on his face, and it was diagnosed as psoriasis. A friend told him that vitamin A was occasionally beneficial for this condition; so he began taking about 25,000 international units of vitamin A per day. After some months the rash disappeared and did not return. At this point he made an extended visit to a foreign country in which extra vitamin A was unavailable. After some months the rash reappeared. On returning to this country, he resumed his consumption of the extra vitamin A and the rash disappeared again.

Does this experiment prove that vitamin A cures psoriasis? Not at all. One example is insufficient for a generalization. It does demonstrate, however, that in this individual vitamin A was effective in removing the rash. Does this incident suggest that you take extra vitamin A if you have a rash on your face? We are in the anecdotal range of confidence and the chances of your being helped are 0%–1%. Even so, it falls in the class of "can't hurt—might help." Why not try it for six months? If your rash goes away, would you be inclined consciously to stop and see if it came back? If it did, what would it prove?

The Effect of Diet on Behavior:
The Allergy and Feingold Hypotheses

Some healthy, active children—sometimes called hyperactive by distraught parents—have become the center of an interesting controversy. One hypothesis states that allergies to specific foods cause behavioral problems. Food allergies are quite rare; an immediate reaction to a particular food occurs in less than 1% of North Americans. Beyond the difficulty of the diagnosis lies the even greater complication of relating the allergy to hyperactive behavior. Many parents lose interest in the allergy hypothesis when they realize the time, expense, and trouble that pursuing it to the end would entail.

Thus, when the Feingold (1975) hypothesis appeared, which stated that hyperactivity resulted from food additives such as artificial colors and flavors, it appealed immediately to thousands of parents at their wits' end in understanding and controlling the behavior of their children. Checking up on the Feingold hypothesis requires monitoring all the foods that children eat to ensure that they are free from additives. Many parents were so pleased with the results that they formed "Feingold Societies" to exchange information on food sources as well as to receive positive reinforcement on the undertaking.

When nutritionist-psychologists set up double-blind experiments, however, they soon discovered that the situation was far more complicated than just a dietary change. The child was receiving far more attention than previously. In addition, this attention was positive rather than negative. The child learned that all these changes in the family's diet as well as his or her own were for his or her benefit. The message was that the family was actually trying to help, not just to criticize. The double-blind experiments came up with an unexpected conclusion: The Feingold diet appeared effective in a fair percentage of trials, due to changes not in diet but in the attitudes of all the participants (Consensus Conference on Defined Diets and Childhood Hyperactivity, 1983).

This example illustrates one of the strengths of science. In evaluating a hypothesis experimentally, scientists often control variables that were not controlled originally. As was demonstrated here, whereas the Feingold diet hypothesis was not confirmed for most children, the experiments demonstrated that the positive results were probably due to the changed psychological factors between parents and child.

Summary

The main objectives of eating may be stated as enjoying well-prepared foods that furnish sufficient but not excess calories for a person's needs, and that also provide sufficient amounts of the essential noncalorific nutrients. The latter two objectives can be met by the application of two quite simple ideas: nutrient density and caloric content of food constituents.

The understanding and use of nutrient density is one of the most valuable applications of science to the purchasing and eating of foods. Fortunately, present-day labels contain information that make it possible to estimate the nutrient density of a number of essential nutrients in your head while shopping. Nutrient density calculations also allow the distinction between junk foods and nutritious foods to be made on a rational basis. Knowledge of the caloric content of the foodstuffs' proteins, carbohydrates, and fats as 4, 4, and 9, kcal/g, respectively, is also valuable and practical.

The four-food-groups-plus-one plan has been developed for people who don't want to make any calculations. One can obtain a healthy diet by eating a variety of foods regularly from each of the four food groups and occasionally from the plus one group.

Table 6A.1 Index of Nutritional Adequacy Food Profiles

Barbecue sauce
Analysis of 1 cup (250 g), which supplies 230 kcal of energy

Nutrient	Unit	Amount	INA	% RDA	0%	10%	20%	30%	40%	50%	60%	70%	80%	90%	100%
Energy	kcal	230.00	1.00	12											*
Protein	g	4.00	0.70	8											*
VA	IU	900.00	1.96	23											*
VC	mg	13.00	1.88	22											*
Thiamin	mg	0.03	0.26	3											*
Riboflavin	mg	0.03	0.22	3											*
Niacin	mg	0.80	0.50	6											*
Ca	mg	53.00	0.51	6											*
Fe	mg	2.00	1.09	13											*

Gelatin dessert, prepared with water
Analysis of 1 cup (240 g), which supplies 140 kcal of energy

Nutrient	Unit	Amount	INA	% RDA	0%	10%	20%	30%	40%	50%	60%	70%	80%	90%	100%
Energy	kcal	140.00	1.00	7											*
Protein	g	4.00	1.14	8											*
VA	IU	0.00	0.00	0											*
VC	mg	0.00	0.00	0											*
Thiamin	mg	0.00	0.00	0											*
Riboflavin	mg	0.00	0.00	0											*
Niacin	mg	0.00	0.00	0											*
Ca	mg	0.00	0.00	0											*
Fe	mg	0.00	0.00	0											*

Olives, pickled, green
Analysis of 4 med, 3 ex lg, 2 gt (15 g), which supplies 15 kcal of energy

Nutrient	Unit	Amount	INA	% RDA	0%	10%	20%	30%	40%	50%	60%	70%	80%	90%	100%
Energy	kcal	15.00	1.00	1											*
Protein	g	0.00	0.00	0											*
VA	IU	40.00	1.23	1											*
VC	mg	0.00	0.00	0											*
Thiamin	mg	0.00	0.00	0											*
Riboflavin	mg	0.00	0.00	0											*
Niacin	mg	0.00	0.00	0											*
Ca	mg	8.00	1.23	1											*
Fe	mg	0.20	1.70	1											*

Popsicle, 3 fl oz size
Analysis of 1 popsicle (95 g), which supplies 70 kcal of energy

Nutrient	Unit	Amount	INA	% RDA	0%	10%	20%	30%	40%	50%	60%	70%	80%	90%	100%
Energy	kcal	70.00	1.00	4											*
Protein	g	0.00	0.00	0											*
VA	IU	0.00	0.00	0											*
VC	mg	0.00	0.00	0											*
Thiamin	mg	0.00	0.00	0											*
Riboflavin	mg	0.00	0.00	0											*
Niacin	mg	0.00	0.00	0											*
Ca	mg	0.00	0.00	0											*
Fe	mg	0.00	0.00	0											*

(Cont.)

Table 6A.1 Cont.

Pudding mix, chocolate, dry form, instant, 4 oz package
Analysis of 1 pkg (260 g), which supplies 325 kcal of energy

Nutrient	Unit	Amount	INA	% RDA	0%	10%	20%	30%	40%	50%	60%	70%	80%	90%	100%
Energy	kcal	325.00	1.00	16											
Protein	g	8.00	0.98	16											
VA	IU	340.00	0.52	9											
VC	mg	2.00	0.21	3											
Thiamin	mg	0.08	0.49	8											
Riboflavin	mg	0.39	2.00	33											
Niacin	mg	0.30	0.13	2											
Ca	mg	374.00	2.56	42											
Fe	mg	1.30	0.50	8											

Sherbert
Analysis of 1 cup (193 g), which supplies 270 kcal of energy

Nutrient	Unit	Amount	INA	% RDA	0%	10%	20%	30%	40%	50%	60%	70%	80%	90%	100%
Energy	kcal	270.00	1.00	14											
Protein	g	2.00	0.30	4											
VA	IU	190.00	0.35	5											
VC	mg	4.00	0.49	7											
Thiamin	mg	0.03	0.22	3											
Riboflavin	mg	0.09	0.56	8											
Niacin	mg	0.10	0.05	1											
Ca	mg	103.00	0.85	11											
Fe	mg	0.30	0.14	2											

Tapioca desserts, apple
Analysis of 1 cup (250 g), which supplies 295 kcal of energy

Nutrient	Unit	Amount	INA	% RDA	0%	10%	20%	30%	40%	50%	60%	70%	80%	90%	100%
Energy	kcal	295.00	1.00	13											*
Protein	g	1.00	0.12	2											*
VA	IU	30.00	0.05	1											*
VC	mg	0.00	0.00	0											*
Thiamin	mg	0.00	0.00	0											*
Riboflavin	mg	0.00	0.00	0											*
Niacin	mg	0.00	0.00	0											*
Ca	mg	0.00	0.06	1											*
Fe	mg	0.50	0.22	3											*

Tapioca desserts, cream pudding
Analysis of 1 cup (165 g), which supplies 220 kcal of energy

Nutrient	Unit	Amount	INA	% RDA	0%	10%	20%	30%	40%	50%	60%	70%	80%	90%	100%
Energy	kcal	220.00	1.00	11											*
Protein	g	8.00	1.45	16											*
VA	IU	480.00	1.09	12											*
VC	mg	2.00	0.30	3											*
Thiamin	mg	0.07	0.64	7											*
Riboflavin	mg	0.30	2.27	25											*
Niacin	mg	0.20	0.13	1											*
Ca	mg	173.00	1.75	19											*
Fe	mg	0.70	0.40	4											*

(Cont.)

Table 6A.1 Cont.

Milk, fluid, whole 3.3% fat
Analysis of 1 cup (244 g), which supplies 150 kcal of energy

Nutrient	Unit	Amount	INA	% RDA
Energy	kcal	150.00	1.00	8
Protein	g	8.00	2.13	16
VA	IU	310.00	1.03	8
VC	mg	2.00	0.44	3
Thiamin	mg	0.09	0.20	9
Riboflavin	mg	0.40	4.44	33
Niacin	mg	0.20	0.19	1
Ca	mg	291.00	4.31	32
Fe	mg	0.10	0.08	1

Milk, fluid, nonfat (skim)
Analysis of 1 cup (245 g), which supplies 90 kcal of energy

Nutrient	Unit	Amount	INA	% RDA
Energy	kcal	90.00	1.00	5
Protein	g	9.00	4.00	18
VA	IU	500.00	2.78	13
VC	mg	2.00	0.74	3
Thiamin	mg	0.10	2.22	10
Riboflavin	mg	0.43	7.96	36
Niacin	mg	0.20	0.32	1
Ca	mg	315.00	7.80	35
Fe	mg	0.10	0.14	1

Eggs, lg 24 oz dz, raw/cooked in shell, whole w/o shell
Analysis of 1 egg (50 g), which supplies 80 kcal of energy

Nutrient	Unit	Amount	INA	% RDA	0%	10%	20%	30%	40%	50%	60%	70%	80%	90%	100%
Energy	kcal	80.00	1.00	4											*
Protein	g	6.00	3.00	12											*
VA	IU	260.00	1.63	7											*
VC	mg	0.00	0.00	0											*
Thiamin	mg	0.04	1.00	4											*
Riboflavin	mg	0.14	3.13	13											*
Niacin	mg	0.00	0.00	0											*
Ca	mg	28.00	0.78	3											*
Fe	mg	1.00	1.56	6											*

Eggs, lg 24 oz per dz, scrambled with milk and butter
Analysis of 1 egg (64 g), which supplies 95 kcal of energy

Nutrient	Unit	Amount	INA	% RDA	0%	10%	20%	30%	40%	50%	60%	70%	80%	90%	100%
Energy	kcal	95.00	1.00	5											*
Protein	g	6.00	2.53	12											*
VA	IU	310.00	1.63	8											*
VC	mg	0.00	0.00	0											*
Thiamin	mg	0.04	0.84	4											*
Riboflavin	mg	0.16	2.81	13											*
Niacin	mg	0.00	0.00	0											*
Ca	mg	47.00	1.10	5											*
Fe	mg	0.90	1.18	6											*

(Cont.)

Table 6A.1   Cont.

Bacon (20 slices/lb, 2 slices raw), broiled/fried, crisp
Analysis of 2 slices (15 g), which supplies 85 kcal of energy

Nutrient	Unit	Amount	INA	% RDA	0%	10%	20%	30%	40%	50%	60%	70%	80%	90%	100%
Energy	kcal	85.00	1.00	4											*
Protein	g	4.00	1.88	8											*
VA	IU	0.00	0.00	0											*
VC	mg	0.00	0.00	0											*
Thiamin	mg	0.08	1.88	8											*
Riboflavin	mg	0.05	0.98	4											*
Niacin	mg	0.80	1.34	6											*
Ca	mg	2.00	0.05	0											*
Fe	mg	0.50	0.74	3											*

Beef, cooked, hamburger (ground beef), broiled, lean
Analysis of 3 oz (85 g), which supplies 185 kcal of energy

Nutrient	Unit	Amount	INA	% RDA	0%	10%	20%	30%	40%	50%	60%	70%	80%	90%	100%
Energy	kcal	185.00	1.00	9											*
Protein	g	23.00	4.97	46											*
VA	IU	20.00	0.05	1											*
VC	mg	0.00	0.00	0											*
Thiamin	mg	0.08	0.86	8											*
Riboflavin	mg	0.20	1.80	17											*
Niacin	mg	5.10	3.94	36											*
Ca	mg	10.00	0.12	1											*
Fe	mg	3.00	2.03	19											*

Beef, cooked, hamburger (ground beef), broiled, regular
Analysis of 3 oz (85 g), which supplies 245 kcal of energy

Nutrient	Unit	Amount	INA	% RDA	0%	10%	20%	30%	40%	50%	60%	70%	80%	90%	100%
Energy	kcal	245.00	1.00	12											*
Protein	g	23.00	3.76	46											*
VA	IU	30.00	0.06	1											*
VC	mg	0.00	0.00	0											*
Thiamin	mg	0.04	0.33	4											*
Riboflavin	mg	0.18	1.22	15											*
Niacin	mg	3.60	2.10	26											*
Ca	mg	10.00	0.09	1											*
Fe	mg	2.90	1.48	18											*

Beef, cooked, steak, broiled, such as sirloin, lean and fat
Analysis of 3 oz (85 g), which supplies 330 kcal of energy

Nutrient	Unit	Amount	INA	% RDA	0%	10%	20%	30%	40%	50%	60%	70%	80%	90%	100%
Energy	kcal	330.00	1.00	17											*
Protein	g	20.00	2.42	40											*
VA	IU	50.00	0.08	1											*
VC	mg	0.00	0.00	0											*
Thiamin	mg	0.05	0.30	5											*
Riboflavin	mg	0.15	0.76	13											*
Niacin	mg	4.00	1.73	29											*
Ca	mg	9.00	0.06	1											*
Fe	mg	2.50	0.95	16											*

(Cont.)

Table 6A.1   Cont.

Beef and vegetable stew
Analysis of 1 cup (245 g), which supplies 220 kcal of energy

Nutrient	Unit	Amount	INA	% RDA
Energy	kcal	220.00	1.00	11
Protein	g	16.00	2.91	32
VA	IU	2,400.00	5.45	60
VC	mg	17.00	2.58	28
Thiamin	mg	0.15	1.36	15
Riboflavin	mg	0.17	1.29	14
Niacin	mg	4.70	3.05	34
Ca	mg	29.00	0.29	3
Fe	mg	2.90	1.65	18

Chicken, cooked, breast, fried, 1/2 breast, bones removed
Analysis of 2.8 oz (79 g), which supplies 160 kcal of energy

Nutrient	Unit	Amount	INA	% RDA
Energy	kcal	160.00	1.00	8
Protein	g	26.00	6.50	52
VA	IU	70.00	0.22	2
VC	mg	0.00	0.00	0
Thiamin	mg	0.04	0.50	4
Riboflavin	mg	0.17	1.77	14
Niacin	mg	11.60	10.36	83
Ca	mg	9.00	0.13	1
Fe	mg	1.30	1.02	8

Frankfurter, heated (8 per lb purchased pkg)
Analysis of 1 frank (56 g), which supplies 170 kcal of energy

Nutrient	Unit	Amount	INA	% RDA	0%	10%	20%	30%	40%	50%	60%	70%	80%	90%	100%
Energy	kcal	170.00	1.00	9											*
Protein	g	7.00	1.65	14											*
VA	IU	0.00	0.00	0											*
VC	mg	0.00	0.00	0											*
Thiamin	mg	0.08	0.94	8											*
Riboflavin	mg	0.11	1.08	9											*
Niacin	mg	1.40	1.18	10											*
Ca	mg	3.00	0.04	0											*
Fe	mg	0.80	0.59	5											*

Sardines, Atlantic, canned in oil, drained solids
Analysis of 3 oz (85 g), which supplies 175 kcal of energy

Nutrient	Unit	Amount	INA	% RDA	0%	10%	20%	30%	40%	50%	60%	70%	80%	90%	100%
Energy	kcal	175.00	1.00	9											*
Protein	g	20.00	4.57	40											*
VA	IU	190.00	0.54	5											*
VC	mg	0.00	0.00	0											*
Thiamin	mg	0.02	0.23	2											*
Riboflavin	mg	0.17	1.62	14											*
Niacin	mg	4.60	3.76	33											*
Ca	mg	372.00	4.72	41											*
Fe	mg	2.50	1.79	16											*

(Cont.)

Table 6A.1 Cont.

Broccoli, cooked, drained, whole stalks, medium size
Analysis of 1 stalk (187 g), which supplies 45 kcal of energy

Nutrient	Unit	Amount	INA	% RDA	0%	10%	20%	30%	40%	50%	60%	70%	80%	90%	100%
Energy	kcal	45.00	1.00	2											*
Protein	g	6.00	5.33	12											*
VA	IU	4,500.00	50.00	113											*113
VC	mg	162.00	120.00	270											*270
Thiamin	mg	0.16	7.11	16											*
Riboflavin	mg	0.36	13.33	30											*
Niacin	mg	1.40	4.44	10											*
Ca	mg	158.00	7.80	18											*
Fe	mg	1.40	3.89	9											*

Pancakes, plain or buttermilk (from mix w/egg, milk)
Analysis of 1 cake (27 g), which supplies 60 kcal of energy

Nutrient	Unit	Amount	INA	% RDA	0%	10%	20%	30%	40%	50%	60%	70%	80%	90%	100%
Energy	kcal	60.00	1.00	3											*
Protein	g	2.00	1.33	4											*
VA	IU	70.00	0.58	2											*
VC	mg	0.00	0.00	0											*
Thiamin	mg	0.04	1.33	4											*
Riboflavin	mg	0.06	1.67	5											*
Niacin	mg	0.20	0.48	1											*
Ca	mg	58.00	2.15	6											*
Fe	mg	0.30	0.63	2											*

Soups, canned, condensed, prepared w/equal vol water, tomato
Analysis of 1 cup (245 g), which supplies 90 kcal of energy

Nutrient	Unit	Amount	INA	% RDA	0%	10%	20%	30%	40%	50%	60%	70%	80%	90%	100%
Energy	kcal	90.00	1.00	5											*
Protein	g	2.00	0.89	4											*
VA	IU	1,000.00	5.56	25											*
VC	mg	12.00	4.44	20											*
Thiamin	mg	0.05	1.11	5											*
Riboflavin	mg	0.05	0.93	4											*
Niacin	mg	1.20	1.90	9											*
Ca	mg	15.00	0.37	2											*
Fe	mg	0.70	0.97	4											*

Note. Adapted from *Nutritional Quality Index of Foods* (pp. 176-541) by R.G. Hansen, A.W. Sorenson, A.J. Witwer, and B.W. Wyse, 1979, Westport, CT: Avi. Copyright 1979 by Avi. Adapted by permission.

VA = Vitamin A   Ca = Calcium
VC = Vitamin C   Fe = Iron

Table 6A.2 Interim Food Guide

The easy way to be sure that one is obtaining all the necessary nutrients is by following a *food guide*. A food guide groups together foods of similar nutrient content and figures out how many servings of each group must be chosen each day to meet nutrient needs. Single meals or whole-day menus may be planned around the food guide. It is a simple solution to an every-day headache.

The list below has been enlarged from older food guides to allow for nutrients about which more is known today. A variety of choices within food groups helps ensure balanced nutrient intake. Eat these foods every day:

Milk Products (protein foods providing calcium) •••••••••••••••••2 servings
One serving is a cup of milk, yogurt, or tofu; 1 1/2 oz of cheddar-type cheese or 1 1/2 cups ice cream. CALORIC RANGE: 80 (nonfat milk) to 375 (ice cream).

Meats, Eggs, Beans, Nuts (protein foods providing iron) •••••2 or 3 servings
One serving is 2 or 3 oz cooked (4 or 5 oz raw) lean, boneless meat, fish or poultry; 2 eggs; 1 cup cooked dry beans, lentils, or tofu; 4 tablespoons peanut butter; 1/2 cup tuna or nuts. CALORIC RANGE: 140 (2 eggs) to 400 (peanut butter).

Grain Products (breads, rice, cereals)••••••••••••••••••••••••••4 to 6 servings
One serving is 1 slice of bread or 1/2 cup cooked cereal, noodles, or rice; 3/4 cup dry cereal; 4 crackers; 1 pancake; 1 roll. Whole grain cereals are preferred because of higher levels of trace nutrients. CALORIC VALUE: 70 calories.

Vitamin C Rich Vegetable or Fruit••••••••••••••••••••••••••••••1 serving
One serving is 1 orange, 1/2 grapefruit, or 1/2 cup orange or grapefruit juice; 2 tomatoes; 1 1/2 cups tomato or pineapple juice; 1 stalk broccoli; 1/2 cup green or red pepper; 3/4 cup raw cabbage, greens, or chili peppers. CALORIC VALUE: 40 calories.

Dark Green Vegetable •••1 serving
One serving is 1 cup cooked broccoli, cabbage, greens, brussels sprouts, or asparagus; 1 1/2 to 2 cups raw dark green lettuce, spinach, or scallions (including tops). CALORIC VALUE: 40 calories.

Potato or Other Vegetable or Fruit ••••••••••••••••••••••••1 or 2 servings
One serving is 1/2 cup corn, beets, potatoes, yams, peas, onion, squash, or green beans; 1/4 cup raisins; 1 peach, apple, small banana, or pear; 4 prunes. CALORIC RANGE: 40 (fruits) to 70 (starchy vegetables).

Fats •••1 serving
One serving is 1 tablespoon oil, margarine, or mayonnaise. CALORIC RANGE: 100 calories (margarine or mayonnaise) to 120 (oils).

Plus Other Foods •••••••••••••••••••••••••••••••••••in Limited Amounts
Use limited amounts of sweets (candy, cookies, cake, sweet rolls, presweetened cereals, soft drinks, etc.); fatty foods (fat crackers, potato chips,

(Cont.)

Table 6A.2   (Cont.)

sauces, gravies, butter, margarine, sour cream, etc.); and *alcoholic beverages* (beer, wines, hard liquors).

NOTE: The food list above provides between 1,100 and 2,200 calories per day, depending on the choices within food groups. Persons who need more calories should choose more or larger servings. Persons who need fewer calories should consider increasing caloric expenditure through increased activity, rather than reducing food intake.

Some Menu Examples

The menus below are based on the Interim Food Guide. They are planned with a small family or single person in mind. Wasting of leftovers is avoided by repeating certain items. For example, tortillas are used in three different ways on three different days.

Breakfast	Lunch	Dinner	Snack
Orange juice Corn tortillas with melted cheese	Tuna sandwich on whole wheat bread Apple Tomato Milk	Tofu stir fry with carrots and broccoli Brown rice Pineapple chunks with bananas	Snack of mixed peanuts and sunflower seeds Milk Crackers
Whole orange, sectioned Split pea soup made with milk Whole wheat toast with margarine	Cottage cheese with chopped onion tops and parsley on romaine Bran muffin	Tacos with romaine, ground beef, grated cheese Cold cooked broccoli with French dressing Pineapple with yogurt	Tuna with mayonnaise on crackers Orange juice
Sliced bananas with milk Cooked egg Whole wheat toast with margarine	Split pea soup made with milk Raw cauliflower and carrots Crackers	Enchiladas made with tortillas, cheese, ground beef or cooked beans, tomato sauce Spinach salad with oil and vinegar Baked apple	Bran muffin Milk

(Cont.)

Table 6A.2 (Cont.)

Breakfast	Lunch	Dinner	Snack
Orange juice Whole wheat French toast with margarine and syrup Milk	Broth with tofu and green onions Brown rice sauteed with chopped vegetables and egg Fresh peach or pear	Sauteed chicken livers in oil Cooked greens Noodles Fruit yogurt	Applesauce Bran muffin
1/2 grapefruit Whole grain hot cereal with margarine and sugar Milk	Chopped chicken liver on whole wheat bread with mayonnaise Sliced green peppers and raw cauliflower	Scrambled eggs with cheese Bulgur or brown rice Corn with margarine Romaine salad with oil and vinegar dressing Baked banana with lemon and sugar	Raisins and nuts Whole wheat toast with margarine Milk

Note. From *The Berkeley Co-Op Food Book* (pp. 72-73) by H. Black (Ed.), 1980, Palo Alto, CA: Bull. Copyright 1980 by Bull. Reprinted by permission.

Table 6A.3 Stability of Various Food Products Under Different Conditions of Storage

Food	Preparation	Signs of Deterioration	Temp. 1	Shelf Life	Temp. 2	Shelf Life
Milk	Powdered	Lumping, strong flavor	40°	24 months	70°	12 months
	Canned	Dark color, fat separation	40°	12 months		
Cheese	Yellow	Mold	30°	2–3 weeks		
Meats	Canned	Bulged can	40°	12 months		
Eggs	Dried	Taste change	40°	12 months	70°	5 weeks
Beans, peas, lentils	Dried	Dried out	40°	Many years		
Nuts	Airtight container	Rancid taste, mold	32°	3–6 months		
Fruits	Canned	Bulged can, dark color	40°	5 years	60°	2 years
and Vegetables	Dried	Loss of color, mold	40°	6 months	32°	1 year
	Frozen	Dried out, color change	10°	6–12 months		
Wheat	Whole kernel, sealed and CO₂	Rancid taste	40°–60°	10 years		
Flours—wheat, rice, rye	Whole grain, milled enriched	Rancid or stale taste	40°–60°	9 months		
Fats and oils include peanut butter	Sealed container	Rancid taste	40°–60°	6 months		
Yeast	Dry, sealed container	Impotent	40°	Many years		
Sugar						
Iodized salt	Airtight container					
Gelatin	Airtight container	Lumpy	40°–60°	Indefinitely		

Note. From "Stability of Various Food Products Under Different Conditions of Storage" by A. Sorenson, April 13, 1977, *Salt Lake Tribune*, Sec. C, p. 1. Copyright 1977 by *Salt Lake Tribune*. Reprinted by permission.

Table 6A.4 Safety Factors and Toxic Effects of Essential Nutrients in Human Diets

Nutrient	Age Group	RDA[2]	Toxic Dose/Day	Period of Ingestion	Safe Daily Maximum	Safety Factor	Toxic Symptoms
Vitamin A	0-1 year	410 RE[a]	> 4,000 RE	2-4 weeks	2,000 RE	10	Hydrocephalus[2]
	Pregnant adult	1,000 RE	> 5,000 RE	6-9 months	4,000 RE	5	Defective CNS of baby
	Adult	800-1,000 RE	> 15,000 RE	years	25,000 to 50,000 IU	10	Anorexia, headache, blurred vision, dry skin[2]
Vitamin D	0-1 year	10 μg	40 μg	years	20 μg	2	Hypercalcemia[3]
	1-12 years	10 μg	25-75 μg		20-40 μg	2-4	Ca deposition in tissues[3]
	Some adults	10 μg	50 μg	21 days	40 μg	4	Cholesterol increase, 10 mg/dl[4]
	Some adults	10 μg	2,500 μg	21 days	40 μg	4	Cholesterol increase, 28 mg/dl[4]
	Most adults	10 μg	25,000 μg	years	—	250?	Diarrhea, headache, nausea[5]
Vitamin E	Adults	10 mg	800-1,600 mg	—	800 mg (estim.)	80-160	Fatigue, hyperthyroidism[6]
			Water-Soluble Vitamins				
Vitamin C	Adult	60 mg	5-10 g? variable	years	1-3 g	50	Kidney stones, oxaluria, uricosuria, cystinuria, G.I. disturbances, nausea, ...[7]

Nutrient	Age						
Thiamin (B₁)	Adult	1.0-1.4 mg	300 mg	—	200 mg	200	None orally[8]
Riboflavin (B₂)	Adult	1.2-1.6 mg	1,000 mg	—	1,000 g	650	None reported[9]
Niacin (nicotinic acid)	Adult	13-18 mg	100 mg	1/2-1 year	500 mg	35	Flushing, headache, nausea, cramps; serum uric acid elevated; liver damage, hyperglycemia[10]
Pyridoxine group (B₆)	Adult	2.0-2.2 mg	2,000 mg	months	1,000 mg	500	Nerve damage[11]
Pantothenic acid	Adult	4-7 mg	> 10,000 mg	weeks	—	1,500	Minor GI upsets[12]
Folacin	Adult	0.4 mg	> 400 mg	5 months	10 mg	1,000	In absence of B₁₂, folacin may mask symptoms of pernicious anemia, but not those of nerve degeneration[13]
Cobalamin (B₁₂)	Adult	3.0 µg	> 3 mg	—	—	> 1,000	None reported[14]
Biotin	Adult	100-200 µg	> 10 mg	6 months	> 10 mg	> 100	None reported[15]
Essential Elements[b]							
Fluoride (9)	1-3 years	0.5-1.5 mg	2.5 mg		2.5 mg	2	Mottled teeth[16]
	4-6 years	1.0-2.5 mg	—		2.5 mg	2	Mottled teeth[16]
	7-18 years	1.5-2.5 mg	—		2.5 mg	2	Mottled teeth[16]
	18+ years	1.5-4.0 mg	> 10 mg	years	4 mg	2	Fluorosis of bone[1]
			> 50 mg	years			Osteosclerosis[1]

(Cont.)

Table 6A.4 (Cont.)

Nutrient	Age Group	RDA	Toxic Dose/Day	Period of Ingestion	Safe Daily Maximum	Safety Factor	Toxic Symptoms
Sodium (11)	Adult	1.1-3.3 g	15 g	Years	10-15 g	7	Possible hypertension[1]
Magnesium (12)	Adult	300-350 mg	6,000 mg	—	4,000 g	18	Muscular weakness[17]
Silicon (14)	—	No human data	—	—	—	—	None reported[18]
Phosphorus (15) P_i	Adult	800 mg	12 g	—	—	15	Possible hypocalcemia[1]
Chlorine (17)	Adult	1.7-5.1 g	> 10 g	years	4-8 g	7	—
Potassium (19)	Adult	1.9-5.6 g	18 g	—	6-10 g	—	Cardiac arrest[1]
Calcium (20)	Adult	800 mg	12,000 mg	Years	3,000 mg	15	Possible hypophosphatemia, fatty stool
Vanadium (23)	Adult	—	2.2 mg	16 months	?	—	Cramps, diarrhea, green tongue[19]
Chromium (24)	Adult	50-200 mcg	—	No human data	Relatively nontoxic to rats	—	None reported[20]
Manganese (25)	Adult	2.5-5.0 mg	No human data	—	5 mg	25-50 (rats)	Anemia, carcinogenic, neurological effects[21]

Element	Group	RDA	Toxic dose	Duration		Ratio	Symptoms
Iron (26)	Adult, female	18 mg	40 mg/kg			6	Liver damage to genetic susceptibles[22]
	Adult, male	10 mg	200-250 mg/kg			—	Death
Nickel (28)		7.5 µg		Well tolerated by rats and monkeys		—	GI irritation[23,24]
Copper (29)	Adult	2-3 mg	100 mg		0.5 mg/kg	40	Vomiting, nausea[1,25]
Zinc (30)	Adult	15 mg	150 mg	Months	30 mg	10	Copper deficiency Decrease in plasma HDL-cholesterol[26]
Arsenic (33)	Rats	30-50 ng/gm diet	70-180 mg fatal dose—human			1250	Nausea, vomiting[27,28]
Selenium (34)	Adult	0.05-0.2 mg	0.5 mg	2 years	0.2 mg	3.5	Nail damage, alopecia, GI disturbances[1,29,30]
Molybdenum (42)	Adult	0.15-0.5 mg	10-15 mg	—	0.5 mg	10	None reported[31]
Iodine (53)	Adult	150 mcg	> 2.0 mg	—	1 mg	7	Goiter, myxedema,[33,34] autoimmune thyroiditis[32]

Note. Table compiled using information from [1]National Research Council (1980); [2]McLaren (1984); [3]Food and Nutrition Board (1974); [4]Fleischman et al. (1970); [5]Briggs (1974); [6]Tsai, Kelley, Peng, & Cook (1978); [7]"Vitamin C Toxicity" (1976); [8]Hayes & Hegsted (1973); [9]Vitale (1976); [10]Miller & Hayes (1982); [11]Schaumburg et al. (1983); [12]Sauberlich (1980); [13]National Research Council (1980); [14]Herbert, Colman, & Jacob (1980); [15]Appel & Briggs (1980); [16]Bhussry (1970); [17]Knochel (1982); [18]Carlisle (1984); [19]Crew & Hopkins (1981); [20]Mertz (1984); [21]Beach, Gershwin, & Hurley (1982); [22]Beutler (1980); [23]Nielsen (1984); [24]Solomons (1984); [25]Allen & Solomons (1984); [26]Solomons & Cousins (1984); [27]Vallee, Ulmer, & Wacker (1960); [28]Nielsen & Uthus (1984); [29]Barbezat, Casey, Reasbeck, Robinson, & Thomson (1984); [30]Combs & Combs (1986); [31]Nielsen & Mertz (1984); [32]Bagchi, Brown, Urdanivia, & Sundick (1985); [33]Wolff (1969); [34]Taylor (1981).

[a]RE = retinol equivalence = 1 µg retinol or 6 µg β-carotene.

[b]The atomic number is listed in parentheses after each element.

Chapter

7

Physical Fitness and Wellness

We stop hiking not because we grow old,
We grow old because we stop hiking.
Finis Mitchell

The material in this chapter will help you

- realize how fitness contributes to wellness;
- understand the different components of fitness; and
- develop an exercise program of your own choice as an essential part of your wellness lifestyle.

In recent years *fitness* has become a household word in the American vocabulary. There are three major reasons for this increase in its popularity as an activity: its connection with protection against heart disease, hypertension, and obesity; its effects on increasing endurance in everyday activities, and its psychological benefits. The role of fitness in avoiding disease is discussed in chapters 8, 9, and 10.

In discussing fitness, we should be clear about its multiple meanings. To many people it means physical fitness as exemplified by aerobics, especially jogging, and the endurance that results from aerobic training. Another type of physical fitness, the development of large, strong muscles, is obtained by training with weights, popularly known as pumping iron. A third type of fitness includes both endurance and strength. Still another type of fitness emphasizes flexibility, as exemplified in ballet dancers and gymnasts.

There are advantages to overall fitness as opposed to specific types such as endurance fitness, strength fitness, or flexibility fitness. Most people engage in a variety of activities in daily living such as housework, carrying a tired child, or washing one's back. Self-esteem is promoted by general competence and not being too specialized. For this reason, I suggest participating in a variety of exercises.

Successful stressor management can be considered as an example of another type of fitness—psychic fitness. As usual, categories such as these give the false impression that each type is separate and distinct from the others. If you have ever worked out for any length of time, you probably experienced psychic benefits from physical fitness and physical benefits from psychological fitness.

Business executives have recently discovered the profitability of being fit. Many business persons take time for workouts before important dinners. A growing number of executives stay only at hotels that have exercise facilities. After a day of intense meetings, business lunches, and cocktail hours, they find that working out is not only relaxing but a means of staying sharp if meetings continue into the evening. Many people find a 30-minute workout before dinner more restful than a 30-minute nap.

George Harris (1986) reports that Dr. Dorothea Johnson, corporate medical director of AT&T's Long Lines Division, sold the idea of Total Life Concept (TLC) to management shortly after the court order that divided the massive AT&T into numerous separate companies. Management feared that the stress of the breakup would result in workers losing faith in the company. But numerous surveys since the TLC program has been instituted have shown the opposite. The workers have better feelings about themselves, co-workers, bosses, and the company itself.

Harris mentions that the Association for Fitness in Business has grown from a few fitness directors in 1974 to over 2,300 professional members in 1986. Harris reports solid research at the University of Pittsburgh has shown that health programs pay off not only in fewer accidents and less absenteeism, but also in a more vigorous, creative workforce.

In the centuries when most people worked at manual labor, it is probable that a higher percentage of the population was fit than at present. Most Americans now work at sedentary jobs to which they are transported in automobiles or other vehicles. High technology civilization has replaced manpower by machine power. If at home, a person's major exercise is toddling from the table to the TV set; little additional energy is expended. Our bodies adjust to this type of existence. We become fatter and less fit. Fortunately, an exercise program can increase fitness at any age.

The Importance of Energy Production

We obtain energy from food. Just staying alive requires some energy. The fact that we remain warm—even when asleep—indicates that we convert food energy into heat. The process of becoming fit and maintaining fitness requires more energy. This extra energy is also converted into heat. The extra heat that is produced represents extra energy that would have been converted into fat if we had not been physically active. Energy usage can be summarized as follows: Some is utilized to maintain life, some is utilized for physical movement, any excess energy is stored as fat. In this chapter I will describe how energy in foods is converted to a chemical that the body can utilize and how this energy is used for muscle movement. In chapter 8 I will describe how extra energy is utilized for fat synthesis. It is obvious that the more energy we use for muscle movement, the less there is left over for fat synthesis.

If you understand the relationships of food as a source of energy, how this energy is converted to the molecule adenosine triphosphate (ATP, the main molecule of biological energy transfer), and how ATP is used for muscle movement and/or fat synthesis, you will become acquainted with how your body works in a new way. You will begin to appreciate how marvelous the human species is. If the equations presented in Table 7.1 and the discussion explaining them is way over your head, feel free to skip them. Understanding these possibly interesting, semitechnical explanations is not essential to benefiting from exercise.

The two previous chapters discussed foods as sources of energy and the function of the enzymes and cofactors that are essential in the release of that energy as ATP. This chapter outlines the pathways of ATP synthesis in muscles from the three major sources of energy in foods. We'll also see how the muscle fibers utilize the ATP in muscle movement and how regular exercise increases fitness. Fitness enhances strength and endurance through modifications of the muscle fibers, as well as improving the efficiency of the energy transport systems.

The Release of Energy From Foods

Before explaining how muscle cells utilize energy, it may be well to mention how they and all other cells obtain their utilizable energy. In other words: How do cells synthesize adenosine triphosphate (ATP)?

Foods obviously include a wide mixture of substances. A detailed list would probably contain thousands of chemicals. The digestive tract and the liver reduce this diversity to a small, relatively constant mixture. A simplification will help in understanding the process. Food constituents can be divided into two groups: those that furnish energy and those that do not. The first group is divided into three major groups: proteins, carbohydrates, and fats. The second group contains the noncalorific essential nutrients like vitamins and elements, and a varied group of dietary fibers, contaminants, toxicants, microorganisms, and so on. Many of these chemicals have been mentioned in chapter 5. The objective in this section is to explain briefly how the potential energy of the calorific nutrients is converted to ATP.

There are two major pathways for ATP synthesis: anaerobic and aerobic. The anaerobic series starts with glucose and ends in lactic acid. It is the fastest route for ATP synthesis and is used for quick, short responses and for heavy work. The aerobic route, which oxidizes either carbohydrates or fats to CO_2 and H_2O, is slower and is utilized for light, endurance-type activities.

Most of the carbohydrates that we eat occur as starch, other high-molecular-weight *polymers*, and sugars. To be absorbed, the polymers must be digested by enzymes in the small intestine into simple sugars. These sugars proceed via the portal vein to the liver, which is able to convert all the natural sugars into glucose. Thus the only sugar present in the general circulating blood under usual conditions is glucose.

Proteins are also large polymeric substances that cannot be absorbed as such. They are digested by enzymes to become a mixture of amino acids in the small intestine. These are absorbed there and, after passing through the liver, enter the general blood supply. Although we think of the main function of amino acids as the building blocks for body proteins, ultimately they are all oxidized. An important step in this process for most of the amino acids is to be converted into glucose. This sugar, whether derived from carbohydrates or proteins, can be oxidized to carbon dioxide and water in cells. The energy that is liberated is transferred to ATP.

Fats are not polymers but are smaller molecules composed of three fatty acid molecules attached to a glycerol molecule. They are called triglycerides and are not soluble in water or aqueous fluids of the digestive tract. For them to be absorbed, some of the fatty acids are split off the triglyceride molecule and the mixture of free fatty acids and *mono-* and *diglycerides* enters the cells of the intestine. These products are then reassembled into triglycerides, combined with proteins, and a new product called *lipoprotein* is secreted into the lymph and, in time, reaches the liver. This organ synthesizes a variety of other lipoproteins, some of which contain cholesterol. These substances will be discussed in chapter 10 in relation to heart attacks. Fatty acids likewise circulate in the blood. As with glucose, fatty acids can be oxidized to carbon dioxide and water in cells with the concomitant synthesis of ATP.

To summarize, mammals, including humans, are able to oxidize the carbon chains of carbohydrates, fats, and proteins to carbon dioxide and water, and to direct much of the energy that is liberated in these reactions into the synthesis of ATP. As far as is known, all living things convert their environmental sources of energy into ATP. Its energy, in turn, is then utilized for synthesis of polymers, for movement, for keeping in touch with the environment, for communication, for reproduction, and for just about everything! It is in this sense that ATP serves as a universal biological currency for energy. A brief description of this process follows.

The Energy Liberated by Oxidation Is Funneled Into ATP Synthesis

Because ATP does not circulate in the blood and is not able to enter cells, each cell must make its own ATP. On a micro scale, it is similar to saying that each person must take responsibility for his or her own wellness. This comparison is not as farfetched as it may seem at first glance. As we shall see, fitness increases the efficiency of the nutrient and oxygen delivery systems to the cells and also increases the efficiency of ATP synthesis. Thus they can synthesize more ATP, which provides more energy for living (i.e., for wellness). By definition, each of the major suppliers of energy in foods must be able to be oxidized in a series of reactions that can be coupled to ATP synthesis. These reactions are presented in Table 7.1.

The first of these routes is called *anaerobic glycolysis* and includes the conversion of glucose to lactic acid. The energy liberated from these reactions is utilized in the synthesis of ATP. None of these reactions require oxygen (O_2); hence the name anaerobic—without air.

Table 7.1   Overall Reactions That Generate ATP*

Net ATP Synthesis	Per Molecule	Per Carbon Atom
Anaerobic: The glycolytic path		
Glucose ($C_6H_{12}O_6$) + ADP + $P_i \rightleftharpoons$ lactic acid + ATP	2	0.33
Aerobic: The coupled phosphorylating respiratory chain		
Glucose + O_2 + ADP + $P_i \rightleftharpoons CO_2$ + H_2O + ATP	30**	5.0**
Fatty acids + O_2 + ADP + $P_i \rightleftharpoons CO_2$ + H_2O + ATP (stearic acid, C_{18})	151	8.7
Amino acids + O_2 + ADP + $P_i \rightleftharpoons CO_2$ + H_2O + ATP (isoleucine)	42	7.0

*These equations are neither complete nor balanced.
**These numbers are corrected for the ATP synthesized anaerobically.
O_2 = oxygen, CO_2 = carbon dioxide, H_2O = water.

You might be puzzled by the terminology and ask, How can one have an oxidation without oxygen? Many years ago chemists defined oxidations as those reactions that involved oxygen directly. Later it was discovered that the same reaction could occur if oxygen was substituted by another chemical. The word *oxidation* was broadened to include these reactions.

The other three series of reactions require oxygen at some stage and are called *aerobic*. Actually, the overall equations as written are somewhat misleading because oxygen does not react directly with glucose, fatty acids, or amino acids, but reacts with other substances that are derived from them. One purpose of writing overall reactions is to emphasize the important reactants and the products that are formed. The three starting materials have been mentioned above. The major product of all three reactions, ATP, now contains the bulk of the potential energy that was originally in the starting chemicals.

It is noteworthy that the yield of ATP from stearic acid, a fatty acid (a typical saturated fatty acid which contains 18 carbon atoms) is about 5 times higher than from a molecule of glucose (which contains 6 carbon atoms). When calculated on the basis of ATP synthesized per carbon atom, the yield from a fatty acid is about 60% higher. These calculations show quantitatively that fat is our most concentrated form of energy. If we stored excess energy as carbohydrate rather than fat, we would probably weigh 2 or 3 times as much as we do now. This extra weight could be a considerable disadvantage when fast or prolonged movement is required. As mentioned above, carbohydrates and most amino acids can be oxidized either anaerobically or aerobically. Fatty acids, on the other hand, can be oxidized only aerobically. The complete oxidation of fatty acids in cells *requires* the presence of some carbohydrate. In contrast, the aerobic oxidation of carbohydrate does not depend on the presence of fat. Although the overall reactions do not suggest it, there is one common pathway of aerobic oxidation for all three energy sources. It is called the respiratory chain.

The Role of Oxygen in Energy Release From Foods

One of the marvels of biochemistry is that it allows a close-up view of the beauties of nature. One such close-up comes from the research that has revealed the role of oxygen in cell respiration. The term *respiration* has classically meant the gas exchange that occurs in the lungs whereby oxygen enters the blood and carbon dioxide is released. The term *cell respiration* refers to the actual reactions that occur in cells that produce the carbon dioxide and utilize the oxygen that has been carried to the cells via the arteries. This series of reactions is called the *phosphorylating respiratory chain* because it couples the synthesis of ATP to the energy-releasing reactions of cell respiration.

It may surprise you to learn that oxygen is actually involved in only one reaction; yet that reaction is essential to maintaining the smooth flow of all the reactions in cell respiration. Without it, all the other reactions of cell respiration stop. The reason that cyanide and carbon monoxide are so lethal is that they interfere with this particular reaction. The brain and heart are so dependent on a regular supply of oxygen that, if they are deprived of this chemical for more than a few minutes, they suffer irreversible damage. Skeletal muscle function, too, is dependent on oxygen supply.

Mitochondria

The enzymes that comprise the phosphorylating respiratory pathway are contained in small particles called mitochondria. These enzymes can complete the oxidation of glucose, lactic acid, fatty acids, and many amino acids to carbon dioxide and water. Because mitochondria are colored red, their number in a muscle fiber helps determine its color. The white, fast-twitch glycolytic muscle fiber contains a minimum of mitochondria; the pink, fast-twitch oxidative fibers contain considerably more; and the red, slow-twitch oxidative, the most. These differences are important because mitochondria provide the most efficient pathway of ATP synthesis and, this in turn, affects fatigability of muscles.

The numbers in Table 7.1 clearly show that the aerobic metabolism of glucose yields 15 times as many ATP molecules per carbon atom as the anaerobic pathway. Stated another way, it means that a cell only has to process 1/15 as many glucose molecules aerobically to obtain an equal number of ATP molecules as would be produced anaerobically. This difference amounts to a significant increase in efficiency. At times, survival as well as wellness may depend on the efficiency by which we synthesize ATP.

Because amino acids in the form of protein make up a much smaller percentage of our diet than either carbohydrate or fat, the energy yield of amino acids is less important than from the other two sources. Incidentally, the carbon chains from most amino acids can be converted to glucose and thus oxidized by either the anaerobic or aerobic pathways.

In summary, I have discussed the synthesis of ATP from the three energy sources in our diet. ATP results from a series of coupled oxidations and phosphorylations. The yield of ATP per carbon atom of substrate has been shown to be considerably greater in aerobic than anaerobic systems. In other words, the aerobic pathway is more efficient than the anaerobic.

The next question concerns how the energy-containing substances and the oxygen are brought to all cells, especially to the voluntary muscles. In this description of the energy supply and transport systems, I'll first describe the components of each and how they function, then follow with how the systems adapt to stimulation, and finally, how training increases their efficiency.

Energy Transport Systems— Cardiorespiratory and Cardiovascular

Oxygen enters the blood from the lungs. When we breathe in (inspire) air, it diffuses to tiny vacuoles called alveoli, which are surrounded by tiny blood vessels called capillaries. The air and blood are in close contact. The reason that we are able to extract the oxygen from the air is that blood contains hemoglobin, the protein that makes blood red, which has the ability to combine with oxygen but not with nitrogen, the major gas in air. The oxygen-rich blood is carried to the heart, which pumps it through the arteries to all the tissues and cells of the body. The cells, in turn, contain myoglobin, another protein that combines with oxygen. As this protein loses oxygen that is used up in the oxidation reactions mentioned above, it accepts more from the oxygen-rich hemoglobin. In this way myoglobin acts as an oxygen reservoir for aerobic reactions in the cell.

To complete the circulatory circuit, recall that the cells in the tissues produce carbon dioxide as a by-product of their aerobic energy production. The oxygen-poor hemoglobin now accepts some of this chemical and carries it via the veins back to the lungs where it is expelled in each expiration. The hemoglobin is now ready to accept another load of oxygen. The whole process of inspiration and expiration is called ventilation.

In this short description of the energy supply and transport systems, we can see how the roles of the heart as a pump, the blood as a pipeline, the lungs as a gas exchanger, and the muscle cells as energy transducers all work cooperatively. Fitness amounts to keeping each of these subsystems operating efficiently. Fitness also includes efficient functioning of the voluntary muscles that do the work.

Types of Muscle Fibers

When I was in my twenties, I used to run with Tom Cureton, a well-known exercise physiologist. His resting pulse was 44; mine was 74. Although he was older than I, he could run a mile under 7 min; I could not. No matter how many times I gritted my teeth and swore to myself that this time I would stay with him for the full distance, I could never keep up with him beyond a half-mile. I used to wonder how it was that fate had given him so much more willpower than me. He had been a distance runner in high school and college, while I had run dashes and high jumped. It was many years later that I learned about the reasons for these differences in natural athletic abilities. The difference between Tom and me was not in our willpowers but in our genes. I had a high proportion of fast-twitch fibers in my muscles, he, of slow-twitch. Since then, the number of fiber types has been expanded to three. The properties of each have been described, and with this information, we can now partially explain the differences in natural athletic abilities in people.

Muscle fibers tend to be long and thin. Some run the whole length of a muscle, while others are much shorter. Some fibers are as thick as a human hair, whereas others are so thin they cannot be seen without a microscope. These physical differences are reflected in their physiological and biochemical properties. The types of fibers and some of their characteristics are shown in Table 7.2. The proportions of the fiber types in our muscles are fixed by our heredity, although training can affect them.

In Table 7.1, I list three types of oxidations that liberate energy from carbohydrates and fats. Table 7.2 shows that each type of oxidation occurs in a specific kind of fiber. The anaerobic glycolytic enzymes predominate in some of the white, fast-twitch fibers, whereas the aerobic glycolytic enzymes predominate in others. Both of these fiber types can form lactic acid from glucose, but the aerobic ones can also utilize oxygen to oxidize the lactic acid completely to carbon dioxide and water and thereby can synthesize considerably more ATP from each molecule of glucose.

Table 7.2 Type and Characteristics of Three Types of Human Skeletal Muscle Fibers

Characteristic	Slow, Oxidative (SO)	Fast, Oxidative, Glycolytic (FOG)	Fast, Glycolytic (FG)
Color	Red	Pink	White
Speed of contraction (twitch)	Slow	Fast	Fast
Strength of contraction	Low	High	High
Fatigability	Least fatigable	Fatigable	Most fatigable
Aerobic capacity	High	Medium	Low
Anaerobic capacity	Low	Medium	High
Size	Small	Largest	Large
Capillary density	High	High	Low
Myoglobin content	High	Medium	Low
Triglyceride stores	High	Medium	Low
Glycogen stores	High	High	High
Phosphocreatine stores	Low	Medium	High

Note. These characteristics have been compiled from *Physiology of Exercise* by H.A. DeVries, 1986, Dubuque, IA: William C. Brown; and *Physiological Basis of Physical Education and Athletics* by E.L. Fox and D.K. Mathews, 1981, Philadelphia: Saunders College.

Anaerobic metabolism, as found in the glycolytic white fibers, requires much less oxygen than aerobic metabolism. Thus, the glycolytic white fibers can function with a smaller blood supply. The two types of white/pink fibers vary in some very important characteristics such as fatigability, size, and capillary density. However, they are similar in their speed and strength of contraction.

In contrast, the red, slow-twitch fibers whose energy is derived primarily from oxidizing fats, as well as glucose, contract more slowly and with less strength than white fibers. On the other hand, these small fibers are fatigue resistant and have a high capillary density. A high capillary density indicates a large blood supply, which can deliver adequate volumes of oxygen to support the aerobic metabolism of these fibers.

The Distribution of Fiber Types in People

Although most of us are unlikely to have our fiber types measured, data on athletes show wide variations in percentage of fiber types in different sport activities. Fox and Mathews (1981) summarize fiber type data from a number of studies on both men and women, both athletes and untrained. Because there was so little difference in the percentages for the two sexes, I'll just mention average ranges.

Percentage fast-twitch fibers in untrained (average?) people are 50%–55%; marathon runners, 20%; long-distance runners, 30%–40%; mid-distance runners, 40%–50%; sprinters/jumpers, 60%–70%; and weight

Table 7.3   Relative Occurrence of Slow-Twitch Fibers in Nine Human Muscles

Name of Muscle		% of Slow-Twitch Fibers	
Scientific	Location	Range	Average
Vastus lateralis	Thigh	35– 65	50
Rectus femoris	Thigh	30– 55	42
Gastrocnemius	Calf	40– 65	52
Tibialis anterior	Lower shin	60– 80	70
Soleus	Below calf	80–100	90
Deltoid	Shoulder	40– 80	60
Biceps brachii	Front upper arm	35– 70	52
Triceps brachii	Back upper arm	15– 50	32

Note. From "Data on Distribution of Fiber Types in Thirty-Six Human Muscles" by M.A. Johnson, J. Polgar, D. Weightman, and D. Appleton, 1973, *Journal of Neurological Science*, **18**, p. 111. Copyright 1973 by *Journal of Neurological Science*. Reprinted by permission.

lifters, 45%–75%. I infer from these figures that some people are naturally stronger than others, whereas others possess more endurance. To give you some idea of the variation in individual muscles, the soleus—the muscle just below the calf—contains 25%–40% more slow-twitch fibers than the other leg muscles. The triceps contains 10%–30% more fast-twitch fibers than the other arm muscles (Johnson, Polgar, Weightman, & Appleton, 1973). Table 7.3 shows the range and percentage of slow-twitch fibers of nine human muscles in average people.

Physical Activity, Energy Usage, and Fiber Types

Let's consider four types of physical activity: at rest; slight; heavy; and light, vigorous. According to Wahren (1977), muscles at rest obtain most of their ATP from fat oxidation. When physical activity commences, different fiber types are preferentially recruited, depending on the type and duration of the exercise.

This pattern of energy usage might be called the default program, to use a computer term. It is the one that is returned to after any type of vigorous exercise is completed and is the one that is in operation at rest. Under these conditions the rate of energy consumption by muscles is minimal. Slight activity like slow walking or window shopping recruits both slow-twitch and fast-twitch, oxidative fibers.

The fast-twitch, white glycolytic fibers are employed in performing heavy work like lifting furniture or weights, shoveling snow, or running a 100-yard dash. If this type of activity is continued for over a few minutes, the fast oxidative fibers may also be recruited. These pink fibers contain sufficient mitochondria to oxidize appreciable amounts of lactic acid—produced by the glycolytic fibers—to carbon dioxide and water, and thus obtain more ATP from each molecule of glucose. For this reason, these oxidative fibers are considered less fatigable than the glycolytic ones.

The third situation refers to muscles doing light, but vigorous, work for long periods. All types of aerobic exercise are included in this category. It includes moving one's body rapidly and consistently, as in fast walking or running/jogging a mile or more. This type of activity is called aerobic (with air) because it stimulates the rate of respiration and also the heart rate.

One significant difference between aerobic exercise and weight lifting lies in their different time frames. Weight lifters need to rest between each set of repetitions. They rest, not because they are lazy, but because this type of exercise fatigues the white muscle fibers that do the work. In contrast, although aerobic exercise recruits the white fibers at the beginning of a session, the red, slow oxidative fibers are gradually recruited as the exercise continues. After about 15 minutes of vigorous cycling, Gollnick (1985) found oxidation of fatty acids provided 80% of the energy.

The differential utilization of the reservoirs of glycogen/fatty acids enables us to deal with a variety of situations. Alternative metabolic pathways are comparable to an automatic transmission that adjusts to load and speed in a car. Low gear corresponds to the use of the strong, fast-twitch fibers that are used to get going but which tire readily. Second gear corresponds to the fast-twitch oxidative fibers. They are also strong and, because of their more efficient oxidative metabolism, have more endurance. High gear corresponds to the use of slow-twitch oxidative fibers that are relatively weak but have the most endurance because they can oxidize fatty acids, our most concentrated form of energy.

Apart from its involvement in aerobic exercise, the shift in the utilization of energy reservoirs from exclusively carbohydrate to a mixture of carbohydrate-fatty acids has survival value. It enables us, as well as other animals, to utilize the most concentrated form of chemical energy that we possess. It also helps conserve the glycogen reserves that are essential for continued muscular activity.

Have you noticed that, as the duration of exercise or activity is extended, the role of oxygen becomes more prominent? Thus far in the discussion of energy supplies and muscle movement, the emphasis has been on the substrate reservoirs for energy and how they are utilized in various kinds of activity. The oxygen transport and supply system also adapts to the body's needs for energy.

Physical Activity and Oxygen Requirement

Most people begin to breathe more rapidly when they work around the house or garden, walk up a hill, or climb up two or more flights of stairs. If the rate of breathing is so fast that it becomes uncomfortable, sensible people stop and rest. It is obvious that when we exert ourselves we expend more energy than when we are resting. We obtain that energy on the spot, as we need it, by oxidizing some of our stored energy reserves of glycogen or fat. The extra oxygen that we require for the exertion is supplied by breathing faster and by increasing not only our heart rate but also our depth of breathing, which is called *hyperventilation*.

The size of the increase in oxygen consumption between resting and different degrees of exertion is impressive. A person sleeping or reclining uses about 200 ml of oxygen per minute. In a 70-kg man (154 lb), this calculates to about 3 ml/kg/minute. A person doing sedentary work or walking slowly uses oxygen about 3 to 4 times faster than while resting, whereas someone doing aerobics, brisk walking, jogging, cycling, or swimming may consume oxygen at 10 or more times the resting rate. These activities make us hyperventilate.

The Relation Between Oxygen Consumption and Pulse Rate

When we hyperventilate, our chests heave as we breathe deeply in and out to get the oxygen we need into the lungs. But to transport the oxygen to the muscles where it is needed also requires that the cardiovascular system function at an increased rate.

The heart pumps about 5,000 ml (approx. 5.3 qt) of blood per minute in a person at rest. Strenuous exercise increases the total blood flow about 4- to 5-fold, and the volume going to the muscles increases about 10-fold. Under these conditions of vigorous exercise, the heart beats faster and also pumps more blood per beat. The pulse rate during strenuous exercise usually increases to well over 100 beats per minute (BPM). The body's response to physical work thus provides a test of the cardiovascular system's ability to provide the oxygen and fuel that the muscles need in order to do the work that they are called upon to do. In summary, the blood can be compared to an endless cafeteria line in which the consumers—the cells—are in fixed positions and the nutrients and oxygen circulate. Cells possess the amazing ability to take out what substances they need from this mixture.

Energy Reservoirs in Muscle

One of the devices that permits these wide ranges of response by muscles is the anaerobic-aerobic dual type of ATP synthesis mentioned above. A second device is the system of energy reservoirs present in muscles. The amount of ATP that is present in resting muscle is sufficient for just a few twitches. The first reservoir for ATP is a chemical called phosphocreatine (PC). There is about 5 times as much PC in a resting muscle fiber as ATP (Edwards, Wilkie, Dawson, Gordon, & Shaw, 1982).

The second reservoir is a carbohydrate polymer called glycogen. It is composed of glucose units. Each glucose unit that is split off can enter the reactions of anaerobic glycolysis that provide energy for the synthesis of ATP. Because glycogen is a bulky molecule, the amount that a muscle can contain is limited; however, recent research has shown that muscle glycogen levels can be influenced significantly by training and diet.

The third reservoir is composed of fats. A small amount occurs in each muscle fiber, but large reserves are found in the fat storage depots. During periods of prolonged exercise, fats are hydrolyzed to fatty acids, which are carried by the bloodstream to the muscle cells. As mentioned above, fatty acids are a more concentrated form of energy than carbohydrates. Their energy, however, can only be liberated by aerobic reactions. A further restriction on the use of fats for energy production is that some carbohydrate must be present in the cell and must also be undergoing aerobic reactions during fatty acids' oxidations. If the glycogen reservoir has been strongly depleted by exhaustive exercise, fatty acid oxidation is also de-creased. The net effect of this carbohydrate-fat relationship is twofold. It increases muscle endurance by utilizing fat, the body's largest store of its most concentrated energy. Secondly, it conserves glycogen so that, except in extreme situations of complete exhaustion, muscles retain some reservoir of energy.

This relationship was epitomized a century ago by Rosenfeld (cited in Krebs, 1966) a biochemist-poet, in the phrase, "Fats burn in the flame of carbohydrates." We now understand the biochemical basis of this re-mark, but because the explanation is somewhat technical, I'll place it in Appendix 7A.

Heavy-Work Exercise Relies Mostly on Fast-Twitch White Glycolytic Fibers

The fast-twitch glycolytic fibers rely on glycolysis as their sole means of ATP synthesis. As shown in Table 7.1, the other product of glycolysis is lactic acid. If it is formed faster than it can diffuse into the blood and be carried away, it will increase the acidity of those fibers. This effect is known to decrease the rate of glycolysis and hence ATP synthesis. These two effects partially explain why the white, fast-twitch glycolytic fibers fatigue most rapidly.

Insofar as the pink oxidative fibers are involved in strength exercise, if they have an adequate oxygen supply, they can oxidize the lactic acid to carbon dioxide and water and obtain additional ATP in the process. For these reasons, the fast-twitch oxidative fibers will not fatigue as readily as the glycolytic type.

Light-Work Exercise Relies Mainly on Slow-Twitch, Red Oxidative Fibers

The slow-twitch oxidative fibers contain more mitochondria than the fast-twitch glycolytic fibers. The reason that the number of mitochondria per cell is important is that they are a key factor in determining the fatigability of muscle fibers. These fibers can completely oxidize glucose residues as well as fatty acids. They synthesize ATP via the phosphorylating respi-ratory chain. This system enables them to utilize their glycogen reserves most efficiently with the result that these fibers are the most fatigue resis-tant of all three types.

The Nervous System Controls the Type of Fiber Recruited

Each packet of muscle fibers contains the same type of fiber: fast- or slow-twitch, but not both. Each packet is innervated by a single motor nerve.

Apparently, the nervous system decides which type of fiber is to be stimulated for a particular type of work or exercise. Have you ever lifted an object that you thought would be heavy, but it wasn't? Or vice versa? In ordinary living, we use slow-twitch aerobic fibers at rest and at the beginning of movements. If we engage in heavy work or exercise, the fast-twitch fibers are recruited. If the work or exercise becomes light, more of the slow-twitch type are recruited as substitutes for the fast-twitch.

Endurance Fitness

The term endurance fitness is used synonymously with Cooper's (1983) term aerobic fitness as used in his numerous books on "Aerobics." As can be seen in Table 7.4, no exercise or activity is completely anaerobic, and, with the possible exception of long-distance running and cross-country skiing, none are exclusively aerobic. The terms aerobic and anaerobic activities signify the major pathways of ATP synthesis; do not take them literally to mean either/or.

By the same token, heavy-work exercise that takes longer than 10 seconds does not derive energy solely from anaerobic reactions. For these reasons, I prefer the term endurance to aerobic exercise and strength to anaerobic exercises.

Endurance fitness is desirable for a number of reasons. First, people who must stop and rest every little while are struggling under a severe handicap. Alternatively, the psychological benefits of being able to complete a long task or a physically active objective that is important to them are immense. Feelings of accomplishment at either work or play make life worth living and contribute to wellness for many people.

Second, aerobic fitness may help avoid premature heart attacks; if they occur, aerobic fitness decreases their severity. Third, aerobic power is also necessary for satisfactory performance of the other types of fitness. Many people curtail their physical activities as they age because they have allowed themselves to become so out of shape that they either can no longer perform adequately, or are afraid of injuring themselves. Maintaining one's endurance fitness will help postpone the "rocking chair" syndrome.

Actually, an aerobic training program amounts to people's subjecting themselves to a safe, regulated amount of stressors at each session. The whole person gradually adapts to this regime by the changes mentioned above. Most importantly, psychological changes occur and general attitude improves as well. These effects are often addictive, and the person begins to look forward to the very activities that were formerly dreaded or avoided.

The degree of aerobic fitness refers to how efficiently the body handles and transports the oxygen from the air to individual cells in which it

Table 7.4   Energy Sources for Various Sports and Activities

Sport/activity	Anaerobic	Aerobic Carbohydrates	Fats
Basketball	H	L	0
Golf (swing only)	H	L	0
Gymnastics	H	L	0
Skiing			
Cross-country	0	L	H
Downhill	I	I	I
Swimming			
100 yd	H	I	L
200 yd	I	H	L
400 yd	L	I	I
Tennis	H	I	L
Running			
100, 220 yd	H	L	0
880 yd	I	H	L
1 mi	I	H	I
2 mi	L	I	I
5 mi	L	I	H
Marathon	-	L	H
Volleyball	H	L	0
Walking, 4 mi/hr	L	I	H
Bicycling (up and down)	H	I	L
Gardening	H	I	L
Bowling	H	I	L
Recreational activities	H	I	L

H = high, I = intermediate, L = low; 0 = zero.

Note. From *Physiological Basis of Physical Education and Athletics* (p. 263) by E.L. Fox and D.K. Mathews, 1981, Philadelphia: Saunders College. Copyright 1981 by Saunders College. Adapted by permission.

indirectly oxidizes glucose and fatty acids and thereby releases the energy that these nutrients contain. To accomplish this complicated task requires the combined efforts of the cardiorespiratory system, composed of the heart, lungs, blood, and associated blood vessels, and the cardiovascular system, composed of the heart, blood, arteries, capillaries, and veins. To avoid repeating these two rather long terms, I'll refer to them both as the aerobic supply system. Aerobic fitness obviously depends on an efficient aerobic supply system. Notice that the heart and blood are members of both systems. The heart pumps the blood, which transports oxygen and energy-containing nutrients, to every cell in the body.

The Measurement of Aerobic Fitness

Scientifically, fitness is defined as *physical working power*, which is measured as the maximum rate of oxygen uptake of which an individual is capable. Because oxygen consumption is directly related to energy expenditure by muscles, which in turn are dependent on the energy supply, we can understand why oxygen measurement serves as an overall indicator of physical fitness.

The measurement of cardiorespiratory fitness was placed on a quantitative basis by Dr. Kenneth Cooper and colleagues at the U.S. Air Force Research Laboratories during the 1960s. In Cooper's first book, *Aerobics* (1968), he describes how the aerobic point system was developed by measuring the oxygen consumption of people as they walked or ran a mile on a treadmill. The faster the subjects ran, the greater their oxygen consumption. For example, someone taking 17.25 ± 2.00 minutes to cover a mile used 7 ml oxygen/kg/minute. This rate was assigned 1 point. A subject jogging a mile in 8 to 10 minutes used oxygen at the rate of 28 ml/kg/minute. This rate was assigned 4 points. The fastest time was assigned 6 points, because the subject consumed oxygen at 6 times the rate of the slowest runner.

In the same experiment, a continuous *electrocardiogram* (ECG) was produced under the same conditions as the oxygen consumption rate. The results made it possible to relate the volume of oxygen used to the amount of exertion—one measure of fitness—and also to evaluate how the heart responded to the stress—a second measure of fitness. In addition, the ECG furnished data on the health of the heart muscle itself under conditions of controlled stress. The treadmill the Cooper group used could be programmed to increase gradually its speed and slope. Thus, at the end of an all-out test, a subject might be running up a 20% grade at a speed of 5 mph. Fitness indeed! Under these conditions, the cardiorespiratory systems of young, extremely fit men could be assessed. This type of maximum effort is only used on subjects whose past history indicates that they won't be injured by the test.

Many subjects, including middle aged, elderly, and the less fit, are tested under submaximal conditions of effort. These tests are just about as informative as the maximal-effort type and do not place the subject under undue risk. Some fitness laboratories use a bicycle-ergometer (work measurement) instead of a treadmill for testing. The workload on these bikes is adjustable, and the oxygen uptake and pulse rate are measured under different intensities of activity. But, there are simpler tests that people can do at home that require only a sturdy box or stairs and a watch with a sweep-second hand.

Measurements of the pulse rate at different conditions of exercise and rest provide valuable information about a person's fitness. The resting pulse rate of a fit person is usually somewhat lower than that of a less fit person. This difference, however, is not very large. A more sensitive test of fitness is that of measuring the pulse rate of people before and after rapidly walking up three flights of stairs or some other standard exercise. The pulse of the fit person will increase to a lesser extent than that of the less fit person. Another measure of fitness is the time required for the pulse to return to its resting value after a specified amount of exercise. The pulse of a fit person will slow down much faster than that of a less fit person. These last two tests show much larger differences between fit and unfit than the resting pulse and are used more frequently.

These simple tests, which require no equipment beyond a watch with a sweep-second hand, are valuable for the person who is out of shape and wants to begin an exercise program that will not be overstressful. Some pulse tests are described in Appendix 7B. The pulse test is also useful for people who exercise aerobically and want to assure themselves that they have reached an adequate, but safe, heart rate.

One of the important advances in health science in recent years is that of placing the fitness of the aerobic supply system on a sound scientific basis. For example, one measure of the efficiency of the heart is how much blood it pumps per beat. This function is called the *stroke volume* and is larger, on the average, in people who exercise regularly than in those who don't. Another measure of efficiency is how much air the lungs can inspire with each breath. This function is called the *vital capacity* and is also larger in people who exercise than in those who don't.

In a classic paper, Dill, Talbot, and Edwards (1930) measured the oxygen consumption per kilogram of body weight of people during a standard run on a treadmill. The person who used the least oxygen (i.e., was the most efficient) was the famous marathon runner, Clarence DeMar. A number of other people were tested before and after aerobic training, and they all showed increases in efficiency.

Other factors affecting blood flow that are important, but less well known, are the increased number of capillaries that form in muscles as a result of aerobic exercise. Fit people tend to have higher hemoglobin concentrations in their blood (Kjellberg, Rudke, & Sjostrand, 1949), and they also have an increased concentration of mitochondria particles that contain oxygen-utilizing enzymes in their slow-twitch muscles (Ingjer, 1978). These changes aid in the more efficient utilization of oxygen.

Efficiency of oxygen usage, like most human characteristics, is affected by both nature and nurture. In other words, there are large differences in efficiency due to heredity (nature). But no matter how high or low one's natural efficiency may be, it can be increased significantly by training (nurture). The importance of a gain in endurance due to a high efficiency of oxygen usage can hardly be overemphasized. It adds a new dimension to what people can do, and how long they can do it, whether at work or play. It's like adding two more cylinders to the power of your car.

As I mentioned in chapter 3, scientists strive for the widest generalizations that the data will support. In a broad category such as aerobic fitness, I have mentioned the use of stress tests, pulse tests, and efficiency of oxygen usage as measures of this type of fitness. It is significant that the results of all three of these tests confirm each other. You may have noticed, however, that all three are active tests. Basically, they are all measuring the same thing: the efficiency of oxygen consumption directly or indirectly, under slightly different conditions. The whole concept of aerobic fitness would be considered more solid if there were some other completely different type of test that could be applied and that also correlated with the conclusions of the three above. Such a test has been developed. It is based on body composition.

Body Composition

Exercise physiologists have used a variety of methods for estimating percentage of body fat. The two most widely used are underwater (hydrostatic) weighing and the use of skinfold calipers. The latest method is called *bioelectrical impedance*. It is based on the finding that electrical conductance is far greater in lean muscle tissue than in fat tissue. With the equipment now available, four electrodes are placed on the right side of the body, on the wrist, hand, foot, and ankle. A painless electrical signal is introduced, and the resistive impedance is measured. The data are fed directly into a computer along with the person's height, weight, age, and sex. The results are printed out immediately in terms of percent fat and total fat weight. The results correlate highly ($\pm$ 5%) with fat composition determined by underwater weighing (Itallie, Segal, Yang, & Funk, 1985). The apparatus is quite expensive, but its ease and accuracy will probably bring it to wide use at fitness centers.

Percentage of Body Fat Is a Measure of Endurance Fitness

What is the connection between percentage of body fat and endurance fitness? The data included in Table 7.5 demonstrate quite conclusively that such a connection exists. Those athletes who engage in aerobic activities to the largest extent are the least fat. The fat content of average Americans gives some idea of how out of shape we are. Even teens are about twice as fat as they would be if fit. I have seen numerous fat amateur tennis players and golfers but never a fat distance runner (an anecdotal observation).

In addition, the connection has a logical explanation. I have mentioned above that fats can only be oxidized under aerobic conditions. A number

Table 7.5   Comparison of Fat Content of Athletes and Nonathletes

Group	Fat (%) Males	Females
Baseball player	11–14	NA*
Basketball player	8–12	15–20
Dancer, ballet	8–15	8–15
Football player	9–19	NA
Gymnast	4– 8	9–24
Runner, distance	6–14	15–19
Skier	7–14	14–22
Swimmer	5– 9	14–26
Tennis player	15	20
Walker, power	8	—
Weight lifter	8–16	—
General population		
15-year-old	12	20
20-year-old	15	25
30-year-old	19 ⎫	30 ⎫
50-year-old	26 ⎬ (10–20)**	33 ⎬ (15–25)**
70-year-old	— ⎭	— ⎭
Obese	Above 40	Above 45

Note. Adapted from *Body Composition and Sports Medicine: Research Considerations in Body Composition Assessments in Youth and Adults* (Report of Sixth Ross Conference on Medical Research, pp. 78-82) by H. Wilmore, 1985, Columbus, OH: Ross Laboratories. Copyright 1985 by Ross Laboratories. Adapted by permission.

*NA = data not available.

**Acceptable ranges of fat content (R. Ruhling, personal communication, 1981).

of organs like the liver, brain, heart, and kidneys can oxidize fats as a source of energy. Yet this usage is too small to prevent people from storing fat if they eat too much and exercise too little. The major potential organ system for fat oxidation occurs in the slow-twitch oxidative muscle fibers of our large muscles. I speak of them as a potential organ system because they are under our voluntary control. These fibers are used preferentially during aerobic exercise, but only then. The bottom line of this discussion is, *if you want to lose fat without also losing muscle protein, which occurs in dieting, you need to engage in regular aerobic exercise.* I'll discuss other aspects of fat deposition in succeeding chapters.

Table 7.6   A Walking-Aerobics Fitness Program for Adults 3 to 5 Times a Week*

Activity Level	Description	Time (Min)	Distance (Mi)
1	Slow walk	40	2
2	Alternate 1/4 mile slow walk, 1/4 mile fast walk	36	2
3	Fast walk	32	2
4	Faster walk	30	2
5	Longer walk	45	3
6	Still longer walk	60	4
7	Continue as long as enjoyable or shift to powerwalking, jogging, bicycling, or other aerobic activities		

*The program assumes level terrain.

I will summarize this section on assessment of endurance (aerobic) fitness by discussing cost and the time it takes. Many hospitals and other health providers have opened fitness or wellness institutes. These centers carry out a variety of tests depending upon an individual's age, gender, and risk factors. The tests offered by two Salt Lake City hospitals are listed in Appendix 7C. Pulse tests that one can do at home are listed in Appendix 7B. If a person doesn't want to bother with any test, he or she can commence a walking program as outlined in Table 7.6. No matter what program or type of exercise one selects, it is advisable to learn to take your pulse rate.

The Importance of Learning to Calculate and Monitor Your Target Heart Rate

Previously, I've mentioned that the aerobic training effect depends on an increased pulse rate. The *target heart rate* represents a range in which training effects can occur but still offers a margin of safety for healthy people. Once you have learned to take your own pulse, you don't have to follow any prescribed routine. If you prefer some exercise that isn't described in any book, you can do it and still be assured that you are in the safe aerobic training range.

The first step is to learn to take your *resting pulse*. This simple procedure requires a watch or clock with a sweep-second hand. The pulse can be taken at the wrist, at the carotid artery in the neck, or over the heart itself. For the wrist, place the second and third fingers of one hand on the opposite wrist (palm up) below the thumb. Count your pulse for 10 to 15 seconds. Multiply by 6 or 4 to obtain the BPM. Some people count for 6 seconds and multiply by 10, but the chances of error are much larger with the short count. Practice sufficiently often to be able to find your pulse readily.

The second step is to calculate your *target heart rate* (THR).

The predicted maximum heart rate (PMHR) = 220 minus your age. The PMHR for a 50-year-old person = 220 − 50 = 170.

Actually, it is not effective or safe to exercise at your maximum heart rate. A suggested range is at 70%–90% of your PMHR. For the person above, the

safe range = 170 x (70%–90%) = 119–153 BPM

A widely used calculation of the target heart rate using 70% of maximum for a 20-year-old is:

Target heart rate = 0.7 (maximum heart rate − resting heart rate)
+ resting heart rate
= 0.7 (200 − 70) + 70
= 91 + 70
= 161 bpm

Keep moving while you take your pulse, as the pulse rate drops rapidly when exercise stops. Cooper (1983, p. 125) suggests that fit people add 10% to their calculated heart rate if it's taken within 20 seconds of stopping.

Developing a Training Program

Most Americans gain weight as they age. Appetites that were acquired during the growing, active years remain relatively constant, while physical activity gradually decreases. The extra weight is due almost completely to fat. For many years the medical profession considered this normal as long as it did not result in obesity. This opinion is now considered faulty by health experts.

Extra fat is deposited, however, even in those people who do not gain weight. The gain in fat is balanced by a loss in protein. People who do not exercise lose muscle and grow weaker as they age. The training effect can delay or reverse these unfortunate, avoidable consequences, but it takes time.

People are not fit or unfit. Fitness represents a continuum, and what I am recommending is that most people can, and should, increase their fitness by engaging in a regular training program. Although I have mentioned athletes as the ideal, I am well aware that not many people over 30 will be motivated to attain that degree of fitness. It is very satisfying, however, to personally experience the increase in fitness that occurs in a regular program. Your muscle fibers are not made of concrete. Neither are your neurons. You are in control of your body, and your muscles can be trained to develop toward increased endurance, increased strength, or both. In addition, what you eat, as well as how much you eat, can affect endurance.

Let's face it. For those people who have not exercised or engaged in an active sport for 5 years or more, I am proposing a change in lifestyle. It will require releasing about 3 hours a week from some present activity to engage in an enjoyable fitness program of your own choosing. Fitness resembles a continuing investment whose dividends increase with time. Some people can tell a difference in a week or so, others in months, and some may take even longer. The premiums aren't in money, but in time. There is little to be gained from an endurance fitness program unless it is kept up for the rest of your life, because the benefits disappear rather rapidly if a certain minimum of physical activity is not continued more or less regularly. There is no guarantee that you will judge the benefits as worth the effort. Most people who stay with a program, however, enjoy the feeling of well-being that fitness bestows and the extra energy and endurance that allow them to participate in activities that they enjoy.

In the pages above I have described some of the differences in muscles and in the energy supply systems due to training. We are now in a position to discuss specific programs, and how to develop safe, enjoyable training procedures that will suit *you*—because you will select them.

Cautions Before Beginning an Exercise Program

If you are over 35, out of shape, and/or overweight, it is advisable to have a thorough physical examination by a physician—preferably one who realizes the importance of exercise—before embarking on an extended activity program. Be sure to tell the doctor that you plan to start an aerobic program. Besides uncovering possible danger, the results will furnish some objective information about what shape you're in at the start. The next step should be a fitness assessment test.

Use of the Heart Rate Target Zone for People in Good Health

If you are in good health with no serious risk factors, you can skip the calculations and use the Heart Rate Target Zone (Figure 7.1), which is

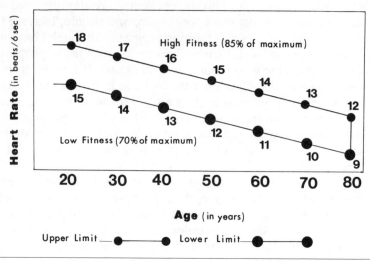

Figure 7.1   The safe heart rate target zone as a function of age and fitness.

suitable for people in the age range 20–80. The chart is based on the equations given above. If you are just commencing, the lower numbers (60%–70% of maximum) will be suitable for your target zone. As time passes, you will find that a certain exercise, at the intensity you have been exercising, no longer stimulates your heart rate to this pulse rate. This change signals that you are more fit and should raise your target rate to a medium level, halfway between the lower and upper figures. In time, you will reach the high fitness level (85% of maximum), and you can maintain high fitness without exceeding this heart rate.

The heart rates listed in Figure 7.1 are calculated from the THR equation above. A widely used test to avoid overexertion is the talk or conversation test. You should be able to carry on a conversation while you exercise. If you cannot, you are stressing yourself needlessly, perhaps dangerously, and probably will give it up because you aren't enjoying it.

Assessment of Aerobic Fitness

The reason for assessment of fitness before beginning an exercise program is to avoid hurting yourself. A middle-aged, slightly overweight person who has not exercised for 5 or more years needs to begin an exercise program gradually. It is dangerous for such a person to exercise at the same intensity as a friend who is already active.

The purpose of the assessment is to find out how much you can exercise to bring your pulse up to a safe maximum without exceeding it. It is important to realize that a safe maximum pulse rate decreases with age.

The strength of the myocardium layer of heart muscle declines approximately at 1% per year after maturity (Brandfonbrener, Lendowne, & Shockin, 1955). This change results in a lowering of the cardiac output in liters per minute. Also, Simonson (1957) found a reduction in size of the lumen in coronary arteries with age. Vital capacity likewise decreases with age (de Vries, 1986).

Bailey (1978), in *Fit or Fat?*, mentioned a woman who was so out of shape that her maximum safe exercise was merely standing still and raising her heels up and down for a few minutes! Imagine what may have happened to her if she suddenly found herself having to climb four flights of stairs. Similarly, the out-of-shape businessman is in jeopardy if he needs to sprint from one airport gate to another while carrying a heavy suitcase. A program of regular exercise provides better protection than an insurance policy in handling sudden exertions.

Fitness assessment tests range from simple step tests that a person can do at home to sophisticated stress tests on programmed treadmills or bicycles in which the subject is monitored by an electrocardiograph. The pulse tests mentioned previously are not useful for diagnostic purposes but only for cardiorespiratory fitness assessment (they are included in Appendix 7B).

Degrees of Fitness

Fitness is unlike conventional beauty, coordination, or musical talent in that the influence of heredity is much less than that of environment. Broadly speaking, almost anyone who is healthy can be fit if he or she desires to be. Here, I need to make an important distinction. People cannot be divided into fit or unfit as distinct categories. Fitness does share with the attributes mentioned above the characteristic of varying in people from one extreme to the other. Like most human characteristics, degrees of fitness form a continuous series.

The aerobics system of conditioning is based on two major principles. The first is that the rate of oxygen consumption must be stimulated by the game, exercise, or physical activity to a certain minimum over the resting rate. The second is that the duration of the exercise must equal or exceed a certain minimum time for the training effect to occur. These two objectives can be met by exercising for 15 minutes 3 times a week in your THR range.

Here we come to the practical aspects of self-assessment tests. You need to start from where you are and proceed sufficiently slowly so that you benefit with pleasure and without discomfort. The less fit you are when you start, the longer it will take to become fit. Don't be competitive about it; accept your unfitness with good grace—after all, it took a long time to get this unfit. Work out an enjoyable program for yourself, but do something!

The Cooper aerobics program is also graded in terms of aerobic points each day and each week. For example, people aged 30-39 who are out of shape are expected to walk 2 miles in 36 minutes 3 times the first week. They earn 11 points for their week's effort. At the end of 6 weeks, they should be walking 2.5 miles in 38 minutes 5 times a week and earning 32 points. After 10 weeks and beyond, they are expected to walk 3.0 miles per day in 44 minutes 5 times a week and earn 33 points. If they continue this program, they will maintain their fitness, or if they prefer, they can shift to other activities to earn 27-32 points a week.

Cooper suggests that an obese person begin by walking 2 miles in 40 minutes 3 times a week. If these times and distances seem too much for you, and you are exhausted after completing a few blocks, don't hesitate to slow down. Many people who begin at this least-fit level are pleasantly surprised at how soon their walking speed improves and they enjoy becoming fit. You should not wear yourself out, however, or feel worse at the end of the exercise than before starting. If this effect occurs, something is wrong. You have exercised too vigorously or discovered that a particular exercise is not suitable for you and should try others.

An important goal of the Cooper group was to determine the number of aerobic points required each week in order to remain fit. They accomplished this objective by examining a group of people who had been exercising regularly for at least 6 months and would be classed as fit by any criterion then available. When their exercises were ranked on the aerobic point scoring system, it was found that the men were exercising at a minimum rate of 32 points per week and the women at 27 points per week.

The point values are more than additive with time. There is a bonus for longer periods of exercise. For example, a person who walks 1 mile in 20 minutes earns 1 point, but if it is continued for 60 minutes, 5 points are earned. The reason for this increase can be best understood by someone who walks or jogs for 1 mile at a comfortable speed one day and then covers 3 miles at the same speed another day. Aerobic points are based on oxygen consumption over the resting rate. It takes a certain time of exercise before a person's rate of oxygen consumption increases very much. The first half mile of a walk or jog does not use as much oxygen as the last half mile.

The Cooper aerobic fitness system is based on a certain minimum effort that is necessary at each session. The more intense the exertion, the shorter its duration need be to accomplish a given number of aerobic points. For example, a woman of 50 who jogs 2 miles in 24 minutes earns 7 points. If she walks 2 miles in 34 minutes, she earns 3 points. She earns 8 points by walking 3 miles in 44 minutes. These point values are based on continuous activity.

Small trampolines have been developed for those people who prefer to exercise at home and are bored with bicycling or running in place. They are easier on joints than jogging on pavements and provide a dog-free environment. They also allow people to exercise in an environment that is less smoggy than the outside air of many cities. It has been estimated that 30 minutes of rebound trampolining is equivalent to 20 minutes of jogging. Records or tapes are available for entire aerobic workouts on minitrampolines.

Aerobic Fitness and Endurance

The changes that occur in the energy supply systems and in the slow-twitch and fast-twitch oxidative muscle fibers in a fitness training program increase the efficiency of oxygen usage. By the same token, these changes also increase endurance. Fit people have more pep and energy and tire less quickly at a given task than less fit or unfit people.

Keeping in Shape by Sports Alone

It is not recommended by Cooper, or any other exercise physiologist whom I have read, that sports should be used as the sole means of keeping in shape. The main reason is that, with few exceptions such as cross-country skiing and swimming, sports do not stimulate muscle groups evenly. Certain muscles are used over and over again, and certain others age neglected. A balanced fitness program should exercise all the muscle groups. Overall fitness will increase your competence at sports. Do not expect sports to contribute to overall fitness.

Sports in which the action is not continuous are ranked much lower in points per minute than those activities that are continuous. Many people, especially tennis players, do not understand why Cooper rates the points for tennis so low. For singles it is only 4.5 points per hour and half that for doubles. The reason is that tennis action is not continuous. Even though players run, hop, jump, and swing during a point, between points and games they walk, often slowly, to a position, or wait up to 30 seconds if an opponent is slow in serving, or longer if the ball must be returned from another court. During these breaks, the heart rate slows down and no training effect occurs. In doubles, the delays are even more frequent and longer than in singles. In contrast, handball, racquetball, squash, basketball, soccer, hockey, and lacrosse are ranked at 9 points per hour of continuous exercise (Cooper, 1983).

In a more recent study, however, Friedman, Rarno, and Gray (1984) tested the physical condition of 28 male singles players, 45–72 years, who played 6–10 hours per week. During an hour of tennis play, heart rates were maintained at a steady-state level between 60%–100% of the age-predicted maximum. Their average fitness level, as measured by maximal oxygen consumption in the treadmill test, was as high as a similar age group who have run 2 1/2 hours per week for 10 years.

The Body as an Engine: Why Warm Up?

In an engine the oxidation of the hydrocarbon fuel produces carbon dioxide, water, and heat in a controlled explosion. Heat production and power production are closely related for the following reason. The gases expand when heated and exert more pressure on the pistons than when the engine is cold. Thus, more power is produced by a warm engine than by a cold one.

The human muscular system responds to heat in a similar way, but for different reasons. As we have seen, carbon dioxide is a waste product in biological oxidations and plays no part in power production. The oxidation reactions are catalyzed by enzymes, and they are affected by temperature. When we sleep in a cold room, our bodies do not cool to room temperature because we produce heat continuously. Yet different parts of our bodies are not all at the same temperature.

We think of 37 °C or 98.5 °F as normal body temperature, but these numbers are average core temperatures and not those of our extremities, which are cooler. When we are quiet in a cool room, our muscle temperatures may drop to about 35 °C (95 °F) or even less. Bergh and Ekblom (1979) found that it takes about 7 minutes of vigorous exercise for muscles to reach their optimum working temperature of 39 °C. During these 7 minutes, the heart rate as well as the oxygen consumption increases significantly. At this higher temperature, the enzymes that form ATP by the oxidation of glucose act more efficiently, as does actomyosin, the enzyme that hydrolyzes ATP and does the work.

If a cold engine is overloaded, it will stall. Similarly, Bergh and Ekblom (1979) also found that abrupt, intensive exercise by a cool body may be associated with an inadequate blood flow to the heart. This situation, even though temporary, can be dangerous. In addition, the chances of damaging cold muscle fibers and connective tissue are much greater than those that have been warmed up by exercises. These exercises should include stretching for flexibility and calisthenics for strength development. Appropriate stretching and calisthenic exercises are included in Appendix 7D.

The Four Phases of a Balanced Aerobics Workout

1. The warm-up. There is more to an aerobics workout than just the aerobics. As the members of an orchestra warm up before a concert, it is advisable for everyone to warm up before engaging in any type of vigorous exercise. The warm-up may commence with light movements such as stretching the hands above the head, twisting the trunk, rotating

the head and neck, and doing partial sit-ups; then proceeding to more vigorous movements as squats, jumping jacks, and running in place, until the pulse rate is definitely elevated for 3–5 minutes. Many joggers/runners start off slowly for the first mile. The objective is to feel warm and loose before commencing any exercise that is vigorous or demanding. Stretching exercises, such as those practiced by Grete Waitz and described in Appendix 7D, are excellent for warm-up and also for cool-down.

2. The aerobic phase. These exercises should bring the pulse into the target range and keep it there continuously for at least 15 minutes, 3 to 4 times a week.

3. The cool-down. The purpose of the cool-down is to prevent blood from pooling in the extremities and to prevent a period of low blood pressure or ventricular arrhythmia that may lead to what is called *post-exercise sudden death*, which occurs at a low but unnecessarily frequent rate after stress tests and aerobic exercise. Dimsdale, Hartley, Gurney, Ruskin, and Greenblatt (1984) found that immediately after exercise ceased, heart rate and blood pressure decreased, while the hormones norepinephrine and epinephrine increased 10-fold and 3-fold, respectively. According to Dimsdale et al. (1984), "The worst possible strategy for exercise cessation would be to have the person abruptly stop exercising and stand" (p. 632). They also cautioned against just sitting around: "The best strategy would be for the work load to be diminished gradually and/or for the subject to rest supine after the exercise" (p. 632). This suggestion fits in well with the Waitz cool-down exercises.

4. Light weight training. As valuable as aerobic exercises may be, they do not exercise all the muscles equally as most of them involve the large leg muscles predominantly. A program of light weight lifting (10-20 minutes) that concentrates on the upper body (e.g., the neck, shoulders, arms, torso, and abdomen) will strengthen and tone these muscles and help decrease the chances of injury in sports or other activities. This program can follow the warm-up, be incorporated in the cool-down, or be engaged in on alternate days.

The Length, Intensity, and Frequency of Aerobic Workouts

The four-phase aerobics workout mentioned above will take about an hour without weight training. If this latter activity is combined with the cool-down, the total time may run somewhat longer. Once you can maintain the 80%–90% target heart rate for 20 minutes, you can keep on a 3-times-a-week schedule. If you choose to rank in the "superior" fitness class, you will need to work out 4 or 5 times a week.

Those people who are used to hurrying through life want to know the minimum time of exercise to earn 10 points. They would prefer to run 1.5 miles in 9 minutes rather than jog 2 miles in 20 minutes. For some people (including myself), running at 6 mph for any appreciable distance is unpleasant. People who set up a rigid time-distance schedule for themselves are not apt to continue unless they enjoy it. Fitness, to me, is not an end in itself, but a condition that will help people enjoy their lives more. Becoming fit and staying fit should not be considered an onerous price to pay for these satisfactions. The fitness activities themselves should contribute to the enjoyment of living, to wellness.

It is possible, of course, to exercise 30 points worth in one day. Exercise physiologists do not recommend this practice as a routine training procedure, and the frequency of most programs is listed at 3 to 5 times per week. Weekend athletes are apt to overstrain and find themselves with sore, stiff muscles a day or so later. People who develop the habit of regular, *enjoyable* exercise 3 or more times a week are more apt to continue than people who knock themselves out once a week.

Cooper, like most other fitness advocates, encourages varied activities to avoid boredom. The objective is not just to stay in shape, but to enjoy it. Exercise programs should be tailored by the individual, based on age, sex, present physical condition, risk factors, and medical problems.

The Cooper aerobics point system is probably the most widely publicized and possibly the most scientifically based fitness program that has yet been devised. It appeals to me both as a scientist and as a person who likes varied activities. Although the point system was worked out based on measurements of oxygen consumption, people soon learn their time and heart target rate numbers and base their workout on their own needs.

Frequency of exercise also affects diet and weight. If you are burning 200 extra kcal per day and are not interested in weight loss, you can consider it as a 200-kcal bonus—an extra degree of freedom to eat what you like—without worrying about your waistline. If you are trying to lose weight, 200 kcal per day 6 times a week adds up to 1200 kcal, or an extra weight loss of a pound every 3 weeks over and above what you would have lost by dieting alone. This, too, amounts to a bonus.

Let's look at frequency from another viewpoint. I consider people who like to exercise as lucky. They not only get health and weight advantages n ~ntioned above, but also enjoy themselves doing it! Although I've not seen data listing people who began aerobic exercise to lose weight or for other reasons, and then became addicted because they enjoyed it or benefited in some way, I've met many people in this category.

Another way of evaluating aerobic exercise is by calculating the calories used. There is a direct correlation between the rate of oxygen uptake and calories consumed. The calories' calculation may be of more interest to the person who is trying to lose weight than that of aerobic points. Pollock, Wilmore, and Fox (1985) list the energy cost of a wide variety of activities (Table 7.7) and of walking or running at different speeds (Table 7.8).

Table 7.7 Energy Cost of Various Activities[a]

Activity	Kilocalories[b] (kcal/min)	Oxygen Uptake (ml/kg • min⁻¹)
Archery	3.7- 5	10.5-14
Backpacking	6 -13.5	17.5-38.5
Badminton	5 -11	14 -31.5
Basketball		
Nongame	3.7-11	10.5-31.5
Game	8.5-15	24.5-42
Bed exercise (arm movement, supine or sitting)	1.1- 2.5	3.5- 7
Bicycling	3.7-10	10.5-28
Bowling	2.5- 5	7 -14
Canoeing (also rowing and kayaking)	3.7-10	10.5-28
Calisthenics	3.7-10	10.5-28
Dancing		
Social and square	3.7- 8.5	10.5-24.5
Aerobic	7.5-11	21 -31.5
Fencing	7.5-12	21 -35
Fishing		
Bank, boat, or ice	2.5- 5	7 -14
Stream, wading	6 - 7.5	17.5-21
Football (touch)	7.5-12	21 -35
Golf		
Using power cart	2.5- 3.7	7 -10.5
Walking, carrying bag, or pulling cart	5 - 8.5	14 -24.5
Handball	10 -15	28 -42
Hiking (cross-country)	3.7- 8.5	10.5-24.5
Horseback riding	3.7-10	10.5-28
Horseshoe pitching	2.5- 3.7	7 -10.5
Hunting, walking		
Small game	3.7- 8.5	10.5-24.5
Big game	3.7-17	10.5-49
Mountain climbing	6 -12	17.5-35
Paddleball/racquetball	10 -15	28 -42
Rope skipping	10 -14	28 -42
Sailing	2.5- 6	7 -17.5

Cont.

Table 7.7 (Cont.)

Activity	Kilocalories[b] (kcal/min)	Oxygen Uptake (ml/kg • min⁻¹)
Scuba diving	6 -12	17.5-35
Shuffleboard	2.5- 3.7	7 -10.5
Skating (ice or roller)	7 -10	17.5-28
Skiing (snow)		
Downhill	6 -10	17.5-28
Cross-country	7.5-15	21 -42
Skiing (water)	6 -85	17.5-24.5
Snow shoeing	8.5-17	24.5-49
Squash	10 -15	28 -42
Soccer	6 -15	17.5-42
Softball	3.7- 7.5	10.5-21
Stair-climbing	5 -10	14 -28
Swimming	5 -10	14 -18
Table tennis	3.7- 6	10.5-17.5
Tennis	5 -11	14 -31.5
Volleyball	3.7- 7.5	10.5-21
Weight training circuit	10	28

[a]Energy cost values based on an individual of 154 lb of body weight (70 kg).

[b]Kilocalorie: A unit of measure based upon heat production. One kcal equals approximately 200 ml of oxygen consumed.

Note. From *Exercise in Health and Disease* (pp. 258-259) by M.L. Pollock, J. Wilmore, and S.M. Fox, 1985, Philadelphia: W.B. Saunders. Copyright 1985 by W.B. Saunders. Reprinted by permission.

Fun and Fitness

There are numerous activities you can select from when looking for fun and fitness.

Walking

Walking as a way of becoming and staying fit has not received as much publicity as jogging. Perhaps it does not need publicity. Davis (1979) quotes the National Center for Health Statistics as showing that in 1975

Table 7.8   Energy Cost of Walking and Running[a]

Activity	MPH	Speed Min/Mi (min:sec)	Grade (%)	Kilocalories[b] (kcal/min)	Oxygen Cost (ml/kg • min⁻¹)
Walking	2.0	30:00	0	2.5	7
	2.5	24:00	0	3.0	8.7
	3.0	20:00	0	3.7	10.5
	3.0	20:00	5	6.0	17.5
	3.0	20:00	10	8.5	24.5
	3.0	20:00	15	11.5	31.5
	3.5	17:08	0	4.2	12.3
	3.5	17:08	5	7.5	21
	3.5	17:08	10	10.0	29
	3.5	17:08	15	13.0	37.5
	3.75	16:00	0	4.9	14
	4.0	15:00	0	5.5	16.1
	4.0	15:00	5	9.0	25.6
	4.0	15:00	10	12.0	35
	4.0	15:00	15	15.6	44.8
	4.5	13:20	0	7.0	20
	5.0	12:00	0	8.3	24
Running	5.5	10:55	0	10.0	29
	6.0	10:00	0	12.0	35
	7.0	8:35	0	14.0	40.3
	8.0	7:30	0	15.6	44.8
	9.0	6:40	0	17.5	49.7
	10.0	6:00	0	19.6	56
	11.0	5:30	0	21.7	62
	12.0	5:00	0	24.5	70

[a]Energy cost values based on an individual of 154 lb of body weight (70 kg).

[b]Kilocalorie: A unit of measure based upon heat production. One kilocalorie equals 200 ml of oxygen consumed.

Note. From *Exercise in Health and Disease* (p. 263) by M.L. Pollock, J. Wilmore, and S.M. Fox, 1985, Philadelphia: W.B. Saunders. Copyright 1985 by W.B. Saunders. Reprinted by permission.

about a third of the U.S. population, 20 years of age and over who reported regular physical activity, chose walking. This percentage was more than twice as high as any other type of exercise.

Suppose a middle-aged, slightly overweight person who has not exercised for many years decides to begin an exercise program but does not know where to begin. For such a person, walking is the easiest, most natural activity that can be suggested. Everyone has walked. There is no new skill to learn. All one needs is the motivation to get out there and start striding.

America has become a nation of inactive people. The President's Council on Physical Fitness has been encouraging citizens to become more active for over 30 years but with mediocre success. Many people begin an exercise program but don't continue it. Several studies have shown that the drop-out rate for walkers is much less than it is for joggers. The reasons are not hard to find. Jogging, especially if practiced on hard pavements, is a dangerous sport. Chris Clegg, an enthusiastic, antijogging walker, has declared "jogging jars joints." *Runners World* magazine, which cannot be accused of an antijogging bias, reported that 60% of runners were disabled by injuries for some period each year. It would seem obvious that if a person picks an activity that is enjoyable, convenient, and not injurious, he or she is more apt to continue it than otherwise. The experience of millions supports walking as that activity.

A Walking Program for Out-of-Shape Adults

The advantages of a walking program have just been outlined. While any kind of walking, even strolling, is more beneficial than stiting at home, a training effect is obtained only under certain minimum conditions. Fortunately, this goal can be approached gradually, as shown in Table 7.6. This walking program is graded. If you don't have any idea about what shape you're in, try the slow walk for 2 miles and time yourself. This first walk will give you a starting point for judging your fitness. If it takes 50 minutes, you can aim for Level 1. If 40 minutes seem too slow, you can start at a higher level.

I suggest that you learn to take your pulse while you walk at the slower speeds, before you get into the training effect range. By the time you come to Levels 4 or 5, your pulse rate should be approaching the 70% target heart rate as shown in Figure 7.1. You now are in command of your own program and can attain higher degrees of fitness at whatever rate seems desirable.

Powerwalking

In ordinary walking, it is difficult to get the heart rate up to the target range. Consequently, even brisk walkers need to walk a long time for aerobic benefits. How to burn more calories per minute, yet safely? Jogging and running aren't the answer. They are too hard on the joints (the knees, ankles, and hips) as well as the shins. A satisfying answer for many people is *powerwalking*, formerly called *racewalking*.

The name racewalking derives from its being an Olympic sport. Most of us aren't interested in racing. We may have seen those funny looking walkers on TV and decided it was not for us. However, in the book, *Racewalk to Fitness,* Howard Jacobson (1980) describes the sport for the average person who wants a safe, aerobic workout that can be done at any convenient time and requires no change of clothes or going to a special place.

Racewalking is defined by the International Amateur Athletic Federation as follows:

Walking is progression by steps so taken that unbroken contact with the ground is maintained. At each step, the advancing foot of the walker must make contact with the ground before the rear foot leaves the ground. During a period of each step when a foot is on the ground, the leg must be straightened (not bent at the knee) at least for one moment, and in particular, the supporting leg must be straight in the vertical upright position (Jacobson, p. 257).

Racewalking actually is ordinary walking with a few special additions that increase the efficiency of movement.

1. The plant. Stand erect with your arms at your sides. Begin to walk by moving your left foot forward and plant your heel at about a 40° angle. Your foot should make a 90° angle with your leg. It is essential that the back edge of the heel strike the ground first.
2. The tilt-step. As the heel strikes, tilt your foot slightly to the outside edge of the shoe and lock your ankle. As the step continues from heel to big toe, the outside edge acts as a rocker and allows for a smooth transition of your weight. Locking the ankle prevents the leg from rotating and avoids runners' knee.
3. Thrust-propulsion. As the left leg pulls forward, the right leg pushes backward until toe-off. This thrust gives forward acceleration. The right leg then swings forward and the right heel is planted.
4. The arm swing. In racewalking, the arms do not hang down and swing with the opposite foot. The arms are bent so that the forearm makes a right angle with the upper arm. This change makes for a shorter pendulum, which, in turn, allows for faster steps than in ordinary walking. The elbows should be held in, close to the body. The loosely clenched fist should come to midchest height at the forward swing. The height of the backswing is determined by how fast you are walking; the faster you walk, the higher your swing.
5. Breathing. Diaphragmatic or belly breathing is the most efficient way of obtaining oxygen while walking. Practice the following

breathing exercise slowly until it becomes reflexive. As you extend your left leg, inhale through your nose and push your stomach out. As you extend your right leg, exhale through your mouth while tightening the rib cage and stomach. Use them as a bellows to force the air out. This 1, 2 cadence is suitable for 15-minute miles and faster. At slower speeds, 15- to 20-minute miles, you can use a 4-count cadence: 1, 2, inhale as left leg, then right leg, extends; 3, 4 exhale as left leg, then right leg, extends.

6. Posture. A powerwalker stands straight up. The spine and head are both erect. Don't look down, but focus the eyes well ahead. Powerwalking will improve your general posture.

7. Warm-up and cool-down. As with all aerobic exercises, a period of calisthenics of 10 to 20 minutes should precede the racewalk and a cool-down of slow walking should succeed it.

At the beginning, don't attempt to walk fast. Emphasize proper technique until each part of each step feels natural. Walk with experienced walkers and have them criticize your form.

Jacobson (1980) suggests that for the first month a beginner practice at a rate of 90-120 steps per minute on an every-other-day schedule. Each day emphasize a different aspect, such as arm-and-leg rhythm, foot placement, heel strike and foot roll, breathing, and upright posture.

As a competitive racer, Jacobson extols the advantages and delights of the racer's life. He devotes much space to improving technique so that a racewalker can go faster. As with most sports, one can go as far as one chooses in this direction. At the very least, I can recommend it as an enjoyable way (for me) to keep fit.

Folk Dancing

What do Americans in leotards have in common with European peasants in their best costumes, American Indians in ornamented dress, and Australian aborigines with painted bodies? They all dance. They all express the rhythm patterns that surround us. Ancient peoples danced. Primitive peoples danced. Preindustrial peoples danced. Technological people are relearning to dance. The need is within us. Let us take up the dances of our forefathers, follow in the footsteps of Zorba, or participate in the aerobic dances. Whatever turns you on the most, just do it; for fun, for relaxation, and for wellness.

Aerobic Dance: A Contemporary Folk Dance

Up until World War I, the bulk of the work done in the world was by manual labor. Despite the hard work in the field or on the construction site, people would gather together after work and on holidays and dance.

Folks put on their ceremonial dress and danced the regional or tribal dances that their forefathers originated generations ago.

Immigrants to the U.S. brought their dances with them, and the traditions were continued in the various ethnic communities and ghettos of large cities. The melting pots—intermarriage and upward mobility—opposed ethnic traditions. The rising young stock clerk wanted to be known as an American, not as a member of an ethnic group. In the cities, folk dancing fell into disfavor except among the older population, and it was not until people realized that something precious was being lost that instruction of the young in folk dancing was recommenced. The various types of social dancing, from ballroom to disco, have not been engaged in by the majority of urban populations. A few years ago it seemed that dancing was on its way out—another fatality of modern civilization.

But something new has developed. Aerobic dancing is sweeping the country, private enterprise has scented profits in sweaty bodies, and numerous programs are now being offered to the public. The aerobic revolution has breathed new life into dancing. The original participants were mostly women 25-35 years old, but gradually older women and men of various ages have been joining in. On this basis, three to four classes a week will provide sufficient exercise to keep a person in condition.

It is interesting to examine aerobic dance as a sociological phenomenon. Like disco, it is done in a group, but each dancer does his or her own thing, without a partner. In keeping with many activities outside the home, there are instructors who have been trained to lead a group in a wide variety of calisthenics, dance steps, and plain old-fashioned exercises to rock music.

Because of the diversity of movements, the music, and the group, aerobic dance is not boring and can even be enjoyable. It is done indoors, which means that dogs, cars, and other people are not problems. Many of the studios provide only the room and the instructor so that costs are minimal. In Salt Lake City, classes are available from 6:00 a.m. throughout the day and into the evening. Some are in private fitness centers, others in school gyms. TV programs for yoga and for calisthenics have long been broadcast. Aerobic dance programs are now available on some PBS stations and video cassettes.

Each session of about an hour is broken up into three parts: a warm-up period of about 10-15 minutes; the aerobic section of 15-20 minutes; and the cool-down, a relaxation period of about 10-15 minutes. Some instructors pause periodically during and just after the aerobic part for pulse taking. For the most benefit, dancers are encouraged to exert themselves—to stretch, to step lively, to keep kicking the legs or waving the arms. They are also warned that if they feel they have overexerted themselves, they should slow down. For safety's sake, it is probably advisable for a person to join a class of a similar age group. As with any aerobic exercise, people who are out of shape should learn the routines slowly and cautiously.

One advantage of these classes is that calisthenic exercises occupy both the warm-up and cool-down periods. These nonaerobic exercises are excellent for maintaining agility, suppleness, and a firm abdomen, as well as for avoiding lower back problems. Although many joggers and cross-country skiers do warm-ups and cool-downs, my impression is that a much wider range of muscles and joints is exercised in dance classes than most people do on their own.

Tai Chi Chuan

This ancient Chinese exercise is practiced daily by millions of people in Asia and a growing number in the U.S. It has been called *walking meditation* because it involves the brain as well as the muscles. It is formal, with set movements, which resemble a slow ballet; many of the movements are similar.

I have participated in Tai Chi for some years and have found it a marvelous waking-up exercise. At the end of a session I feel warm, graceful, and relaxed, and my joints feel well lubricated. The exercise takes approximately 15 minutes and definitely stimulates the pulse rate. Kurland (1981) measured the oxygen consumption of subjects while they were performing Tai Chi and concluded that their energy expenditure was equivalent to walking slowly. In addition, Tai Chi includes dynamic relaxation, encourages good posture, and reduces stress and tension by a combination of mental exercise and physical movement. People with arthritis or other joint problems may need to modify some of the leg-bending movements.

To conclude this section, I can suggest that, no matter what shape you are in as you read these lines, there is a safe, pleasant, and enjoyable conditioning program in which you may participate. You can develop one for yourself or with the help of professionals. For further information, consult the fitness books by Cooper (1983) and Sharkey (1984).

I should also specify that a fitness program will not handcuff you to a jock who will force you to do things you don't like. It's not like dieting. You are in control of your own program. If it becomes boring, you can change it at any time. Once the habit becomes established, if you miss a session, or a week, or even longer—as for an illness—you will realize that it's not the end of the world. You pick up where you left off and go on from there. If you are typical, you will soon look forward to the sessions as adding fun and variety to your life.

Aerobic fitness not only helps protect against heart attacks, it also contributes to wellness in a variety of subtle ways. A fit, well person has the energy to engage in activities beyond the minimum to stay alive. Such people do not merely exist, they live.

Physical Changes in Aerobic Training

As mentioned in the introduction to this chapter, aerobic fitness is estimated by measuring the maximal oxygen uptake under conditions of
maximal, aerobic work. Degrees of fitness have been set up depending
on the efficiency of oxygen usage. You might wonder, what is the connection between maximum oxygen uptake and efficiency of usage? Under
conditions of maximum exertion, the amount of oxygen uptake becomes
the limiting factor. In a stress test, both are measured, and the oxygen
consumed per unit of work done is taken as a measure of the efficiency.
Fitness is thus defined as the ratio of the rate of oxygen intake per kilogram per minute to the rate of working under maximal conditions. It has
subsequently been established that the ratio is also valid under submaximal conditions. A person who can do a given amount of work using
less oxygen than another person is considered more fit. Training increases
efficiency. How does it come about? It is dependent on both the energy-
utilizing system (the muscle fibers) and the energy-supplying systems
(the cardiorespiratory and cardiovascular systems).

Fox and Mathews (1981) summarize the changes in the muscle fibers
due to 12 weeks of training as an 80% increase in myoglobin content and
a 100% increase in ability to oxidize both glycogen and fats. In 6 months
the number of mitochondria—where these aerobic enzymes are located—
doubled. The storage of both glycogen and fats in the muscle fibers was
also increased. As we saw in Table 7.1, aerobic oxidations are 15 times
more efficient in ATP synthesis than anaerobic, and this number increases
to 25 when fats are oxidized.

These changes increase the efficiency of oxygen usage as follows: Myoglobin functions as the intracellular reservoir of oxygen. The more of it
that is present in the cell, the more efficiently the oxygen can be utilized.
It is somewhat similar to having water piped into a house compared to
having a well outside. There may be an almost unlimited supply of water
in each case, but the difference lies in the delivery systems. If a sudden
need for water develops in the house, such as dousing a small fire, it is
much more efficiently met by filling a pan from the tap than having to
go outside for each panful.

The major changes in the cardiovascular system due to training are an
increased heart size, a decreased heart rate both at rest and at a given
work level, an increased stroke volume, and an increased blood volume
and total hemoglobin. To spell out the connections, the increased heart
size is due to thicker, stronger *ventricular muscles*, which result in the increased stroke volume, which, in turn, results in a lower heart beat per
minute both at rest and when stimulated. The heart muscle is working
more efficiently.

It is interesting that total blood supply to muscles does not increase
during exercise or due to conditioning, but the number of capillaries per

muscle fiber does increase. This result brings more blood in intimate contact with the muscles, and so the supply of both oxygen and energy is augmented.

The question of whether there is a conversion of fiber types during training has been investigated ever since the differences in muscle fibers were first discovered. Present data do not support an actual conversion from slow-twitch to fast-twitch or vice versa. What has been observed is an increase in fast-twitch oxidative fibers and a decrease in fast-twitch glycolytic fibers (Saltin et al., 1977). This change represents an increase in the number of mitochondria—the site of oxidative metabolism—in fast-twitch fibers. Whether this change results from an actual conversion of fiber types of reflects a change in the rate of synthesis of the two fiber types is not known. In either case, the change does explain the increased oxidative capacity, and thus the increased efficiency of ATP synthesis, of muscle fibers from trained people.

The chest muscles respond to ventilatory training by also becoming more efficient, which allows them to do their work using less oxygen than by untrained ventilatory muscles. This decrease in oxygen consumption by ventilatory muscles allows more oxygen to become available to the skeletal muscles. The effective lung volume also increases during training, which, of course, results in more oxygen being processed per breath.

In summary, an increased efficiency has been demonstrated in each of the three major systems that are involved in aerobic exercise: the skeletal muscles themselves, the cardiovascular system, and the cardiorespiratory system. The summation of these changes results in the increased endurance that is the hallmark of trained, fit people.

Strength (Anaerobic) Fitness

Just as the term aerobic fitness refers to activities and exercises that stimulate the slow-twitch oxidative fibers, the term anaerobic fitness refers to activities and exercises that stimulate the fast-twitch fibers. These exercises include weight lifting, certain sport activities like running short distances, shot-putting, discus throwing, and flexibility training.

If anaerobic fitness, however, were confined to a few athletes, it would have no place in a book for a general audience. Actually, the large muscles of all humans, especially those in the upper legs, arms, and back, contain a high percentage of anaerobic muscle fibers. Table 7.2 contains the percentages of slow-twitch muscle fibers in various muscles and fast-twitch by difference. It is obvious that anyone interested in general fitness should keep the muscles in shape that are involved in good posture and a strong back. In addition, muscular strength is useful around the house. It's handy to be able to unscrew a tight jar lid or replace a frayed belt on a vacuum cleaner without calling a neighbor who works out.

Body Changes in Weight Training

A group of college students was enrolled in a weight-training experiment that met twice a week for 10 weeks. Wilmore (1974) found that they all gained strength in the biceps, grip, shoulders and chest, and legs. The percentage increase in the women was greater than the men in all categories but the biceps. The subjects showed no change in total body weight; lean body weight increased about 1%, whereas absolute body fat decreased about 1%.

The large muscles, of course, are exercised in warm-up and cool-down exercises described in the aerobic section. Without resistance in these exercises, however, these muscles hardly grow in size at all. In fact, even in the weight-training experiment, Wilmore found the largest increase of males was slightly less than 1/2 inch in shoulder girth. The largest increases among the women were about 0.2 inch in biceps, chest, and shoulders. It is obvious from these figures that the large increases in muscle mass that one sees in magazines and movies demands a long-term, hardworking schedule by men. By the same token, women who pump iron will find it difficult to increase their muscle girth to a degree that is unattractive.

Many people, especially women, seem satisfied with a strictly aerobic exercise program that includes the anaerobic warm-up and cool-down. For those who choose to include a strength training program, I'll mention some valuable tested procedures.

Strength Training Procedures: The Overload Principle

In the sixth century B.C., Milo of Crotona became the strongest man in Greece by carrying a calf on his shoulders every day until it grew to a full-sized cow, which he carried the length of the stadium at Olympia. Milo inadvertently discovered what is now called the *overload principle*. It states that the strength and endurance of a muscle will improve only when it performs at or near its maximum capacity. That is, at work loads that exceed those normally encountered. For continued improvement, the overload must be increased as the muscle gains strength, as in Milo's experiment. This modification of the overload principle is called *progressive resistance exercise*.

Research has also demonstrated that overloading is specific. The only muscles that increase in strength are those that are exercised. How can these insights be applied by a person who is not a competitive athlete but merely wants to stay in shape? In answering this question, I'll assume that the person is engaging in an aerobics program but wants more defined and stronger muscles than such programs provide. The statements above furnish a basis for developing an individual program. It would include applying the overload principle to the major muscle systems of the body until a desirable state of strength and endurance was attained, as defined by the person. The second part of the program consists of maintaining this desirable state.

I'll introduce the topic of how to increase muscle strength by explaining the three common types of overloading. They are (a) isometric contraction (constant length), a static contraction in which neither the muscle nor the resistance moves; (b) isotonic contraction (equal tone or tension), the muscle can lengthen or shorten as it moves; and (c) isokinetic (equal speed), over the full range of motion. Each type has advantages and disadvantages (De Vries, 1986).

The isometric method was first described in 1953 by Hettinger and Mueller. They showed that a maximum training effect could be obtained from a single 6-second isometric contraction a day against a specified resistance. Muscle strength improved at an average rate of 5% a week. The idea of a fast workout appeals to many people, but it turns out that for maximum effect each joint should be exercised at three to four angles 5 times a day, which reduces the time-saving factor. In addition, isometric exercise increases blood pressure, which excludes it from cardiac rehabilitation programs or adult exercise programs.

Fox and Mathews (1981) consider isokinetic training programs the most suitable for improving strength and endurance for athletic performances. The speed of movement can be varied depending on the sport. Isokinetic equipment is used by many coaches but is not widely available in commercial gyms.

Isotonic and isokinetic procedures have the great advantage of working the entire range of motion in one contraction. The isotonic method was placed on a sound scientific basis by DeLorme and Watkins (1951). It is based on the idea of repetition maximum (RM): the maximum weight that a muscle can lift over a given number of repetitions (10 RM = 10 repetitions). They suggested the following program for increasing muscle strength.

Set 1   10 repetitions at a load of 1/2 10 RM
Set 2   10 repetitions at a load of 3/4 10 RM
Set 3   10 repetitions at a load of 10 RM

Subsequent research by Berger (1962) showed that three sets, each with a 6-RM load, resulted in the greatest increase in strength when performed 3 times a week for 12 weeks.

Some Strength-Training Generalizations

1. In strength-training programs, the size and strength of muscles increase proportionately. The size (diameter) of fast-twitch increases, not the number. Strength is related to quantity of muscle, not to quality (De Vries, 1986).

2. Progressive weight overloading is considered the most effective strength-training procedure developed so far. It is suggested that each muscle group be trained on an every-other-day basis. In a given session, it may be desirable to alternate between arm-chest and leg-abdominal exercises.
3. Strengthening exercises do increase both speed and power of contraction. For maximum effect, every contraction should be made throughout the full range of motion. If full motion is practiced routinely, flexibility will be increased as well as strength. The data demonstrate that the term *muscle bound* has no basis in fact.
4. A variety of specific sport skills like running, swimming, tennis, jumping, and throwing can be increased by appropriate weight-training programs. A skier, for example, may work for extra strong thighs.
5. Low repetitions with high resistances result primarily in strength increase, whereas high repetitions with low resistances result primarily in increased endurance. Both strength and endurance can be increased by a program using intermediate resistance and intermediate repetitions.

Effects of Strength Training on Muscle Fibers and Energy Sources

Strength training is similar to endurance training in that many physical changes occur, but the changes are quite different in the two types. In strength training, most of the effects are found in the muscles themselves and fewer in the energy-supply systems.

The most obvious effect, and I suspect the main reason for its popularity among young men, is the increase in size of the large muscles. When these muscles are viewed through a microscope, the white, fast-twitch fibers are seen to have increased in diameter, for which the technical term is *hypertrophy*. The numbers of these fibers as a percentage of the three fiber types have also increased, which leads to the hypothesis that they have split and divided whereas the slow-twitch type have not. Because these fibers contain the least number of mitochondria, the concentration of these oxidative particles in the whole muscle has decreased. The concentrations of the energy-containing ATP and CP both increased significantly in resting white fibers as a result of strength training.

The Specific Effects of Strength-Training Methods

Much of the research on training methods has been done with the objective of aiding athletes to improve their performance. There is no question that this objective has been successful. Records continue to be broken in both track-and-field and swimming events. Successful training methods focus on the muscles, the movements used, and the duration of specific events. Notice that these events are for individuals, and training can be highly specialized.

However, I want to emphasize that use of the overloading principle for gain in strength-fitness will not by itself increase cardiorespiratory fitness. In a 16-week study of high-intensity Nautilus training, Hurley et al. (1984) observed a 44% increase in strength, but body weight and percent fat did not change. Maximal oxygen uptake—the measure of aerobic fitness—did not change. Heavyweight lifters do huff and puff during their brief sets of repetitions, and their heart rate increases; but in this study the volume of oxygen intake was no greater than that produced by walking at 4 miles per hour. Hurley et al. explain the "huffing and puffing" of weight lifters as being due to a decrease in stroke volume of the heart. In other words, the heart has to beat more often because the volume of blood that it pumps per beat decreases markedly during heavy exercise. At this relatively low level of oxygen intake, one has to exercise a full hour to obtain an aerobic effect. Many weight lifters do not come close to 60 minutes of continuous heavy exertion in a single workout.

What about team competition like football and basketball in which individual positions require different abilities and both aerobic and anaerobic endurance is necessary? These endurance characteristics, except for the degree of fitness, are much closer to that of the lay public than that required by a sprinter or a pole-vaulter. I suggest that for all-around, nonspecialized living, a person should engage in both endurance and strength exercises. The two objectives are not incompatible; they complement each other.

Mixed Fitness Training: Endurance and Strength

Most adults who are interested in fitness are not athletes. Readers may have the impression from my separation of aerobic and anaerobic programs that the results are quite distinct, aerobics leading to cardiorespiratory fitness and anaerobics leading to skeletal-muscle fitness. Fortunately, there are programs in which the two objectives can be easily combined.

One such program is mentioned in the 4 stages of an aerobics workout, in which Stage 4 consists of lifting weights. Actually, if a person desires to keep muscles in tone without an increase in size, lifting of light weights can be substituted for some of the cool-down exercises of Stage 3. This objective can also be realized by a program called interval training.

Interval Training

By necessity, anaerobic programs like lifting of heavy weights require rest periods. Aerobic programs, however, usually involve continuous exercise. Swedish workers (Astrand, Astrand, Christensen, & Hedman, 1960) have demonstrated that rest periods during aerobic workouts can increase endurance significantly. A subject could work for an hour intermittently, whereas he became exhausted in 9 minutes of continuous work. His physical work was over 3 times greater per hour when he worked intermittently compared to continuously. His pulse rate reached 204 bpm, and his blood lactate concentration reached 150 mg per 100 ml when he worked continuously, but only reached 150 bpm and 20 mg per 100 ml when he worked intermittently. These numbers indicate that most of the energy came from aerobic metabolism during the intermittent work regime and from anaerobic metabolism during the continuous regime. In this connection, recall the much greater efficiency of the aerobic compared to the anaerobic pathway in energy release. These results and many others support high-intensity interval training as a means of developing both endurance and strength in a single workout.

Fartlek

Who says the Swedes are always somber? They invented *fartlek*, meaning speed play. It involves alternating slow and fast running in which neither the work nor relief intervals are precisely timed. It is actually a form of interval training because both aerobic and anaerobic capacities are developed. It amounts to alternating sprinting, jogging, and walking (preferably out of doors) as the mood dictates, and includes a 10-minute jog warm-up and a slightly longer jog cool-down.

Circuit Weight Training

Circuit weight training is the term used for a type of light weight lifting that is almost continuous. It differs from heavy weight lifting in that the different exercises are performed at 40% of a 1 RM at each station. In an experiment carried out by Gettman, Ward, and Hagan (1982), a group of men and women in their mid-thirties participated in a 12-week program to determine whether circuit weight training by itself or in combination with a running program produced desirable changes in aerobic fitness, muscular strength, and body composition.

In the circuit weight-training program, 10 weight-training exercises were performed in three circuits of 12-15 repetitions in 30 seconds each. A 15-second rest period was allowed after each group of repetitions at each station. The running program was similar except that a 30-second run on a track replaced the rest period between stations.

When compared to a control group that didn't exercise, both of the circuit weight-training groups showed significant improvements in three components of fitness compared to the controls: Aerobic fitness increased about 15%, as measured by an increase in maximum oxygen uptake; muscular strength increased about 20%; and body fat decreased about 3.5%.

Maintenance of Fitness

As just mentioned, general fitness can be attained by a suitable program that combines both endurance and strength training. After a desirable degree of fitness has been reached a person may not want to progress to higher levels and may wonder if continuation of the program is required, or if not, where, and how much to cut down. It may surprise you to learn that anaerobic-strength fitness is maintained at a much lower energy expenditure than is required to gain it. De Vries (1986) estimates that strength can be maintained by as little as one set at 1 RM once a week on each muscle group. However, I suggest that out-of-shape, middle-aged and older people approach 1 RM cautiously. Prudence suggests one set at 4-6 RM for starters. Aerobic fitness maintenance requires a minimum of three 15-minute workouts a week at whatever target heart rate and fitness level that is desired. According to Cooper, longer workouts do not increase fitness but are useful in weight reduction.

General Fitness Notes

As mentioned above, weight lifting or short, hard exercise results in an increase in strength of the fast-twitch glycolytic muscle fibers and in their greater endurance at heavy work. A number of factors are responsible for these changes. The muscles tend to contain more glycogen—their primary fuel reserve—than less fit fibers and therefore can work longer. Also, they are thought to become more resistant to the effects of lactic acid on lowering their efficiency of working. Another factor concerns the changes in the fast-twitch oxidative fibers. They develop more mitochondria and thus are able to oxidize more of the lactic acid to produce more ATP—the immediate source of energy for muscle work.

Retention of Fitness

Berger (1962) found that the strength gained during a 3-week isotonic training program was not lost during a subsequent 6-week period of no training. Waldman and Stull (1969) found that, after a lapse of 12 weeks of no training, 70% of elbow flexion strength was retained. Ceasing of aerobic exercises, however, results in fairly rapid loss of fitness. In about 2 months, a person who stops aerobics will be out of shape.

Fortunately, for fit people whose schedule does not permit workouts 3-5 times per week, reducing workout frequency to 2 times per week maintains fitness (maximum $\dot{V}O_2$) for a 10-week period. Workouts as infrequent as once a week retard but do not prevent loss of fitness (Fox & Mathews, 1981, pp. 333-338).

Working Out at Home, in the Gym, or at an Aerobic Dance Studio

Some people prefer to work out in the privacy and convenience of their own living quarters. Others like the variety of equipment, camaraderie, motivation, and instruction available at commercial establishments. For those readers who are considering buying their own equipment, I can recommend articles in *Consumer Reports* in the past few years on rowing machines and home gyms (8/85); exercise bikes (8/86); running shoes (10/86); and ski exercisers (11/86). Before paying hundreds of dollars for your own equipment, I would suggest using a variety of them at a gym for a long enough time so that your choice is based on experience, and also that you know how to use what you plan to buy.

Adaptation of the Human Body to Type of Exercise

An interesting anecdotal experiment concerns a world-class U.S. weight lifter who, at the age of 25, decided to give up weight lifting and take up long-distance running (De Vries, 1986). After 3 years of training, he ran a marathon in 3 hours, 3 1/2 minutes. Within this period his weight had gone from 226 to 162 lb; his strength (total snatch, clean and jerk) had decreased by almost 200 lb (730 vs 534 lb); but his effective strength was greater (3.23 vs 3.30 lift weight per pound of body weight).

Take a Break!

What sedentary worker hasn't had the doldrums, the yawns, the blahs hit him or her in midafternoon from time to time, or even daily? One or more of the exercises shown in Appendix 7E will help get your blood flowing and the mist out of your eyes, and will evaporate the fog in your brain. They aren't aerobic, but if you are unable to leave your computer, they may stimulate you even longer than an erotic film.

To summarize, a general fitness maintenance program should include an aerobics section as described by Cooper and others and an anaerobics section for the maintenance of strength and agility. Both types contribute to an attractive appearance.

Waking Up Exercises

People's responses to waking up in the morning (or whenever) are probably as varied as their personalities. In my limited observations, I have come to the conclusion that some people wake up much faster than others. For those who wake up slowly—say 15 minutes or more before they can utter "good morning"—I will be brash enough to suggest waking-up exercises. They needn't be very vigorous. Again, the speed and the amount of exertion should be determined by you as to what makes you feel awake, alive, and friendly after about 15 minutes.

My own exercises are of two types: those done standing up that maintain flexibility and those done lying supine that are primarily for the back. I do the standing ones first and fairly slowly, at a comfortable speed for me. A number of these are tai chi warm-ups. They make me feel graceful as I perform them. I have never had a back problem although I am aware that my back is weaker than it used to be. About 20 years ago my back began to ache on a long automobile trip. It was at that point that I began these present exercises of slow, limited motion sit-ups. I attribute my lack of back trouble to having done these daily all these years. I expect that by now you are aware that my experience does not provide evidence that these exercises will help you in any way. I suggest them as among the things that probably won't hurt and may help. These types of exercises are shown in Appendix 7F.

Aerobic Exercise and the Elderly

It is common knowledge that most people become less active physically as they age. There are many reasons for this decrease in activity: injuries; illnesses, such as arthritis, that make movements painful or difficult; impairment of vision, hearing, and touch; lack of companionship; depression; inability to accept declining performance in a sport; danger of falling on ice or snow in the winter; a self-image that no longer includes activity as a regular thing to do.

There is a growing awareness among the elderly that much of their stiffness, aches, and pains are not necessarily related to growing old, but to inactivity. Older people are discovering that activity will aid them in enjoying their lives. Aerobic activity and muscular exercise are as important, if not more so, to people past 70 as to people under 50. Many people in this upper-age group have never exercised and do not know how to begin. If you are at all disabled or have medical problems, talk to your doctor first, and secure his or her ok on what you should or should not do. Remember, the purpose is to expand your activities, not restrict them by injury.

If you are past 70, free-living, with or without a companion, and would like to commence an exercise program, I would suggest inquiring at a senior citizen center, church, or community center for the time and place of a fitness exercise class. If you have any medical or personal restrictions, talk to the instructor before the first class. If you live in a retirement home, there may be such a class already going. If not, inquire about starting one. Talk to your friends about starting or joining such a class. There is power in numbers!

The success of an exercise class can be measured in a number of ways. One of the most important is the feeling that the exercises are fun. You should feel better, be more cheerful, stand up straighter, be more aware of your body, and feel more playful—but not necessarily all at once or every time. In general, the participants should feel better at the end of a session than at the beginning. The exercises should be paced slowly enough so that no one feels rushed.

Mall Walking

Many people who have begun to walk regularly find they are stymied in the winter by snow and ice and in the summer by heat. Walking in malls in the morning before the stores open provides a neat solution to these problems and is also sufficiently popular to lead to friendly sociability.

Psychological Benefits of Aerobic Exercise in Middle-Aged People

Blumenthal, Williams, Needels, and Wallace (1982) assessed the effects of aerobic exercise on a group of healthy, middle-aged adults. Sixteen subjects engaged in a regular program of walking-jogging for 10 weeks and were compared to a matched, sedentary, control group. All subjects took a variety of psychological tests such as Profile of Mood States, the State-Trait Anxiety Inventory, and a retrospective questionnaire on self-perceptions of change. The exercisers exhibited less state and trait anxiety, less tension, depression and fatigue, and more vigor than the controls.

Apart from these subjective feelings, aerobic exercise has been found by Dustman et al. (1984) to improve a number of important psychological functions in a group of average sedentary people of both sexes, aged 55–70 years. The subjects were divided into three groups: a control group, which remained sedentary; an aerobic exercise group; and a nonaerobic exercise group. The aerobic participants, after a warm-up, engaged in fast walking or jogging to stimulate their hearts to a safe target rate 3 times a week for 4 months. The nonaerobic, strength-flexibility group also exercised for about an hour 3 times a week.

All three groups were tested before and after the exercise program. They were given eight neuropsychological tests. Response time, visual organization, memory, and mental flexibility improved significantly more in the aerobic group compared to the others. Together, these tests can be considered a measure of cognitive ability. There were no differences in depression scores, visual acuity, or sensory thresholds among the groups. The authors suggest that in the aerobic group, improved transport and utilization of oxygen occurred in the brain and enhanced cerebral metabolic activity. I consider this work as justifying aerobic activity as long as physically possible.

Passive Exercises

It is my impression that some people are more concerned with their appearance than with their health and fitness. Americans want to look attractive in bathing suits, but they don't want to work for it. Men want to look muscular without exercising, and women want a good figure, also without exercises. Affluent people will pay large sums to look attractive as long as the activity does not involve sufficient physical exertion to produce sweat. The long-term popularity of massage, spas, and special baths in many parts of the world suggests that humans dislike vigorous physical activity.

The latest fad, called "passive exercise," has recently come to the U.S. from Europe. According to the *Wall Street Journal* (Zonana, 1982), the technique generates thousands of tiny electric shocks to stimulate muscle contractions in flabby parts of the body. Passive exercise is billed as "the civilized way to streamline your body." One young San Francisco lawyer is quoted as saying, "I don't care how I get the body I want. If one method hurts less than another, I'll choose the less painful" (p. 1). Another client had tried biking, jogging, and weight lifting but could "never get into it." After 13 shock treatments, he said, "My waist is three inches smaller" (p. 1).

I am continually amazed at how many people treat their bodies like the paint job on their cars. It doesn't matter what's underneath as long as it looks good. Self-deception is the cruelest ruse of all. Passive exercise purveyors claim that the treatments can tone muscles and remove fat from the midsection. Health professionals scoff at these false promises. Even the purveyors, however, do not state that the shock treatments will improve the cardiovascular system.

Compliance

Many people have not exercised to any extent for so many years that the very idea of getting out there in some kind of an outfit that exposes their legs and torso is out of the question and absurd. Also, the fact that exercise cannot promise them anything definite for weeks, if not months, is another deterrent. They are so used to not feeling well for so many years, and to popping a pill when they feel worse than usual, that to speak to them in terms of becoming aware of one's body in a positive sense is like speaking a foreign language. Of course, they are aware of their bodies; they feel punk most of the time. The message they are getting from their bodies is, "Use me as little as possible." These people have created vicious cycles for themselves. They act as if they were miserable but will only admit it to a good friend, who, by definition, listens sympathetically and does not offer advice. Can these people be helped? Or are they like alcoholics, who may despise themselves but cannot be reached until they admit they cannot trust themselves to take a single drink?

An interesting example of compliance was obtained on the participants in the brain function exercise experiment by the Dustman group (1984) mentioned previously. When the experimental results were published, the participants were sent a reprint, thanked for their cooperation, and informed that aerobic exercise did have a beneficial effect on the brain. They were also encouraged to keep exercising (R. Dustman, personal communication, 1986). Four years later, they were contacted by mail as to their exercise habits (recall that they all had been sedentary before participating in the experiment). The return rate of replies was very high—25 out of 27. The compliance data were very interesting and surprising. Sixty-seven percent of the aerobic exercise group were still working out at least 3 days a week—an impressive compliance. But, what was more surprising was that 53% of the nonaerobic exercise group were now working out aerobically on a regular basis. It is also interesting that, of the group that was exercising 4 years later, 80% were females and 44% were males. This experiment deserves to be repeated with thousands of participants.

Sometimes a small thing, like taking a walk, leads to new possibilities and, if the walking becomes frequent, serves as a path to a positive view of living and an altered lifestyle. Think of something enjoyable, convenient to do, and easy on the joints, and do it regularly for a month, alone, with a friend, or in a group, whichever appeals to you the most. Be careful in what you choose. If you do not find it enjoyable and stimulating, you will probably not continue. There are many paths to fitness, but they share one thing in common: They are self-sustaining on a long-term basis only if each person has found an activity or group of activities that more than repays the effort in psychological benefits.

Body Awareness

By body awareness, I mean that the signals that have originated in the muscle–nerve junctions are transmitted to the spinal cord and finally to the brain, where they may become conscious feelings. We don't understand how these signals are translated into positive feelings and attitudes like self-esteem, self-confidence, unflappability, calmness, willingness to share emotions with others, caring, and loving, but millions of people have experienced these benefits. It is no longer a secret but a well-recognized path towards wellness.

Another aspect of body-awareness concerns muscle tension. A host of biofeedback studies has demonstrated that many people are not aware of the tensions of their own muscles (Brown, 1974; Stern & Ray, 1980). In fact, Gaarder and Montgomery (1981) state: ''This is the fact that anxiety cannot exist in the presence of deep muscle relaxation'' (p. 19).

The body awareness that I am referring to is not dependent solely on muscle relaxation. It can be more accurately described as an awareness of muscle tone or strength as the basis of positive feelings, or of flabbiness or weakness as the basis of negative feelings. Feldenkrais (1972), in *Awareness Through Movement* and in subsequent books, has vividly demonstrated many practical applications of awareness in developing alternate pathways of signal conduction after injury of arms or fingers.

As conditioning proceeds, a person becomes more aware of muscle-nerve feedback. Once it is sensed as a continuing phenomenon, the last hurdle has been surmounted and compliance becomes easy because fitness has become self-rewarding. The person is on a path toward wellness.

Fitness, Endurance, Fatigue, and Recovery

Tests of fitness are of two types: those that measure strength and those that measure endurance. Fatigue is involved in both situations directly or indirectly. In weight-lifting or sprinting competitions, each competitor makes one attempt at a time with sufficient rest in between for recovery. The reason for this protocol is to rule out fatigue as a factor. On the other hand, endurance is usually measured by how long it takes a person to become fatigued, or to lose force (Edwards, 1981). Thus endurance and fatigue are like the two sides of a coin. The subject of fitness can be approached from either side: those factors that increase endurance or strength or those factors that are responsible for fatigue and how they relate to fitness. Fatigue is thus basic in understanding both fitness and endurance. Fatigue also includes a quantitative assessment of endurance. For these reasons, I'll introduce the subject of endurance with a discussion of fatigue.

Fatigue, like most other physiological phenomena, is gradual. It increases with duration of exercise or work until a maximum is reached, which is called exhaustion. Recovery from fatigue is also gradual and is complete when maximal strength or endurance is regained. As we shall see, if specific muscles are exercised, fatigue can be quite specific. Yet, if certain muscles play an important role in the metabolism of the whole body, like the inspiratory muscles, their fatigue can result in general fatigue. Boredom and other disaffections of the nervous system also can exert a general effect.

Factors Affecting Fatigue of Fibers
Utilizing the Anaerobic Glycolytic Energy System

This energy transduction system occurs exclusively in the white, fast-twitch glycolytic fibers that are used in such activities as weight lifting, heavy work, or sprinting. These are the fibers that are used in activities requiring strength. They are the strongest of the three fiber types, and they are also the most fatigable.

Muscle research has established two factors that correlate with fatigue in these fibers. The first is a decrease in the glycogen pool, the major energy reservoir. The other is an accumulation of lactic acid, the end product of anaerobic glycolysis. Sahlin (1982) carried out an interesting experiment in which he measured the drop in tension (a measure of fatigue) in white fibers that had been repeatedly stimulated electrically and had accumulated considerable lactic acid, compared to nonstimulated fibers that had been incubated in a solution of carbonic acid (H_2CO_3). The hydrogen ion concentration (pH) was the same in both samples; so was the drop in tension. The increased acidity in both samples inhibited the reactions of glycolysis, which are necessary for the synthesis of ATP. The experiment demonstrated that lactic acid contributes to muscle fatigue not by some specific reaction but because it increases acidity. Lactic acid also inhibits the contraction process by preventing the interaction between actin and myosin to form actomyosin, thereby decreasing the release of energy from ATP. (Estimates of the major pathways of ATP synthesis in muscles of a number of sports and in a variety of recreational activities were presented in Table 7.4.)

Factors Affecting Fatigue of the Fibers Utilizing the Aerobic Glycolytic Energy System

These pinkish fibers are also strong but contain sufficient mitochondria to carry out the complete oxidation of glucose, first to lactic acid and then to carbon dioxide and water. This capability decreases fatigability in two ways: First, it helps prevent the accumulation of lactic acid; and second, the oxidation of the acid results in the production of additional ATP. With continued exercise, however, the glycogen reservoir becomes depleted, and the supply of oxygen and other necessary substances may be insufficient to maintain force, which is the definition of fatigue.

Factors Affecting Fatigue of Fibers Utilizing Aerobic Oxidation of Carbohydrate and Fat (SO Fibers)

These slow-twitch fibers are weaker than the other two types but, because they contain more mitochondria, are red in color. They are able to oxidize completely both carbohydrate and fat. In addition to providing the most ATP per carbon atom of substance oxidized (Table 7.1), the fat also spares glycogen. As a result, these fibers are the least fatigable of the three types. Like the FOG fibers, they are also dependent on the blood supply for oxygen and nutrients.

Correlations Between Fiber Types, Metabolic Pathways, Strength, and Fatigability

It is interesting that there are three major pathways to release the *potential energy* from carbohydrates and fats (Table 7.1) and that each fiber type utilizes one of them as its major energy source for the synthesis of ATP. The FG fibers are the strongest, use the anaerobic pathway, which is the least efficient, and are the most fatigable. They are also the greatest producers of lactic acid. The FOG fibers are intermediate in strength and in fatigability, whereas the SO fibers are the weakest but the least fatigable. On encountering correlations like these, biologists search for reasons. I'll offer a few here for your critique. They are based on the assumptions that both strength and endurance are necessary for human survival and that glycogen depletion and lactic acid accumulation are major factors affecting fatigue.

The fast, strong fibers are useful in emergencies. To use Cannon's (1939) term, they are the muscles we use in fight or flight. Their synthesis of ATP requires no oxygen (i.e., is independent of a blood supply), at least on a temporary basis. They are easily fatigable because their route of ATP synthesis, anaerobic glycolysis, uses large amounts of glycogen per molecule of ATP synthesized, and one of the products of the reaction, lactic acid, slows down glycolysis. The FOG fibers provide the first backup. They are not as strong as the FG type but are much less fatigable. They use glycogen more efficiently by completely oxidizing its product, lactic acid, to carbon dioxide and water. These reactions not only prevent the accumulation of lactic acid but also yield additional ATP. For endurance activities, the SO fibers are recruited. Although weaker than the other two, they can continue working for hours due to their ability to utilize fat oxidation for ATP synthesis and thus spare their glycogen store. They can also oxidize lactic acid for ATP synthesis.

Recruitment of Fiber Types

Fox and Mathews (1981) have outlined the gradual shift in fiber recruitment in running races of different distances. They class a 100-m race (10 seconds duration) as 100% anaerobic, using FG fibers exclusively. For 200 m (20 seconds), the ratio shifts to 90:10 anaerobic (FG):aerobic (FOG), whereas at 1500 m (3 minutes, 45 seconds), the ratio is close to 50:50. By the end of a 5000-m race (14 minutes), the ratio is anaerobic: aerobic (20:80) and for a marathon (2 hours, 15 minutes and longer), the ratio is 2:98. These figures do not reveal the fact that in the longer races fat becomes the major source of energy (Gollnick, 1985).

I have used foot racing in these examples because the type of metabolism has been measured and some data on the causes of fatigue are available. In applying these ideas to everyday living (e.g., working around the house and doing sedentary work), I suspect that a majority of activities that people engage in utilize mostly anaerobic pathways and but a small percentage of aerobic oxidation of glycogen (glucose). If this presumption is correct, it suggests that ordinary endurance would be furthered by some form of mixed anaerobic-aerobic exercises.

In addition to these metabolic factors in muscle fibers that are known to affect fatigue, various parts of the nervous system have been implicated in fatigue awareness. The details remain to be worked out. The neuromuscular junction is probably involved. The higher nerve centers are known to receive feedback impulses from the muscles, which can affect the conscious control of fatigue (Enoka & Stuart, 1985).

The Value of Fatigue

Because ATP is the direct source of energy for muscles and CP is its first reservoir, one might expect that fatigue would be due to a decrease in the concentration of these two phosphagens in muscle fibers, which would correspond to the decrease of force. This expectation holds to some extent in fatigued muscle. Bergstrom (1967) found a large decrease in PC concentration and a smaller decrease in ATP concentration after 10 minutes of high-intensity exercise. This result was confirmed by Brooks, Nunnally, and Bodinger (cited in Brooks and Fahey, 1984), who used the sophisticated noninvasive technique of nuclear magnetic resonance (NMR). This technique also showed an increased acidity in the fatigued muscle.

Saltin (1981) studied glycogen levels in fiber types and reported that, at exhaustion, both fast-twitch and slow-twitch fibers were depleted. Although not measured in this experiment, lactic acid is commonly found in high concentrations in exhausted or highly fatigued muscle.

To summarize, fatigue results in changes in a minimum of four muscle constituents: a depletion of glycogen, the major energy reserve; an increase in lactic acid, the main product of anaerobic glycolysis; a small decrease in ATP concentration, the direct source of energy for muscular work; and a large decrease in PC, the energy backup for ATP. Can these four facts be combined into a reasonable hypothesis to explain fatigue? To me the most puzzling result was the retention of appreciable amounts of ATP in exhausted muscle.

Sahlin (1982) suggested that acidosis acts as a safety mechanism to protect the fibers from total ATP depletion, which might result in cell death. The only muscle cells that have been found to be devoid of ATP are those in rigor mortis. I might add here that muscle cells, in common with all other living cells, utilize ATP for a variety of functions essential to their own survival. Because there may be conditions in which muscle cells are overstimulated to such an extent that, if they responded, all their ATP would have been utilized, Sahlin's suggestion makes good sense. It's better to be exhausted than dead, assuming, of course, that one has a safe place to rest.

Endurance

The changes that occur in the energy supply systems and in the slow-twitch and fast-twitch oxidative muscle fibers in a fitness-training program increase the efficiency of oxygen usage. By the same token, these changes also increase endurance. Fit people have more pep and energy and tire less quickly at a given task than less fit or unfit people. Actually, an aerobic training program amounts to people subjecting themselves to a safe, regulated amount of stress at each session. The whole person gradually adapts to this regime by the changes mentioned above. Most importantly, psychological changes also occur, and general attitude improves as well. These effects are often addictive, and people begin to look forward to the very activities that they formerly dreaded or avoided.

As mentioned above, weight lifting or short, hard exercise results in an increase in strength of the fast-twitch glycolytic fibers and in their greater endurance at heavy work. A number of factors are responsible for these changes. Fit fibers tend to contain more glycogen, their primary fuel reserve, than less fit fibers and therefore can work longer.

The Effects of Supplementary Carbohydrate Intake on Endurance

The timing of carbohydrate intake can effect endurance of people who expect to exercise for periods of 2 hours or more. If glucose is ingested an hour before exercise, its uptake by tissues is stimulated by insulin to such an extent that a mild hypoglycemia results. A greater dependence on muscle glycogen occurs, which, in turn, decreases endurance to a greater extent than when no carbohydrate is ingested (Costill, 1985).

Costill (1985) also reports some interesting results for people who hike or backpack more than 2 hours consecutively. The experiment involved cyclists who were exercising at 50% of capacity (50% of $\dot{V}O_2$max) for 4 hours. One group received 43 g (1.5 oz) sucrose just before and at 1-hour intervals during the exercise. The control group received no sugar. The blood glucose of the sugar-fed group was consistently higher than the controls. Apparently the higher concentration of blood glucose resulted in more entering the muscle and sparing glycogen. Glycogen depletion in the vastus lateralis muscle was significantly higher in the control group than in the sugar-fed group. To test endurance, at the end of the 4-hour cycling, the subjects performed at maximum capacity until exhausted. The sucrose-fed group exercised 45% longer than the controls.

In another experiment lasting 3 days, in which the subjects exercised aerobically and continuously for 2 hours each day, the effects of diet on muscle glycogen content was measured. Subjects consuming a low-carbohydrate diet (40% kcal) showed a progressive decrease in muscle glycogen—from 120 mmol/kg before exercise to 20 mmol/kg at the end of the third day. Comparable figures for those consuming a high-carbohydrate diet (70% kcal) were 120 mmol/kg at the start and 100 mmol/kg of glycogen at the end of the third day.

These experiments provide impressive evidence that consuming a high-carbohydrate diet will significantly increase endurance for active people. I wonder what effect such a dietary change would make on the average, out-of-shape American who consumes a high-fat (40% kcal) diet. I don't know of any experiment yet performed to answer this question, but anecdotal accounts from friends who have recently changed to lower fat, higher carbohydrate diets uniformly mention their increased energy and endurance.

How to Speed Up Recovery From Fatigue

It is widely believed that the best way to overcome muscular fatigue is to go to bed and sleep. This prescription may be psychologically satisfying, but it is mostly myth. Rest should follow an adequate cool-down. A recovery program should take into account the kind of exercise that made us tired. Also, knowledge of what has become depleted or changed in the muscle fibers that were used in the exercise is useful. Recovery can be speeded up or retarded, depending on what we do when the physical stress ends. For example, long duration aerobic exercises affect the slow-twitch muscles primarily.

Bonen and Belcastro (1976) measured the lactic acid concentration in runners who had just completed a 1-mile run. After 20 minutes of rest, its concentration in the blood had decreased to about half. In contrast, if the runners had exercised lightly, either continuously or intermittently, for only 10 minutes, the lactic level had also decreased to about half. After 20 minutes of light exercise, however, blood lactic acid had decreased to one-fifth of its concentration at the end of the run. This experiment furnishes a valid reason for a cool-down, but the length of it is probably longer than most runners realize is necessary. It is also noteworthy that a continuous jogging cool-down reduced lactic acid somewhat faster than interval jogging. In another experiment, these researchers found that, for optimum lactic acid removal, trained people should cool-down at a higher rate of oxygen consumption than untrained people. Although this experiment did not measure fatigue directly, the increased rate of lactic acid disappearance resembles that in the interval work-rest experiment mentioned previously (Bonen & Belcastro, 1976). Factors other than lactic acid accumulation are also responsible for fatigue. Even so, it appears that the less lactic acid that accumulates, or the quicker it is removed, the faster the recovery from fatigue.

The role of the central nervous system in recovery from fatigue was demonstrated in a series of clever experiments by Setchenov (cited in Brooks & Fahey, 1984). He observed that if a muscle of one limb was exhausted by exercise, recovery was faster if the opposite limb was exercised moderately (active pause) during the recovery period. Asmussen and Mazin (cited in Brooks & Fahey, 1984) took this interesting observation one step further and showed that an effective active pause could also consist of mental activity. This interesting approach to recovery is attributed to facilitatory impulses arising in the nervous system. Physical work doesn't have to be mindless if you think instead of daydream during pauses.

Use of Fatigue as a Marker

For people starting an exercise program, fatigue can be used as an indicator of when to stop. The time it takes to recuperate after exercise is a good guide at any age. Some signals of overfatigue are the following: (a) breathing and heart rate are still accelerated 10 minutes after the end of exercises, (b) marked weakness or fatigue after a 2-hour rest period, (c) restlessness and poor sleep at night, and (d) feeling tired the day after exercising.

Flexibility

Flexibility refers to the range of motion of limbs or body parts about a joint or joints. It commonly decreases with aging, and I suspect that many people accept increasing joint stiffness as another of the afflictions of old age. Although most occurrences of joint stiffness are automatically blamed on arthritis, many of them result solely from lack of exercise. Maintenance of flexibility is important for graceful movement in walking, running, standing, and even in sitting down and standing up. Nonathletes as well as athletes will benefit from flexibility exercises.

The joints of babies tend to be quite flexible, but school children become less flexible up to the ages of 10 to 12, after which flexibility improves in young adulthood. Flexibility after 25 gradually decreases unless specific exercises are practiced regularly. In general, women are more flexible than men from youth to old age. As with most other characteristics, flexibility of specific joints is strongly affected by heredity. Topflight hurdlers who depend on hip flexion are born, not made.

Flexibility is limited by bones and soft tissues. Muscle tissue as such does not limit flexibility, but it is strongly influenced by connective tissue, which covers muscles and also attaches them to ligaments and tendons. Connective tissue is composed of collagen, a protein that turns over very slowly and becomes more rigid with age. The increase in rigidity can be slowed by stretching exercises. These exercises are of two types: static and dynamic. Some flexibility exercises are described in Appendix 7F.

Delayed Muscle Soreness

One common aftereffect of fatigue, especially if little-used muscles are involved, is soreness appearing a day or two after the exercise. As might be expected of a very common phenomenon, there have been many hypotheses to explain this delayed stiffness. Abraham (1979) considered three major hypotheses: muscle spasms in the sore muscles, structural damage to the muscles themselves, and damage to the connective tissue that surrounds the muscles. He devised experiments to evaluate each one in people who had exercised in a way to produce sore muscles. He found evidence to support only one—that of connective tissue damage. Because collagen, the protein that comprises connective tissue, turns over very slowly, Abraham's conclusion seems very reasonable.

More recently Sjostrom and Friden (1983) examined muscle biopsy samples with the electron microscope and found evidence of fiber damage in muscles subjected to exhaustive eccentric exercise. In contrast to concentric exercise, in which the muscle is shortened during the work, eccentric exercise occurs with the muscles extended, as in the thigh muscles when walking downhill. People who have hiked down long, steep grades have learned from painful experience about the stiffness resulting from eccentric exercise. Under these conditions, the muscles are extended and the connective tissue does not absorb all the force, with consequent damage to the muscle fibers themselves.

As we age, crossbridges due to chemical reactions form in connective tissue, and it literally becomes stiffer and more rigid. People over 60 who have not been physically active should be conservative in becoming active. If you overdo and ache for a week, you may conclude that it is too late to commence an active program. It is for this reason that I recommend a walking program on a level surface as the starting exercise for such people. With the possible exception of swimming, it is less apt to make you stiff and sore than any other type of exercise. When you can walk 4 miles in an hour without becoming exhausted, you are in a position to consider more vigorous exercises if you feel the urge.

I advocate the lifting of light weights for healthy people of all ages. However, if you have never done it or have not for years, start in with very light weights of 2-10 lb, and just do a few repetitions on a variety of muscles for a week or two. It may be advisable to do it under the supervision of a trained person who knows how easy it is to overdo. Remember, 60-year-old connective tissue just doesn't have the stretch of 20-year-old or even 40-year-old tissue.

Handling Stiffness

Most active people get stiff from time to time, whether from an especially exhausting hike or workout or from engaging in a new activity. For example, I called a friend to play tennis, but he had a sore back from golf! There are two ways of responding to ordinary muscle stiffness of the arms or legs: by cutting down on or cutting out exercise for a day or two until it feels better, or by ignoring it and working through it. Duration seems almost independent of what you do. For myself, if it really hurts, I cut down. Aspirin often helps.

Your answers to the following questions will give you some idea of your general knowledge about aerobic exercise. The more you know about sports and exercises, the more independently you can safely develop your own program, if you choose.

Test Your Aerobics I.Q.

1. People should be able to carry on a conversation while they are exercising aerobically.

    ___ Yes ___ Maybe ___ No

2. Localized exercise or spot reducing can reduce fat in specific areas of the body.

    ___ Likely ___ Unlikely

3. In order to have a beneficial exercise routine, a person should exercise vigorously once a week.

    ___ Likely ___ Unlikely

4. Exercise is of little value in weight reduction because relatively few calories are burned during an exercise session (for example: 11 hours of walking are required to burn a pound of body fat).

    ___ Correct ___ Incorrect

5. The minimum amount of time an adult needs to engage in endurance exercise per session to improve heart and lung endurance is:

    ___ A.   5-14 minutes per session
    ___ B.   15-24 minutes per session
    ___ C.   25-34 minutes per session

6. The minimum number of times per week an adult needs to exercise to improve heart and lung endurance is:
   ___ A. **1-2 times per week**
   ___ B. **3-4 times per week**
   ___ C. **5-6 times per week**

Answers to Aerobics Quiz

1. **Yes.** This is referred to as the "talk test" and can help a person monitor the intensity of exercise. People exercising should feel that their heart and lungs are working but they should be able to converse at the same time.

2. **Unlikely.** Muscles can be toned and firmed through exercises designed for one body part but the fat will not be reduced. The best way to decrease fat stores is through aerobic exercise.

3. **Unlikely.** Exercising once a week may be more harmful than beneficial. The "weekend athlete" will not improve cardiovascular endurance if he or she does nothing else the remainder of the week.

4. **Incorrect.** Besides the calories burned in aerobic exercise, the metabolic rate is elevated for several hours after. In addition, aerobic exercise aids in appetite control.

5. **B.** Depending on the research study, 15-24 minutes is the minimum amount of time a person must be exercising at a proper intensity to improve heart and lung endurance. Warm-up and cool-down periods are not included in the aerobic time.

6. **B.** The beginning exerciser should start with three sessions per week. The person will increase cardiovascular fitness and then plateau after several weeks. To further improve fitness, four sessions per week or a higher pulse rate will be necessary.

Summary

Fitness is advocated in this chapter as an end in itself and as a contributor to wellness. Endurance exercises help keep the cardiorespiratory and cardiovascular systems in good shape and also aid in weight control. Strength and bending exercises keep the musculature fit and contribute to flexibility of the joints. I suggest aerobic walking as a safe, convenient and pleasurable long-term program.

Well people require lots of energy for the things they want to accomplish. Fitness permits them to utilize the energy that is in their food as

efficiently as their hereditary endowment allows. In addition, fitness contributes to wellness in what can be termed somatopsychic pathways. By
this I mean that fit people in general are less anxious, more relaxed, and
have greater self-esteem than the less fit. This conclusion is supported
by many controlled experiments.

Appendix 7A
Explanation of the Phrase "'Fats Burn in the Flame of Carbohydrates''

Fatty acids are not oxidized directly but are first combined with coenzyme
A and then broken down, two carbon atoms at a time, to the small
molecule, acetyl coenzyme A. Practically all the fatty acids found in foods
contain an even number of carbon atoms so that stearic acid-C-18 forms
9 molecules of acetyl coenzyme A, eicosapentaenoic acid (EPA) forms
10 molecules of acetyl coenzyme A, and so forth. Similarly, glucose is
converted to two molecules of pyruvic acid, which, in turn, is metabolized to acetyl coenzyme A. As far as is known, there is no chemical or
biological difference between the acetyl coenzyme A molecules that are
formed from fats and those that are formed from carbohydrates. Why
is it, then, that the further metabolism of the acetyl coenzyme A from
fats requires concomitant metabolism of carbohydrate whereas the acetyl
coenzyme A derived from glucose does not? The answer to this question
lies in the next step in the metabolism: the entrance of the acetyl group
from acetyl coenzyme A into the citric acid cycle.

The citric acid cycle, also called the tricarboxylic acid cycle or the Krebs
cycle, is a multienzyme system located in mitochondria which converts
the acetyl group of acetyl coenzyme A into carbon dioxide and hydrogen
atoms. In entering the cycle, each acetyl group combines with a molecule
oₓ oxalacetic acid to form citric acid. This acid is then converted consecutively into six other acids—as shown in Figure 7A.1. In these reactions,
the two carbon atoms of the acetyl group are converted into two molecules
of carbon dioxide; and oxalacetic acid is reconstituted, which can then
combine with another molecule of acetyl coenzyme A to keep the cycle
turning. In these reactions, the cycle itself is acting as a catalyst in the
oxidation of acetyl groups.

The names of the acids of the citric acid cycle are listed in Figure 7A.1,
as well as the two reactions in which carbon dioxide (CO_2) is liberated
and the four oxidation reactions, each of which liberates two hydrogen

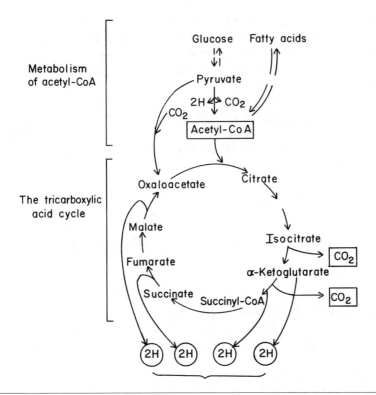

Figure 7A.1   Electron transport and oxidative phosphorylation (ATP synthesis).

atoms. It is worth emphasizing that practically all the carbon dioxide that you expire with every breath is produced in these reactions. The hydrogen atoms eventually react with oxygen to form water in another series of enzymatic reactions that is called the phosphorylating respiratory chain. These reactions, which also occur in mitochondria, are the source of much of the ATP that is used in muscle movement. With insufficient oxygen these reactions slow up or stop, and the organism may die.

The citric acid cycle may also be slowed or stopped by a decrease in concentration of one or more of the acids which it contains. This decrease occurs by side reactions that "drain off" the acids of the cycle. For the sake of simplicity, I have not listed these side reactions, but they are discussed in biochemistry textbooks. Now we can begin to interpret Rosenfeld's metaphor. The *flame* refers to the turning of the cycle, which is the first step in the final oxidation of carbohydrates and fats.

We are now ready to consider an important distinction between fatty acid oxidation and carbohydrate oxidation. Both sources of energy form acetyl coenzyme A. The crucial difference is due to the fact that pyruvic acid can react to form oxalacetic acid as well as acetyl groups. Whenever the concentration of one or more of the cycle acids gets low, this reaction can form more oxalacetic acid and keep the cycle going. Recall that pyruvic acid can be formed from glucose—a carbohydrate. Fatty acids feed into the cycle only as acetyl coenzyme A, which does not serve to replenish the acids of the cycle when their concentrations are lowered by side reactions.

This explanation, then, gives the biochemical reasons why fatigue occurs when the glycogen reserve of muscles is used up. Without a noncycle source of oxalacetic acid, which can come only from carbohydrate in muscle, fats cannot be oxidized at a rate to produce sufficient ATP to maintain muscle movement.

Appendix 7B
Pulse-Monitored Step Tests

These tests all require measuring your pulse after a definite amount of exercise. Rodahl (1966), in *Be Fit for Life*, describes a number of short, easy pulse tests. The first he calls hopping in place. It consists of jumping up and down on the floor 20 times. The feet should be raised at least 1 inch from the floor. Stop and remain standing for exactly 1 minute; then count your pulse for exactly 15 seconds. Pulse beats under 17 score 3 points; 17-20, score 2 points; 21-23, score 1 point; and pulse beats over 23 score zero points.

Rodahl's second test is a stair climb. In this test, you climb 10 steps of a flight, 5 times, up and down, as rapidly as possible. Two points are earned if the task was completed in less than 15 seconds, and no points if it took over 30 seconds. The pulse is taken for 15 seconds immediately on stopping. Thirty beats or less scores 2 points, 31-35 scores one point, and over 36 beats scores no points.

The third task is a step test. With shoes off, you step up and down on a chair or piano bench 18 inches high once every 2 seconds for 1 minute. On stopping, count your pulse immediately for 15 seconds. If the pulse exceeds 37 beats, score 1; 31-37, score 2; 25-30, score 3; and under 25, score 4.

For men under 50 a total score of 9 on the three tests is considered excellent, and a score of 3 is poor. For women under 50, excellent and poor are 8 and 2, respectively. For men over 50, excellent is 8 and poor is 2, and for women over 50, comparable scores are 7 and 1.[1]

---

[1]These scores are approximations since Rodahl included more tests.

According to Kraus (1972), a simple test is to find out how many flights of stairs a person can walk up without getting winded. He states that a healthy adult should be able to manage four or five at a moderate pace without feeling any strain at all. This judgment includes people over age 65.

Calculation of Target Pulse Rate

According to the *Guidelines for Graded Exercise Testing and Exercise Prescription* established by the American College of Sports Medicine (ACSM, 1980), factors such as "1) type of exercise, 2) age, 3) functional capacity, 4) health, 5) risk factors, and 6) symptomatology" must be considered before a laboratory evaluation and exercise program can be developed for an individual.

The ACSM Guidelines list the following primary risk factors for coronary vascular disease:

- 35 years of age, or older
- hypertension
- *hyperlipidemia* = serum cholesterol over 250 mg/dl
- cigarette smoking
- *ECG abnormalities* (consult an M.D. for guidance)

Secondary risk factors are the following:

- family history of coronary artery disease
- obesity
- physical inactivity
- diabetes mellitus
- *hyperuricemia*
- certain kinds of Type A behavior

Using 85% of the safe, maximum heart rate (HR) as the top limit for exercise, subtract 10% for each primary risk factor and 5% for each secondary risk factor. For example, John Jones is 40 years old, has not been physically active, is slightly obese, has a blood pressure of 150/90, and a resting heart rate of 80 beats per min (bpm). His safe, maximum exercise target heart rate (HR) can be calculated as follows:

85% - standard, safe, maximum HR with no risk factors
30% - sum of Jones' risk factors
55% - Jones' calculated safe maximum HR

His safe, maximum exercise target heart rate would be

  220   - the maximum HR for anyone
  − 40   - his age
  <u>180</u> bpm - age-predicted maximum HR
  − <u>80</u> bpm - resting HR
  100 bpm - uncorrected HR due to exercise—HR reserve
  × <u>.55</u> bpm - safety factor based on risk factors
   55 bpm - corrected HR due to exercise
  + <u>80</u> bpm - resting HR
  135 bpm - his safe, maximum exercise target HR

His safe, exercise target heart rate range would be

$$135 \pm 10 \text{ bpm} = 125\text{–}145 \text{ bpm}$$

Appendix 7C
Professional Fitness Evaluation

The Fitness Institute, located at Latter Day Saints (LDS) Hospital in Salt Lake City, Utah, offers two types of fitness evaluation. Evaluation A includes a bike fitness test (not a diagnostic test to detect coronary artery disease); underwater weighing for body fat analysis; blood analyses for total cholesterol, HDL, LDL, glucose, and blood count; cardiovascular and orthopedic screening, interviews, and recommendations for weight and stress management and nutrition for $235.

Evaluation B ($350) is similar except that the bike fitness test is replaced by a treadmill test with resting and exercise electrocardiogram (ECG) that assesses cardiovascular fitness and does detect coronary heart disease.

The Life Center, at Alta View Hospital, Sandy, Utah, offers similar tests and checkups, a health hazard appraisal, and discussion of and recommendations for adopting a wellness lifestyle. Cost, $75.

Appendix 7D
Grete Waitz's Warm-Up

Grete Waitz (1985), the Norwegian Silver Medalist in the Marathon, attributes her lack of injuries to using these 11 exercises before and after working out.

1. The grapevine. With legs shoulder length apart, reach for the sky, first with one hand, then with the other, for about 10 seconds.
2. Waist twists. Keeping legs shoulder length apart, reach hands to one side. Twist, keeping your face forward, 10 times to each side.
3. Hamstring stretch. Sitting on the floor with one leg straight and the other bent so that the sole touches the inner thigh, slowly reach for the toes of the extended leg and hold for 10 seconds. Repeat 2 times on each leg.
4. Groin stretch. Keeping your back straight and the soles of your feet together, bend forward from the waist and gently push your knees apart. Hold for 10 seconds and repeat 2 times.
5. Cross pull. On the floor, cross your right leg over your bent left knee. Wrap your left arm around your right knee and pull it toward your chest, twisting your upper body to the right as you look over your shoulder. Hold for a count of 10 and keep it gentle.
6. Quad stretch. Lying flat on your back, bring your heels as close to your buttocks as possible. While touching your heels, raise your hips off the floor. Hold for 10 seconds, inhaling as you rise. Repeat twice.
7. Calf and hamstring stretch. On your back, pull one knee onto your chest with both hands and then extend the leg straight up. Hold for 10 seconds and then lower the foot to about 4 inches from the floor. Flex your foot for about 10 seconds to get a calf stretch, then lower it to the ground. Repeat with the other leg.
8. Lower and upper back. With arms straight out to the sides while on your back, draw knees up to the chest. Roll knees to one side, turning your head the other way. Hold for 10 seconds. Repeat 3 times on each side.
9. Stomach strengtheners. On your back with your knees bent, feet flat on the floor, cross your arms on your chest and slowly rise halfway. Hold for a few seconds and repeat 5 times. Gradually work up to 10.
10. Upper power. For women: Do a modified push-up with knees bent on the floor. For men and stronger women: extend the legs. Push up 5 to 10 times. Keep the back straight.
11. Spine builder. Face down, lift your left leg and right arm for a few seconds. Do three on each side.

Repeat all 11 after a workout.

Note. From "Grete's Great Warm-Up" by G. Waitz, 1985, *Health and Fitness Magazine*, pp. 36-42. Copyright 1985 by *Health and Fitness Magazine*. Reprinted by permission.

Appendix 7E
Take a Break!

The following program—developed by Denise Austin, an exercise consultant in Alexandria, Virginia—is endorsed by the American College of Sports Medicine. It is suggested that people do these exercises on chairs without wheels.

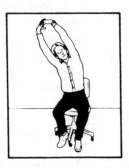

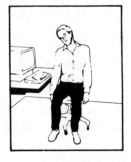

Side Stretch. Interlace your fingers. Lift your arms over your head, keeping your elbows straight. Press your arms backward as far as you can. Then slowly lean to the left and then to the right until you can feel stretching.

Neck. Let your head drop slowly to the left, then to the right. Slowly drop your chin to your chest, and then raise your chin as high as you can. Turn your head to the left, return it to the normal position, and then turn it to the right.

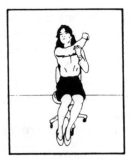

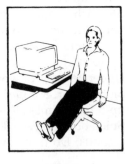

Middle-Upper Back Stretch. Raise your right arm and grasp it below the elbow with your left hand. Gently pull your right elbow toward your left shoulder as you feel the stretch. Hold for five seconds. Do both sides.

Quadriceps. Bring your legs straight out in front of your body, and then hold them in that position for five seconds. Make sure you are sitting up straight. Relax. Repeat.

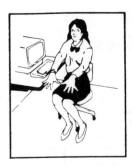

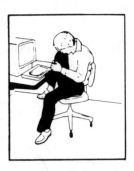

Fingers. With palms down, spread your fingers apart as far as you can. Hold for the count of five. Relax. Repeat.

Knee Kiss. Pull one leg to your chest, grasp with both hands, and hold for a count of five. Repeat with opposite leg.

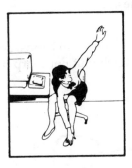

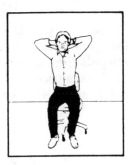

Windmill. Sit in a chair. Place your feet apart on the floor. Bend over and touch your right hand to your left foot with your left arm extended up. Alternate sides repeatedly.

Pectoral Stretch. Grasp your hands behind your neck and press your elbows back as far as you can. Return to starting position, then drop your arms and relax. Repeat.

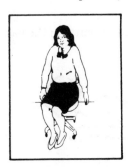

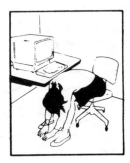

Shoulder Roll. Slowly roll your shoulders forward and backward five times in a circular motion using your full range of motion.

Back Relaxer. Sit on chair. Bend down between your knees as far as you can. Return to upright position, straighten, and relax.

Appendix 7F
Back Exercises

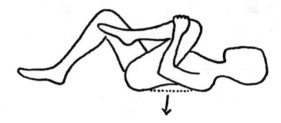

Back Flexion
(single knee to chest)

1. Lie on back with knees bent.
2. Bring one knee up towards chest, grasp knee with hands, and pull towards chest until you feel a good stretch (but not sharp pain) in the back muscles.
3. Relax, allow elbows to straighten.

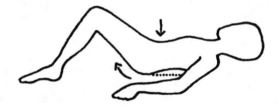

Pelvic Tilt

1. Lie on back with knees bent.
2. Tighten the stomach muscles and flatten the small of the back down against the floor.

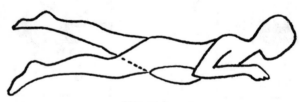

Hip Extension

1. Lie on stomach with legs straight, feet over edge of table. (Place pillow under stomach to relieve strain on back.)
2. Lift leg up approximately 10 inches.
3. Lower leg slowly and relax.

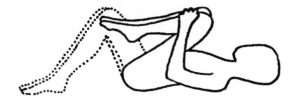

Double Knee to Chest

1. Lie on back with knees bent.
2. Keep small of back flat; bring knees up towards chest.
3. Grasp knees with hands and pull back towards chest until you feel a mild stretch in the back muscle.
4. Relax; allow elbows to straighten.

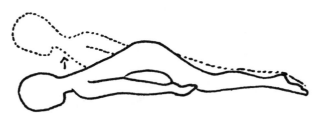

Trunk Lift

1. Lie on stomach with one pillow placed directly under the stomach. Keep arms at sides.
2. Raise the head, shoulder and back up as high as possible; also raise the arms (do not hold your breath).
3. Lower to the floor and relax.

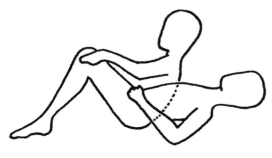

Partial Sit-Up

1. Lie on back with knees bent, placing hands on thighs.
2. Roll chin towards chest, then lift shoulders up off floor.
3. Continue curling trunk upwards until fingertips can touch the tops of the knees.
4. Slowly uncurl body down to floor; relax.

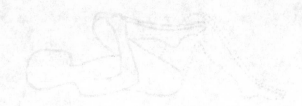

Chapter

8

Food, Wellness, and Weight Control

A scientific breakthrough of major significance has been the recognition that many problems long attributed to aging are, in fact, infirmities that could be avoided if people would only be more active.

C. Carson Conrad
President's Council on Physical
Fitness and Sports

This chapter will help you

- understand why overweight/obesity is such a serious medical problem;
- recognize why going on a diet is generally unsatisfactory for long-term weight loss;
- incorporate regular endurance exercise into your weight-control program; and
- keep your weight in line.

Food affects wellness both positively and negatively. Most people enjoy a good meal, and this is enhanced by the sociability of friends. The sharing of food as a token of friendship extends throughout recorded history. The coupling of holidays and feast days is no coincidence. All of these social activities, in which food plays a role, can contribute to individual wellness.

However, the long-term consumption of certain foods that may be deficient in one or more essential nutrients can result in illness for an individual or a group. One reason that beriberi was endemic in the Orient for years was that the people would not eat brown rice, and the remainder of the diet was unable to supply a protective amount of vitamin B_1 (thiamin). Certain vitamins are unstable and, even though they are present in the food supply, may be destroyed or removed in food processing or in meal preparation.

Food can also contain substances in toxic quantities, either naturally occurring, as grain grown in seleniferous soils, or toxins produced in some stage of storage or preparation, as aflatoxins in peanuts. Certain foods may not be tolerated by some people because of lack of enzymes to digest particular substances. Seventy percent of black American adults develop toxic symptoms if they drink milk; they lack the enzyme lactase, which hydrolyzes lactose, the major sugar of milk (Bayless, 1976).

The amount of food consumed over a long period can also affect health. An extreme in either direction often has serious consequences. Obesity results from overeating and anorexia nervosa from undereating. Neither condition represents the actions of a well person.

Concept of Desirable Body Weight

In recent years a previously uncommon type of malnutrition has become widespread in developed countries. I am referring to overweight/obesity. In past cultures members of the nobility and ruling classes could assure themselves of a plentiful food supply, and possibly were large in girth as an obvious demonstration of their rank. In addition, famine and/or epidemics could strike suddenly at any time, and past experience showed that fat people survived to a greater extent than thin. Although the Greeks, following the advice of Hippocrates, may have recognized the disadvantages of obesity, this wisdom was forgotten or ignored for many centuries in Europe. In contrast, peasants, workers, and slaves seldom had enough to eat. Self-control was unnecessary. Food consumption was dictated by the culture and the environment.

Significant change has occurred in food production and distribution in the past 50 years due to the application of technology to agriculture. The masses in some parts of the world can afford excess calories on a regular basis for the first time in history. This bonanza has not been without disadvantages. Sugar has become a cheap source of calories, and for many years meat was also. People have tended to overindulge in the consumption of favorite foods, and as a result, the overweight population has skyrocketed. In the technological age, each of us needs to learn a new skill. It is how to eat for wellness.

Obesity is usually considered a personal problem that affects the health of an individual. In a different approach, Hannon and Lohman (1978) have calculated the overall energy cost of overweight in the United States. The excess fat that American adults carry amounts to 2.3 billion lbs. The energy saved by dieting to reach optimal weight is equivalent to 1.3 billion gals. of gasoline. The annual energy savings from this source alone would be sufficient to supply the annual residential electricity demands of Boston, Chicago, San Francisco, and Washington, D.C.

A consensus panel (Burton, Foster, Hirsch and Van Itallie, 1985) recently assembled by the National Institutes of Health on the health implications of obesity, discussed the prevalence, distribution and dangers of obesity in the U.S. As reported by Kolata (1985a), slightly over a quarter (26%) of the adult population is considered obese. Among black women between ages 45 and 55, 60% are obese, compared to 30% of white women in the same age range. The difference is attributed to social pressure in the more affluent group. Apparently with the food supply seemingly assured, the self-confident, well-to-do people, with an assist from a multitude of advertisers, are opting for the lean, youthful appearance. The lean cuisine and lean beef are now in.

The 1983 Edition of the Metropolitan Weights Tables

Since 1959 the weight standard for Americans has been the Metropolitan Life Insurance Company's table of *Desirable Weights for Ages 25 to 59*. The chart was based on the longevity of policy holders of different weights. The old table was reviewed and reevaluated in 1983, and a new table has been introduced (Metropolitan Life Insurance, 1983). It shows increases in weight for height based on lowest total mortality. The weights are not associated with reduced incidence of disease but only with mortality (Entmacher, 1983). It is interesting that the headings have also been changed for the following reason. "Because the words 'ideal' and 'desirable' mean different things to different people and have created confusion, these terms will no longer be used in referring to Metropolitan's height and weight tables. The new tables are a health education tool—a guideline" (p. 16). Another reason for the withdrawal of the terms *ideal* and *desirable* is that total weight is not a measure of fatness, and fatness is the culprit in shortening life. The public needs a measure of fatness that is as simple, accurate, and convenient as weighing.

Body Mass Index

A simple, approximate way to estimate fat content is by calculating what is called the body mass index (BMI) as equal to the weight (W) divided by the square of the height (H^2): BMI $= W/H^2$. A Nomogram relating

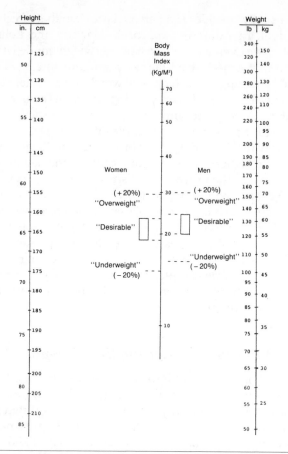

Figure 8.1   Nomogram for body mass index. *Note.* From ''A Nomograph Method for Assessing Body Weight'' by A. Thomas, D. McKay, and M. Cutlip, 1976, *American Journal of Clinical Nutrition, 29*, pp. 302-304. Copyright 1976 by *American Journal of Clinical Nutrition.* Adapted by permission.

BMI to overweight/obesity is shown in Figure 8.1. To use the nomogram, place a straight edge from the weight column on the left to the height column on the right, using pounds-inches or Kg-cm. The line will cross the BMI line for most people between acceptable and obese. This quick and easy method will give you an approximation of your fat status.

Smoking is another confounding factor on the relation of weight to mortality. The Framingham survey uncovered the perplexing correlation between low body weight and early mortality. On examining the data in more detail, it was found that many underweight men were also cigarette smokers. The subjects were not dying from underweight but from smoking (Garrison, Feinleib, Castelli, and McNamara, 1983). It is for this reason, as discussed more fully in chapter 10, that I prefer the 1959 tables, as shown in Tables 8.1A and 8.1B.

The Effects of Dietary Restriction on Longevity of Rodents

Rats are widely used in nutrition research because their requirements and physiological responses to dietary variables are remarkably similar to humans. In these two sections I'll review two interesting and relevant types of experiments with rodents: the first about food restriction, the second about the effects of taste on appetite and thus on weight control.

Fifty years ago McCay, Drowell, and Maynard (1935) fed just-weaned rats a diet adequate in essential nutrients but low in calories. They observed that their life-span was significantly lengthened. Their rate of aging was slowed, and, in addition, the number of spontaneous tumors was significantly less than those of the rats that ate a normal diet. In an extension of this work, Weindruch and Walford (1982) compared the average life span of a strain of underfed middle-aged mice to those which were fed the usual amounts of chow. The underfed mice lived significantly longer than the controls—41 months versus 34 months ($p < .01$). The mice were not exercised. I am not suggesting underfeeding for humans, but I think that these results are interesting relative to the increased mortality of obese people compared to normal-weight people. On the basis of these and other studies, it is easy to see why Hirsch calls obesity a disease (cited in Kolata, 1985a).

Factors Affecting Adult Weight

Many people, no matter how hard they try to stay thin or become thin, never quite seem to manage it. Thousands of overweight people have gone to fat farms or participated in experiments in hospital wards where their diets were closely controlled and lost weight—large amounts, in fact. They have been exercised, lectured at, exhorted, tutored, and otherwise encouraged to control their calorie consumption; but on their home turf, 95% gain back those precious pounds quite promptly. What is the problem here? A need for calories beyond a matter of willpower? A lack of self-control? A need for calories beyond human understanding? Or a subtle difference in metabolism that has not yet been identified? Recent research on weight control suggests that differences in metabolic efficiency may be involved. Most people produce a certain amount of heat from the calories they consume. Other people are more efficient in their usage of excess calories; they utilize them to synthesize fat rather than dispose of them as heat.

One of the factors that may be involved is in the fat cells themselves: their numbers and size. Kolata (1985b) has summarized the work of Jules Hirsch and colleagues at Rockefeller University who have observed that the fat cells of normal-weight people tend to remain the same size unless they overeat or are starved. Even if people stuff themselves for weeks in an experiment, and their fat cells increase in size, the cells will return to normal size when the people return to their usual diets and revert to their usual weights. This type of response has been labeled the *set point* by researchers on weight control. In contrast, the fat cells of obese people are twice the size of those of normal-weight people. When these people lose weight, their fat cells become tiny, as if they were being starved. Their set point is set too high. The question these results have raised is, how do the fat cells communicate their status to the nervous system, which in turn affects appetite and weight?

In studying the metabolism of obese people who had lost weight in the hospital, Hirsch and colleagues, according to Kolata (1985b) made another very interesting observation. Although their weight had been brought down to normal, their metabolism had not. They were marvels of efficiency. Their caloric need to maintain their weight was 25% below normal. In other words, if they consumed as many calories as people of their same weight but who had never been fat, they would gain weight while the never-fat people would not.

The Rockefeller researchers have also studied the question of where fat is lost when people lose weight. One woman who had an excess of *gluteal* fat lost 15% of her body weight, but none from her hips and thighs. A man with much abdominal fat halved his weight but kept his paunch. These results suggest that all fat depots are not alike. The work opens up exciting possibilities in exploring the differences. The report of this work (Kolata, 1985b) does not state whether these subjects were exercised. The results also suggest to me that the best way to control obesity is to avoid it in the first place. I realize that this suggestion may come too late for many readers.

Source of Calories Influences Weight

Animal experiments have demonstrated quite conclusively that the source of calories in a diet can affect body weight independently of its total caloric content. Also, appetite is significantly affected by the composition of the diet. Both rats and humans tend to become obese on foods they like.

Energetically speaking, a calorie from protein equals a calorie from carbohydrate equals a calorie from fat. In other words, a calorie from one source is equivalent to a calorie from any other. This statement is called the *equivalence principle*, and it serves as the basis for most quantitative diet calculations.

What is not widely understood, even by many nutritionists and diet counselors, is that the equivalence principle does not apply without qualification. Blaxter (1971) summarized the results of many studies on the efficiency of storage of foodstuffs by various species as follows: carbohydrates, 62%–77%; protein, 64%–74%; and fats, 79%–85%. These percentages show quite clearly that fat in the diet is stored at a significantly higher efficiency than either carbohydrate or protein. The key word in the sentence above is *stored*. These percentages hold only for animals that are gaining weight.

In a similar experiment, Schemmel (1976) compared the amount of energy in a high-fat and a low-fat diet that was required to obtain a weight gain of one gram. With the Osborne Mendel strain, the rats required 50% more energy to lay down a certain amount of depot fat on the low-fat, high-carbohydrate diet than on the high-fat, low-carbohydrate diet. Calculated another way, rats fed the high-fat diet were 2 1/2 to 3 times as efficient in storing fat than those on the low-fat diet. These results confirm those mentioned above. Herberg, Döppen, Major, and Gries (1974) also observed that male NNRI mice fed a high-fat diet gained more weight than those fed a high-carbohydrate diet even though the total calorie intake of the high-fat group was less. Comparable results have been obtained by Sims et al. (1973) in humans. Lean adults were furnished excess calories as mixed diets (i.e., high-carbohydrate, low-fat). At an intake of 8,000 kcal/day, the subjects gained far less weight than could be accounted for by the excess calories. In contrast, Sims (1976) readily induced weight gain with a relatively small increase in dietary fat. Thiebaud et al. (1983) infused healthy human subjects with a lipid-glucose-insulin solution and measured the energy cost of fat or glucose storage. They found that lipid storage from lipid has a much lower energy cost than lipid storage from glucose.

Swaminathan et al. (1985) studied the thermic effects of different types of meals in obese and lean subjects. There was little difference in thermic effects of glucose and protein in the two groups. Fats, however, provided some interesting, significant differences. Obese subjects showed very little increase in metabolic rate following ingestion of fat ($-0.9 +2.0\%$) compared to that in lean subjects ($14.4 + 3.4\%$). Similar differences were found with mixed meals containing all three energy sources. This difference—which may have a hereditary basis—may explain the easier weight gain of some people compared to others on similar diets.

What is the explanation of these anomalous results? Have nutritionists found an exception to the first law of thermodynamics? No, not at all. As often happens with an unexpected result, the answer is interesting. It is also important as it includes an often ignored point. There is more to calorie counting than the energy released in metabolism. Less energy is required in converting dietary fat to body fat than in converting dietary carbohydrate or protein to body fat. This difference, which may be appreciable on high-fat diets, means that more energy becomes available for additional fat synthesis.

Individual (Genetic) Differences in Responding to a High-Fat Diet

Schemmel and Mickelsen (1974) found that the effects of high-fat diets in rats were subject to strong genetic differences. One strain of rat on a high-fat diet gained 55% more than when fed a low-fat, grain diet, but a second strain only weighed 14% more on the high-fat diet. It appears that rats, like people, vary in their efficiency in storing dietary fat as body fat. Some people can eat almost anything and stay thin. Others seem to get fat when they even think about a cream puff. The reasons for these differences are as yet unknown.

High-Sugar Diets

A person may be full but still eat an enticing dessert or ask for another cookie or sweet. If appetizing fare is available, people tend to overeat. A common explanation is that we like sweet foods because we have a sweet tooth. Experiments have demonstrated that a newborn baby will smile if a few drops of a sucrose solution are placed on the tongue. Because most sweet foods are not poisonous, it is possible that mankind's sweet tooth has developed and persisted because of its survival value. It should not be surprising then to learn that sugar is the additive used in largest amounts by food processors. It is interesting that sucrose, which had been dissolved and offered as a supplement, resulted in more obesity than a diet high in solid sucrose. Kanareck and Hirsch (1977) also found similar effects when weanling rats were allowed free access to sugar solutions.

High-Fat Diets

The obesity-promoting effects of high-sugar diets in rats are modest compared to high-fat diets (Allen & Leahy, 1966). What may surprise you is the statement that humans also have a fat tooth. Because fat does not have the distinctive flavor of sugar, it is not as obvious that we like some foods because of their fat content. Take meat, for example. For years, USDA grading of beef has been based on fat content. Prime grade contains more fat than choice grade, which, in turn, is fatter than good grade. How often do you voluntarily eat a piece of dry toast, or a baked potato that has not been drowned in butter, margarine, or sour cream? Dips, nuts, most snack foods—all are fatty.

Supermarket Diets

Sclafani and Springer (1976) carried the variation in food composition as affecting food consumption a giant step further by offering rats a variety of foods, which the scientists called a Supermarket Diet. In addition to the regular chow, the rats were given, on an *ad libitum* basis, the following foods (in parentheses after each food are the fat and sugar percentage by weight, respectively): chocolate chip cookies (19, 72), salami (37, 0), cheddar cheese (32, 0), bananas (2.6, ?), marshmallows (0, 82), milk chocolate (34, 57), peanut butter (48, 9), and sweet condensed milk (9, 54). The rats that were fed this mixture were a strain that previously had not gained much extra weight on a high-fat diet. On the supermarket fare, however, they outgained their chow-fed controls by 269%! Is it any wonder then that foods that are rich in both sugar and fat are practically irresistible?

These results lead to some rather interesting comparisons. Apparently the gustatory delights of rats and humans are very similar. Given access to unlimited amounts of a high-fat diet, rats become obese. Oscai (1982) fed rats a high-fat diet (42% of calories from fat) and compared their weights at 60 weeks to those fed rat chow—a low-fat diet (18% fat). Both groups had unrestricted access to food. The body weight, as well as the percentage of carcass fat of the group fed the high-fat diet, was over twice that of those who ate the low-fat diet.

The American diet at 40% of calories from fats can be considered a high-fat diet. Therefore, it is not surprising that estimates of obesity of Americans vary from 20% to 40% of the population. It appears that, for both rats and humans, a high-fat diet results in more obesity than from other types. Another similarity between these two species is that the average American does not exercise much more than a rat in a cage. As was mentioned in chapter 7, aerobic exercise 4 to 6 times a week at an average of 200-300 kcal per session, will help permit partaking of favorite (i.e., fatty, sweet) foods, and yet avoid the flab.

Balancing the Human Energy Equation

Fit people keep their energy equation in balance. When intake chronically exceeds outgo, it leads to obesity. When outgo chronically exceeds intake, it leads to emaciation. Obesity is far more common in developed countries than emaciation, and it is only the former that will be discussed here.

People who regularly eat in excess over their requirements for physical activity are following a pattern that is unhealthy. I think that I am justified in calling it an abnormal pattern from the increased risk of a number of diseases associated with obesity. Even a partial list is a long one and includes hypertension, stroke, heart disease, diabetes, gout, arthritis, hernias, and varicose veins. Maintaining wellness while afflicted with obesity or one or more of these conditions is not an easy task.

For some reason, most people, including physicians, ascribe *obesity* and *overweight* to overeating. Weight loss through dieting has received an undue emphasis for many years. As a result of the publicity, the public's interest in dieting seems insatiable. At the time this sentence is being written, three diet books are included on the nonfiction national bestseller list. Unfortunately, dieting as the way to weight control doesn't work very well for most people. They shift from one diet to another (or say they do), lose a few pounds, and gain them back again. This approach has been called the *rhythm method of girth control.*

Even the grossly obese, those who seek medical help for their problem and endure extreme dietary restriction under supervision in a hospital or diet farm for long periods, usually regain their weight after returning home. Follow-up studies have shown that compliance with the diet is obtained in only about 5% of patients. Still, the search for appetite regulation goes on. A New York man has invented a fork that contains red and green lights in the handle that alternately flash at preset times. When the red light is on, he lays the fork down. The device has helped him slow down his eating, and he has lost over 60 lbs. with its use (Guyon, 1981). Would such a device work for you?

Kraus and Raab (1961) emphasized physical inactivity as a contributing factor for many of the ills of technological people. Fourteen years later, Burkitt and Trowell (1975) attributed the rise in these same diseases to dietary changes, especially a decrease in dietary fiber. It is my impression that the diet book made a much bigger splash among physicians and health popularizers than did the book urging increased physical activity. The reason usually given for emphasizing diet rather than physical activity to achieve weight loss is that exercise does not use up many calories. A pound of fat is equivalent to 3,600 kcal. To utilize this much energy by running or walking would require running or fast walking for about 8 hours. A realistic goal for most people: The time required can be divided into 1 period, 4 to 6 times per week. The time factor has led many people to discard all forms of exercise as effective in weight control and thus emphasize dieting. This reasoning is oversimplistic in that it disregards other effects of aerobic exercise such as its influence on appetite, its long-term heating effect, which uses calories for hours after the activity has been concluded, and the positive psychological effects of exercise that aid in appetite control.

The Kraus and Raab (1961) thesis has a long and honorable history. Hippocrates advocated a long walk in the early morning for depressed people and a brisk walk before dinner for the overweight. To quote dicta, no matter how notable the originator, is still relying on anecdotal information and is therefore suspect. During the past 25 years, however, certain nutritionists and exercise physiologists have published data on controlled studies that are quite convincing about the effects of aerobic exercise on weight control.

Do Fat People Eat Too Much?

Jean Mayer (1975), a noted student of obesity and its causes, states that "people frequently become obese not because they eat more than thinner people but because they are less active than the slender" (p. 65). Pollock, Wilmore, & Fox (1975) have summarized 28 studies that relate physical activity to changes in body weight and percentage fat in people between 19 and 57 years. They point out that a moderate jog for 30 minutes or a brisk walk of 45–60 minutes per day will utilize 300-500 kcal. On the basis that a pound of fat represents 3,600 kcal, a person exercising 5 days a week would lose a pound of weight approximately every 10 days. This rate of weight loss amounts to 36.5 lb per year! Remember, all this can be accomplished without any change in diet! A modest dietary change, such as eating one less piece of buttered toast, one less can of beer, or one less sweet a day—each equivalent to 100 kcal—would increase weight loss another 25% or a total of 45 lb per year.

Gwinup (1975) studied the effects of walking on a group of obese women. Their diet was not restricted. Weight loss was directly related to time spent walking. He reported that a minimum program for weight loss included continuous walking for 30 minutes per day at least 3 days a week, and of sufficient intensity to expend at least 300 kcal per session.

Bailey (1978) in Fit or Fat suggests that fat people who begin to exercise regularly should not be concerned about their weight: They are replacing fat by muscle and this change contributes to fitness. In contrast, in weight loss by dieting alone, lean body mass (muscle) is lost as well as fat and water.

Dahlkoetter, Callahan, and Linton (1979) examined both sides of the energy equation in an experiment with 44 obese women. They averaged 39 lb overweight per person. The subjects were divided into four groups: controls, eating habits (diet), exercise, and a combination diet-exercise group. The importance of aerobic exercise in energy utilization was explained to the latter two groups. Behavioral modification techniques were employed with the three experimental groups initially and each week during the 8-week duration of the experiment. This study is important in that, in addition to measuring weight changes, physical fitness of all subjects was also determined.

Weight loss by the diet and exercise groups was similar (7 to 8 lb) after 8 weeks, and both groups stayed at that plateau during the next 24 weeks. The combination diet-exercise group, however, lost an average of 13 lb during the first 8 weeks, and continued to lose weight, although at a slower rate, for the second 8 weeks. The results showed that exercise alone was as effective as diet alone in achieving weight loss, but that the two together were considerably more effective than either one separately. Percentage of fat loss was not calculated. Waist and thigh circumferences—a measure of fat—decreased in all the experimental groups, but the largest decrease was found in the combination exercise and behavior modification group. No significant differences were found between the control and experimental groups in skinfold thicknesses and in biceps, bust, and hip circumferences.

As might be expected, fitness of the diet group, as measured by a step test, number of sit-ups per minute, and resting pulse rate, was not improved. Fitness of the exercise and combination groups improved significantly, and the improvement was maintained during the subsequent 8 weeks. Blood pressure fitness was normal for all four groups (123/78, systolic/diastolic) initially, and decreased statistically significantly in the diet, exercise, and combination groups compared to the control. Social adjustment—as measured by a questionnaire—of the three experimental groups all showed improvement, but there was no difference among them. An interesting sidelight of this experiment is that there were no dropouts.

The Effects of Exercise on Appetite

The idea that exercise stimulates appetite is very widely believed. Many people reason as follows: Exercise is a good way to gain weight, not lose it. If I use up a hundred calories by exercising but stimulate my appetite to eat an extra 150, I'll gain weight. And so they would if their logic followed reality. But does it? Do scientific studies confirm or refute the folklore?

Surprisingly, research can be cited on both sides. Some types of exercise increase appetite and others do not. Some are useful for people wishing to gain weight and some for those trying to lose weight. It is important to recognize the difference so that you can choose the type that will aid you in your objective.

It is essential to make a few distinctions if we are to look at this question scientifically. In the first place, some exercises, like weight lifting, resemble hard physical work very closely. Because these exercises increase strength, they are called strength exercises. Other exercises, like jogging, walking, swimming, and most sports, involve moving the body through air or water. This group is called endurance exercise. Both types of exercise place a stress on the person, but the overall effects, including those on appetite, are very different.

A weight lifter or manual laborer moves heavy mass through space on a discontinuous basis. One who pumps iron will carry out a certain number of repetitions and then rest. Workers likewise rest at intervals to avoid exhaustion. Their pulse rate increases during the weight-moving phase but decreases during the resting phase.

Endurance exercises, on the other hand, are continuous, or almost continuous, for 15 minutes or more. The pulse increases and stays elevated for the entire period. Oxygen is utilized for the release of energy from both carbohydrates and fats. Is it reasonable to expect that these two types of exercise should affect appetite in different ways?

Before attempting to answer this question, I should discuss the place of sedentary workers in this scheme. Many people who engage in light work, such as housewives and desk workers who garden or golf on weekends, believe that they are active enough to keep in shape. Unfortunately, this hope is unrealistic. A goodly proportion of these people are also overweight. Sedentary workers tend to overeat and are relatively fatter than those whose work is more physically demanding (Mayer, Roy, & Miha, 1956). Apparently, the appetite control mechanism in the brain doesn't function very efficiently at low levels of physical activity. I feel that I cannot overemphasize the fact that the only exercise that is useful in controlling appetite is the aerobic type carried out continuously for a minimum of 15-20 minutes. An explanation of this difference has so far eluded nutritionists. Research on appetite has demonstrated that it is controlled by a large number of feedback systems. The actual control center is thought to lie in the hypothalamus or near it. The appetite control center or appestat is sensitive to a number of factors such as the concentration of glucose in the blood, to a variety of hormones, and to neurotransmitters in the brain that affect mood. At the present time it is not known which of these regulatory factors respond differently to endurance exercises compared to strength exercises.

Strength Exercises Increase Appetite

The body adapts to the stress of hard work by building large muscles. These people are strong, and to accomplish the work they are called upon to do, they eat a lot. A classical example of how hard, physical labor increases appetite was reported by Karvonen, Pekkarinen, Metsala, and Rautanen (1961). The scientists measured the diets of Finnish lumberjacks and found that their daily intake averaged over 4,700 kcal. These men were not obese, despite consuming almost twice as many calories as more sedentary workers.

Thus, if an overweight, sedentary person is considering an exercise program and wants to lose weight, scientists can suggest what type of exercise to avoid: the heavy-work, weight-lifting kind. Can science also suggest a type of exercise that is helpful in weight loss? It is the endurance type.

Endurance Exercises Do Not Increase Appetite

In the studies that I have mentioned previously, endurance exercise programs resulted in weight loss. It is reasonable to assume that appetite was not increased, but because food intake was not measured, some other factor may have become responsible for the results. Fortunately, this assumption has been checked in a number of other studies.

Dempsey (1964) measured the food intake of young men who engaged in endurance exercise for an hour a day—enough to result in considerable weight loss. Their food consumption did not increase. Similarly, two experiments at the University of Illinois in which middle-aged men jogged 3 days a week found that the men's fitness increased, but not their appetites (Holloszy, Skinner, Toro, & Cureton, 1964; Skinner, Holloszy, & Cureton, 1964). Similarly, in two separate studies, Woo, Garrow, and Pi-Sunyer (1982a, 1982b) exercised obese women aerobically at 110% and 125% of their sedentary energy expenditure. The spontaneous caloric intake of the subjects did not increase at either level of exercise. Subjects who exercised at the higher level consistently lost about 2 lb per week during the 7-week experiment.

It thus appears that the type of exercise is important in appetite regulation and therefore in weight control. The distinction is between the effects of endurance exercise and strength exercise on appetite. Why should the latter increase it and the former not? At the present, scientists can't answer this question.

The process of conditioning is really one of adaptation. The muscles respond to the demands placed on them by both macroscopic and microscopic modifications. The changes are quite different in the two types of conditioning: endurance and strength.

Muscle mass increases as a result of heavy work. A weight lifter develops big muscles. If you see a man with bulging biceps, you can be pretty sure that he either is a weight lifter or uses his arms for lifting heavy objects at his work. In terms of energy generation, these large, *hypertrophied* muscles have not changed significantly from those of an unfit person whether the biceps are 8 inches or 18 inches. These large muscles utilize carbohydrates as the major energy source. Large muscles are strong, but they don't necessarily have the capacity for continuous work.

Muscles that are conditioned for continuous activity are not much larger than unconditioned muscles. To find the difference between the two types of muscle, the tissue must be looked at with an electron microscope or tested for the activity of certain enzymes. Numerous studies have demonstrated significant increases in the number and size of mitochondria and in particular enzymes as a result of aerobic exercise (Holloszy & Booth, 1976). Greater endurance results from the ability of conditioned muscle to use oxygen more efficiently than unconditioned muscle. The greater rate of oxidation means that carbohydrate oxidation is increased, as well as that of fatty acids and lactic acid.

As exercise continues, the use of fats as energy source increases. This effect may sound technical and trivial, but it isn't. In the first place, with fat as the fuel being burned, the very substance that is in excess in overweight people is being utilized. In the second place, and this is a fact of profound significance, fats cannot be oxidized anaerobically. White muscle fibers, with their low number of mitochondria, cannot oxidize many fatty acids. These fibers rely on the anaerobic utilization of carbohydrate for their energy supply. In endurance exercises, red fibers, which can oxidize fats, are recruited; fat becomes the preferred fuel to provide ATP.

Dieting Without Exercise: The Cruel Way to Weight Loss

Now we are in a position to understand why weight loss by diet alone is so inefficient and difficult. In the absence of much physical activity, appetite remains large or may even increase; and if weight is actually lost, lean muscle tissue is included as well as fat.

People need a measure of fatness that is as simple, accurate, and convenient as weighing. No such method is available as yet. Weighing has the disadvantage of not distinguishing between muscle and fat. Two people may each weigh within the normal range of the weight tables, but one may be twice as fat as the other. A person who diets to lose weight assumes that the weight lost is fat. If they haven't exercised, they have probably lost valuable muscle tissue as well. A dieter who loses muscle becomes weaker. As the person senses this effect, it becomes a block to further dieting. In the interconnected systems that we call body and mind, signals are being sent from the muscles to the brain with feedback messages that this program is self-destructive.

High-Fat, Low-Carbohydrate Diets Decrease Appetite and Also Endurance

Apart from exercise, appetite can be affected by what a person eats. In the high-fat Atkins diet (Atkins & Linde, 1978), calories are not restricted because the diet itself tends to decrease appetite. It is not so well known, however, that high-fat diets also decrease endurance.

Bogardus, LaGrange, Horton, and Sims (1981) measured the endurance of obese, untrained women on either of two weight-loss diets providing a daily intake of 830 kcal. The high-fat diet contained 64% fat and 1% carbohydrate, and the low-fat diet contained 29% fat and 36% carbohydrate. Both diets contained 35% protein. Endurance was estimated by measuring the time to exhaustion on cycling at about 75% of maximum oxygen uptake. At the start of the experiment, there was no significant difference in the endurance of the two groups. At the end of 1 week, and after 6 weeks on the diets, the endurance of the low-fat group had not changed, whereas that of the high-fat group had dropped to about a third of the low-fat group.

The researchers also measured the glycogen content of the large thigh muscle (vastus lateralis) and found that it correlated very highly with endurance. Subjects on the high-fat diet lost half their muscle glycogen in a week. These results are important in the design of combined diet-exercise programs for untrained, obese subjects. Those on a low-fat, restricted-calorie diet performed well at a variety of work loads, whereas those on the high-fat, calorie-restricted diet did not.

Endurance Exercise Assists in Fat Loss

For the overweight person who desires to reduce, endurance exercise eases the pain of dieting. No outlandish, exotic, unbalanced, unappetizing, boring, and possibly dangerous diet is necessary or even suggested. Many people have lost weight solely by walking; many others have learned to cut down on the number and size of their portions and have lost weight faster. Finally, remember that the desirable objective is fitness, not weight loss. If you understand your goal and the path to achieve it, you are less apt to flounder and lose your way.

Many people who have persevered on their diet and have lost considerable weight are disappointed at the result. They don't look any better than before. This result is predictable. Weight loss by caloric restriction alone is due not only to loss of fatty tissue but also to some loss of muscle. The percentage of fat does not change as much as desired. Muscles remain flabby. Aerobic exercise, on the other hand, with or without caloric restriction, increases lean muscle mass and decreases fatty tissue. The cosmetic effect is positive. The person looks leaner, more fit, and more attractive. In this connection, spot reduction techniques by specific exercises for thighs, arms, and waist have not been shown to be effective. The important thing is to exercise for the training effect and let the fat come off where it may. What exercise can do is to keep the muscles and connective tissue firm so that the fat does not accumulate in unattractive, flabby masses.

Fat deposition is under hormonal control. It is obvious that sex hormones play an important role in the location of the fat depots. In addition, the blood level of the male sex hormone, testosterone, is temporarily increased due to exercise in both sexes, and it aids in the maintenance of muscle tissue (Metivier, 1983; Shangold, Gatz, & Thysen, 1981). Other hormones play an important role in fat metabolism. One result of aerobic exercise is an increase in *epinephrine* and *norepinephrine* in the blood. These two hormones, called *catecholamines*, aid in mobilizing fat that is used for energy. In weight loss by dieting alone, these hormonal responses are not called upon and both fat and muscle tissue decrease.

Effects of Dietary Feedbacks on Eating Behavior

Messages flow in a continuous stream from the digestive system to the brain. They are independent from those originating in the muscles and differ in some important respects. The stomach, for example, informs the brain of its fullness through the nervous system as well as by hormone secretion. After a certain period of emptiness, the stomach sends signals that we interpret as hunger pangs. It is time to eat. After eating a certain amount, we become aware of being full and stop, or should stop. The mechanisms that generate these intermittent feedback signals are not well known, but we do know that if malfunctioning occurs, extreme thinness or obesity may result.

Other feedbacks to the brain originate in taste buds and odor sensors. Receptors in these cells can often distinguish between spoiled and safe foods. When they haven't, other sensing mechanisms in the stomach can stimulate involuntary rejection of its contents. These safeguards have strong survival value.

Does a person eating a healthful diet in healthful amounts receive frequent, long-term, feedback signals, similar to what he receives from being fit? Probably not. The lack of feedback from both adequate and inadequate nutrition places the nutrition path to wellness in a separate category from the other.

Malnutrition Provides No Feedback

Do we receive feedback signals of our nutritional status on a long-term basis? Does a person on a deficient diet sense the inadequacy before any symptoms are noticeable? I have not heard or read of any. The onset of symptoms or clinical signs is usually the first indication that something is wrong. The most common cause of hypercholesterolemia is a diet high in cholesterol and saturated fat. The first observable symptom of this risk factor may be a heart attack that is fatal. Sudden death seems too high a price to pay for a diet that contained unhealthful components. A diet may contain carcinogens that give rise to a cancer and a slow, painful death. No symptoms may become evident until the disease process is well advanced.

Another very common example of a nutritional situation with no feedback, or in which the feedback is inadequate to control behavior, is that of chronic, slight overeating. The person may ignore the satiety signals or, if he or she is a fast eater, may have overeaten before the signals were received by the brain.

A person who is eating too much can acquire information about weight directly from a scale, a determination of percentage of fat, appearance minus clothes in a full-length mirror, or friends' comments ("You're picking up a little weight, aren't you?"). In contrast, someone who is receiving far less calories than is required soon becomes aware of hunger pangs and gradually becomes weaker unless food is eaten.

Weight Loss Tactics

There are numerous partial solutions for the moderately overweight person who wants to lose weight and shape up. The first does not even concern diet. It is to increase endurance activity on a regular basis. Choose something that you like to do and let the positive feelings help you to accomplish the dietary objectives. As I see it, endurance activity is the main source of positive feelings that is under the individual's control. Use it to your own benefit.

The second partial solution should be the resolve not to go on a diet. As I've written before, a weight-loss diet directs one onto a circular path that leads nowhere. What is needed—and this is more than a semantic trick—is a program of dietary management. Consider the food you eat in the same dispassionate, objective way as you do your budget. If you can balance your monetary budget, you can balance your energy budget. They both deal with income and expenditure whether it be dollars or calories.

A popular and often effective route to dietary management is by means of behavior modification based on cognition. Control of behavior is dependent on analysis; that is, to find those actions and habits that contribute to the present unsatisfactory eating behavior. After these habits are identified, they can be modified, and control of food ingestion becomes possible. These procedures are described by Stuart (1985) in *Act Thin, Stay Thin*. A number of individual and group programs for weight control are available. These include Weight Watchers, TOPS (Take Off Pounds Sensibly), Overeaters Anonymous, and others. Learning food intake management, like aerobic exercising, is often more easily accomplished on a long-term basis, as well as more pleasant as part of a group. Urban, technological man and woman are enthusiastically participating in dance-aerobic classes with specific goals under professional supervision for a fee. Neighborhood and church-centered aerobic activities are also being organized.

Effects of Fiber on Appetite and Weight Loss

In 1976, Heaton commented that carbohydrate refining makes the consumption of starch and sugar quicker, easier, and less satisfying. As a natural obstacle to food ingestion, fiber adds effort to eating. Nutritionally, the role of fiber may be to act as a natural preventive to overnutrition.

Since that time nutritionists have found that not all fibers decrease appetite equally, as the following experiment illustrates.

Krotkiewski (1984) added a palatable, granulated guar gum preparation (10 g twice a day) to the diet of obese subjects. Their body weights were significantly reduced in a 10-week experiment, even though they were told to maintain their ordinary eating habits. The average loss in body weight was 4.3 kg (9.5 lb), of which 2.5 kg (5.5 lb) was fat ($p < .01$). A slight reduction in total cholesterol was also found. Commercial wheat bran, another type of fiber that does not affect appetite, was used as a control. The subjects were asked to rank their hunger from ''no desire to eat'' to ''unbearable hunger.'' Significant decreases in hunger were found, particularly in the two meals following ingestion of the guar gum.

Dietary fiber can also act as an energy diluent in high-energy density diets. Duncan, Baron, and Weinsier (1983) compared the effects of low-energy density and high-energy density diets on satiety, energy intake, and eating time among obese and nonobese subjects. All subjects were allowed to eat to satiety at each meal over a 5-day period without the subjects knowing that the amount of food eaten was the main objective of the experiment. Satiety was attained on the low-energy density (high-fiber) fare at a mean energy intake about one-half that of a high-energy density (low-fiber) diet (1,570 vs. 3,000 kcal/day). In this experiment, fiber was not added as a supplement but was present in a low-fat diet as fresh fruits, vegetables, whole grains, and dried beans.

Practice Gustatory Sensualism

Predatory animals and some people, especially teenage boys, eat as though the purpose of eating is to get it over with as soon as possible. In the wild, rapid eating may be necessary; but in the well-fed developed countries, it is not. I remember, as a boy, watching middle-aged women dally with their forks as they lunched and thinking what a waste of time it was. Now I advocate slow eating, especially for people who are trying to control their weight. This statement should include most adults.

There are two reasons for this suggestion, the first one having a physiological basis, the second, psychological. Table sugar, of all our common foods, is probably the most rapidly digested and absorbed. It takes 10-20 minutes for these processes to furnish sufficient glucose in the circulating blood to affect the appestat, the postulated mechanism in the hypothalamus portion of the brain, which detects the sugar and sends messages to the cerebral cortex that we are less hungry and that we should slow down or stop eating. Fast eaters can devour 500 kcal or more in 20 minutes or less, and by the time they get the message, they have overeaten.

If you agree with me that eating should be an enjoyable pastime, then the psychological factor becomes a logical necessity. Why not expand your enjoyment by a factor or 2, 5, or 10? The slower you eat a favorite food, the longer your enjoyment. Since discovering this principle, I have eaten chocolate candies by tiny pieces and moved each bit around on my tongue to salvage every last bit of flavor I can muster for as long as possible. I might suggest that you practice this technique in private until it can be accomplished unostentatiously. I have learned to extend enjoyment of a piece of Godiva chocolate to 5 minutes and make one M&M last 60 seconds. This practice also works for prime rib, baked potatoes, and even vegetables!

Weight Control by the Elderly

In general, elderly people are less active than when they were younger. Consequently, they require fewer calories, but their essential nutrient needs do not decline. If anything, they increase because of lower efficiency of absorption or increased need, such as for calcium. The elderly, like other groups, can meet their essential nutrient requirements without consuming extra calories by eating high-nutrient-density foods (see chapter 6). Weight control for the elderly is also aided by daily long walks at as fast a tempo as is comfortable.

As shown in Table 7.5, the increase in average fat content as people age is not a consequence of aging per se, but occurs because many people become less physically active as they grow older, but their appetites remain constant. I suspect that watching TV for hours a day contributes to less activity in many age groups. Latin, Johnson, and Ruhling (1987) measured the fat content of 25 North American males aged 56 to 70. The average fat content as measured by underwater weighing was 22%. The range was 16%–35%. One man of 57 measured 16% fat, and another of 67 measured 17%. Both of these people are aerobically active most days of the week. Neither one is on a diet. They are two healthy, unfortunately atypical, Americans.

Latin et al. also developed an equation to calculate the lean body weight and thus the percentage of fat in males. Two simple measurements are all that are required: the total weight in kilograms and the abdominal girth in centimeters. By use of the equation, the percentage of fat can be calculated with an error of 3% compared to the underwater method. Here is the equation and a sample calculation. Similar equations are not available for women.

1. Calculate the lean body weight (LBW)

   LBW (kg) = 36.594 + 1.0325 (Wkg) − 0.5916 (G_a cm)

   Wkg = total weight in kg

   G_a = abdominal girth in cm

2. Calculate the percentage fat

$$\text{Percent fat} = 1 - \frac{\text{LBW}}{\text{Wkg}} \times 100$$

3. To calculate the percentage fat of a 70-kg man whose LBW is 50 kg

$$\text{Fat \%} = (1 - \frac{50}{70}) \times 100$$

$$= (1 - 0.71) \times 100$$

$$= 0.29 \times 100$$

$$= 29\%$$

Fitness: A Major Step Toward Weight Control

Pollock, Wilmore and Fox (1978) summarized the effects of endurance exercise on weight loss. There was little correlation between weight loss and loss of fat. For example, Pollock et al. (1976) measured the effects of endurance exercise on men 49 to 65 years. After 20 weeks of a walking-jogging program for 30 minutes per day, three days a week, there were significant increases in maximum oxygen uptake, and decreases in resting heart rate, diastolic blood pressure, body weight, fat, and waist measurements compared to nonexercised controls. There was no change in body weight or percentage fat in the control group, while the exercise group lost 2.6 pounds of weight ($p < .05$), and 3.5 pounds of fat ($p < .01$). What is the reason for fat loss exceeding total body weight loss? The average exerciser had gained a pound of muscle.

The evidence that I have reviewed has brought me to the conclusion that dieting has been overemphasized as the way to slimness. I agree with Bailey (1978) that fat loss, not weight loss, is the proper goal. Losing 20 to 50 lb by diet alone seems an endless road to overweight people. They become discouraged and quit. Physical activity offers a new approach in which weight loss ceases to be a criterion of success. For many people an exercise program will commence the important process of replacing fat by muscle. This change in metabolism, by mechanisms we do not yet understand, in time improves the psyche and decreases appetite.

Even so, there are three qualifications about weight loss and exercise programs that need to be stated. The first is that they are not 100% successful, especially if long-term compliance is included in the evaluation.

Another qualification is concerned with the nonexercise portions of the program such as personal attention, involvement with the program, and effective leadership. These factors may affect compliance independently of the aerobics. Finally, most of the studies have involved a small number of subjects for a limited time period, with sometimes inadequate control groups, so that the degree of credibility is not as high as might be desired compared to other types of prospective intervention studies. Despite these shortcomings in proof of effectiveness, your chances of long-term successful weight loss are much higher in a combined endurance exercise and diet program than in dieting alone.

It is common knowledge that many fat people suffer from a negative self-image. They are caught in a vicious cycle. They eat because they are miserable, and they are miserable because they overeat. Physical activity offers a way to break out of the cycle. The well-known positive psychological effects of regular physical activity, such as a walking program, will help in improving a person's self-image, and this, in turn, will reinforce the motivation to continue.

In concluding this discussion on exercise and weight control, I am impressed by the superior effectiveness of exercise over diet alone in attaining and maintaining a desirable weight. I further want to emphasize that heroic measures are not required for "normal," overweight people to achieve their objectives. I have placed the word normal in quotation marks to indicate that many people gain weight in their twenties and thirties because they are busy with earning a living and getting ahead. They may also have an income that allows them to eat all the thick steaks or whatever else appeals to them for the first time. They have gradually added 10–20 lb without being aware of it, or dismiss it by thinking that they can lose it at any time. I want to alert those people that now is the time. The longer they live as overweight/obese, the harder it will be to lose it; and the effect the extra pounds will exert as a risk factor for many diseases inexorably increases. Also, many overweight/obese people adjust to their condition by cutting out activities they formerly enjoyed with the excuse that it is due to aging. In my opinion, this type of attitude and the behavior that results decreases the chance for wellness. I believe that normal people can and will make the effort to lose weight when they become aware of the facts presented in this chapter and in chapters 9 and 10 on the dangers of overweight. On the other hand, I also recognize that some people are compulsive eaters for deep-seated psychological reasons and will not be able to control their weight until these problems are resolved.

The key to weight control lies in two words: regularity and patience. If you are terribly out of shape, it may take months to reach the minimum intensity for the training effect. But—and this is perhaps the only place in this book that I can make a sweeping generalization—if you stay with the program as outlined above (Pollock et al., 1978), you will gradually become fit, build muscle instead of accumulating fat, and feel better than you have in years: You will start walking the paths to wellness.

Eating a Healthy Diet

The term *healthy diet* sounds simple and innocuous, but it isn't. A person might think that nutrition research would have progressed to the point of defining a healthy diet by the year 1985, but it hasn't. This was the year that the RDA book was to be revised and the latest values published. In October, the media were informed in a letter from Frank Press, Chairman of the National Research Council, to James B. Wyngaarden, Director of the National Institutes of Health, that a Research Council Committee on Dietary Allowances was unable to agree with a panel of independent reviewers and the Food and Nutrition Board on the interpretation of scientific data on which the RDAs for a number of vitamins are based. Critics denounced a draft as purely academic and a threat to welfare programs; the authors would not compromise on a revised version. The National Research Council was trying to avoid what has been called "the fiasco of 1980," quoted by Marshall (p. 420) in publicizing differing interpretations of nutrition-health data.

This controversy illustrates the handling of scientific conclusions when they affect the public interest. In this example the participants are nutritionists of high repute. They do not disagree about the data, only about its application to public programs. As reported by Marshall (1985), two major issues were debated. The first concerns the objectives of the RDAs. From their inception in 1941 the RDAs have been "designed for the maintenance of good nutrition of practically all healthy people in the U.S." This objective has been discussed in chapter 5.

Henry Kamin, the chairman of the committee to reevaluate the RDAs wanted to "reexamine original assumptions and calculations and try to rebuild RDAs from the ground up" (p. 420). D. Mark Hegsted, professor emeritus of Nutrition, Harvard Medical School, objected to Kamin's decision to define minimal nutrient requirements, rather than set broad standards for good health (p. 420). Apparently many committee members, as well as myself, think that the objectives of the RDAs should not be changed without first obtaining a broad expression of opinion from nutritionists and other people involved in applying the RDAs to public programs.

The second issue was concerned with the Kamin committee's recommendation to lower the RDAs for vitamins A and C. Many nutritionists think the RDAs for these two vitamins should not be changed unless new data justifies a decrease. No such data were offered.

It was decided, in view of the widespread disagreement, that a wider consensus would be sought before the next revision of the RDA book would be published. At this date (May, 1987) no such statement has appeared. Thus, the 1980 RDA Table 5A.1 remains the most recent recommendation on nutrient intake.[1]

It is interesting that this table includes only one source of energy—that of protein. What lies behind the omission of fat and carbohydrate from the RDA energy chart? In the first place, protein occupies a unique function in our diets. Besides furnishing calories, proteins contain the dietary essential amino acids, without which growth and development will not occur. From their discovery many years ago, a tremendous research effort has been supported in identifying all the essential amino acids, both qualitatively and quantitatively, and their proportions in a wide variety of proteins. The requirements of infants, children, adolescents, and adults have been determined. In short, we know a great deal about the protein requirements of the human race.

Although there is also an essential fatty acid, the fact that extra carbohydrate can be converted to fats implies that there is no important difference between them as source of calories. The assumption has come under question, but no general consensus has yet been reached. Two differences have been mentioned: the stimulating effect of fats on appetite so that people tend to overeat, and the greater efficiency of fat deposition from fats than from carbohydrates, so that overeaters of fats lay down even more fat. High-fat diets also decrease endurance. Whether high-fat diets make people more susceptible to atherosclerosis and cancer compared to equal-caloric diets high in carbohydrates is actively being investigated.

---

[1]Olson and Hodges (1987) and Olson (1987) suggest a new term, Recommended Dietary Intakes (RDI), for vitamins C and A. They recommend daily intakes of 40 mg (60 mg) and 30 mg (50 mg) for vitamin C for adult men and women respectively. Amounts of the 1980 RDAs are given in parenthesis. The lower value for the RDIs is mainly due to the selection of a smaller body pool size than formerly used. Olson recommends RDIs for vitamin A of 700 μg (1,000 μg) and 600 μg (800 μg) respectively for men and women. Olson justifies the lower recommendations, especially for women, as less apt to cause reproductive abnormalities. Undoubtedly, these recommendations will be fully discussed before the publication of the next RDA book.

In a practical sense, the term healthful diet is used in the health professions as one that will help prevent, and not induce, a disease. I suspect that many laypeople use the term with this meaning also. The two major diseases in the U.S. at present are heart disease and cancer. In each, nutrition acts as a risk factor. Overweight/obesity is the most prevalent nutritional disease, and even though it isn't known how many people die from it directly each year, there is little doubt that it contributes to the incidence of heart disease, cancer, diabetes, and high blood pressure.

The Beginnings of the Diet–Heart Hypothesis Controversy

Most of the research on diet as a risk factor for heart disease and on the pathological effects of obesity has been carried out since World War II.

By 1961, the American Heart Association thought the data sufficiently strong to recommend a diet lower in saturated fatty acids and cholesterol, and higher in polyunsaturated fatty acids than the usual American diet. This recommendation was given qualified approval in 1972 in a joint statement by the American Medical Association Council on Foods and Nutrition and the Food and Nutrition Board of the National Academy of Sciences. These groups supported the role of diet as a risk factor but suggested that it be implemented by physicians in counseling patients rather than by urging dietary modification for the general public. At about that time, Gortner (1975) published a chart that showed no relationship between per capita consumption of beef, eggs, and butter and deaths from heart disease over the period 1900-1970. Recall that ecological data of this type have the lowest credibility of any kind of survey (see Table 3.1).

These differences of opinion among the experts received even more publicity after the McGovern Senate Select Committee on Nutrition and Human Needs (1977) suggested seven dietary guidelines. These goals applied not only to the prevention of atherosclerosis and hypertension but also to cancer, diabetes, and cirrhosis of the liver. In terms of nutrients, the dietary goals are contrasted to those of the present American diet in Figure 8.2. In terms of foods, accomplishing the goals would require eating more fresh fruits and vegetables, whole grains, vegetable oils, fish, and fowl, and decreasing the consumption of red meats, whole milk and products containing it, most cheeses, eggs, table sugar, and salt. These recommendations are based on the assumption that you are now consuming the current American diet as outlined in Figure 8.2. These changes are detailed in the following "Dietary Guidelines for Americans."

Dietary Guidelines for Americans

1. Eat a variety of foods daily. This recommendation suggests daily consumption from the four food groups, and a person should eat a variety of foods from within each group.
2. Maintain ideal weight.
3. Avoid too much fat, saturated fat, and cholesterol. Choose lean cuts of meat and low-fat dairy products, trim fats from meats, cut down on fried foods, and eat eggs in moderation. Read labels carefully so that polyunsaturated fats (PUFA) can be increased over the saturated fats (SFA).
4. Eat foods that retain their original starch and fiber contents in preference to those in which these components have been removed: for example, whole-grain products over white flour and white rice. Eat more fresh green and yellow vegetables of all types and also legumes such as peas and beans.
5. Decrease sugar intake by consuming less table sugar, syrups, and candies. Buy canned fruits in light syrup rather than heavy. Most fresh or dried fruits have a sweet flavor due to their sugar content, but the bulk of the fruit is composed of cellulose and other fibers. In addition, the nutrient densities of noncalorific nutrients in a fruit are much higher than in a candy bar.
6. Keep salt consumption to a reasonable level. Always taste a food before you salt it. A touch of salt may be all you need. Become aware of the salt content of processed and snack foods. Refer to Table 9.2 for the salt content of some processed foods.
7. Consume alcohol in moderation, if at all. More than two drinks a day of alcoholic beverages can lead to serious metabolic problems over a period of years. Pregnant women should consult their pediatricians as soon as possible about alcohol consumption.

Needless to say, these recommendations created a storm of controversy, notably from the Food and Nutrition Board and the American Medical Association. The latter organization stated (1979), "It cannot be *assumed* [italics added] that the proportions of saturated and unsaturated fat and the levels of cholesterol in the diet are of universal importance. For healthy people, moderation in fat intake should become the rule of thumb." The Food and Nutrition Board (1980) responded to the dietary goals with a lengthy critical statement about them and included its own dietary recommendations entitled *Toward Healthful Diets*.

First, the Food and Nutrition Board stated that it considers single, inclusive recommendations to the public regarding intakes of energy, fat, protein, cholesterol, carbohydrate, fiber, and sodium as scientifically unsound. Second, it noted that the population of the U.S. has never been healthier. Even so, the two diseases, cancer and heart disease, account for about two-thirds of the deaths of adults. They are both multifactorial diseases. Is it justified to single out diet for special emphasis? Third, the diet–heart hypothesis is based on epidemiological research, which establishes correlations but not cause and effect. The board believes that more conclusive data than that obtained from epidemiology alone are required before dietary recommendations are justified.

Obesity, however, is recognized by the Food and Nutrition Board as the most prevalent form of malnutrition in the U.S. and has been identified as a contributory cause of a variety of diseases. According to the Food and Nutrition Board, recommendations on the importance of avoiding obesity are justified. For adult Americans, the board recommended a diet

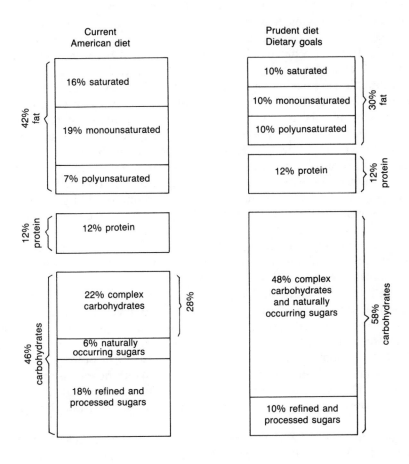

Figure 8.2 Percent of calories from different nutrients. *Note.* From *Dietary Goals for the United States,* prepared by the Senate Select Committee on Nutrition and Human Needs, 1977, Washington, DC: U.S. Government Printing Office. Copyright 1977 by U.S. Government Printing Office. Reprinted by permission.

containing a variety of foods selected from the four food groups. Energy intake should be adjusted to avoid overweight. An increase in exercise aids in weight control and weight loss. Intake of low-nutrient density foods (e.g., sugars, alcohol, fat, and oils) should be reduced preferentially in weight-loss diets. Salt should be used in moderation, between 3 and 8 g per day. The Food and Nutrition Board suggestion, however, leaves the following decisions up to the individual: (a) how much fat, (b) what kind of fat (i.e., the P/S ratio), (c) how much carbohydrate, and (d) what kinds of carbohydrate (i.e., the starch/sugar ratio and the unrefined/refined starch ratio). Does the suggestion, "Keep your weight in line," mean that these four questions can be ignored safely? I think not for the following reasons.

First, the board's suggestion ignores the effect that the total fat/total carbohydrate ratio has on the nutrient density of the total diet. It was shown in chapter 6 that fats and sugars act as nutrient diluents and make the obtaining of an adequate diet more difficult. Second, if a person continues to eat a typical American high-fat diet and not gain weight, total calories from carbohydrates must be restricted. What are consequences of this restriction? One consequence is that the carbohydrates consumed should have a high-nutrient density, especially in the B-vitamins. In practice, this objective also entails a low consumption of table sugar, which has a nutrient density of zero, and a high consumption of fresh fruits and vegetables. Another consequence is that refined carbohydrates must also be restricted for two reasons: They tend to have a low-nutrient density, and secondly, they are low in dietary fiber. A majority of Americans are probably affected by diet as a risk factor for diseases and as the direct source of calories for overweight/obesity. The fat/carbohydrate ratio is important in both of these situations.

The P/S ratio of fat is independent of the total calories ingested. The ratio is important in affecting blood cholesterol levels for many people. A low ratio, as in red meats and whole milk products, tends to raise blood cholesterol in many people. Fowl and fish both have higher P/S ratios than red meats and contain less total fat as well. In other words, the keep-your-weight-in-line dictum does not spell out the means to achieve it, but a person who accomplishes it and still ingests an adequate diet is conforming to the prudent diet that the Food and Nutrition Board has criticized.

For both the Food and Nutrition Board and the Senate Select Committee and their consultants, areas of agreement on the constituents in a healthy diet for adults would include the following guidelines:

- The RDAs.
- The consumption of a variety of foods from each of the four food groups.
- Energy intake to keep weight in line. This objective involves emphasis on high-nutrient density foods (i.e., ingestion of sugars and fats should be low for adult sedentary workers).
- Protein intake in the range of 10%–12% of total calories.
- Moderate use of salt.

Areas of disagreement include the following:

- The fat/carbohydrate ratio calculated as percentage of total calories.
- The importance of the P/S ratio.
- The cholesterol content of the diet.

Stated in this manner, it becomes obvious that the area of disagreement is mostly concerned with fats—the amount and types. You might wonder why this topic should create such controversy. The reasons become clear when we move from fat to the sources of fat. The main foods that contain the bulk of our fat and cholesterol are meats, eggs, and dairy foods. If everyone cut down on these foods, it would have large economic repercussions on U.S. agriculture and the U.S. food industry. Actually, the U.S. diet is changing in the direction of the dietary goals.

The Food and Nutrition Board sidestepped the fat issue by leaving the decisions on fats and carbohydrates up to the individual. The Senate Select Committee recommendations (1977) and the dietary guidelines I listed above are more specific about reducing fat consumption, especially saturated fats and cholesterol. In practice, the disagreement seems more apparent than real. Are people more apt to cut down on fatty animal foods if the changes are spelled out for them rather than making a general recommendation that will require the individual to come to the same conclusions? Perhaps a survey should be made to determine how many Americans know enough about nutrition at the present time to answer the four questions listed above for themselves. Perhaps it is useful for them to have the specific dietary changes spelled out.

Another aspect of the Food and Nutrition Board's criticism of the dietary goals concerns the board's call for more conclusive data before alerting the public to the possible dangers of the present American diet. In my opinion, this criticism is not a scientific one, but one of judgment. It raises the question of how conclusive the results and conclusions of epidemiological experiments need to be before the federal government is justified in recommending them to the public. Many of the goals are based on research that falls in categories 4 and 5 of Table 3.1, which are not very conclusive. A question that needs to be asked at this point: How soon, if ever, will results of more conclusive dietary experiments be available? My guess is that it will take a minimum of 20 years and probably longer, if ever. In the meantime, should the data presently available be ignored? My judgment says no. I see no harm, and possibly considerable value, in the U.S. government recommending the prudent diet with qualifications to adults. To me, the recommendation supports a general objective of this book, which is to encourage people to take responsibility for their own health practices, including their diets.

The noncaloric essential nutrients can be obtained in amounts as suggested by the RDAs by selecting high-nutrient-density foods from the four food groups plus one. Dietary fiber is not mentioned explicitly in the prudent diet, but adequate intake can be obtained if one interprets the term unrefined carbohydrate to mean derived from whole grains and fresh vegetables.

Toward Wellness Diets

Did it strike you as odd, or even inconsistent, that this long discussion on healthful diets was concerned mostly with avoiding disease? Actually, to many people, including physicians, health means nothing more than the absence of disease. I have labeled this section "Toward Wellness Diets" to highlight the difference in meaning between the two terms. Wellness accentuates the positive, not merely the absence of the negative.

In this sense, we know very little about diet's contributions toward wellness. The only diet that I confidently say contributes to wellness is milk for a baby from a well-nourished, well mother. The subject of food and mood is in its infancy. A special diet for endurance-type athletes is being developed. I can imagine that, in the years to come, special diets for studying, listening to music, looking at art, and love-making will be available at the friendly supermarket.

At the present time, we probably know more about diets for exercise than any other type. For the team, the big steak before a football game is "out." A light meal high in carbohydrates and low in fat is "in." The reasons for these changes, how different types of exercise affect appetite, and how food is converted to the energy actually used by muscles were discussed in chapter 7.

For those readers who desire more specific information, consult the Food Guide from the Berkeley Co-Op (Black, 1980) in chapter 6 (Table 6A.2). The following cookbooks utilize these dietary guidelines:

American Heart Association Cookbook by R. Eshleman and M. Winston, 1984, Ballantine Books, New York.

Rotation Diet by M. Katahn, 1987, Bantam Books, New York.

The New Laurel's Kitchen by L. Robertson, C. Flinders, and B. Ruppenthal, 1986, Ten Speed Press, Berkeley, CA.

Summary

Weight control has become an objective for many people since the close relationship between overweight/obesity and a variety of chronic diseases has been publicized. Unfortunately, the role of dieting in weight control has been overemphasized. People on diets tend to be miserable; they are hungry all the time. Those with great willpower stick it out until the desired weight is lost, and then most of them gain it right back again. Long-term weight loss depends on behavior modification: the control of calorie input. Behavior modification should also include information and thus motivation concerning caloric usage. A consideration of the energy equation reveals that energy output is also a factor in weight control.

Many people who want to lose weight don't exercise because they have heard that it takes a lot of exercise to use up the calories contained in one piece of pie. It is also common knowledge that exercise increases appetite. Exercise is thus dismissed as self-defeating. Both of these statements represent half-truths. Several studies have demonstrated that endurance exercise does not increase appetite, and with many people it actually decreases it. A person who engages in aerobic exercise regularly at the rate of 200-300 kcal/day, at the very least, can eat an occasional piece of pie without gaining weight. Thousands of people who had difficulty with weight control by diet alone have found that with endurance exercise as an adjunct, they feel better, are less hungry, and gradually attain their objective of a desirable weight.

Table 8.1A Suggested Body Weights for Height for Adults

Suggested body weights[1] for height for men 25 years of age and over

Height[2] Feet	Inches	Small Frame	Medium Frame	Large Frame
5	2	112-120	118-129	126-141
5	3	115-123	121-133	129-144
5	4	118-126	124-136	132-148
5	5	121-129	127-139	135-152
5	6	124-133	130-143	138-156
5	7	128-137	134-147	142-161
5	8	132-141	138-152	147-166
5	9	136-145	142-156	151-170
5	10	140-150	146-160	155-174
5	11	144-154	150-165	159-179
6	0	148-158	154-170	164-184
6	1	152-162	158-175	168-189
6	2	156-167	162-180	173-194
6	3	160-171	167-185	178-199
6	4	164-175	172-190	182-204

Suggested body weights[1] for women 25 years of age and over

Height[3] Feet	Inches	Small Frame	Medium Frame	Large Frame
4	10	92-98	96-107	104-119
4	11	94-101	98-110	106-122
5	0	96-104	101-113	109-125
5	1	99-107	104-116	112-128
5	2	102-110	107-119	115-131
5	3	105-113	110-122	118-134
5	4	108-116	113-126	121-138
5	5	111-119	116-130	125-142
5	6	114-123	120-135	129-146
5	7	118-127	124-139	133-150
5	8	122-131	128-143	137-154
5	9	126-135	132-147	141-158
5	10	130-140	136-151	145-163
5	11	134-144	140-155	149-168
6	0	138-148	144-159	153-173

Note. From *How to Control Your Weight* by the Metropolitan Life Insurance Company, 1960, New York: Author. Copyright 1960 by Metropolitan Life Insurance. Reprinted by permission.
[1]Weight in pounds, according to frame (in indoor clothing).
[2]Height with shoes on (1-inch heels).
[3]Height with shoes on (2-inch heels).

Table 8.1B   Growth Standards for Children

Height and weight of children 4-18 years of age

Age	Girls Height (in.)	Girls Weight (lb)	Boys Height (in.)	Boys Weight (lb)
4	40.7	36.1	40.8	36.1
5	43.4	40.9	43.4	40.3
6	45.9	45.7	45.9	44.7
7	47.8	51.0	48.1	50.9
8	50.0	57.2	50.5	57.4
9	52.2	63.6	52.8	64.4
10	54.5	71.0	54.9	71.4
11	57.0	82.0	56.4	78.9
12	59.5	94.4	58.6	86.0
13	62.2	105.5	61.3	98.6
14	63.1	113.0	64.1	111.8
15	63.8	120.0	66.9	124.3
16	64.1	123.0	68.9	133.8
17	64.2	125.8	69.8	129.8
18	64.4	126.2	70.2	144.8

Note. From "Some Physical Growth Standards for White North American Children" by F. Falkner, 1962, *Pediatrics, 29,* p. 448. Copyright 1962 by *Pediatrics.* Reprinted by permission.

Chapter

9

Blood Pressure and Wellness

It is the function of medicine to help
people die young as late as possible.
Old Greek Adage

The information in this chapter will help you

- control and/or avoid hypertension;
- understand the interplay of the risk factors
  in hypertension—a multifactorial disease;
  and
- realize the beneficial effects of regular aerobic
  exercise on blood pressure.

The fact that blood, a liquid, occurs in the body under pressure has been known to mankind since someone killed the first warm-blooded animal aeons ago. When an artery is cut—even a small one—the blood spurts out like water from a garden hose. Descriptions of battles when men fought with swords and battle axes speak of the blood of the victim engulfing the victor. It is really not surprising that a warrior who had just cut off his opponent's head would be exulting at his victory rather than wondering why the blood shot up so high.

The physiological significance of blood pressure was not realized until Harvey discovered the circulation of the blood in 1628. For the first time, the function of the heart as a pump was demonstrated. For the first time, the mythological idea of the heart as an organ of emotion was replaced by a physiological one.

Although Harvey postulated that the blood circulated, no one knew how until Malpighi in 1661 discovered the capillaries that connect the arteries and the veins. The full circuit was now mapped; the pathway of the blood from the right heart through the tissues and back to the left heart was described. The heart provided the pressure, or the driving force, for the circulation of the blood.

The first man actually to measure blood pressure was Stephen Hales, an English clergyman. In 1732 he described the following experiment (Evans, 1949):

> In December I caused a mare to be tied down alive on her back. Having laid open the left crural Artery about three inches from her belly, I inserted into it a brass Pipe, whose bore was one sixth of an inch in diameter; and to that, by means of another brass Pipe which was fitly adapted to it, I fixed a glass Tube, of nearly the same diameter, which was nine feet in length: Then untying the Ligature on the Artery, the blood rose in the Tube eight feet three inches perpendicular above the level of the left Ventricle of the heart: But it did not attain to its full height at once; it rushed up about half way in an instant, and afterwards gradually at each Pulse twelve, eight, six, four, two and sometimes one inch: When it was at its full height, it would rise and fall at and after each Pulse two, three, or four inches. (p. 609)

The predecessor of the present cuff for measuring blood pressure was invented by Rivi-Rocci in 1896. The cuff fits over the upper arm and can be inflated until the arteries are constricted to such an extent that blood flow stops. The cuff is then gradually deflated until the reader begins to hear the flow of blood by means of a stethoscope placed on the lower arm. The maximum pressure attained in the arteries as the blood is pumped out of the heart is called the systolic pressure (SP). The minimum pressure that occurs between beats of the heart is called the diastolic pressure (DP). Blood pressure is greatest in the large arteries closest to the heart. As the arteries divide and grow smaller in diameter, pressure decreases. It is lowest in the small *arterioles* and *capillaries*, and remains low in the veins that return the blood to the heart.

Blood Pressure Measurements

Because blood pressure is affected by such a variety of stimuli (e.g., emotions, time of day, time since last meal, recent exercise, etc.), it is advisable to standardize as many of these factors as possible no matter who measures your blood pressure or where it is measured. In a large study of Western Electric employees in Chicago, Souchek, Stamler, Dyer,

Paul, and Lepper (1979) concluded that the mean of three readings on the right arm, taken at one sitting, was a more accurate measure of blood pressure than one, and well worth the extra time. Some physicians and clinics routinely have a person sit quietly for 5 minutes before a measurement is taken.

In recent years more elaborate electronic devices record the pressures and the two are recorded as a printout. In addition, home devices are now available. Consumer Reports (1979) comments on three types and rates various products. One general suggestion for home measurers of blood pressure is to have your device checked in your doctor's office so that the two agree. There is enough variability in readings so that, if you change doctors, it is advisable to double-check each time.

What Is Hypertension?

Blood pressure varies from person to person and even in the same person from time to time. Your blood pressure is higher when you are standing than sitting, which in turn is higher than when you are lying down. Blood pressure is apt to be higher when a person is nervous or stressed. Yet, despite all these variations, the medical profession has suggested standard conditions that allow comparison of blood pressure readings of one person over a period of years and between groups of people. These conditions include placing the cuff on the right arm, and having the person seated and at rest for 5 minutes. Blood pressure should be measured three times and the readings averaged.

Blood pressure is an example of a continuous variable. There is no gap between normal pressure and hyper pressure. The distinction is similar to that between tall and short people. We say that a person 4 feet in height is short and one 7 feet in height is tall. When the height of a large number of people is measured, it is found that there is a continuous variation between the shortest and the tallest. Blood pressure measurements have given similar results. The distinction between normal blood pressure (normotension) and high blood pressure (hypertension) is arbitrary, but necessary because of its medical importance.

In the U.S. a recent large-scale hypertension detection and follow-up program (HDFP) included measurement of over 178,000 people between 30 and 69 years (Daugherty & Entwisle, 1983). The cutoff between normal tension and hypertension was made at a diastolic pressure of 95 mm Hg and systolic pressure of 140 mm Hg. With these definitions 14% of the population has diastolic hypertension and 30% had systolic hypertension. In this population, about twice as many black people had hypertension as whites.

The Importance of Detecting Hypertension

The worldwide use of the blood pressure cuff on millions of people has resulted in a gradually increasing awareness by public health workers that high blood pressure of even moderate degree is a serious condition that requires prompt control. No matter how well a person may feel, long-term wellness becomes an impossible objective for someone with uncontrolled high blood pressure. The reasons behind this statement will be presented in this chapter.

One reason for the concern of the medical establishment is that hypertension gradually increases unless it is treated early. Another reason is that the disease has no symptoms. In fact, claims have been made that hypertensive people may have stronger feelings of well-being than normotensives. These factors lead to the denouement. A person may have never felt better in his life one day and suffer a debilitating stroke or heart attack the next. In this sense, hypertension is possibly the most insidious chronic disease of them all.

Beneficial Effects of Controlling Hypertension

The data linking hypertension to heart disease and stroke are quite convincing. Some of the most conclusive data comes from the long-term Framingham study. In this work, normotensive blood pressure was defined as having *systolic/diastolic* pressures below 140/90 mm mercury; mild hypertensive, in the range 140/90 to 160/95; and definite hypertensive, above 160/95. Over a period of 18 years, the incidence of cardiovascular disease was 6 times higher in hypertensive men than in those with normal blood pressures. In women the ratio of heart disease was about 10 times higher in the hypertensive group (Kannel & Sorlie, 1975).

Since 1972 the incidence of death from stroke in the U.S. has declined by 42%—a magnificent decrease for a 10-year period. Although there are many possible reasons, epidemiological experts consider the decrease in hypertension as one of the most potent. Hypertension research workers suggest that treating the 35 million Americans in the mild category may lower the stroke deaths still more.

The findings of the 5-year Hypertension Detection and Follow-Up Program (HDFP) were published in 1979 (HDFP cooperative group, 1979). This research represented the results of a randomized trial of the effects of medication on 10,940 patients with differing degrees of high blood pressure in 14 communities in the U.S. Five-year mortality from all causes was 17% lower for the treated group than for the controls ($p < .01$) and 20% lower ($p < .01$) for the subgroup with diastolic blood pressure of 90 to 104 mm Hg at entry. This subgroup was considered to have mild hypertension. These results suggest that there is a large potential for saving thousands of lives yearly by identifying and treating hypertensive people from both sexes, blacks and whites, in the age range 30 to 69 years.

The Joint National Committee on Detection, Evaluation, and Treatment of High Blood Pressure (1984) summarized the recommendations for physicians of a number of previous studies, including the HDFP. In addition the committee addressed the use of nonpharmacological therapies, especially for people with mild hypertension. The reason for a nonmedication therapy stems from the undesirable side effects of the antihypertensive drugs. Here we have an example of a medical condition in many patients responding to nondrug therapy. I discuss it here as an example of what people can do for themselves when they take responsibility for their own health.

First and foremost, the blood pressure of a person with mild hypertension needs to be monitored regularly, at least once a month, by a physician, clinic, or at home, so that the effectiveness of the therapy can be evaluated. There is a strong correlation between body weight and blood pressure. Weight reduction often results in a substantial decrease in blood pressure, even if ideal body weight is not achieved.

Other factors that are under the control of the individual that may postpone or avoid long-term medication are: the salt content of the diet, alcohol consumption, fat consumption, smoking, and amount of exercise. The studies that established these factors as risk factors for hypertension are mentioned in the next few pages. Kolata (1979) refers to James Hunt, University of Tennessee Medical School, who estimates that at least 85% of patients can achieve normal blood pressure by nondrug measures. To determine which factor or factors are responsible for an individual's hypertension will require a carefully monitored, long-term self-experiment.

U.S. blacks develop hypertension at an earlier age than whites. Thus young black people comprise a main target group for screening for hypertension and commencement of prompt therapy for those who require it. Hypertension in the U.S. is so widespread and can begin at such an early age than many physicians suggest screening of all children at 3 years of age. The parents of young children with average diastolic values above 80 mm Hg should develop a therapeutic program with their physician.

Does this suggestion of universal screening represent an example of medical overconcern, that is, of hypochondria on a national scale? I think not. Hypertension has been recognized by the medical profession as a major risk factor for stroke, heart disease, and kidney disease. It contributes to the 500,000 cases of stroke yearly and to over a million heart attacks. Many of these diseases could be avoided or postponed for years if blood pressure were controlled. Accomplishing this objective will require first, that those people who are at risk from high blood pressure be identified; and second, that they be educated to continue an appropriate form of therapy. Considerable progress has been made in attaining the first objective. Through widespread publicity, the percentage of adult hypertensives who are unaware of it has dropped from 50% in 1970 to 25% in 1980.

Attaining the second objective will be more difficult. It amounts to convincing people who are not sick in the usual sense to change their diets and lifestyles, or to take some form of medication for the rest of their lives. To many people, this type of therapy doesn't sound sensible. The rationale for this suggestion will occupy much of the rest of this chapter.

Role and Control of Blood Pressure

Pressure is necessary for the blood to circulate to bring oxygen and nutrients to all the cells of the body. If the blood stops circulating due to a heart attack, a blockage of a major artery to an essential organ, or a loss of large volumes of blood due to an injury, a person may die or suffer severe incapacitation.

There are two major factors that determine the magnitude of the blood pressure: the cardiac output, or the volume of blood that the heart pumps at each contraction; and the resistance within the circulatory system.

The volume of blood is maintained relatively constant by the liquid we imbibe every day, which should amount to a minimum of eight full 8-oz glasses, and the volume of urine excreted by the kidneys. Obviously, if the kidneys become less efficient or are damaged, blood pressure may increase or decrease. The resistance within the circulatory system is controlled by a number of mechanisms. It appears that it is this resistance factor to which the various dietary and drug therapies are directed. The term *essential hypertension* is used when the cause of the condition is unknown.

It is interesting to realize that, although all the blood in the body is under pressure, the pressure varies from organ to organ and from time to time. For example, if a person has just eaten a large dinner, more blood will flow to the digestive organs to aid digestion. A person who exercises will build up extra pressure in the muscles so that extra nutrients can be brought to them and side products can be removed. This redistribution of the blood supply according to need explains why a person who exercises vigorously soon after a meal has muscle cramps. Some blood is withdrawn from the stomach muscles and rerouted to the skeletal muscles. The blood supply is insufficient for both sets of muscles and one or the other may go into a spasm, cease to function, and become painful. If a person is swimming, an episode of cramps can have serious consequences. The one organ in which the blood pressure is relatively constant is the brain. Whether we are asleep, daydreaming, or concentrating, its blood supply hardly varies.

The physiological control of blood pressure does not occur in the arteries, but in smaller vessels called arterioles, which carry the blood to the tissues. The arterioles have a strong muscular coat that can expand and contract. When they contract, the diameter of the arteriole decreases and the blood pressure goes up. As might be expected, the expansion and contraction process is complicated. It is governed by the nervous system, hormones, and local influences. High blood pressure represents a condition in which one or more of the controlling factors is not working correctly.

It may surprise you to learn that the kidney plays an important part in controlling blood pressure. I'll briefly describe how the kidney functions in the control of blood pressure because much of the therapy of hypertension acts on the kidneys. The kidneys synthesize a *proteolytic* enzyme called *renin*, which is secreted into the blood. There, it meets a protein, *angiotensinogen*, which is synthesized in the liver. Renin hydrolyzes angiotensinogen to form three peptides called *angiotensins*. One of the angiotensins stimulates the *adrenal cortex* to secrete *aldosterone*, a steroid hormone that, in turn, acts on the kidneys to increase retention of sodium ions and water (i.e., to increase blood pressure). A diuretic-type drug stimulates the kidneys to excrete more urine. This fact makes clear why diuretics are usually the first therapy in the control of high blood pressure.

Angiotensin also stimulates the sympathetic nervous system to release the *neurotransmitter norepinephrine*, which—you may recall from chapter 4— is released during stress. This hormone increases blood pressure by constricting the arterioles. Here, we have a direct connection between stress responses and hypertension. It has been discovered recently that renin and the angiotensins are also synthesized in the brain. This finding provides another possible mechanism for how human stress influences blood pressure.

Before discussing the human data on hypertension, I think it advisable to review the research that has used rats. The rat model is not subject to the limitations of human research, and from this work we can begin to understand the interactions of suspected risk factors under standard conditions of diet and environment.

Hypertensinogenic Effects of Diets High in Sodium Chloride on Rats

Meneely, Tucker, Darby, and Auerbach (1953) fed rats different amounts of sodium chloride as the sole variable in an otherwise wholesome diet. They found that chronic ingestion of salt regularly produced a type of hypertension in the rat that appeared to duplicate human hypertension. Rats were fed three ranges of sodium chloride. The lowest level corresponds to 1–10 g per day for man. Rats ingesting these amounts of salt never became hypertensive. The moderate excess range, corresponding to 14–28 g per day produced hypertension and shortened life in some of the rats. The highest level of sodium chloride consumption, equivalent to 35–49 g per day for man, produced definite hypertension in most of the rats. This amount equals that consumed in Northern Japan, possibly the highest average consumption in the world.

Meneely and colleagues found another significant similarity between rats and humans in these experiments. Not all the rats on the high-salt diet developed hypertension. For example, the mean systolic blood pressure for the low-salt-fed animals was 122 m of mercury. The average pressure for the moderate salt group was 130 with a range from 114–160. At the high level of sodium chloride ingestion, the mean pressure was 152 with a range from 125 to 205. It is worth noting that this large variation was obtained on a rat population that had been inbred for many generations.

Meneely et al. made still other observations on rats that are of interest to humans. The rats that developed hypertension on the high-salt diets were more likely to show significant changes in their electrocardiograms late in life, and they also showed an elevated serum cholesterol.

Of all the adverse effects of sodium chloride on rats, the most sensitive index was that of survival. The slopes of the survival curves were related to the levels of dietary salt. For example, rats ingesting a moderate excess of salt, equivalent to the U.S. average, began to die at a faster rate after 17 months. Taking 10 days for a rat as equivalent to one year in humans, 17 months corresponds approximately to age 51. At the highest level of salt intake, the life-shortening effect amounted to 32 years.

Another interesting finding of the Meneely group was that adding salt to the diet of old rats did not raise their blood pressure as much as adding the same amount of sodium chloride to the diet of young rats. This finding could be readily explained by the observations made at autopsy of the young and old rats. The small arteries and arterioles in the kidneys, pancreas, and testes showed more fatty degeneration of the muscle cells of the rats fed extra salt since weaning. A noted pathologist, Dr. Ernest Goodpasture, examined the tissues of rats fed the high-salt diet and found a similarity between the lesions present and those seen in human malignant hypertension—a severe form of essential hypertension.

The Meneely group also studied the protective effect of potassium chloride on the toxic effects of excessive sodium chloride in the diet. When extra potassium chloride was added to the diet of rats receiving moderately excessive sodium chloride, they still developed hypertension, but there was a tremendous improvement in survival. Extra potassium chloride added to the diets of rats receiving the highly excessive dietary sodium chloride that had been shown to produce the highest blood pressures resulted in moderate rather than severe hypertension.

Dahl (1972) and colleagues at the Brookhaven National Laboratory took these observations a giant step further. They interbred some of the rats that did not develop hypertension on the high-salt diet, and similarly interbred those that did develop hypertension. After a few generations, they had two completely different strains of rats: one extremely sensitive to increased salt intake, and the other resistant to it.

In summary, the rat experiments have been very valuable in demonstrating the complex relationship between salt content of the diet, the age of the rats, and their genetic makeup. Some strains are resistant to high sodium chloride, others develop hypertension readily on moderate levels of salt. Young rats are more sensitive to extra salt than older ones. This observation has two important consequences. Once hypertension had been initiated, it became self-perpetuating even though the salt content of the diet was lowered. Secondly, when hypertension is initiated by raising the salt content of the diet in rats of different ages, the life expectancy of young rats is reduced considerably more than that of older rats.

The finding of fatty arterioles in hypertensive rats provides a partial explanation of their high blood pressure. Finally, the ameliorating effect of potassium chloride in diets high in sodium chloride suggests that other dietary factors besides salt may play a role in the degree of hypertension that develops, and thus on longevity.

Risk Factors for Human Hypertension

The epidemiological approach to the control and prevention of chronic human diseases includes the identification of risk factors for each disease. Risk factors are defined as habits, lifestyle practices, hereditary susceptibility, dietary insufficiencies and excesses, and the possible effects of stress on the statistical probability of a person's acquiring the disease. In practice, a list of all possible risk factors is compiled, epidemiological data on each is collected, and those with significant correlations to the disease are studied further. The risk factor concept includes investigating possible mechanisms between an acknowledged risk factor and physiological factors that are known to be active in the disease process. Risk factors for human hypertension are of two types: alterable and nonalterable. Although they can be separated for the sake of discussion, there are interactions among the risk factors of both the alterable and nonalterable types (see Table 9.1).

Analysis of the risk factors for hypertension is not just complicated by its being a multifactorial disease; hypertension is more accurately described as an interdependent multifactorial disease. For example, the black box that we call hereditary susceptibility interacts with salt consumption, age, obesity, and stress.

Table 9.1 Risk Factors for Hypertension

Nonalterable Risk Factors	Alterable Risk Factors
Hereditary, family	Diet
Heredity, ethnic group	Weight
Age	Aerobic fitness
Sex	Alcohol
	Stress management

Nonalterable Risk Factors

The idea of risk factors evolved during the early years (1949) of the classical Framingham study of the epidemiology of heart disease. In the course of that work, which will be described in some detail in the next chapter, risk factors were correlated with the subsequent incidence of coronary heart disease in the community. Risk factors are useful in predicting how many people in a given population will develop symptoms or die from a particular disease within a certain time period. For example, the Framingham study found that men with hypertension between the ages of 30 and 49 were at twice the risk of developing coronary heart disease in the following 20 years. This information is important for both physicians and the public to know, but it is subject to a serious limitation.

Heredity—A Unique Type of Risk Factor. The limitation is that the predictions based on risk factors do not apply to individuals. The reason for this important qualification is that the probabilities of developing heart disease or hypertension are based on the average person in the study, and no individual is average in all respects. Thus a person's hereditary susceptibility or resistance to the disease is averaged out in the usual epidemiological studies. The advantage of neglecting heredity is that it allows the effects of personal risk factors such as age, smoking habits, and overweight to be calculated in the predictions of the incidence of the disease in a population.

But most people are more interested in what affects their own chances of avoiding a disease than in the probabilities as an impersonal statistic. My impression is that many people are playing the odds. They are taking a calculated risk that they can enjoy their cigarettes or their thick steaks and not be subject to unpleasant medical consequences. They may or may not know the odds as an impersonal statistic. They certainly don't know the odds as applied to themselves as individuals. The odds vary widely from person to person. If, however, a physician could say to a beefy man with hypertension, ''You have a 90% chance of having a stroke or heart attack in the next 5 years because both your parents had hypertension and died in their sixties," instead of "You have double the chances of having a heart attack in the next 20 years compared to all men of your age with hypertension," I expect the impact would be far greater, and the person would shape up far more conscientiously.

To obtain the data that will permit a physician to make a statement on an individual's probabilities is well worth the effort. It would require research into family history, causes of death, or, if parents are still living, their chronic diseases or lack of them. Obtaining information on a person's heredity can provide a unique view into that person's resistance or susceptibility to a number of chronic diseases. It also possesses the strong advantage of identifying susceptible individuals, often before they develop symptoms of hypertension or heart disease.

Another unique feature of heredity as a risk factor is that it cuts across, or influences, all the others. The close relationship between hereditary susceptibility to salt in the diet and hypertension is quite well known. Less well known is the hereditary relationship between short psychic stress and rise in blood pressure. I suspect that there are many other hereditary relationships that investigators will discover. At the present stage of knowledge, our genes, our susceptibility or resistance to a wide variety of conditions and diseases, are encased as in a black box. Through research at many centers, thin beams of light are beginning to dispel the blackness.

Genetic research in rats has recently demonstrated that the gene that is partly responsible for salt-induced hypertension codes for the synthesis of a hormone that is known to be involved in human hypertension (Rapp, 1983). Other evidence that there is a strong genetic component in human hypertension comes from research on twins. The blood pressure of identical twins remains close in the same environment whereas that of nonidentical twins may vary widely under the same conditions.

Research in molecular genetics is utilizing genes made in the laboratory as probes to identify and isolate defective genes in a person's cells. With this approach scientists will be able to predict some time in the future those people who will develop hypertension on a moderately high-salt diet. Still further down the road, it may be possible to replace a defective gene with an effective one. When this possibility becomes routine, commonplace, and cheap, it will usher in a new age in the prevention of diseases.

Age. Heredity, gender, and age are nonalterable risk factors, but age is different from the other two in that it changes continuously. In some cultures blood pressure does not increase with age. Even in the U.S. many elderly people do not exhibit hypertension. These exceptions indicate that aging per se is not a risk factor. Rather, aging allows the effects or risk factors that affect the physiological functioning of the circulatory system to express themselves over time. This view helps explain why blood pressure keeps increasing with age in many people. The longer a risk factor such as overweight is allowed to act, the more pronounced is its effect. We are fortunate that, by controlling a risk factor such as overweight, many people are able to stop the increase, or even decrease their high blood pressure.

Hypertension in some people begins at a relatively young age—during their 20s and 30s. According to Kaplan (1980) it is characterized by increases in both diastolic and systolic pressures. This increase is thought to be due to a thickening of the smaller vessels (arterioles) that retards the flow of blood. In midlife an interesting change occurs: The diastolic pressure levels off in many people, whereas the systolic keeps on increasing throughout life. The systolic increase is interpreted as due to hardening of the large arteries (*arteriosclerosis*, which will be discussed in chapter 10). In this interpretation, hardening of the arteries is a causative factor in systolic hypertension and is the reason that hypertension is an important risk factor for heart disease in the elderly.

Gender.   Studies of excess mortality in the U.S. among both men and women have shown that the higher the blood pressure, either diastolic or systolic, the greater the chance of dying (Kaplan, 1980). Significant increased mortality starts at systolic pressures in the range 138–147 mm, and diastolic pressures of 88–92 mm. In males with systolic pressures of 158–167 mm and diastolic pressures of 98–102 mm, there was a doubling of the death rate compared to those in the normal range. According to the Pooling Project Research Group's (1978) surveys and calculations, there are at least 20 million people in the U.S. with mild hypertension. Without therapy, the excess mortality of both sexes over the range 88–102 mm diastolic blood pressure adds up to 4 million men and 3.2 million women over a 20-year period.

Alterable Risk Factors

Although salt consumption has received the most publicity as a risk factor for high blood pressure, survey data demonstrate that overweight/obesity affects more people. For this reason, I will discuss it first.

Obesity.   The effects of obesity as a risk factor for hypertension start at an early age. Higgins, Keller, Metzner, Moore, and Ostrander (1980) measured the blood pressure of over 2,000 people under age 20, and repeated the measurement 13 years later. They reported that the most significant correlation with the development of hypertension later in life was fatness. The correlation was higher in women than in men and became higher with increasing age. Here we have another example of the importance of weight control in adolescents and young adults. In the nationwide community hypertension evaluation clinic screening program of over a million Americans, Stamler, Stamler, Riedlinger, Algera, and Roberts

(1978) found that overweight people had incidence rates of hypertension 50% to 300% higher than others. The incidence in the overweight was relatively higher in the 20–39 age group than in the 40–64 age group.

In another study, Stamler et al. (1980) measured the effects on blood pressure of moderate weight loss achieved by improvement in eating and exercise habits in middle-aged men with mild hypertension (diastolic pressure, 90 mm). There was a significant correlation between change in weight loss and decrease in blood pressure. It appears that, for many people, weight reduction alone is sufficient for decreasing blood pressure.

Sodium Chloride (Salt) Consumption. In reading the popular literature on hypertension, I frequently get the impression that an author is saying that if we all cut down on salt the problem will go away. The solution to hypertension is not that simple. In chapter 6, I presented Mertz's curve (Figure 6.3), which showed the relationship between toxic consumption of an essential nutrient and the range of optimum consumption. The numbers are known for salt consumption in many human societies and some of these are presented in Figure 9.1. It is tempting to conclude from the straight line between the Eskimos, with the lowest daily intake, and the Northern Japanese, with the highest, that salt consumption is the major, if not the sole, factor contributing to hypertension. Consumption ranges from about 5 g p er day for Eskimos to about 27 g per day for Northern Japanese. As I've mentioned in chapter 3, ecological data show average intakes of whole populations. There are so many uncontrolled variables in data of this type that it is suitable only for providing suggestions for further research. How do these figures compare to the requirements for sodium and chlorine and the RDAs for these elements?

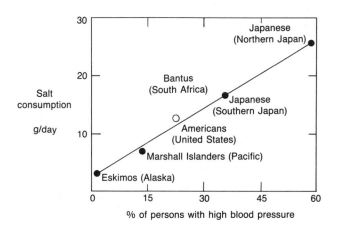

Figure 9.1 Relation between salt consumption and prevalence of hypertension in six societies. *Note.* From "Salt and Hypertension" by C.K. Dahl, 1972, *American Journal of Clinical Nutrition,* **25,** p. 237. Copyright 1972 by *American Journal of Clinical Nutrition.* Reprinted by permission.

The Sodium Chloride Requirements of Humans. Sodium chloride (common table salt), as the name suggests, is composed of the two elements sodium (40%) and chlorine (60%). Both sodium and chlorine are essential elements; there is no question that we need some of both in our diets. The actual physiological requirement for salt is only about 550 mg per day. Persons who add no salt whatever to their food would still be consuming adequate amounts of these essential elements. Estimation of the RDA for adults for each element gives 1.1–3.3 g per day for sodium and 1.7–5.1 g per day for chlorine. These figures calculate to an RDA for sodium chloride of 3.8 g per day.

The Sources of Salt in the U.S. Diet. Most of us have friends who add salt to their food before they even taste it, or we observe people in restaurants who salt their food as though there were an imminent shortage. In actuality, however, the major source of salt in foods is not added by people at the table but is present in processed foods. Approximately two-thirds of the salt that Americans consume is present in processed foods as an additive. Table 9.2 lists the sodium content of some popular foods and meals.

Table 9.2   Sodium Content of Selected Food Types

Item	Serving	Na$^+$ Content* (mg)
Beverages		
Beer (4.5%)	12 oz	18
Wine	3.5 oz	< 10
Coffee (brewed)	6 oz	2
Cafe Vienna	6 oz	94
Instant mocha	6 oz	48
Tea (brewed)	8 oz	19
Soft drinks	12 oz	30-80
Gatorade	8 oz	123
Tang (orange)	3 tsp in 6 oz H$_2$O	1
Candy	1-2 oz	25-100
Hershey's milk chocolate	1 oz	26
Processed Cereals		
All Bran	1 oz (1/3 cup)	320
Cheerios	1 oz (1-1/4 cup)	307
Corn Flakes (Kellogg's)	1 oz (1-1/4 cup)	351
Grape-nuts	1 oz (1/4 cup)	197
Product 19	1 oz (3/4 cup)	325
Quaker 100% Natural	1 oz (1/4 cup)	12
Raisin Bran (Kellogg's)	1.3 oz (3/4 cup)	269
Special K	1 oz (1-1/3 cup)	265

(Cont.)

Table 9.2 (Cont.)

Item	Serving	Na$^+$ Content* (mg)
Shredded Wheat 'n Bran (Nabisco)	1 oz (1-1/3 cup)	0
Wheaties	1 oz (1 cup)	354
Wheat germ (toasted)	1 oz (1/4 cup)	1
Snack food		
Cheetos cheese puffs	1 oz	368
Lay's potato chips	1 oz	207
Rold Gold pretzel sticks	1 oz	875
Doritos tortilla chips	1 oz	180
Prepared meals		
Beans & beef in tomato sauce, Campbell's	8 oz	1150
Oriental beef, Stouffer's	9-1/8 oz	1175
Vegetable beef stew, Stouffer's	10 oz	1675
Beef stroganoff w/noodles, Stouffer's	9-3/4 oz	1300
Cannelloni, beef w/tomato sauce, Mrs. Smith's	8-1/4 oz	1660
Chicken a la King, Campbell's	8 oz	897
Chicken & dumplings, Banquet	8 oz	1298
Chicken pie, Stouffer's	10 oz	1530
Chile con carne w/beans, Stouffer's	8-3/4 oz	1265
Chop suey, beef w/rice, Stouffer's	12 oz	2040
Chop suey, beef, Banquet	8 oz	1334
Enchiladas, beef, Van de Kamps	4 enchiladas	1481
Beans & franks, Banquet	10-3/4 oz	2153
Chicken dinner, Banquet	17 oz	3562
Meatloaf dinner, Banquet	19 oz	3649
Mexican dinner, Swanson	18 oz	1938
Veal parmagian, Banquet	11 oz	2527
Macaroni & cheese, Green Giant	8 oz	1163
Sausage pizza, Stouffer's	6 oz	1320
Ravioli, beef in sauce, Campbell's	1 ravioli (1 oz)	80
Fried rice w/chicken, LaChoy	4 oz	1153
Spaghetti w/meat sauce, Stouffer's	14 oz	1970
Spaghetti w/meatballs, Banquet	8 oz	1334
Sweet & sour pork, LaChoy	8 oz (1 cup)	1693
Turkey w/gravy & dressing, Swanson	9-1/4 oz	1396
Turkey pie, Banquet	8 oz	1017

Note. Data from *Food Values of Portions Commonly Used* (pp. 21-33) by J.A. Pennington and H.N. Church, 1985, Philadelphia: J.B. Lippincott. Copyright 1985 by J.B. Lippincott. Adapted by permission.

*Multiply the sodium (Na$^+$) content by 2.4 to obtain the salt (sodium chloride, NaCL) content.

Table 9.3   Sodium Content of Some Processed Foods

Food	Serving	Sodium
Green Giant green beans (frozen)	1/2 cup	255 mg
Ritz crackers	1 oz	200 mg
Spam	3 oz	1025 mg
Campbell's cream of mushroom soup	1/2 cup	550 mg
Swanson lasagna (frozen)	1 serving	855 mg
Planters cocktail peanuts	1 serving	117 mg
Pepperidge Farm white bread	1 serving	117 mg
Lay's potato chips	1 serving	191 mg
Jell-O instant pudding and pie filling	1 serving	404 mg
Heinz dill pickles	1 serving	1137 mg
Campbell's tomato juice	1 serving	292 mg
Oscar Mayer bacon	1 serving	302 mg
Herb-Ox instant beef broth	1 serving	349 mg
Wish Bone Italian dressing	1 serving	315 mg
Stouffer's chicken breasts (frozen)	1 serving	715 mg
Kraft American Singles	1 serving	238 mg
Bumble Bee chunk white tuna	1 serving	628 mg
Country Pride homogenized milk	1 serving	130 mg
Chef Boyardee beefaroni	1 serving	1186 mg
Oscar Mayer bologna	1 serving	672 mg
Beef	1 serving	381 mg
Heinz tomato ketchup	1 serving	154 mg
Skippy creamy peanut butter	1 serving	167 mg
Campbell's beans and franks, canned	1 serving	1050 mg
Swanson TV dinner	1 serving	1152 mg

Note. From *Food Values of Portions Commonly Used* by J.A. Pennington and H.N. Church, 1985, Philadelphia: J.B. Lippincott. Copyright 1985 by J.B. Lippincott. Adapted by permission.

Most people have no idea of the salt content of processed foods. Most commercial cakes and pies contain large quantities of salt. It is probably reasonable to assume that most processed foods will be high in salt unless labeled otherwise. Table 9.3 lists the salt content of a number of well-known processed foods.

The major sources of salt in home-cooked foods are grain products, dairy products, and mixed protein dishes. A list of high-salt foods includes anchovies, bacon, caviar, processed cheese, canned fish, french fries, frankfurters, ham, herring, smoked or salted meats, salted nuts, olives, pickles, potato chips, pretzels, and sausage.

A number of low-salt cookbooks are now available in bookstores, and some progressive restaurants are now featuring low-salt dishes. As I have said before, if food entrepreneurs realize that there is a demand for low-salt products, they will be supplied. Consumer Reports (1984) lists some low-salt foods:

- B & G Bread and Butter Pickles,
- Delmonte Whole Kernel Corn,
- Fleischman's Margarine,
- Planter's Dry-Roasted Peanuts,
- DelMonte Tomato Sauce,
- Peter Pan Creamy Peanut Butter,
- Campbell's Chicken with Noodles,
- Campbell's Chunky Vegetable Beef Soup,
- Chicken of the Sea Chunk Light Tuna,
- Borden Lite-Line American Processed Cheese, and
- Herb-Ox Chicken Flavor Broth and Seasoning.

Prices of low-salt foods may be higher than the standard versions.

Baby foods have until recently been salted to suit the tastes of parents, not babies. The amounts present were even more excessive for the child than is found in most adult foods. An FDA directive makes it now possible for parents to purchase low-salt baby foods. It is believed that the taste for salt is not inborn but is acquired. By adolescence it is firmly established. Don't penalize a baby by feeding it a high-salt diet! Although unproven, it is thought that excessive intake of salt starting from an early age may later help induce hypertension in many people.

In addition to hypertension, other pathological conditions in which excessive salt intake is suspected are swelling of the extremities, especially the legs; headaches due to edema (swelling) of the tissues in the head; congestive heart failure; and premenstrual tension (bloating and irritability). For those people who may wish to cut down on salting their food at table, the substitutes listed in Table 9.4 may be helpful.

It is unfortunate for consumers that most food labels do not list the actual amounts of salt that the product contains. The present practice of listing ingredients in order of concentration is of little value to people trying to control their salt intake. Who could guess that a serving of Wheaties contains 365 mg of sodium and one of Nutrigrain contains 255 mg, unless the values are listed on the containers?

Not All Sodium Salts Induce Hypertension. For the past 30 years or so the scientific dogma has considered the sodium ion (Na^+) as the causative agent in high-salt hypertension. Kurtz and Morris (1983) have recently questioned this conclusion. They point out that practically all the research on salt has been carried out with sodium chloride. A few preliminary communications have reported, both in patients and in salt-sensitive rats, that oral feeding of sodium bicarbonate induced a lesser increase in blood pressure than that induced by equivalent amounts of sodium chloride. Still,

Table 9.4 Salt Substitutes

Meat, Fish, and Poultry

Beef	Bay leaf, dry mustard powder, green pepper, marjoram, fresh mushrooms, nutmeg, onion, pepper, sage, thyme
Chicken	Green pepper, lemon juice, marjoram, fresh mushrooms, paprika, parsley, poultry seasoning, sage, thyme
Fish	Bay leaf, curry powder, dry mustard powder, green pepper, lemon juice, marjoram, fresh mushrooms, paprika
Lamb	Curry powder, garlic, mint, mint jelly, pineapple, rosemary
Pork	Apple, applesauce, garlic, onion, sage
Veal	Apricot, bay leaf, curry powder, ginger, marjoram, oregano

Vegetables

Asparagus	Garlic, lemon juice, onion, vinegar
Corn	Green pepper, pimiento, fresh tomato
Cucumbers	Chives, dill, garlic, vinegar
Green beans	Dill, lemon juice, marjoram, nutmeg, pimiento
Greens	Onion, pepper, vinegar
Peas	Green pepper, mint, fresh mushrooms, onion, parsley
Potatoes	Green pepper, mace, onion, paprika, parsley
Rice	Chives, green pepper, onion, pimiento, saffron
Squash	Brown sugar, cinnamon, ginger, mace, nutmeg, onion
Tomatoes	Basil, marjoram, onion, oregano

Soups

Bean	Pinch of dry mustard powder
Milk chowders	Peppercorns
Pea	Bay leaf and parsley
Vegetable	Vinegar, dash of sugar

Salads

Oil and vinegar plus spices to taste

Low-salt commercial salad dressings

Note. From *Cooking Without Your Salt Shaker* (pp. 12-13) by the American Heart Association, 1978, Cleveland, OH: Author. Copyright 1978 by the American Heart Association, N.E. Ohio Affiliate. Reprinted by permission.

the *assumption* has been made that the chloride ion (Cl^-) is inert—that *all the hypertensive effects are due to sodium ion.*

Kurtz and Morris checked this assumption by feeding rats other sodium salts than chloride. They found that hypertension could be induced with high intakes of sodium as sodium chloride but not with equivalent amounts of sodium bicarbonate (common baking soda), sodium ascorbate (the salt of ascorbic acid, Vitamin C), or a combination of the two. The difference in blood pressure could not be attributed to differences in potassium, weight gain, or caloric intake. It is interesting that the rats given sodium chloride excreted more calcium in their urine than those given sodium bicarbonate. Similar results have been reported by Whitescarver, Guthrie, and Katchen (1984).

These results contradict the present opinion that sodium ion in any form should be restricted in the diet. Apparently sodium-containing food auxiliaries like monosodium glutamate, a widely used flavor accelerator (Accent), and sodium ascorbate, for heavy users of vitamin C who may use it to obtain a nonacid urine, are not hypertensinogenic. The work also suggests that food processors experiment with other sodium-containing flavoring agents than sodium chloride.

In concluding this discussion of salt as risk factor for hypertension, it appears that many, but not all, people are affected by a high-salt diet. Personal experiments can be valuable in a situation like this one. There are two types of experiments that I suggest, although there are probably others just as useful. Suppose that you are in the age range 28–33, are not overweight, are fairly active, but your diastolic blood pressure is in the high normal range (84–88 mm). You may have no idea of your salt consumption but would like to reduce your diastolic pressure to 80 mm or below. If you have control of your diet (i.e., eat home-cooked meals most of the time), you may make a conscious effort to markedly decrease your salt intake for a few weeks. Have your blood pressure taken at weekly intervals starting at the beginning of the low-salt diet and see if it changes. A low-salt diet can be very tasty and appetizing if some of the salt substitutes in Table 9.4 are used.

The second experiment may be easier to carry out. It involves eating a high-salt diet. Consciously eat more salty foods than usual (like those listed in Tables 9.2 and 9.3). Again, have your blood pressure checked at weekly intervals. If your pressure remains constant, you may be one of those who doesn't have to watch their salt intake, and your high-normal blood pressure may to due to other factors.

As a cautionary measure, parents with hypertension, or those descended from families in which hypertension has frequently occurred, should have the blood pressure of their children checked annually from the age of 3.

Alcohol Consumption. Klatsky, Friedman, Siegelaub, and Gerard (1979) studied blood pressure in relation to alcohol consumption in 84,000 people of both sexes and three races. There was no difference between nondrinkers and those who drank two or fewer drinks a day. Men and women who imbibed more than three drinks a day had higher systolic and diastolic blood pressures ($p < 10^{-6}$ to $p < 10^{-24}$). This group also showed higher incidence of pressures of over 160/95. The association of blood pressure and drinking were independent of age, sex, race, smoking, coffee use, former heavy drinking, educational attainment, and obesity. The authors concluded that "the findings strongly suggest that regular use of three or more drinks of alcohol per day is a risk factor for hypertension" (p. 1194).

Additional Suggested Dietary Risk Factors for Hypertension

In addition to the four risk factors discussed above, researchers are busy investigating a number of others. McCarron, Morris, and Cole (1982) have suggested that hypertension may result from a dietary calcium deficiency. The conclusions were based on a small sample of people, and the results need independent confirmation on a much larger number of subjects before calcium deficiency can be accepted as a legitimate risk factor. In the meantime, people can assure themselves of adequate calcium intake by consuming plenty of low-fat dairy foods.

A recent symposium on calcium and hypertension, chaired by Drs. Draper and Robison (1986), demonstrated the complexity of the subject. In general, the symposium revealed that calcium may be inversely similar to sodium in that there may be a population of hypertensives whose hypertension can be controlled by an increase in dietary calcium.

Low-Potassium Levels.   Although low-potassium intake has not received as much publicity as low calcium, the case for low potassium as a risk factor is considerably stronger. Meneely reviewed (1973) six reports confirming the effects of low-potassium intake resulting in hypertension in both rats and humans. As mentioned previously, the incidence of hypertension in Northern Japan is one of the highest in the world. This condition has been related to their high-salt intake. Sasaki (1962) noticed that one village in that area had a much lower rate of hypertension than another. He found that the salt intake was similar, but the people in the village with the lower amount of hypertension ingested more potassium.

Iacono and Dougherty (1983) have noticed a correlation between polyunsaturated fats (PUFA) in the diet and hypertension. In two small incompletely controlled studies, one in the U.S. and another in Finland, they reported a decrease in blood pressure after increasing the ratio of PUFA to saturated fats in the diet.

Bulpitt (1982) cautions against overemphasis of any one dietary factor as a risk factor, as total calories, carbohydrate, total fat, sodium, and potassium intakes are all interrelated. There are no published long-term studies in which all of these variables have been measured.

Stressors.   Sometime ago I was having my blood pressure checked by a nurse whom I know and who had taken it many times previously. While adjusting the cuff and getting ready to take the measurement, she mentioned a sensitive social question that she knew I was interested in, and we discussed it for a minute or so. To the surprise of both of us, my pressure was 140/95 mm Hg, the highest it had ever been. I had not been aware that the discussion had excited or depressed me in any way. She said, "Oh dear, I shouldn't have brought up this topic. I'll go away for a few minutes and retake it without saying a word." She did, and the reading was now my average of 126/82. This incident illustrates that a person may be affected by psychic stressors without being aware of it.

Sharp, temporary increases in blood pressure, as happened to me, are well-known phenomena. These responses are under the control of the sympathetic nervous system and the secretion of the catecholamine hormones. It is part of the fight-or-flight response first emphasized by Cannon many years ago. Because fight-or-flight behaviors are inappropriate in present society, the question is raised, Do these responses, which are not followed by the evolutionary-developed primitive behavior of fight or flight, in time lead to more less permanent hypertension? Present knowledge does not allow a yes or no answer to this question, but some interesting insights are available. Falkner (1981) administered mental arithmetic tests to adolescents from hypertensive families and normotensive families. Those from families with a predisposition to hypertension showed higher heart rates and higher and more prolonged increases in blood pressure than the normotensive controls. In this study, about 75% of the youngsters with a family history of hypertension displayed signs of a hyper-responsiveness to the psychic stimulus. Falkner (1981) followed up this interesting study with one of salt loading on similar subjects. Those with a family history of hypertension also showed a hyper-response to this stressor.

Light, Koepke, Obrist, and Willis (1983) went a step further by using young (aged 18–22) male students as subjects. They were divided into a high-risk group, those with borderline systolic hypertension or a parental history of hypertension, and a low-risk group, who had neither borderline hypertension nor a parental history of the disease. A control group, composed of both high-risk and low-risk subjects sat and read for 5 hours. All subjects drank 1 l of water during the first hour and 0.2 l every 30 minutes for the next 4 hours. The urine volume was measured, and its content of sodium was determined. During the fourth hour, the experimental subjects engaged in competitive games for small stakes. Degree of stress was estimated by continuous monitoring of heart rate and frequent blood pressure readings. The high-risk subjects differed from the low-risk subjects during the games in two significant responses: Their heart rates increased considerably more, and their sodium excretion decreased, whereas sodium excretion did not change in the low-risk subjects. All but one subject who showed a large sodium retention had a hypertensive parent. This result strongly suggests that repeated stressors on susceptible subjects can result in chronic hypertension.

This research demonstrates clearly the effect of psychic stress on kidney function in high-risk human subjects. The relation between increased heart rate and decreased sodium excretion suggests that the sympathetic nervous system mediated both. The increased understanding of the mechanism of the two responses will aid in developing better therapies for high blood pressure than are now available. This conclusion has already been demonstrated in dogs. Thus the interconnected relations among heredity, salt retention, stressors, and high blood pressure are becoming clearer.

Effects of Exercise on Blood Pressure

Some of the connections between exercise and weight control were discussed in the previous chapter. The increased susceptibility of overweight people to a number of diseases, including hypertension, is now widely recognized. Insofar as aerobic exercise aids in weight reduction, it might also be expected to aid in reducing hypertension; and so it does, as shown below. In contrast, heavy weight exercise tends to increase blood pressure.

Endurance (Aerobic) Exercise
Decreases Hypertension in Many People

Hagberg et al. (1983) placed a group of hypertensive sedentary adolescents in an aerobic exercise program for 6 months. Both systolic and diastolic blood pressure decreased significantly with training. In a larger study, Cade et al. (1984) enrolled 105 patients with established diastolic hypertension in an aerobic exercise program of running 2 miles a day for 3 months. In 58 patients who were not taking medication before the exercise program, mean blood pressure decreased by 15 mm Hg. Of 47 patients on medication, 24 were able to discontinue it. In the group still taking medication, mean blood pressure decreased from 120.9 ± 28.8 mm Hg to 104.4 ± 17.9 mm Hg.

In a presentation to the American Heart Association (Haglund, 1986), 19 males with an average blood pressure of 135/94 mm Hg were divided into two groups. The first group exercised aerobically for 10 weeks of treadmill/stationary bicycling, in which their heart rates stayed in the 65%-80% target range, for 30 minutes 4 times a week. Their diastolic (but not their systolic) pressure dropped an average of 9.6 mm Hg. None of the nine placebo exercisers, who did stretching and light calisthenics 4 times a week, lowered their blood pressures significantly.

Strength-Type (Anaerobic) Exercise Increases Hypertension

Ewing, Irving, Kerr, and Kirby (1973) studied the effects of the static isometric exercise of pressing a handgrip at 30% of maximum in 15 adult, untreated, hypertensive patients. Arterial blood pressures increased significantly in all subjects. In a similar experiment, Lind and McNicol (1967) measured an average increase of 45 mm Hg systolic and 40 mm Hg diastolic when their subjects pressed a handgrip at 50% maximum. These experiments clearly demonstrate that hypertensive or cardiac rehabilitation patients should not engage in isometric exercises.

Factors Involved in the Higher Prevalence of Hypertension in U.S. Blacks

The National Heart, Lung, and Blood Institute of the National Institutes of Health (U.S.) subsidized a 5-year Hypertension Detection and Follow-Up Program whose objective was to study the effectiveness of anti-hypertension therapy in reducing mortality on over 150,000 hypertensive people. At the beginning of the program, before any therapy was commenced (Daugherty, 1983), 43% of the black male subjects (30–69 years) had diastolic blood pressures over 90 mm Hg as did 25% of the white male subjects. Beyond the actual percentages, other differences in hypertension between blacks and whites have been observed. Young blacks tend to go from a normotensive condition to a hypertensive one in just a few years. Whites became hypertensive more slowly.

Another significant difference between the two groups lies in the severity of hypertension. About 75% of white subjects had mild hypertension with a diastolic pressure of less than 105 mm Hg, whereas only 57% of the black patients had mild hypertension. U.S. black people are almost twice as likely to have severe hypertension as whites. Are these large differences due to hereditary influence? Or are other factors involved? In the process of evaluating risk factors, we will see how they interact and make a shambles of simple, monofactorial answers.

Many years ago, Donnison (1929) reported on the blood pressure of 1,000 black men in Kenya. He found that the mean pressures were similar to those of whites in Europe and the U.S. A recent study of the blood pressures of blacks on three Caribbean Islands found a relatively low prevalence of hypertension. The population on St. Kitts, which had the highest average of the three, still showed a lower incidence of high blood pressure than has been found in U.S. blacks (Khaw & Rose, 1982). Thus it does not appear that the higher prevalence of hypertension found in U.S. blacks has a hereditary basis. The data suggest that environmental factors are probably responsible. It seems likely that the impact of a particular risk factor on a specific population will be dependent on the presence or absence of other risk factors.

Diet may influence the greater susceptibility of U.S. blacks to hypertension. The sodium and potassium contents of diets of blacks and whites were estimated by urine analysis in Evans County, Georgia, in 1961 and again in 1968 (Grim et al., 1980). The data suggest that the sodium content of the diets of blacks and whites were similar, but that the potassium content of the black's diet was significantly less than the white's. Langford and Watson (1975) measured the sodium and potassium intake of over 600 black high school girls in Mississippi. The ones with hypertension had a higher ratio of sodium to potassium in their urine. These results suggest that the higher prevalence of hypertension in blacks compared to whites may be due to differences in potassium consumption. As mentioned above, low dietary potassium has been suggested as a risk factor for hypertension. It is possible, however, that blacks are more susceptible to the hypertensionogenic effects of sodium than whites (Weinberger et al., 1982).

Lactose Intolerance May Lead to a Calcium Deficiency

Dr. Bayless (1976) of Johns Hopkins University estimated that more than 30 million U.S. Americans may have a hereditary lactose intolerance due to the lack of the enzyme lactase. This group is mostly made up of blacks, those with a southern European or Mideastern background, and Asians. Most of these people do not tolerate milk or ice cream well because these foods contain appreciable amounts of lactose. These same products are also the chief sources of calcium in many people's diets. Fortunately, the organisms in yogurt contain a lactase enzyme. Kolars, Levitt, Aougi, and Savaiano (1984) reported that autodigestion of lactose makes yogurt a well-tolerated dairy product for lactase-deficient persons. Thus it is possible that, if calcium lack contributes to hypertension, people with lactose intolerance can supplement their diets with yogurt rather than taking a calcium supplement in pill form.

Stress as a Hypertension Risk Factor

It was reported at a recent symposium that black populations in Africa and on Caribbean Islands have a similar range of blood pressures to U.S. whites. Fewer black farmers and fishermen who live in villages had hypertension compared to those who live in cities. Most U.S. blacks are city dwellers at present. Dr. Watkins (1984) suggested that the urban and rural differences may be due to the stress of daily living. Dr. Gerald Thompson, Chief of Medicine at Harlem Hospital, New York, commented that socioeconomic factors may be involved in these differences between blacks and whites in prevalence and in severity of hypertension. He believes that blacks living in the U.S. are under greater stress than whites.

In this connection, Harburg, Schull, Erfurt, and Schork (1970) studied two groups of black people in Detroit. The investigators found a relationship between annual income and number and severity of social and personal stressors. People living in the lower income area were exposed to considerably more environmental stressors than those in the higher income area. Thirty-one percent of the residents in the high-stress area had hypertension (defined as 160+ mm mercury systolic and/or 95+ mm diastolic) compared to 18% in the low-stress area ($p < .04$). There was no significant difference in mean weight or age between the two groups. No other hypertension risk factors were measured.

The complexity of blood pressure control is made very clear by these studies of U.S. blacks and whites. The data show the interplay among the factors of heredity, salt content of the diet, potassium content of the diet, socioeconomic status, and stress. Some of the other risk factors mentioned above may also be involved in the greater incidence of hypertension in U.S. blacks.

Other Nonmedical, Antihypertensive Therapies

The list of risk factors mentioned in the pages above implies that a hypertensive person might be able to control the condition by changing diet, controlling stress, exercising more, and losing weight. In addition, still other therapies for controlling hypertension have been suggested.

Wallace, Silver, Mills, Dillbeck, and Wagoner (1983) measured the systolic blood pressure of 112 subjects, 35–64 years, who practiced Transcendental Meditation, and compared them to a matched group that did not practice this form of meditation. The blood pressure of the transcendental meditators was significantly less than the controls. The difference was independent of diet and exercise patterns but was related to the length of time the person had meditated. Those who had meditated over 5 years had significantly lower blood pressures than those who had meditated less than 5 years.

Biofeedback and relaxation was studied by Engel, Glasgow, and Gaarder (1983) as a means of reducing systolic blood pressure. Patients who received the behavioral treatments achieved and maintained reductions in blood pressure for at least 18 months. Patients who had been receiving diuretic therapy were able to maintain reduced pressure for at least 9 months after discontinuing medication.

In 1981 the First International Conference on the Human/Companion Animal Bond was hosted at the University of Pennsylvania. Dr. Aaron Katcher, the conference chairman, is known for his observation that people's blood pressure decreases when they pet their dogs. In contrast, blood pressure usually goes up when people talk to one another. Blood pressure even decreases when a person watches a tank of tropical fish (Helyar, 1981).

A Step-By-Step Nonmedical Program for Reducing High Blood Pressure

Suppose a person, age 35, has mild hypertension (140/90) but wants to avoid taking medication for it. Let us suppose further that the person is chubby, does not exercise regularly, smokes, drinks alcoholic beverages daily, and consumes a typical American diet, which contains 40% fat calories and moderate amounts of salt. As you may realize, all of these have been mentioned as risk factors or possible risk factors for hypertension. Are some more important than others? What course of action is feasible?

Harlan et al. (1984) have analyzed the data on hypertension from the National Health and Nutrition Examination Survey (NHANES-1), which examined a representative sample of over 20,000 U.S. people aged 1–74. Correlations with increasing blood pressure were made in decreasing order with age, body mass index (BMI), and pulse rate for both men and women, and blacks and whites. The identification of these three variables as major risk factors suggests a number of tactics for reducing blood pressure.

The correlation coefficient between age and hypertension is the largest of any. The reason for age ranking as the number one is that it includes all the legitimate risk factors like overweight, lack of fitness, years of smoking, and so forth, whose effect on blood pressure increases with age. In those cultures where blood pressure does not increase with age, we also find that overweight does not increase with age either. In this sense, age represents the summation of all the lifestyle habits that contribute to hypertension.

Thus the first objective for an overweight person with mild hypertension at any age is weight control. Because a high pulse rate suggests lack of fitness, the second objective might be to commence an aerobic exercise program. Such a program will not only help to control both of these variables and save people from a stroke or cardiovascular event later in life, but it will also add to their enjoyment of living within a short time.

Although this survey did not find a correlation between high blood pressure and salt consumption, many others have. Kaplan (1980) suggests a moderate reduction in salt intake to about 5 g/day. This reduction can be readily accomplished by not adding salt to food at table, omitting heavily salted foods like pickles and pickled meats and vegetables from your diet, and not consuming processed foods that contain much added salt.

A handy booklet that contains information on the caloric and sodium content of over 6,000 foods is titled *The Barbara Kraus Sodium Guide to Brand Names and Basic Foods* (Kraus, 1984). It contains analyses for sodium of many fresh, canned, and frozen fruits and vegetables. For example, a cup of boiled fresh green peas contains 3 mg of sodium; a cup of canned, 401 mg; and a cup of frozen, 184 mg. Cutting down on salt requires more knowledge than most people have at their fingertips. It takes an effort but it can be done. Fortunately, a number of food processors are marketing low-salt products. If the demand is great enough, their numbers will increase.

Other dietary modifications include additions of low-fat dairy products as calcium sources, and more fresh fruits and vegetables to insure an adequate intake of potassium. If these dietary, weight control, and aerobic exercise modifications have not restored the person to normotension in 6 months, I would further suggest a cumulative program in which other risk factors are controlled as additions to those already mentioned. If you drink more than the equivalent of 3 oz (2 drinks) of 80-proof whiskey a day, cut back on this level. Take the Stress Questionnaire in chapter 4 and, if your score indicates that your stress level is high, begin a program of stress management.

These suggestions may strike you as quite a change in lifestyle for the relatively benign condition of mild hypertension. I can assure you, however, that mild hypertension may gradually change to medium and then to severe, and if left untreated, the effects may lead to many more major changes in lifestyle than I have mentioned. Lund-Johansen (1980) studied subjects with untreated, borderline hypertension for 10 years. He found that, almost without exception, the mild condition had changed into the classic pattern of primary hypertension. The blood pressure of the normotensive control group did not change over this period. Black people should be screened more frequently than white, or they may be suddenly found with extremely high blood pressure and die before therapy has become effective. If what I have written is unconvincing, visit a nursing home and observe the lifestyle of people there who have had strokes. Imagine yourself in that wheelchair as your lifestyle for the terminal years of your life.

For some hypertensive people, none of the nonmedical suggestions listed above may have been effective in controlling their blood pressures. For these people, long-term drug therapy under direction of a physician becomes necessary. Drug therapy for mild hypertension often utilizes diuretics, which may prevent, or at least delay, the onset of more severe hypertension. But even diuretics have undesirable side effects, such as greater excretion of potassium, that may involve some changes in dietary habits. People on diuretic therapy should eat more potassium-rich fruits or take potassium supplements, and have occasional monitoring of potassium levels in the blood. If drug therapy can be avoided by the dietary, exercise, and stress control regimens outlined above, it is worth it.

Therapy for Hypertension:
A Lifelong Commitment

As mentioned above, untreated hypertension may gradually increase, and as the years go on serious symptoms may appear. The coronary arteries become damaged and the plaques occupy more and more area. This effect is the basis for hypertension's being a major risk factor for heart attacks. If the affected arteries are in the brain, a stroke often results. If the arteries are in the kidneys, they function less effectively and kidney failure may develop.

The reason for the gradual development of one or more of these serious pathological conditions is that the causative factors continue to act on the sensitive tissues, and the extent of the damage progresses inexorably. The therapies I have mentioned are not cures, even though they prevent hypertension from worsening. *This is the reason they must be continued for life.* If therapy is discontinued, the pathological processes are enabled to wreak their damage again. It has been estimated that a man of 35 with mild hypertension who does not receive therapy, possibly because he does not know that he has the condition, will have his life shortened an average of 16 years for this reason alone.

Summary

The syndrome of chronic hypertension has such serious consequences that everyone's blood pressure should be checked a minimum of once a year. Those people in the mild range (125/85-140/95 mm Hg) should be checked more frequently. It is estimated that up to half of hypertensives who are also overweight might regain normotensive status by weight loss alone.

There are a wide number of possible risk factors (dietary, stress, hormonal, and hereditary) that may act singly or in concert as contributors to hypertension. Tests are being developed to identify those people in each group so that therapy can be individualized. In the meantime, a number of drugs have been demonstrated to be effective in the control of hypertension. Untreated high blood pressure becomes progressively greater with time, so it is suggested that hypertensives be identified and therapy commenced as soon as possible.

IF YOU HAVE NEVER HAD YOUR BLOOD PRESSURE MEASURED OR IF IT HAS BEEN LONGER THAN A YEAR SINCE IT WAS LAST MEASURED, DO IT TODAY.

10

Wellness and Your Heart

It is often necessary to make a decision on the basis of knowledge sufficient for action but insufficient to satisfy the intellect.

I. Kant

This chapter will help you

* understand the risk factors for heart disease and how to reduce them;
* calculate the cholesterol content of your diet and its effect on serum cholesterol, and
* realize the role of certain personality characteristics on the incidence of heart attacks.

An electronic technician had his first attack of angina at age 39. In the next 8 years he had three major heart attacks. The last one left him so weak that his family was informed that the end was near. As a last-ditch measure, his physician suggested a heart transplant. At age 47 he was flown to Stanford Medical School where the famed team working with Dr. Norman Shumway replaced his heart. The operation and hospital costs totaled about $75,000. These were paid by his group insurance and by a federal grant to Stanford.

He is one of the lucky ones. Four years later he is well enough to tend a garden, go deer hunting, and take daily walks. He has had to retire from his job and takes about a dozen different pills 6 times a day. The side effects of the medication include fragile bones and susceptibility to many infections from the immuno-suppressant drugs that keep his body from rejecting the transplanted heart. His diet is restricted to lean meat, fruits, and vegetables. Foods high in cholesterol, sugar, and fat are prohibited. He is well pleased with the outcome because he is alive and can play with his grandchildren, whom he would not have known without the transplant. Still, does his restricted lifestyle appeal to you?

Although much of this chapter is concerned with heart disease and how to increase your chances of avoiding it, the program I will outline also has a positive objective—adding to your wellness. The program includes a discussion of personal value systems and their role in the enjoyment of life. Many North American males postpone this type of self-analysis until after they have had a heart attack. Such men can and do achieve considerable wellness, but they are living under a cloud. The fear of death was their basic motivation for changing their lifestyles. I ask the question: Why wait? Analyze your value system now, before a heart attack. Live your life under the blue sky of wellness.

Definition of Coronary Heart Disease (CHD)

There are numerous diseases of the heart of which coronary disease is but one type. Coronary heart disease (CHD) is often defined as any one of three conditions (Kannel, Dawber, Kagan, Revotskie, and Stokes, 1961). The first is *myocardial infarction*, or death of a portion of heart tissue due to a sudden decrease in the blood supply. The connection between this event and the growth of fatty deposits in the artery, called atheromas, will be described shortly. The second is *angina pectoris*, or sharp pains in the chest with a feeling of suffocation and impending death. The pains are of brief duration and are often precipitated by exercise or excitement. Angina pectoris is found more commonly in women than men. An attack is seldom fatal but indicates a serious condition of the heart. The third is *sudden death*, which is often attributed to heart disease when no other cause was evident. Sudden death may result from a massive death of heart tissue, called an infarct, or from other causes. With the increase in coronary intensive care units and speedy, competent ambulance units, the number of deaths from smaller infarcts has decreased in recent years.

The ultimate questions about heart disease might be stated as follows: What are its causes and how might they be avoided by an individual? It may take 50 years, or longer, for scientists to obtain answers to these questions. At the end of World War II, however, medical scientists realized that they could obtain proximate answers to the question by studying the habits of people in different parts of the world using epidemiological procedures.

As I mentioned in chapter 3, epidemiological studies involve large numbers of people. This provision immediately affects what variables can be controlled, and what measurements can be taken. In this usage the word *variable* acquires a special meaning. It doesn't mean something that varies, which is beyond the control of the investigator. It means a factor that varies between two groups. For example, if the incidence of heart disease is being measured in a population, and the disease rate of the men is measured separately from that of the women, then the sex difference is called a variable. Similarly, if smokers are compared to nonsmokers, smoking is considered as a variable. A variable may represent a quantitative difference, as when men who smoke over a pack a day are compared to those who smoke less. To sum up: What variables are measured and how precisely they are measured is determined by the objectives of the research and how much is known about the effects of a particular variable when the study is commenced.

The Search for Risk Factors

A risk factor is usually defined as a personal or cultural habit, a dietary constituent, a hereditary condition or tendency, or any other long-term factor that tends to increase a person's chances for acquiring a disease. Hopkins and Williams (1986) have discussed many possibilities that have been suggested or investigated as risk factors for heart disease. I'll list some of the widely publicized ones here:

- elevated blood concentrations of cholesterol;
- triglycerides;
- glucose;
- low-density lipoproteins;
- uric acid;
- insulin;
- high blood pressure;
- smoking of cigarettes;
- a particular type of abnormal electrocardiogram;
- overweight;
- an elevated pulse rate;
- Type A behavior;
- a variety of stresses;
- a diet high in fat, sucrose, or refined foods;
- a diet low in fiber, vitamin B₆ (pyridoxine), or magnesium; and
- lack of exercise.

It is obviously impossible for all the suggested risk factors to be investigated in any one study. In planning an experiment, the epidemiologists list which ones they will measure, which criteria of heart disease they will use as end points, what population they will be studying, how the subjects will be selected, how long the study will last, what factors they will attempt to keep constant, and so forth. In some respects the situation resembles a murder on a wealthy person's estate with twenty-odd guests present, all of whom are suspects. In a murder mystery the detective sifts the clues from the extraneous facts and observations and suspicions of the suspects and gradually narrows the possibilities to the one who "done it."

A team of epidemiologists is comparable to a detective, but with most chronic diseases, there is more than one murderer (i.e., risk factor); also, there is no assurance that all the risk factors have been identified. In addition, it is possible that two risk factors, each of which is rather weak, may, in combination, become a potent pair. For people who like to solve mysteries, scientific research provides the most intriguing puzzles imaginable.

It was recognized from the outset that epidemiological data would not identify the causes of heart disease. What the scientists were seeking were statistically significant correlations between one or more of the risk factors that were studied and cardiovascular events.

The distinction between risk factor and cause can be readily appreciated by the example of a person jaywalking across a busy street. It is obvious that the risk of getting hit by a vehicle increases with the amount of traffic. Yet, if a person were killed by being hit by a car, we would not say that crossing the street was the cause of the death; being hit by the car might be called the precipitating cause and a broken neck the medical cause.

To summarize: The various factors that epidemiologists have found to be associated with different diseases should be regarded as risk factors, not causes. This distinction is important. Identification of causes will require many more years of scientific investigation. For example, cigarette smoking is a risk factor for both lung cancer and heart disease, but it is very likely that the causes for the two diseases resulting from smoking are quite different. Epidemiologists actually measure possible risk factors such as dietary habits, customs, food ingredients, and smoking habits, and it is these factors that are correlated with the incidence of the disease under investigation. Risk factors are not causes of disease, and the public should realize the importance of this distinction.

The Modern Epidemic of Coronary Heart Disease— The Search for Reasons

The word *epidemic* means a significant increase in the occurrence of a disease. Epidemics due to infections are usually of short duration. The classic epidemics of history seldom lasted more than 2 years at most.

Is it correct to speak of the present widespread occurrence of CHD in developed countries as an epidemic? Strictly speaking, it is not. The concept of heart disease as a separate entity has been distinguished in just the past 35 years. The incidence of CHD has been high during this entire period, but comparative data from 60 to 100 years ago are lacking. Without a standard of comparison, there is no basis for the claim that there has been a huge increase in heart disease in recent years. Even so, most public health authorities believe that there has been such an increase. Evidence to support this conclusion comes from the present difference in the incidence of heart diseases between *developed* and *underdeveloped* countries. In general, it is much higher in the former. By using the usual criteria of what is meant by the term developed, the United States was an underdeveloped country 80 years ago. Another example concerns urban-rural differences in many countries. In South Africa, for instance, heart disease is much more common among the urban Bantu people than among those living on farms.

An encouraging sign is that the mortality from CHD in North America has been declining slowly for the last 20 years. Epidemiologists are not yet agreed on explanations for this desirable trend, but it does suggest that people are responding to the publicity about the disease.

One important clue toward discovering the causes of CHD is the relationship between incidence of atherosclerosis and age in various countries. In the U.S., for example, a study of autopsy records in Minnesota (White, Edwards, & Dry, 1950) found a 3.5 times increase in men of different ages. At age 35 there was a 20% incidence, and at 55 there was a 70% incidence. The occurrence of signs of atherosclerosis was lower in women at both ages: 10% at age 35, 20% at age 55, and 38% at age 65. From these figures one might think that CHD is a normal process that accompanies aging in both sexes.

Data from Japan show that this idea is unsound. Kimura (1956) carried out measurements in Kyushu and found that there was 0% atherosclerosis in both sexes at age 35. The incidence in males was below 10% at age 65, and in women it was about 5%. Other studies confirm the conclusion that CHD is not a necessary associate of old age (Stamler, 1978).

In comparing Japanese with North Americans, researchers have not controlled the hereditary factor. Perhaps the Japanese are less subject to CHD than Americans. This possibility, too, has been checked by comparing the incidence rate of CHD of Japanese men living in Japan, Hawaii, and Los Angeles (Kato, Tillotson, Nichaman, Rhoads and Hamilton, 1973). These studies confirmed the low rate in Japan. In Los Angeles the rate was similar to that of Caucasian Americans in the same economic bracket and in Hawaii the rate was intermediate. What variables were responsible for these differences?

In searching for the causes of CHD, the studies mentioned above have eliminated aging and heredity as general agents. Environmental factors, such as diet, remain a large area of possible contributors. Support for diet as an important factor came from an unexpected source: studies of the incidence of heart disease in Northern European countries during World War II (Malmros, 1950).

Risk Factors and the Individual

The heredity of groups has been excluded as a general risk factor. This statement means that there seems to be no difference in innate susceptibility to heart disease in any one ethnic group or nationality. As far as is known, blacks, whites, Orientals, North Americans, Japanese, English, Bantus, and so on, as members of Homo sapiens, have the same tendency to resist the disease or acquire it.

Risk factors for heart disease, by definition, increase the chances of developing the disease. The risk factor concept has grown out of epidemiological studies of populations and thus apply to the average person. Because not everyone who smokes and has hypertension or hypercholesterolemia dies from heart disease, it becomes obvious that individuals differ in their susceptibility to these risk factors. Many smokers will die prematurely, whereas others will puff away into their eighties. These differences probably have hereditary basis. If you quit smoking, it is because you assume that you are average in your resistance to the pathological effects of inhaled smoke. Actually, your genetic background determines whether you are very susceptible, average, or resistant to the chemicals in smoke.

Is there any way for a person to tell where he or she stands on the resistance scale to a particular risk factor? Family histories can furnish a good deal of information about that. If one or more of your parents and grandparents died from a heart attack, your chances of developing the disease are considerably greater than someone whose family history is clear of it. As I mentioned in chapter 7, tests are being developed to determine whether a person is likely to become hypertensive if he or she consumes extra salt. Similar tests may be developed to predict if an individual is sensitive to cholesterol or fats in the diet. Certain types of abnormal electrocardiograms also have hereditary basis.

Would it be worthwhile for each person to become aware of his or her resistance or susceptibility to the risk factors for major diseases? The costs would be considerable. Who would pay for it? Would persons ever smoke or eat an appetizing, high-fat meal if they knew that their lives might be shortened thereby?

Diet and Heart Disease

Ordinarily one would not imagine that death rates make for interesting reading, but to epidemiologists they provide leads for further research.

Following World War II, the mortality statistics for a number of European countries showed a marked drop in fatalities among civilians in diseases like diabetes and heart disease during the war years (Malmros, 1950). It was during this same period that food was rationed, especially fats and sugar. The Malmros paper plotted national consumption of various foods against incidence of disease. In Sweden, Finland, and Norway the death rate from coronary artery disease dropped precipitously from 1939 to 1942-43. During these years, the consumption of total fat, eggs, butter, and milk also declined precipitously. In the U.S., however, where consumption of dairy products and eggs increased during the war, the death rate from heart disease continued to increase. The data suggest rapid, significant correlations between diet composition and heart disease. What was the connection?

It is important to recognize that, although the Malmros study was a pioneering landmark in correlating diet and heart disease in humans, it didn't prove anything. If you refer to Table 3.1, you will see that this work falls in Category 5, ecological studies. There are too many uncontrolled, unmeasured variables in studies of this type for them to serve as more than signposts for further research. With this important limitation in mind, we can recognize that these correlations still have an important function.

In the United States two broad approaches were initiated to obtain answers to the question of whether heart disease was related to diet. One approach involved collecting data on causes of death and consumption of various foods in many countries of the world, underdeveloped as well as developed. One of the most thorough investigations of this type was the International Cooperative Study on Epidemiology of Cardiovascular Diseases Seven Country Study under the direction of Ancel Keys (1970). In this study about 12,000 men, aged 40-59, from various socio-economic groups, were observed intermittently for 10 years. They were natives of the following countries: Greece, Italy, Japan, Yugoslavia, the United States, Finland, and the Netherlands.

The Seven Country Study was experimental and prospective. Diet intake was estimated by recall and average diets were analyzed for type of fat but not for cholesterol content. These characteristics place it in Category 4 of Table 3.1, and thus its conclusions carry a higher degree of credibility than those of Malmros.

There was a significant positive correlation between saturated fat content of the diet, serum cholesterol concentration, and mortality due to heart disease over a 10-year period. The Seven Country Study not only supported the diet-heart hypothesis, but also was among the first to suggest that all fats are not alike in their physiological effects on the cardiovascular system. Those men who regularly consumed a diet high in saturated fats had a much higher rate of heart disease than those whose diet contained larger amounts of monounsaturated or polyunsaturated fats.

The objectives of these studies, as well as many others all over the world, were to enlarge the knowledge concerning the factors that contributed to heart disease. Clinical observations and collection of histories by physicians on their patients, epidemiological correlation between death rate from heart disease and diet, such as that of Malmros mentioned above, and scientific experiments on animals together had suggested a large number of factors that might influence the incidence of heart disease. The dietary variables that were measured, as well as lifestyle habits such as smoking, alcohol consumption, and amount and type of exercise, would be subjected to an extensive statistical analysis. High positive correlations would suggest that a particular factor contributed to heart disease; a consistent negative correlation would suggest that the factor might protect against heart disease; and intermediate or low correlations would suggest that there was no connection. I want to emphasize that in the early 1950s when these studies were being planned, they were acknowledged as fishing expeditions. Although the factors being measured were suspected as contributing to heart disease, a lot of guesswork was involved in their selection.

The fact that the studies mentioned above were on a worldwide basis suggested answers for the following questions: Why should Finnish farmers have the highest rate of heart disease in the world and Japanese workers one of the lowest? How do the risk factors for Americans, Japanese, Eskimos, and the Maasai of Africa compare? The possibility that answers to these and other questions might be forthcoming was breathtaking. It was recognized from the outset that epidemiological data of this type would not answer questions about the causes of heart disease but identify those personal, environmental, and physiological factors that increase the risk of heart disease.

Another prospective study has been carried out in Framingham, Massachusetts, a suburb of Boston. This town was selected as the site for a long-term project in public health because it seemed typically American. Its citizens are largely middle class and are descended from the usual mix of European hereditary backgrounds. The objectives of the study were publicized in advance, and about 7,000 adult citizens of Framingham were selected at random to furnish a valid cross section of the population. An additional 10% were permitted to volunteer for the study. The unique aspect of the Framingham project is its long-term nature. It was originally set up to study its population for 20 years. The results obtained at that time seemed so valuable that the project was continued for another 10 years.

The subjects of both sexes who were selected had never had a heart attack. They were given physical examinations, which included weight measurements and electrocardiograms (ECGs). This latter procedure provides objective evidence of how the heart is functioning. In addition, such habits as smoking (kind and amount), average daily consumption of alcohol, degree of physical activity, and types of food eaten were documented in considerable detail. No attempt was made to influence the lifestyle of these people. In fact, it was assumed that no significant change in their habits would occur for the duration of the project. The Framingham study falls into Category 4 of Table 3.1, but the results are especially valuable because of its long-term nature.

In the 6-year follow-up, it became apparent that there were large differences in the incidence of CHD in this population, especially among the middle-aged males (Kannel et al., 1961). The habits of the group who suffered a heart attack before age 50 were carefully examined. This group of men had many similar habits. They were moderate to heavy cigarette smokers and were physically inactive; they overate, as evidenced by varying degrees of overweight; and their diets were high in cholesterol, saturated fats, refined carbohydrates, and salt. The clinical findings in this group were also similar. Their serum cholesterol values were high—as defined in this study, over 250 mg/dl. They tended to have hypertension—defined as systolic/diastolic blood pressure greater than 140/90 for either term. Many had also developed abnormal ECGs. Because this group of men had more heart disease than the average, their habits and clinical findings were considered as possible predictors of disease.

Sophisticated statistical analysis was required to determine which of the personal habits and clinical findings correlated sufficiently highly with the appearance of CHD to warrant considering them as significant risk factors. This exercise in statistics narrowed the field considerably. In the original evaluation, after 6 years had elapsed, only four risk factors were positively identified. They were an elevated blood cholesterol, as defined above; hypertension, as defined above; cigarette smoking, especially over a pack a day; and an abnormal ECG.

These four risk factors have stood the test of time in the Framingham study. After 20 years, they are the only ones that show statistically significant correlations with heart disease in that population. Furthermore, these four risk factors gained considerable credibility when they were tested as predictors of heart disease in the seven European countries that had been studied by Keys and colleagues (Keys, 1970). It is interesting that the European incidence of CHD was somewhat lower than the U.S. correlations predicted, thus suggesting that other factors than these four are operating in the U.S. One such risk factor that was not measured in the original Framingham study—that of psychological stress—has recently been measured extensively in both North America and Europe and found to meet the rigid statistical criteria of the specific risk factor (Friedman & Rosenman, 1974). As time goes on it is likely that other risk factors will be identified.

The risk-factor concept has had many practical applications. The finding of one or more risk factors present in a person allows a physician or a well-informed health technologist to calculate the degree of risk. In other words, the increased probability that someone with one, two, or more risk factors will develop CHD can now be calculated with some degree of assurance.

The identification of risk factors has provided the scientists who are searching for the definite causes of CHD with a starting point for their studies. For example, what are the sources of elevated blood cholesterol? To what extent are risk factors influenced by environmental events or by hereditary background? How does smoking affect arteries? If a person who is at risk reduces one or more of his or her risk factors, are his or her chances of developing CHD lessened? Does his or her age influence the probabilities? Data bearing on these and related questions are now becoming available.

Identifying the risk factors for heart disease is primarily an activity of epidemiologists. It is an empirical procedure, and, as I've mentioned, decisions are based on the magnitude of correlation coefficients between particular suspected risk factors and the incidence of one or more disease processes related to atherosclerosis.

The next step in the long road of understanding the causes of atherosclerosis is that of studying the process of atheroma growth. This study includes identifying what initiates it and what contributes to its growth, classifying the steps in the process and relating them to the chemical composition at each stage, and finally, a very important practical aspect, determining to what extent the process of atherosclerosis can be reversed.

The Development of Atherosclerosis

The word atherosclerosis is derived from two Greek words and literally means hardening of the atheromas. Much of the research on heart disease has been directed towards understanding the origin of atheromas and the processes involved in their growth and hardening. But recall that the atheromas are growing and hardening inside of an artery, so the entire artery hardens. This process is called arteriosclerosis, hardening of the arteries. There are other causes of arteriosclerosis than atherosclerosis, but the latter is the most common.

The discovery that many of the U.S. soldiers who died in the Korean War had fatty streaks in their arteries was one of the first widespread indications that atherosclerosis has its beginnings many years before a heart attack or a stroke occurs. Fatty streaks have even been found in children as young as 10 years. Medical scientists now believe that fatty streaks are the forerunners of the atheroma, which in Greek means gruel; atheromas are mushy deposits in the lining of an artery.

Analysis of the components of the fatty streaks has shown that they do not contain cholesterol. It is deposited later as the atheroma increases in size, hardens, and changes into a plaque. The plaque grows by its inter-action with blood platelets and their constituents and with low-density lipoproteins, which contain cholesterol. The final stage includes calcification, which enlarges and hardens the plaque. If the obstruction becomes so large that it occludes the flow of blood in a coronary artery, the heart tissue in that area will die from lack of oxygen.

As Figure 10.1 shows, a fatty streak may be present in the midteens, progress to a fibrous plaque by age 30, calcify during the forties, and culminate in an infarct around age 60. If the occlusion occurs in a cerebral artery, an artery supplying the brain, a portion of the brain dies, and the person is said to have a stroke or a cerebral infarct. A stroke is often accompanied by a paralysis of varying extent and duration.

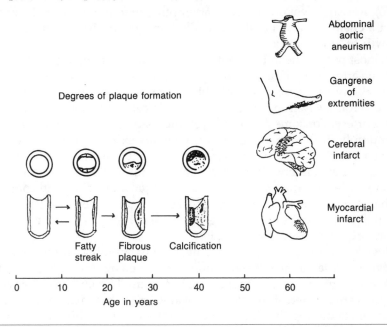

Figure 10.1   Diagram of the development of atheromas and their clinical end points.

Causative Factors in Atherosclerosis

The description of atherogenesis (i.e., the production of atheroma) and its consequences raises a host of new questions. I'll mention a few of them and the current hypotheses to explain the growth of atheromas because knowledge of the process will probably, in time, lead to new therapies and more effective preventive measures than we have at present. Research of this type serves as a necessary prelude to the development of a rational therapy. At the present time there are three main hypotheses that serve

as guidelines for research to explain the initiation and growth of atheromas. I'll outline them very briefly.

The Response to Injury Hypothesis

Over 100 years ago the famous German pathologist Rudolph Virchow
suggested that atherogenesis was initiated by injury to *endothelial cells* that
form the lining of the arteries. Atherogenesis refers to the growth of
plaques (atheroma) from this lining. The injury hypothesis, as modified
by recent research, states that plaques form in response to recurrent injuries to endothelial cells in arterial walls. These cells may be damaged
by mechanical, chemical, immunologic, or toxic factors (Ross & Glomset,
1976). Research workers are now attempting to find out how risk factors
start a chain of events that eventually damage arteries and induce the
growth of atheromas.

In most people the injured cells are replaced, the lining remains intact,
and the artery stays clear. In some people, however, the injured cells lose
their ability to keep large molecules, such as lipoproteins containing
cholesterol, away from the smooth muscle cells that compose the bulk
of the artery. For some reason not yet understood, the muscle cells begin
to multiply. If the blood chronically contains excess lipids, a condition
termed *hyperlipidemia*, the proliferation of the muscle cells continues, and
a plaque that contains cholesterol begins to form. The plaque also contains a variety of other substances such as lipids, proteins, and complex
carbohydrates. Later on, calcium deposits are found. These deposits make
the plaque harder, and reversing plaque size becomes much more difficult with the onset of calcification.

Ross and Harker (1976) at the University of Washington have shown
in monkeys that, if the initiating injury is followed by chronic hyperlipidemia, the plaques continue to increase in size until finally the classic condition of atherosclerosis results. The plaque finally becomes large enough
to diminish or stop the flow of blood to the heart. Without a source of
oxygen or nutrients, a portion of the heart dies. The person suffers a heart
attack or, technically speaking, has an infarct.

Ross and Harker believe that chronic hyperlipidemia, which is often
due to low-density lipoproteins (LDL), may not only prevent regression
of the atheroma, but may also serve as the initial injury factor. Other factors, such as the chemicals contained in cigarette smoke or the effects
of hypertension, may contribute to the continued growth of atheromas.
The response-to-injury hypothesis does emphasize the importance of
keeping the concentration of low-density lipoproteins in the blood from
rising throughout life. Because these are the major cholesterol-containing
substances in the blood, we can see the link between high levels of blood
cholesterol and the process of atherogenesis.

The Monoclonal Hypothesis

In contrast to the injury hypothesis, which had its beginnings over a century ago, the monoclonal hypothesis stems from modern genetics (Benditt, 1977). Very briefly, this idea divides the process of atherogenesis into three stages. First, a mutation in an artery wall cell is postulated. The mutated cell divides, and its offspring form a *clone*. This change is called the initiation stage. Second, some factors promote the multiplication of the mutated cells, which, if continued, form a plaque. Finally, the plaques accumulate lipid, calcium, and clotted blood to form a thrombus.

One advantage of the monoclonal hypothesis is that by postulating a mutation it relates atherogenesis to tumor formation. Plaque growth is suggested as an example of the growth of a benign tumor. This idea is supported by some epidemiological data collected by E. L. Wynder (1976), which show a correlation between the incidence of heart disease and that of colon cancer in 20 countries. As I have mentioned previously, such correlations provide interesting leads for further research. They should not be understood as anything more than a suggestion that the two conditions share common causative factors.

The key question that the monoclonal hypothesis must answer is whether the known factors associated with the development of atherosclerosis are capable of causing mutations. Many factors do. Cigarette smoke, for example, contains chemicals that are metabolized by the liver and by artery-wall cells into active *mutagens*. Cholesterol, a long-term villian in heart attacks, can be metabolized to a derivative with tumorigenic properties. Thus, although the monoclonal hypothesis is far from proved, it provides a new way of looking at the data and has suggested many new experiments with which to investigate the factors leading to cardiovascular diseases.

The Clonal-Senescence Hypothesis

A third hypothesis to explain why smooth muscle cells proliferate in plaque formation is called the clonal-senescence hypothesis. Martin and Sprague (1973) suggested that the number of muscle cells is regulated by inhibitors, but that as a person ages, the cells producing the inhibitors manufacture less of them. This decrease allows smooth muscle cells to proliferate, and atheromas then form. One of the interesting aspects of this hypothesis is its emphasis on the role of aging in atherosclerosis. But, as I have mentioned, atherosclerosis is not inevitable. Certain habits can prevent it, and other habits can accelerate it.

In conclusion, scientists have identified the main events in the formation and growth of plaques. The causes behind these events are being investigated, but they have not yet been identified. With further research, it is hoped to be able to explain the role of the known risk factors in atherosclerosis in the initiation and growth of plaques.

So far we have discussed the risk factors for CHD on a qualitative basis. To be really useful in applying them to the people of a large country like the U.S., however, quantitative data are required and have been collected. Substituting the quantitative data into equations has allowed epidemiologists to obtain answers to interesting questions like the following: Are risk factors of equal importance in contributing to the incidence of CHD? Do they act independently? How is their influence affected by diet, age, and sex?

Risk Factors

As I've mentioned, the Framingham study began in 1949. The 6-year follow-up was published by the Framingham group in 1961 (Kannel et al., 1961). Recall that all participants showed no signs of heart disease at the beginning of the study. After 6 years, the incidence of CHD was 36/1,000 (3.6%) in the group of males aged 40-59 at the start and who had not developed any risk factors in the interim. The incidence of coronary heart disease among those with one risk factor averaged about 3 times higher compared to those with none. Incidence varied from slightly over 3-fold for those with high cholesterol; a 2- to 2.6-fold increase for those with hypertension; and a 2- to 3-fold increase for those with abnormal ECG. In other words, these three risk factors were of approximately equal importance.

In the 6-year period over 30% of the population had developed at least one risk factor and about 7% showed two. The rate of heart attacks in males aged 40-59 who showed two risk factors after 6 years was almost 6 times higher than the no-risk-factors population. For those few men who had developed all three risk factors (0.6%), the subsequent CHD incidence rate was 50%. Half the men in this group had a heart attack!

Women in the 40-59 age group were less subject to CHD. The ones who remained without risk factors during the 6-year period had a heart attack at about half the incidence rate of the men. This figure doubled for those with one risk factor and doubled again for those with two. Another difference between the sexes was that in women the predominant form of CHD was angina pectoris without physical damage to the heart, whereas in men heart damage was more common than the symptom of angina by itself.

At the 20-year follow-up the relative importance of the various risk factors was calculated. The first three risk factors for cardiovascular disease were the same for men and women, ages 45 to 74. I will list them in the order of the strength of the relationship between the risk factor and the cardiovascular event: hypertension, serum cholesterol concentration, and abnormal electrocardiogram indicating *left ventricular hypertrophy* (ECG-LVH). The fourth, for men, was cigarette smoking. For women, the fourth was diabetes (Kannel, 1983).

Kannel also calculated the relative risk of developing heart disease over the 20-year period in relation to the number of risk factors that men had at the start of the study. Setting the incidence of heart disease for those with no risk factors at one (1.0), he calculated that for one risk factor the chances were 1.6 times higher; 3 times higher for those with two risk factors; and 4 times higher for those with three risk factors at the beginning.

The consistency of the risk factors as well as their cumulative effects on heart disease in the long-term Framingham study emphasize the importance of their early control in reducing the incidence of coronary heart disease in the U.S. The results are probably applicable to other countries with high rates of the disease. Two cautions should be mentioned in applying these conclusions. It should be remembered that these calculations apply to populations, not to individuals. Secondly, the ranking of the risk factors mentioned above applies only to those that were measured in the Framingham study. Other risk factors, stress for example, were not evaluated in the Framingham experiment.

I have mentioned the importance of hypertension as a risk factor for both coronary heart disease and stroke in the previous chapter. At this point, we will turn our attention to the second most important risk factor: serum cholesterol concentration.

It is significant that both the response-to-injury and the monoclonal hypotheses explicitly mention cholesterol as one of the chief factors that contributes to atheroma growth. The factors affecting blood cholesterol concentration have probably received more publicity than all the other risk factors involved in atherosclerosis, and yet the role of diet as a factor in atherogenesis is one of the most controversial.

The controversy over the relationship between diet, cholesterol, and heart disease is informative to examine because it has its roots in science, national dietary habits, and economics. Basically, the controversy revolves around the following question: What degree of credibility is necessary for the Federal government to advocate that the American people change their diets away from red meats, eggs, and high-fat dairy products, and towards a larger proportion of fowl, fish, cereal grains, and vegetables? I'll take up the scientific questions first and the political-economic ones later.

Factors Affecting Blood Cholesterol Concentration

Cholesterol is a fatty substance that is synthesized in a number of tissues. The liver is the major site of synthesis. Cholesterol has had a bad press in recent years, and sometimes I get the impression from popular articles that it should be avoided completely in the diet, and further that we might all be better off if we didn't have any in our bodies. Actually, cholesterol is an essential substance that has many functions. It serves as the starting point for the synthesis of sex hormones and bile acids. It is present in all the membranes of mammals and probably acts as an insulator in the brain. Its presence in eggs and milk suggests that young, growing animals require more than they can make. Complete vegetarians (vegans) who consume no animal products, and thus no cholesterol, synthesize it from amino acids, carbohydrates, or fats.

The blood cholesterol concentration of most adults remains constant over long periods of time. It responds slowly to changes in diet with respect to both total calories and diet composition. It is well known that a diet high in saturated fats tends to raise blood cholesterol.

The constancy of blood cholesterol concentration serves as an excellent example of the dynamic steady state as described in chapter 4. Although the total concentration doesn't change, the individual molecules of cholesterol in the blood turn over at a rapid rate. The situation can be outlined quite simply as follows:

$$\text{Rate of addition} \rightarrow \left[\begin{array}{c} \text{steady state} \\ \text{blood cholesterol concentration} \end{array} \right] \rightarrow \text{rate of removal}$$

To understand the dynamics of blood cholesterol concentration, we need to know three things. First, where does it come from? The sources are known: it comes from the diet and biosynthesis in tissues, mostly in the liver. Second, what factors influence its steady state concentration? Third, what determines its rate of removal from the blood? These factors are diagrammed in Figure 10.2.

Factors Affecting Cholesterol Synthesis

It has been known for many years that animals can synthesize cholesterol from any type of foodstuff—proteins, carbohydrates, or fats. These three foods are all sources of energy, and in the reactions of energy release they all form a *common intermediate*, a substance called acetyl coenzyme A. This substance is also the starting point of cholesterol synthesis and fatty acid synthesis. As Figure 10.3 illustrates, acetyl coenzyme A is a key compound in metabolism. If people's energy intake is in balance with their energy utilization, most of the acetyl coenzyme A that is formed is oxidized to carbon dioxide (CO_2) and water (H_2O), and the remainder is used to form sufficient cholesterol and fatty acids to replace those which are excreted or used in other reactions of metabolism.

If, however, energy intake is in excess of that which is utilized, the extra energy is stored as fat. The fatty acids of this depot fat are synthesized from the excess acetyl coenzyme A. In some people who are

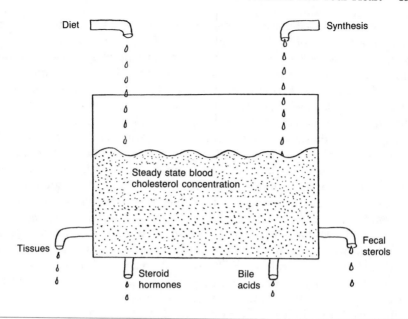

Figure 10.2   The major factors that determine the steady state concentration of blood cholesterol.

Sources of Energy

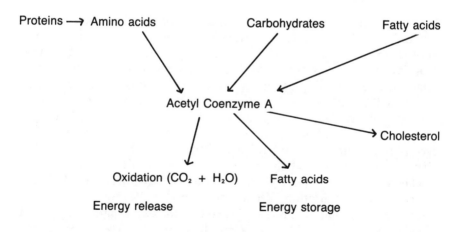

Figure 10.3   The key role of acetyl coenzyme A in metabolism.

overweight—that is, are storing fat—some of the extra acetyl coenzyme A is also converted to cholesterol. We now have a basis for understanding the correlation between overweight and a high blood cholesterol concentration.

The rate of cholesterol synthesis in the liver is also known to be affected by the amount of cholesterol in the diet. People who consume mixed diets of foods derived from both animal and plant sources consume cholesterol directly. The average North American diet, for example, contains about 600 mg of cholesterol per day. Now, it is known that the rate of synthesis of cholesterol by the liver is influenced to some extent by the amount of cholesterol in the diet. Diets high in cholesterol reduce cholesterol synthesis in the liver. This effect, however, only occurs at quite high dietary intakes of cholesterol. The liver does compensate for a high cholesterol intake but not sufficiently to offset the high intake. People who consume large amounts of cholesterol (600 to 1,000 mg/day) very frequently are found to possess a high blood concentration of cholesterol.

Apart from the amount of cholesterol in the diet, the percentage that is absorbed is also affected by the amount of fat in the diet. More cholesterol is absorbed from high-fat diets (40% of total calories) than from low-fat diets (20% of total calories). An explanation of this difference is based on the insolubility of cholesterol in watery solutions, such as would be formed in the intestine from low-fat meals. As the fat content of a meal is increased, the cholesterol that it contains is more readily dissolved in the fat, and thus a higher proportion of cholesterol is absorbed.

Dietary Factors Affecting the Steady State Concentration of Cholesterol in the Blood

If everyone has the same factors that affect the steady-state concentration of blood cholesterol, how is the large difference from one person to another explained? Two major factors are probably diet and heredity. Many vegans, who consume no cholesterol, have a blood cholesterol level of as low as 140 mg/dl. In contrast, many meat-eating North Americans' blood analyzes at 300 mg/dl or higher. But even people on similar diets can show differences as large as 100 mg/dl. These differences reflect variations in amount and type of fat ingested, as well as in the amount and type of fiber. The claims in Dr. David Reuben's book, *The Save Your Life Diet* (1976), on the blood cholesterol lowering effect of wheat bran has not been confirmed in many additional studies, but other types of dietary fiber are effective. Mathur, Khan, and Sharma (1968) fed chick peas to people on a high-fat diet. Bile acid excretion increased significantly, and blood cholesterol dropped from 206 mg/dl to 160 mg/dl. Diet is also known to affect the amount and species of bacteria present in the intestine. These bacteria can influence the amount of sterols excreted in the feces.

Hereditary factors probably govern the amount of dietary cholesterol absorbed from the gut, the rate of synthesis of cholesterol by the liver and other organs, and the blood:tissue distribution of cholesterol. The net effect of all of these factors helps determine the steady state concentration of blood cholesterol. It appears that dietary modifications are the most practical means of lowering blood cholesterol.

Apart from the amount of fat in the diet, the type of fat that it contains also influences the total concentration of cholesterol in the blood. By the type of fat, I mean the degree of saturation-unsaturation of a triglyceride. An explanation of these terms follows, and I've also included a few examples of fatty acids of different degrees of unsaturation.

The fats we eat contain fatty acids combined with glycerol. The product is called a glyceride, or, more technically, a neutral triglyceride. In this discussion, however, we need only to consider the structures of the fatty acids. A fatty acid contains a carboxyl group (COOH) at one end. A chain of carbon atoms of varying length is attached to it. The following are some examples of different types of fatty acids:

CH_3COOH Acetic acid, the acid found in vinegar, a C_2 saturated fatty acid

$CH_3CH_2CH_2CH_2CH_2CH_2CH_2CH_2CH_2CH_2CH_2CH_2CH_2CH_2CH_2CH_2COOH$ Stearic acid, a saturated C_{18} fatty acid (often abbreviated as SFA or S), occurs as a fat in animal and vegetable fats

$CH_3CH_2CH_2CH_2CH_2CH_2CH_2CH_2CH=CHCH_2CH_2CH_2CH_2CH_2CH_2CH_2COOH$ Oleic acid, a C_{18} monounsaturated fatty acid (often abbreviated as MUFA), occurs in animal and vegetable fats

$CH_3CH_2CH_2CH_2CH_2CH=CH\ CH_2CH=CH\ CH_2CH_2CH_2CH_2CH_2CH_2CH_2COOH$ Linoleic acid, a C_{18} polyunsaturated fatty acid (often abbreviated as PUFA or P), occurs in vegetable oils

In saturated fatty acids (SFA), all the available positions on the carbon atoms are filled by hydrogen atoms. We say that all the carbon atoms are saturated because they cannot hold any more hydrogen atoms. In some fatty acids, however, the carbon atoms are surrounded by less than the maximum number of hydrogen atoms. We speak of them as being unsaturated. The number of unsaturated carbon atoms varies from zero in stearic acid, and two in oleic acid, to four in linoleic acid.

One method of estimating the amounts of the different fatty acids in different substances is to look at the fats when they are at room temperature (70 °F, 21 °C). Meat fats become solid at room temperature, whereas mono- and polyunsaturated fats, as in olive oil and corn oil, respectively, remain liquids. Observe the fat in a broiler pan after cooking a steak or a chicken. As it cools, the beef fat solidifies, whereas the chicken fat will remain liquid. This difference in physical property is directly related to the fatty acids each type of fat contains. In the example above, the P/S of beef fat is about 0.1, whereas that of chicken fat is 0.78 (U.S. Department of Agriculture, 1976). The reason for explaining the structure of fatty acids in this much detail is that, as major constituents of our diets, they

Table 10.1   Composition of Some Fats, Oils, and Spreads

Type of Fat (1 Tablespoon)	Kcal	Cholesterol	Fat Content				P/S
		mg	Total	SFA	MUFA	PUFA	
			grams				
Butter	123	36	13.9	8.7	4.7	0.5	0.06
Lard	116	12	12.8	5.0	6.4	1.4	0.28
Mayonnaise, soybean	99	8	11.0	1.6	3.7	5.7	3.6
Margarine, corn oil							
Lightly hydrogenated	120	0	13.6	2.0	5.0	4.0	2.0
Moderately hydrogenated	120	0	13.6	2.2	4.9	3.7	1.7
Crisco	106	0	12.0	3.2	5.3	3.5	1.1
Vegetable Oils							
Coconut	120	0	13.6	11.8	1.6	0.2	0.02
Corn	120	0	13.6	1.7	3.9	8.0	4.7
Cottonseed	120	0	13.6	3.5	3.0	7.1	2.0
Olive	119	0	13.5	1.3	10.4	1.8	1.4
Palm	120	0	13.6	6.7	5.6	1.3	0.2
Peanut	120	0	13.5	1.2	2.3	4.3	1.8
Safflower	120	0	13.6	1.2	3.3	10.1	8.4
Sesame	120	0	13.6	1.9	6.0	5.7	3.0
Soybean	120	0	13.6	2.0	3.7	7.9	4.0
Sunflower	120	0	13.6	1.4	3.3	8.9	6.4
Wheat germ	120	0	13.6	2.6	2.5	8.5	3.3

Note. Adapted from *Food Values of Portions Commonly Used* (pp. 62, 63, 141, 142, 199, 200) by J.A.T. Pennington and H.N. Church, 1985, Philadelphia: J.B. Lippincott. Copyright 1985 by J.B. Lippincott. Adapted by permission.

affect how much cholesterol is present in our blood serum. The poly-unsaturated/saturated ratio (P/S ratio) is now being included on the labels of many high-fat products. Table 10.1 lists the composition of some fats and oils. Most vegetable oils—with the exception of palm and coconut—have P/S ratios larger than 1.0.

In this connection, it is not safe to assume that, because margarines are made from vegetable oils, they all have high P/S ratios. People prefer a fat that spreads rather than runs over the food. For this reason, the oils, which are liquids, because they contain many polyunsaturated fatty acids, are reacted with hydrogen gas, which changes many of the double bonds to single bonds. The product is now a solid at room temperature and, by the addition of a yellow dye, resembles butter in appearance. The process is called hardening because the more hydrogen that is added, the harder the product at room temperature.

The amount of hydrogen that is added also affects the P/S ratio. Many people will pay a premium price for a product with a high P/S ratio, and margarines containing corn oil or safflower oil with P/S ratios of 2:1 or even 4:1 have been hydrogenated the minimum amount to yield a solid product. The cheaper margarines, made from the less expensive soybean and cottonseed oils, generally have P/S ratios of 1:1 to 1.5:1. For comparison, butter, which is a natural product, has a P/S of 1:15.

Margarine was invented by a French chemist named Mege-Mouriez. He won a prize offered by Napoleon III for an imitation butter. Beef tallow was used as starting material. The original margarines had a pearly lustre and were named after the Greek word *margarites* meaning pearl. Why should the French have been interested in an artificial butter? At the time, their empire was expanding into tropical regions. In a warm climate without refrigeration butter goes rancid quite quickly—much more rapidly than meat. It is possible that in the rather elaborate procedure developed by Mege-Mouriez some of the unsaturated fats were removed, which would confer even greater storage stability on the product.

Rancidity develops in fats due to the reaction of unsaturated fatty acids to the oxygen of the air. The products are called *peroxides*, which are chemicals that, in turn, react with other components in the fat to form non-edible products. The high P/S margarines now on the market could be expected to become rancid even faster than butter if they are not kept at refrigerator temperatures. Some corn oil margarines are fortified with vitamin A and also with beta-carotene as coloring material. Burton and Ingold (1984) state that both of these compounds can act as anti-oxidants, although they have not been tested for this function under the conditions of margarine storage. The reason that natural oils such as corn oil, or soybean oil, remain edible even when stored at room temperature for long periods is due to the presence of vitamin E, an antioxidant that prevents peroxide formation.

Margarines are now made exclusively from vegetable oils and contain no cholesterol as do butter and lard. It is somewhat amusing to see that there are imitation margarines on the market. These products have had air stirred into them to lower the fat content. They contain 50 to 70 kcal a tablespoon instead of 100. They are required by law to be labeled "imitation margarine" to indicate their lower fat content. Their P/S ratios may vary from 1.7 to 4.5, depending on the source of oil and the degree of hardening.

The P/S Ratios of Fats Strongly Influence the Steady State Blood Cholesterol Concentration

The liver seems very efficient in converting saturated fatty acids into cholesterol. Saturated fatty acids, which comprise the majority of the fats of red meats and dairy products, tend to raise the blood cholesterol concentration. On the other hand, the monounsaturated fatty acids, which occur in olives, peanuts and their oils, avocados, and also in red meats, do not affect the blood cholesterol concentration very much at all. On the other hand, polyunsaturated fatty acids in the diet actually lower the blood cholesterol concentration. Common sources of these fatty acids are corn, soybean, safflower, and sunflower oil; nuts; and many species of fish.

These effects of the three different types of fatty acids were observed in the Seven Country Study of Keys and colleagues (Keys, 1970). The investigators found that people in the Mediterranean countries had a much lower average blood cholesterol concentration than those from Northern Europe, even though they consumed about the same amount of total fat. To what was the difference due? Southern Europeans use a lot of olive oil in their cooking (e.g., in salads, for frying, etc.), and the main fatty acid in olive oil is oleic acid, which is monounsaturated.

In contrast, the Northern Europeans' chief source of cooking fat was butter, and they also drank large quantities of whole milk, which is not only high in total fat (50% of total calories) but also in saturated fat (66% of total fat). The P/S ratio of dairy fats is about 0.05.

Although the P/S ratios of the overall diets were not measured, it was considered probable that the Mediterranean diet was significantly higher than the North European. Further, it was postulated that this difference was responsible for the lower blood cholesterol concentration in the south, and that this difference was in turn responsible for the lower rate of heart attacks there. Fortunately, these hypotheses were amenable to experimental testing.

Keys, Anderson, and Grande (1957) at the University of Minnesota carried out small-scale experiments on humans in which the dietary fats were controlled both in amount and in degrees of saturation/unsaturation. The data were regular enough for them to develop an equation by which they could calculate a change in blood cholesterol concentration from the P/S ratio of the diet and the amount of cholesterol in the diet. These well-regulated experiments confirmed their hypothesis that a diet high in saturated fats and low in polyunsaturated (i.e., a low P/S ratio) increased the blood cholesterol concentration. Preformed cholesterol in the diet also increased it. For the first time, it now became possible to calculate the effects of the chief dietary contributors to blood cholesterol quantitatively. The overall conclusions were confirmed by others, although the original equation has been modified. In the examples that I will present on how to reduce blood cholesterol by dietary means, I will use the equation of Mattson, Erickson, and Kligman (1972) for the calculations.

Jackson et al. (1984) varied the P/S ratio of diets to normal subjects to 0.4, 1.0 or 2.0. After 2 weeks on each diet they measured a reduction in total blood cholesterol of 6% and 12% on the two higher P/S ratio diets compared to the lowest. There was no change, however, in the HDL/LDL ratios among the three diets. This short-term experiment suggests that diet alone is insufficient to raise the HDL/LDL ratio. Non-dietary factors however, can accomplish this desirable objective.

Nondietary Factors That Influence the Steady State Concentration of Blood Cholesterol

Cholesterol does not occur freely in the blood. As a fatty substance, it would float in such a watery medium and gunk up the entire blood-transport system. To avoid this complication, the liver synthesizes special proteins that contain both fats and proteins. These lipoproteins associate with cholesterol and make it soluble in blood plasma. Two of these transport proteins, called high-density lipoprotein (HDL) and low-density lipoprotein (LDL), are involved in the distribution of cholesterol to the tissues that do not make it and in cholesterol excretion. Most of the blood cholesterol occurs in the LDL fraction.

Recent research has discovered that the two lipoproteins have different functions. LDL acts as an errand boy delivering cholesterol to the tissues, whereas HDL functions in the excretion of cholesterol. Thus a high HDL/LDL ratio indicates an efficient excretory mechanism for cholesterol. The results of many surveys have suggested that people with a high HDL/LDL ratio are less prone to heart attacks than those with a low ratio (Castelli & Levitas, 1977; Miller, Thelle, Forde, & Mjos, 1977; Hulley, Cohen, & Widdowsom, 1977; Schwartz, Halloran, Vlahcevic,

Gregory, & Swell, 1978). For these reasons LDL and HDL analyses are considered by many physicians as being of greater diagnostic significance than analyses for total cholesterol.

The HDL/LDL ratio can be changed in the desired direction by either raising the amount of HDL or lowering that of LDL. Regular aerobic exercise has been shown to increase the HDL/LDL ratio (Enger, Herbjornsen, Erikssen, & Fretland, 1977; Lehtonen & Vikari, 1978). Hartung, Foreyt, Mitchell, Vlasek, and Gotto (1980) measured HDL and LDL levels in three groups of free-living middle-aged males: marathon runners, joggers, and physically inactive men. Their diets were estimated. This work would fall in Category 4 of Table 3.1. The results showed that marathon runners had the highest HDL levels (65 mg/dl), followed by the joggers (58 mg/dl), and the inactive men had the lowest (43 mg/dl). Dietary factors did not appear to influence significantly the HDL concentration. Total cholesterol varied in the three groups in mg/dl as 188, 205, and 211, respectively. A more conclusive experiment would require a controlled diet for the three groups as well as measuring the lipoproteins as affected by the duration of the exercise regime.

Moderate consumption of alcohol has been reported by Castelli and Levitas (1977) and Yano, Rhoads, and Kugan (1977) to elevate HDL levels. David Kritchevsky (personal communication, 1982), a well-known researcher on cholesterol in animals, has humorously remarked, "Now I run from bar to bar." Weight loss by overweight men raises HDL/LDL primarily by decreasing LDL levels.

It is estimated that approximately 1 in 500 of unselected children have some form of hereditary, familial hyperlipidemia. These children represent a group of people who are at high risk of developing atherosclerosis in later life. They account for at least 5% of all heart attacks in persons under age 60 (Kolata, 1983). Children whose parents or siblings have diagnosed hypercholesterolemia should have their blood cholesterol checked early in life and, if the value is elevated, should be placed under the care of a physician-dietician. The therapy recommended by Glueck and Stein (1979) includes (a) dietary cholesterol should not exceed 300 mg/day; (b) total fat should not exceed 35% of total dietary energy; and (c) types of fat should be equally divided among saturated, monounsaturated, and polyunsaturated.

The Role of High-Density Lipoproteins

I have already mentioned a possible role of HDL in the excretion of cholesterol. The question of the synthesis of HDL particles remains to be discussed as well as the role of these particles in the actual excretory process. For this description, I have to go back and mention even fatter particles than LDL. As you might suspect, they are called very low density lipoprotein (VLDL). These particles are very rich in triglycerides, and there are enzymes in blood plasma that hydrolyze these fats. As this process occurs, some of the proteins of the VLDL are transferred to other particles to form HDL.

There seems to be little doubt that high levels of HDL help protect against CHD. This statement is supported by empirical as well as direct data. For example, HDL levels are low in cigarette smokers, the obese, and in diabetics; all of these groups are subject to high rates of CHD.

The data indicate that the cholesterol that is carried back to the liver in HDL particles is the direct source of bile acids, derivatives of cholesterol that are stored in the gall bladder and excreted in the gall via the intestinal tract. The bile acids are not merely excretory products. They are very important in the absorption of fats and the fat-soluble vitamins. A high proportion of the bile acids is reabsorbed in the intestine, returned to the liver, and used over again. This circulation of the bile acids from the liver to the gall, to the intestine and back to the liver, is called the *extra-hepatic circulation*. Some of the bile acids that are not reabsorbed in this circulation are excreted via the stool. This route is the major one by which cholesterol is metabolized and excreted. It is suggested, but not proved, that people who consume high-fat diets reabsorb more bile acids from the extra-hepatic circulation and thus maintain their blood cholesterol at higher levels than is desirable.

Dietary Cholesterol Compared to Saturated Fats

Many research results have demonstrated that the higher the blood cholesterol, the greater the risk of a heart attack. It thus behooves a person who is concerned with maintaining a low serum cholesterol concentration to know what the major food sources of cholesterol are. To this end I have constructed Table 10.2, which lists the cholesterol content of some common foods. Because cholesterol can also be readily synthesized from saturated fats, I have also listed the fat content of these foods, their P/S ratios, calories per serving, and the contribution to blood cholesterol made by fats and by the preformed cholesterol in those foods.

I'll illustrate the practical application of these figures by presenting the situation of an American male who has a blood cholesterol level of 250 mg/dl. He has been advised to lower it by diet to the 200 mg/dl level. His objective is to lower his cholesterol by 50 mg/dl with minimum change in his diet. Table 10.3 lists some of the foods that he consumes daily.

From this analysis, it can be seen that his cholesterol intake is not excessive and is somewhat below the American average. The contributions

Table 10.2   Fat and Cholesterol Content of Some Common Foods and Their Contributions to Plasma Cholesterol

Food	Amount Per Day	Calories	Calories From Fats	P/S	Cholesterol Content	Plasma Cholesterol Contribution		
						From Fatty Acids	From Cholesterol	Total
		kcal/day	*%*		*mg/serving*	*mg per 100 ml*		
Eggs	1 50 g	80	68	< 0.1	250	1.5	12.5	14.0
Fats and oils								
Butter	30 g	215	100	< 0.1	18	7.9	3.7	11.6
Margarine								
Regular	30 g	215	100	1.5	0	4.5	0	4.5
Corn oil	30 g	215	100	2.0	0	−2.6	0	−2.6
Oil								
Safflower	30 g	265	100	9.1	0	−7.2	0	−7.2
Fruits								
Orange juice	1 cup (diluted 1 + 3) 120 g	120	0	0	0	0	0	0
Apple	1 150 g	70	0	0	0	0	0	0
Avocado	1 280 g	370	90	0.7	0	—	0	—
Grains								
Bread, white	1 slice 25 g	70	13	0.6	0	0	0	0
Oatmeal	1/4 cup 60 g	32	14	—	0	0	0	0
Rice, instant	1/4 cup 40 g	45	0	—	0	0	0	0
Fish								
Haddock, breaded, fried	1 fillet 85 g	140	32	1	56	0.2	3.3	3.5
Shrimp, canned	85 g	100	9	—	128	0.3	5.4	5.7

Food	Measure	Weight							
Meats									
Beef steak									
Lean and fat	1 serving	100 g	330	73	< 0.1	100	5.6	4.5	10.1
Lean only	1 serving	100 g	145	32	< 0.1	90	3.1	4.0	7.1
Chicken									
Breast	1 serving	100 g	140	29	2.0	72	1.5	3.5	5.0
Lamb, chop									
Lean and fat	1 serving	100 g	330	75	< 0.1	100	5.6	4.5	10.1
Pork, chop									
Lean and fat	1 serving	100 g	330	73	0.25	25	5.6	4.5	10.1
Milk and cheese									
Milk, whole	1 cup	300 ml	160	50	< 0.1	25	3.4	1.6	5.0
Milk, skim	1 cup	300 ml	90	1		7	0	0.4	0.4
Cheese									
Cheddar	1 cup	40 g	160	70	< 0.1	64	4.2	1.9	6.1
Cottage	1 cup	115 g	120	35	< 0.1	12	1.5	0.8	2.3
Cottage, low-fat, 2%	1 cup	115 g	100	18	< 0.1	10			
Yogurt									
Whole milk	1 cup	227 g	140	48	< 0.1	29	2.5	1.1	3.6
2% milk	1 cup	227 g	127	22	< 0.1	14	1.2	0.5	1.7
Vegetables									
Beans, common varieties	1 cup	125 g	30	trace	0	0	0	0	0
Potatoes									
Baked	1 medium	100 g	90	trace	0	0	0	0	0
Chips	10 pieces	20 g	115	72	2	0	-2.5	0	-2.5
French fries	12 pieces	60 g	150	43	2	0	-1.5	0	-1.5
Miscellaneous									
Brownies, with nuts, mix	1 serving	20 g	85	42	1	0	0	0	0
Ice cream	1 scoop	32 g	60	47	< 0.1	19	1.1	0.7	1.8
Peanut butter	1 tbsp.	16 g	95	76	1	0	0	0	0

Note. Compiled from "A Perspective View of Dieting to Lower the Blood Cholesterol" by H.M. Whyte and N. Havenstein, 1976, *American Journal of Clinical Nutrition,* **29**, p. 785; and *Home and Garden Bulletin No. 72, Nutritive Value of Foods* (pp. 5-39), 1971, Washington, DC: U.S. Department of Agriculture, U.S. Government Printing Office.

Table 10.3   Fatty Foods in Subject's Present Diet

Food/Day	Cholesterol Content (mg)	Contribution to Plasma Cholesterol From Fatty Acids (mg per dl)	From Cholesterol	Total/Day
Egg, (1)	250	1.5	12.5	14
Beef, lean and fat (8 oz, 220 g)	200	12.4	10.0	22.4
Milk, whole (2 cups)	50	6.8	3.2	10.0
Butter (1 oz, 30 g)	18	7.9	3.7	11.6
Total	518	28.6	29.4	58.0

to his blood cholesterol are almost equally divided between that from fatty acids and that from preformed cholesterol. Minimal dietary changes to help him accomplish his objective might include decreasing his egg consumption to one every other day; changing from 8 oz of regular beef every day to 6 oz of lean beef every other day, and substituting low-fat fish or fowl 3 times a week; changing from whole milk to 2% fat milk or skim milk; and substituting corn oil margarine for butter. These changes, and their calculated effects on his blood cholesterol, are listed in Table 10.4.

The dietary changes listed will decrease the daily cholesterol intake to about 235 mg per day, somewhat less than half of the original intake. These same alterations will also lower the contribution of fats to plasma cholesterol levels. The net result is a reduction of blood cholesterol of about 50 mg/dl. The magnitude of this decrease is similar to those obtained in experiments with humans where the diet was carefully controlled (Mattson et al., 1972).

One advantage of calculating the contributions to plasma cholesterol of fats and cholesterol separately is that it shows the major contributors explicitly. The important role of dietary cholesterol is made clear by these calculations. It explains the emphasis on cutting down on egg yolks; eating lean beef, pork, or lamb; substituting fowl and fish on a regular basis, drinking low-fat milk; and substituting high P/S margarine for butter.

The conclusion drawn above, that reduction in dietary saturated fat and cholesterol can reduce plasma cholesterol concentrations, has been accomplished numerous times in experiments with both animals and humans. The key question then remains: Will reduction of blood cholesterol help prevent heart attacks in middle-aged men?

Table 10.4 Effects of Changes in Subject's Diet on Plasma Cholesterol Concentration

Food/Week	Total Cholesterol Content (mg)	Contribution to Plasma Cholesterol/Week (mg per dl)		Contribution to Total Plasma Cholesterol	
		From Fatty Acids	From Cholesterol	Per Week	Per Day
Egg (4 servings)	1000	6.0	50.0	56.0	8.0
Beef, lean (24 oz, 675 g, 4 servings)	360	12.4	16.0	28.4	4.0
Chicken (1 serving)	72	1.5	3.5	5.0	0.7
Fish (1 serving)	56	0.3	5.4	5.7	0.8
Vegetarian (1 serving)	0	-10.5 (est.)	0	-10.5	-1.5
Milk, 2% (14 cups) or	210	7.8	10	17.8	2.6
Milk, skim (14 cups)	98	0	4.5	4.5	0.6
Margarine, corn oil (30 g)	0	-18.2	0	-18.2	-2.6
Total[1]	1700 (1590)	0 (-8)	85 (79)		12 (10)

[1]Totals given are for diet including 2% fat milk. Numbers in parentheses represent the additional decrease if skim milk is substituted for 2% milk.

Human Experiments to Check the Diet–Heart Hypothesis

A significant decrease in cardiovascular mortality rates was found in two studies carried out in hospitals. With both experiments the dietary changes included a decrease in saturated fat and cholesterol in the experimental group. In the Los Angeles Veterans Administration study (Dayton, 1970) a significant decrease of 31% in fatal atherosclerotic diseases was found in 8.5 years in a group of men whose average age was 65.5 years at the start of the experiment. Similar results were obtained in a Finnish mental hospital (Turpeinen, 1979). The men showed a 53% decline in coronary heart disease mortality and the women 34%, over two 6-year periods compared to the control group. In both hospitals the patients did not have control of their own diets, and thus the composition of the food that was eaten was decided by the physicians in charge.

I interpret these results to mean that cholesterol can indeed be lowered significantly by dietary changes if the experimental diet is consumed consistently. Both of these experiments fall under Category 2 of Table 3.1. The conclusions have a high degree of credibility for the subjects that were studied. One nagging question that surrounds experiments of the type that utilizes subjects confined in a hospital, prison, boarding school, and the like can be stated as follows: How representative of the population at large is the population in the study? The fact that two very dissimilar hospital populations reacted similarly to diet changes does increase confidence in the conclusions over one study by itself, but remnants of the nagging question still remain.

Attempts to Change Dietary Habits

To avoid the uncertainties and disadvantages of using hospital patients as subjects, two large-scale intervention trials have been carried out with free-living, normal subjects.

Oslo and the Multiple Risk Factor Intervention Trial (MRFIT)

The Oslo primary prevention trial lasted 5 years and included over 1,200 men, aged 40-49, who had never had a heart attack (Hjermann, Holme, Velve Byre, & Leren, 1981). They were considered coronary-prone because they all were very hypercholesterolemic (av. 322 mg/dl) and smoked cigarettes. The U.S. experiment was called the Multiple Risk Factor Intervention Trial (MRFIT), included over 12,000 subjects, lasted 8 years, and cost $110 million (MRFIT Research Group, 1982). In addition to the two risk factors mentioned above, some subjects were hypertensive (a well-recognized risk factor for heart disease) and were given diuretics to control it.

In both experiments the men were randomized into two groups: a control group and an intervention group. The control group was informed of the objectives of the study, but no measures were taken to change their dietary or smoking habits. The intervention group was counseled repeatedly during the trial about the dangers of hypercholesterolemia and how it could be controlled by dietary means. The group members were also advised to quit smoking. The results of the two experiments turned out to be surprisingly different.

The Oslo intervention group averaged 13% (43 mg/dl) lower in serum cholesterol over the 5-year period than the control group. A complicating factor was observed in the first few months of the experiment. The serum cholesterol concentration of the control group dropped as precipitously as the intervention group! The 5-year incidence of CHD in the intervention group was 47% lower than the control group—a statistically significant difference ($p = .028$). The control group's values then leveled off, whereas the intervention group's continued to decrease. In addition, incidence rates of all cardiovascular events and sudden coronary death were also reduced significantly (42% and 72%, respectively). Death from all causes was reduced by 31%, but this figure was not statistically significant.

An important assumption that is made in experiments of this type is that the control group does not change its habits during the course of the experiment. This assumption was not met in either section of the Oslo study: 25% of the counseled group reported cessation of smoking, but 17% of the control group also quit. The differences in the incidence of CHD might have been even wider and more significant if the control group had remained more constant, or if 100% of the counseled group had stopped smoking.

In the MRFIT study (MRFIT Research Group, 1982) the experimental group was composed of hypercholesterolemic smokers (253 mg/dl). It was further subdivided into those who were hypertensive and those who were normotensive. The hypertensives were treated with diuretic drugs. The normotensives were, of course, not treated. This subdivision led to some important unanticipated results.

A 7.1% reduction in mortality from CHD was found in the intervention group that was counseled to cut down on saturated fat and cholesterol and to stop smoking, compared to the control group that was not counseled. Although this result was in the same direction as that obtained by the Oslo experiment, the difference was too small to be statistically significant. Two reasons for this disappointing result were found in a detailed examination of the data. The first was similar to that found in the Oslo experiment. The control group had changed its habits over the experimental period in the same direction as the intervention group. For example, the serum cholesterol levels of the intervention group dropped to 233 mg/dl by the end of the experiment, only slightly below the 240 mg/dl of the control group. Similarly, intervention had decreased smoking from 60% to 35%, but the control group had also decreased from 60% to 45%.

In this connection, it is relevant to mention that there was a large reduction in deaths from heart disease in the U.S. during the 1970s, the same years that the MRFIT study was in progress. The specific reasons for this reduction are not known, but it is possible that a large number of U.S. men decreased their risk factors voluntarily. This effect of the control group's not remaining constant in its habits over the course of the 8-year experiment is a recognized hazard of this type of large-scale, long-term experiment. It is for reasons like these that these studies fall under Category 4 of Table 3.1. They have a fairly low degree of credibility unless the p value is considerably less than $p = .05$, which was not found in the MRFIT experiment.

The second flaw was exposed by the mortality data. Total deaths in the intervention group were slightly higher than those in the control group. This unexpected result suggested that, because there was a reduction in deaths from heart attacks, there must have been an increase in deaths from other causes. What other factors may have been increasing mortality? Again, further examination of the data showed that the higher death rates were found in the group of hypertensive men who had been taking diuretic drugs to lower their blood pressure. This disturbing observation suggests that the diuretic drugs in the dosages used may have contributed to the higher death rates in the hypertensive group.

The two diuretics used in the study, chlorthalidone and hydrochlorthiazide, are very widely used in the control of hypertension in the U.S., and their effects are being looked into very carefully. When asked how he would advise the physicians of men who are taking these drugs to control their hypertension, Dr. Friedewald, Associate Director for Clinical Applications at the National Heart, Lung, and Blood Institute, replied that the patients should be given an electrocardiogram (ECG). If certain abnormalities are found, the diuretic dosage should be reduced to very low levels or possibly a different type of hypertensive drug should be administered (Kolata, 1982).

Do these inconclusive, unanticipated results mean that the MRFIT experiment wasted a lot of money? One response to these results suggested that perhaps the lifestyle–heart disease connection wasn't "all that it's cracked up to be"(Nutrition Today, Jan./Feb. 1983, p. 20). In my opinion these doubts are unfounded. In the first place, the experiment was not a direct test of the diet–heart hypothesis; other variables, like cigarette smoking and hypertension, were included. In the subset of normotensive, hypercholesterolemic, cigarette smokers, the CHD rate was 49% lower in the intervention group compared to the controls. This result compares well with the Oslo data. One limitation of this particular MRFIT result is that it is based on a relatively small population. In the second place, the data brought out unexpected side effects of two diuretic drugs that had been very widely used. Although these effects undoubtedly decreased the value of the MRFIT experiment, they contributed considerably to knowledge that is important in the control of hypertension.

In summary, the hospital experiments provide the most conclusive data that support the diet–heart hypothesis. In this controlled environment, the subjects had no choice but to eat the experimental diets. It is likely that a large-scale diet experiment with free-living subjects will not be undertaken in the foreseeable future because such an experiment was discussed and shelved in favor of the MRFIT. In addition, the cholesterol reductions of the intervention group were disappointing despite the repeated counseling and urging of the subjects to cut down on saturated fats and cholesterol. As mentioned above, the control group reduced their blood cholesterol levels voluntarily almost as much as the intervention group.

I suggest that the categories and credibilities listed in Table 3.1 are useful in evaluating and comparing the results and conclusions of different types of experiments. The lower category of the free-living, intervention experiments suggests to me that they not be given equal weight to the hospital experiments. This line of reasoning leads to the conclusion that diet can influence blood cholesterol concentrations and lower incidence of heart disease if the prescribed diet is followed consistently. Conversely, the MRFIT results illustrate the limitations of experiments in which the diet is not controlled.

The Lipid Research Clinics
Coronary Primary Prevention Trial

With this background from the MRFIT experiment, the Directors of the next study, the Lipid Research Clinics Coronary Primary Prevention Trial (LRC-CPPT) (1984a, 1984b), had little choice but to try a different method of reducing serum cholesterol—one that would yield larger decreases in the experimental group and larger differences between the groups.

In this experiment, also conducted by the National Heart, Blood, and Lung Institute, cholesterol reduction was achieved by use of a synthetic resin called cholestyramine. This resin absorbs bile acids in the digestive tract. Recall that cholesterol is converted to the bile acids in the liver. They are stored in the gall bladder and secreted into the digestive tract to aid in the digestion of fats. Normally, about 90% of the bile acids are reabsorbed from the digestive tract, return to the liver, and are resecreted in the bile. This cycling of the bile salts is called the *entero-hepatic circulation*. The bile salts that are not reabsorbed are excreted in the stool. This pathway serves as the major route of cholesterol excretion.

Swallowing a resin that absorbs the bile salts and is excreted with them prevents a certain proportion of the bile salts from recycling, and thus results in their greater excretion. Because more cholesterol is converted to bile salts if their concentration is lower, the net effect of cholestyramine treatment is one of lowering the blood cholesterol concentration.

It is worth noting that this experiment assumes that the cholestyramine method of lowering blood cholesterol is equivalent in all respects to lowering it by diet. The assumption seems reasonable, but, because the reduction in blood cholesterol is achieved by a different mechanism than by dietary means, other differences may appear if the two procedures could be compared directly.

Cholestyramine is used as a drug in the treatment of certain types of hyperlipidemia (high serum cholesterol concentrations). It has some undesirable side effects like nausea, constipation, and interference with absorption of some of the fat-soluble vitamins. For these reasons, its use requires surveillance by a physician.

In the experiment with cholestyramine, over 3,800 men aged 35–59, who showed no symptoms of heart disease, and with an average blood cholesterol of 265 mg/dl, were randomized into two groups. One-half received the resin cholestyramine, the other half a placebo. The percentage of smokers was the same in both groups, as was their average blood pressure, which was normal. Thus no hypertension-reducing drugs were administered, nor were the subjects encouraged to quit smoking or modify their diets appreciably. The study was of the double-blind type. That is, neither the subjects nor the doctors who examined them knew whether they were taking the active agent or a placebo.

The strategy paid off. After 7 years, blood cholesterol had decreased 10% in the cholestyramine group versus 4% in the control group. There was a 19% reduction in risk ($p = .05$) in the primary end point, defined as definite coronary heart disease death and/or nonfatal heart attack. Three other types of coronary heart disease endpoints were reduced similarly. There was no difference, however, in all cause mortality, due primarily to more accidental and violent deaths in the experimental group. These were considered as chance occurrences.

Now I must discuss the question of how the data were reported and what conclusions were drawn. The accepted procedure for publication of scientific research is by publication in a respected journal. If the results have direct bearing on the public interest, it is common to hold a press conference *at the time* (my italics) of publication. In contrast, the LRC-CPPT briefing occurred a full week before the publication of the work in *The Journal of the American Medical Association* (Lipid Research Clinics Program, 1984a, 1984b). The reason given for this procedure was to prevent leaks of incomplete or distorted information.

To me, an even more serious error was in the wording of the conclusions. The one from the scientific paper reads, "The LRC-CPPT findings show that reducing total cholesterol by lowering LDL-cholesterol can diminish the incidence of CHD morbidity and mortality in men at risk for CHD because of raised LDL-cholesterol levels. This clinical trial provides strong evidence for a causal role for these lipids in the pathogenesis of CHD." (p. 351). A second conclusion states, "The LRC-CPPT results give a clear and consistent picture of the relationship of the primary end point, CHD incidence, to changes in cholesterol levels." (p. 373).

In contrast, the conclusion presented in the press briefing was, "In summary, the LRC-CPPT is the first study to demonstrate *conclusively* (my italics) that the risk of coronary heart disease can be reduced by lowering blood cholesterol." (Nutrition Today, 1984, p. 25). In my opinion, and in the opinion of many nutrition experts, as presented in Nutrition Today (1984), this last conclusion is unjustified and misleading to the American public. In the first place, there are so many uncontrolled variables in epidemiological experiments (as discussed in chapter 3) that it is next to impossible to demonstrate any conclusion conclusively. Secondly, when a conclusion is established conclusively, by definition, the consensus of experts accepts it, instead of attacking it as vigorously as occurred. In summary, I think that the American public—which paid for this research—is entitled to a more objective presentation of the results and conclusions than they received from the LRC-CPPT press briefing.

The authors suggest that even though direct cholesterol lowering by diet was not accomplished, the results support the diet–heart hypothesis. They also suggest that the results would apply to younger men, those with lower cholesterol levels than the men in this study, and hypercholesterolemic women. Valuable results might be obtained if one or more of these hypotheses were to be checked by experiments.

Due to the side effects, the expense, and the general bother, no one is advocating that this drug be used on a wide scale. I will conclude the discussion of these experiments by quoting Dr. Irvine Page (1983), a long-term researcher in this field. "The public should be urged to eliminate the risk factors; they have nothing to lose and probably much to gain" (p. 12). I agree. The question becomes: How can hypercholesterolemic individuals reduce their blood cholesterol? For those who seriously want to reduce their blood cholesterol levels, I have outlined dietary changes that can accomplish this objective with a minimum of martyrdom. In fact, healthful diets and cookbooks detailing how to buy and prepare tasty, appealing dishes and meals that are low in saturated fat and cholesterol have become quite popular among cooks who prefer cooking for two than for one. A list of these is presented at the end of the chapter. In general, this cuisine is known as the *prudent diet.*

The High-Fat North American Diet

If I were asked to name the one biggest flaw in the American diet, it would have to be its high-fat content, especially its high proportion of saturated fat. In 1971-72 the U.S. Government surveyed the diet of over 28,000 persons in the age range from 1 to 74 years. Dietary intake was estimated from a 24-hour recall and a questionnaire and has been extrapolated to cover the whole U.S. population. Data on the fat, cholesterol, and sodium intake have been published by Abraham and Carroll (1981). I'll briefly summarize the fat intake for adults aged 18-64, of both sexes. Percentage of total calories from fat calculated to 37%.

With few exceptions, the traditional diet of mankind through the ages has ranged from 10% to 25% in calories derived from fat. Fats contain over twice as many calories per unit weight as carbohydrates or proteins, thus a high-fat diet, such as the American, can be considered a concentrated diet. It is obvious that it is more difficult not to overeat when partaking of a concentrated diet rather than a minimally processed, diluted, high-carbohydrate diet. This fact, coupled with the low amount of aerobic physical activity engaged in by most Americans, goes a long way toward explaining the prevalence of overweight and obesity in the U.S.

The fat-in-food problem can be made manageable most easily and applied in the supermarket and kitchen if it is divided into three smaller goals: (a) reduce total fat in the diet from an average of 40% to 30%; (b) increase the proportion of polyunsaturated fatty acids (PUFA) compared to saturated (SFA) to 1:1; and (c) decrease cholesterol consumption from about 600 mg per day to 300 mg or less.

Reduction of the fat content of the diet from 40% to 30% or lower, involves more than spreading the margarine less thick on the morning toast, or using 1 tablespoon of whipped cream on the pumpkin pie instead of 2. As a first step, it would probably be valuable to know the major sources of fat in the American diet.The major source of fat is meat (25%), followed by dairy products (15%). These two sources furnish almost half the American dietary fat. For teens of both sexes, the percent of fat from these sources is even higher (45%). If your diet is typical of the U.S. diet, reduction in the consumption of red meats and high-fat dairy products would result in a lower intake of total fat as well as of saturated fats.

How to Reduce the Fat Content of the Diet

It is not necessary to become a vegetarian to reduce your fat consumption. Cutting down does not mean cutting out. For example, you can reduce your meat consumption from 2 or 3 times a day to 1 time daily. Also consider the fat content of various cuts and types of meat (Brody, 1981). There is a wide variation here. Meats containing 75% or more of total calories as fats are bacon, choice cuts of beef, frankfurters, pork sausage, spareribs, untrimmed pork loin and ham, luncheon meats, and canned meats. In the intermediate 40% to 75% range, we find rump and lean cuts of beef, lamb chops and veal, and trimmed lean cuts of pork. Chicken roasted with skin contains considerably more fat (50%–75%) than that roasted without skin (30%–40%). Dark meat of roast turkey lists at 30%–40% calories from fat, but the white meat comes in at less than 20%. Small chickens contain less fat than older, larger birds. Broilers have less than 10% fat compared to roasters at 12%–18%. Fish and seafood that have been breaded or fried are found in the 30%–40% range, but broiled fish generally contain less than 30% of its calories from fat.

Milk and milk products are also available in a wide range of fat content. Whole milk (3.5% fat) furnishes 49% of calories as fat, 2% milk furnishes 36%, and skim milk 2%. Cottage cheese can be purchased with low-fat content (19% of calories) and yogurt likewise. As shown in Table 10.5 there is a tremendous range in fat composition in popular cheeses. Hard and processed cheeses average 65%–75% of calories from fat. A few

Table 10.5   Fat Content of Various Cheeses

	Fat Percentage	
Cheese Type	Wt/Wt	Kcal
American		
Process	32	75
Cheese spread	21.1	66
Blue	29	74
Brie	28	75
Camembert	25	73
Cheddar	33	74
Cottage		
Creamed	4.5	41
Low fat, 2%	1.9	19.5
Mozzarella		
Regular	21.6	69
Part skim	15.9	56
Ricotta		
Regular	13	67
Part skim	8	50
Swiss	28	66

Note. From *Food Values of Portions Commonly Used* (pp. 16-17) by J.A.T. Pennington and H.N. Church, 1985, Philadelphia: J.B. Lippincott. Copyright 1985 by J.B. Lippincott. Reprinted by permission.

cheeses contain less than 20% of calories as fat. Some of them are St. Otho, beer cheese, hand cheese, low-fat ricotta, gammelost, and sapsago.

We think of butter, cream, and rich desserts as containing lots of fat, and they do. But fat, usually saturated fat, is hidden in dozens of other foods that we ordinarily don't think of as high in fat. A few foods with fat content calculated as percentage of total calories are: hot dogs, 80%; hamburgers, 64%; Danish pastry, 56%.

Helen Black (1980) of the Berkeley Co-Op has calculated the fat content of some typical meals. Bacon and eggs with a skimpy amount of butter on the toast contains 55% of calories as fat. In contrast, shredded wheat, whole milk, and orange juice calculates to 18%. With 2% fat milk, the overall fat content reduces to 15% and with skim milk to 7%. Lunch, composed of a peanut butter sandwich, whole milk, and an apple, contained 48% calories as fat, mostly from the peanut butter. The schoolboy's classic of hamburger, french fries, and a milk shake came out at 43% calories as fat. A dinner of hamburger stroganoff on rice calculated to 44%. If the sour cream is substituted by low-fat yogurt, the fat calories drop to 30%.

In chapter 6 I listed the results of a study by Wyse et al. (1976), who carried out an interesting calculation of the effect of preparation of potatoes on their fat content (Table 6.7). A baked potato contains no fat, and 161 g (about 6 oz) provides 160 kcal of energy. About a third of the total weight of french fried potatoes is fat, and only 55 g (2 oz) are required to furnish 150 kcal. Potato chips are even fattier. The fat content now comes to 72% on a weight basis, and 26 g (about 1 oz) contains 150 kcal.

If the fat content is converted to percentage calories from fat, to be comparable to the other percentages I have cited, the numbers are even more startling. Fat furnishes 43% of the calories in french fries and 63% of those in potato chips.Few, if any, people eat baked potatoes without butter or sour cream, so to make the comparison realistic I'll add the calories in a pat of butter. One pat (5 g) contains 36 kcal, all from fat (USDA, 1976). Adding 36 to 150 gives 186 kcal total, and a fat percentage of 19. Two pats would raise fat calories to 32% of total kcal, still appreciably lower than fries or chips. If you add a tablespoon (15 g) of half-and-half sour cream to a baked potato, you are adding 16 kcal of fat, enough to bring total fat calories to 10%. On the other hand, you can add a full ounce (28 g) of whole milk yogurt, which contains only 8 kcal from fat, and the baked potato combination now calculates to 5% of the kcal from fat. You can drown the potato in yogurt made from skim milk and still not have to worry about fat calories.

How to Reduce Saturated Fat Intake

Another aspect of the fat story concerns the degree of saturation. Saturated fatty acids are the major precursors of cholesterol and tend to raise the concentration of cholesterol in the blood. Monounsaturated fatty acids in the diet neither elevate nor depress blood cholesterol, whereas polyunsaturated fatty acids actually depress blood cholesterol concentration. These are important differences; a high blood cholesterol is considered as a risk factor for cardiovascular disease. Most meat, meat products, and whole milk dairy products contain a high proportion of their fats as saturated fatty acids. For example, percentages of saturated to monounsaturated to polyunsaturated fatty acids in beef and dairy products are approximately 56:40:3.

Fatty acid composition and P/S ratio for a variety of foods are presented in Table 10.2. Beef and dairy products have a P/S of only 0.04; pork is somewhat higher at 0.35. Chicken and other fowl are in the range 0.55, but most fish contain such a high percentage of PUFA that the P/S is 1.5. Vegetable oils vary widely in P/S. One should not assume that this whole group has a high value of P/S. They vary from cottonseed oil at 0.02 to safflower oil at 7.1.

Red meats and high-fat dairy products furnish a high proportion of their calories as fats, and these fats have low P/S ratios. For these reasons the prudent diet restricts the use of red meats, butter, yogurt made from whole milk, ice cream, heavy cream, sour cream, and cheeses made from whole milk or cream.

The Prudent Diet

The prudent diet was developed and publicized by Dr. Joliffe and nutritionists in the Health Department of the City of New York during the 1950s for the use of members of the Anti-Coronary Club (Christakis et al., 1966). The diet targets fat as a major contributor to heart disease. The average American diet contains approximately 40% of total calories as fat; the prudent diet recommends 30%. The average diet has a P/S ratio of 0.3; the prudent diet recommends 1.0. During the 14 years that the diet was in operation, the incidence of heart attacks among members of the Anti-Coronary Club was less than half the expected rate. A reduction of this size is impressive even though the experimental population was not chosen randomly and diets were not measured. The subjects were instructed in the principles of the diet and agreed to conform to it while they participated in the experiment. The book *The Prudent Diet* by Bennett and Simon (1973) is filled with delicious recipes that follow the principles of the diet and contains many hints on selecting low-fat foods. It directly addresses the question of how to eat less fat, especially saturated fat.

As a substitute for these high fat-containing foods, the prudent diet suggests unrefined foods that are high in complex carbohydrates. Examples of such foods are whole grains, all types of fresh vegetables, and fresh fruits. If these foods are used to bring the fat content of the diet down to 30% of total kilocalories, a number of desirable consequences follow. Recall that carbohydrates contain only 4/9 of the kilocalories per unit weight as fat. Thus, these foods automatically decrease energy intake, which helps keep one's weight in line. Second, unrefined foods contain a large amount of their original dietary fiber. This undigestible material provides bulk to the diet. A person who eats high-bulk foods will feel full without ingesting a large number of kilocalories. Dietary fiber makes for slower eating, which is also considered desirable for most of us. In addition, dietary fiber helps prevent constipation without the use of drugs. Finally, the prudent diet furnishes sufficient vitamins such that supplements are unnecessary. Remember, the prudent diet is not a vegetarian diet. It substitutes complex carbohydrates, fiber, and vitamins for high-fat foods.

Oat Bran and Mega-Niacin Supplements for Lowering Blood Cholesterol

Anderson et al. (1984) supplemented the diets of 20 hypercholesterolemic men with oat bran or beans for 21 days. These food materials are rich in water-soluble fibers. Both supplements decreased total blood cholesterol by 19% ($p < .0005$). The major decrease with both supplements was on LDL (low density) cholesterol.

The vitamin niacin was given in large doses (7-8 g/day) in the large-scale Coronary Drug Project (Coronary Drug Project Research Group, 1975) that lasted for 10 years with more than 8,000 subjects with previous heart attacks. Patients receiving niacin experienced significantly lower mortality than those on placebo or five other drugs. Unfortunately, however, there were unpleasant side effects that ruled out its widespread use.

In a smaller, shorter study, Alderman et al. (1986) slowly increased the dosage from 100 mg/day to 2,000 mg/day. Side effects were again noticed, but they were transient in all but three subjects. The results on blood cholesterol levels were impressive: Total cholesterol fell by 16% and HDL rose by 41%. The investigators suggested that this promising therapy be administered under a physician's direction. Hoeg, Gregg, and Brewer (1986) suggest that niacin be used as the first choice of drugs for reduction of LDL cholesterol.

Additional Risk Factors for Coronary Heart Disease

I have spent many pages detailing the role of cholesterol as a risk factor for heart disease. As you have seen, it is a complicated subject because of the relationship of blood cholesterol to diet: It can be raised by diet and it can be lowered by diet. It exists in the blood in multiple associations with lipoproteins, some of which are considered advantageous, others a threat.

In addition, there is no one concentration of blood cholesterol above which it is generally agreed that it acts as a risk factor, and below which that it does not. Most North Americans are in the range 200–300 mg/dl. All that can be said is that there is some risk at the lower end and considerably more at the upper. Finally, the large-scale epidemiological experiments of recent years have not led to very conclusive results that middle-aged men at the high end would be less susceptible to heart attacks if they decreased their blood cholesterol levels.

Extra Vitamin D as a Contributory Risk Factor for Heart Disease

Any dietary constituent or other condition that tends to increase serum cholesterol may be considered as a contributory risk factor. Blood cholesterol increase is one of the side effects of excess intake of vitamin D. Fleischman, Bierenbaum, Raichelson, Hayton, and Watson (1970) gave seven subjects 1,000 IU of vitamin D each day in addition to their normal diet. After 21 days, the average increase in blood cholesterol was 10 mg/dl ($p < .05$). In four subjects the serum cholesterol rose from 10 to 81 mg/dl, whereas in three subjects it did not change. A survey of infarct patients in Norway found that their average vitamin D intake was 6 times the RDA and significantly higher than age-matched controls (Linden, 1977).

The vitamin D–cholesterol hypothesis was checked in Norwegians in a 4-year prospective study by Vik, Try, Thelle, and Forde (1979). Serum samples from 23 men in the Tromso heart study who had developed myocardial infarctions were analyzed for 25-hydroxy-vitamin D, binding protein for vitamin D, cholesterol, and triglycerides. The values were compared to age-matched controls who had not developed heart attacks. No significant differences in serum levels were found in the vitamin D metabolite and its binding protein or in blood pressure. Serum cholesterol concentration was significantly higher ($p < .05$) in the patients and triglycerides even more so ($p < .0025$). These data do not support the high dietary vitamin D-cholesterol hypothesis.

The data linking vitamin D intake to cardiovascular disease in humans are insufficiently conclusive to place excess vitamin D as a definite risk factor, but they are suggestive. The risks of taking a supplement that contains vitamin D clearly seem to outweigh the benefits. I suggest that each person inventory his or her vitamin D consumption and limit it to a maximum of 400 IU per day.

Because of its close relationship to diet, the cholesterol question has received enormous publicity in the popular press for the past 20 years.

Almost everyone is interested in food and most people are as interested in health; the media has provided an all-out response. In addition, the food industry, which is one of the major industries in the country, has a huge stake in people's eating habits. If research results suggest a change away from red meats, for example, the meat producers are interested in not only how sound the data may be, but also how many people will follow the recommendations and whether the grading of meat itself will be affected.

For these reasons, my discussion of cholesterol as a risk factor has been lengthy. But do not equate length with importance. I repeat: The four major risk factors are approximately of equal importance. Recall that hypertension was given a chapter by itself. The two remaining risk factors for heart disease, cigarette smoking and obesity, are also important predictors of heart attacks, but I will discuss them in far less space.

Other dietary constituents, such as insufficient calcium, magnesium, and selenium, have been suggested as risk factors from time to time, and I will also discuss what is known about them. The latest recognized risk factors, stress and overweight, are just now emerging as independent risk factors. These two can also act as contributory risk factors.

In concluding this discussion of risk factors, it is necessary to state that there is a good probability that the list is yet incomplete. Even though the incidence of heart attacks is decreasing in the U.S., it is still the main killer of middle-aged men, and additional risk factors will probably be identified.

Abnormal ECG Pattern

An abnormal electrocardiogram (ECG), indicative of *left ventricular hypertrophy*, is ranked as the third strongest risk factor in the Framingham 20-year follow-up. This type of hypertrophy often results from chronic, untreated hypertension. It is quite distinct in causation and significance from the left ventricular hypertrophy observed in some athletes.

Abnormalities in the ECG pattern attain greater significance with advancing age. The incidence of sudden death doubles in men aged 45-54 with abnormal ECG-LVH patterns compared to controls. But in older men aged 55-64, who exhibit an abnormal pattern, their risk of sudden death is 12 times greater than for men of the same age with a normal pattern. An abnormal ECG of this type indicates major coronary artery obstruction. Such people should be under medical surveillance.

Cigarette Smoking

Cigarette smoking has been identified as a consistent, strong risk factor for heart disease in all the studies in which this habit has been measured.

There is far more unanimity about the dangers of smoking than there is about the dangers of blood cholesterol. In the Framingham study, for example, those who smoked a pack or more a day were twice as likely to suffer a heart attack as nonsmokers.

Cigarette smoking has received wide publicity as a major risk factor for lung cancer. Unfortunately, it is not as widely known that cigarette smoking is responsible for more deaths per year due to heart disease than due to cancer. According to Dr. Jesse Steinfeld (1984), formerly Surgeon General of the U.S., smoking is the number one public health problem in this country. He states that smoking is involved in more than 350,000 premature deaths per year: 170,000 from coronary heart disease, 130,009 from cancer, and 50,000 from chronic, obstructive lung disease.

One of the encouraging statistics in recent years is that among U.S. adult men, the number of smokers has decreased from 38% to 33% between 1980 and 1983. The number of smokers among women, however, has decreased much less, from 29.8% to 29.0% during the same period. These figures have some interesting implications for male–female longevity predictions. There seems to be a widespread belief that women live longer than men because they are the stronger sex. Enstrom (1984) has calculated that the life expectancy of North American women exceeds that of men by 6.2 years at age 35. Among nonsmokers, the difference in longevity is about 4 years. Thus smoking may explain about half of the male/female differences in longevity up to the present. In fact, Miller and Gerstein (1984) suggest that, if accidental deaths are also taken into account, there is very little difference in longevity between the sexes.

Statistics on Smoking, Coronary Heart Disease, and Mortality. A number of studies have shown that there is a dose-response relationship between number of cigarettes smoked, number of years a person has smoked, and risk of coronary heart disease. Risk decreases when a person quits smoking. A serious complication of smoking is that it acts synergistically with other risk factors for heart disease and with exposure to airborne pollutants, such as asbestos, to severely decrease longevity. Sudden cardiac death is more common among smokers than nonsmokers. Two-packs-a-day smokers run 8 times the risk of dying from *atherosclerotic aortic aneurisms* than nonsmokers.

Lung Disease. Cigarette smoking is a major cause of lung diseases such as bronchitis and emphysema in both sexes. Smokers miss more days from work and stay longer in hospital for respiratory illnesses than nonsmokers (Steinfeld, 1984).

Effects of Smoking on Women. Women who use oral contraceptive pills are at higher risk of myocardial infarction if they also smoke. Among 55 women who had a heart attack before age 50, the proportion of smokers was 89% compared to 55% among nonsmokers ($p < .001$) (Surgeon

General of the U.S., 1979). In another study, women who smoked about two packs a day but who were not on the pill had an infarction rate 20 times higher than nonsmokers. About 14% preterm deliveries in the U.S. are to mothers who smoke. Smoking mothers have about twice as many low-birthweight babies as nonsmokers.

Smoking Magnifies the Risk in Coronary-Prone Families. As mentioned above, the synergistic effect of smoking with other risk factors or other environmental conditions is well recognized. It is also recognized that the members of some families have a tendency to develop early coronary disease. Hopkins, Williams, and Hunt (1984) have examined the prevalence of the risk factors of smoking, hypertension, hypercholesterolemia, obesity, diabetes, and stroke on the incidence of early coronary disease in Utah families with known susceptibility to heart disease compared to controls with no documented susceptibility.

The investigators found a magnified risk of smoking among the first degree relatives of those who had died of coronary disease by age 45. These effects of smoking were unique; they were not shared with the other risk factors in this group of people. In other words, if you have a close relative who died of a heart attack before age 45, smoking will increase your risk of having a heart attack 3 times higher than it would be for the general population.

How Smoking Leads to Heart Attacks. Because smoking is such a popular habit, many lives could be saved if it could be made less dangerous. If we knew what chemicals in cigarette smoke were poisonous, it might be possible to remove them by some means and place the habit in the same innocuous category as chewing gum or drinking weak tea.

A number of carcinogens have been identified in tobacco smoke, but discussing them is not relevant here. The two chemicals identified to date as contributory risk factors in heart disease are nicotine and carbon monoxide. How each leads to heart damage can be paraphrased from Ben Franklin in the line, A little poison may breed great mischief.

The effects of nicotine on the heart are indirect. Nicotine stimulates the discharge of the catecholamines epinephrine and norepinephrine. Heart rate and blood pressure both are increased by these hormones. As a result, cardiac oxygen demand is increased but not its supply. Blood platelet adhesiveness is also increased. This effect can lead to vascular obstruction that results in *ischemia*, a deficiency of blood circulation to the heart. Arrhythmias that may lead to a fatal fibrillation are also favored.

The effects of carbon monoxide are also indirect and just as lethal. This gas displaces oxygen from hemoglobin so that the major effect is hypoxia (a lack of oxygen) for an organ that needs a continuous supply in order to function. The heart cells shift to anaerobic glycolysis to synthesize ATP, lactic acid accumulates, and the excess acid depresses cellular contractility.

In addition, heart mitochondria are very sensitive to oxygen lack, and their ability to synthesize ATP by aerobic reactions is impaired. Heart damage is the end result. You may recall from chapter 7 that a muscle can only work for a very limited time under anaerobic conditions. When it becomes exhausted, people are forced to rest. The heart muscle responds similarly, but the result may be fatal. All organs and tissues of our bodies are dependent on a beating heart to provide them with the oxygen and energy supplies for their aerobic metabolism. If only part of the heart dies, it is called a myocardial infarction, and if the person is lucky, he or she may recover from it.

A person may have developed a degree of atherosclerosis that partially restricts blood flow to the heart, but not sufficiently to result in a heart attack. Smoking, by acting through the mechanisms mentioned above, may be the last straw, which results in an infarction.

Filter-tip cigarettes that remove much of the tar and nicotine have become very popular in the U.S. and Canada. Many smokers believe that they have decreased their risks of disease by smoking this type. What is the evidence on this question? Steinfeld (1984) states that there is no good evidence that smoking low-tar and nicotine cigarettes protects a smoker from cardiovascular diseases. But what about reducing the risks? Castelli et al. (1981) found no difference in the incidence of heart disease in the Framingham study between the smoker of regular cigarettes and the smoker of filter-tip cigarettes.

Hammond, Garfinkel, Seidman, and Lew (1976), in a large-scale, 12-year study, recorded the number of deaths from CHD in men and women who smoked both low-tar and nicotine (low T/N) and high-tar and nicotine (high T/N) cigarettes. When the subjects were matched according to the number of cigarettes smoked per day, the deaths from CHD were consistently lower (about 14%) among the low T/N smokers than among high T/N. However, the deaths from CHD were 737 among the low T/N smokers who smoked 20-39 cigarettes a day, and 671 among the high T/N smokers who smoked 1-19 cigarettes a day ($p < .05$). Heavy smoking more than offsets the effects of low T/N for CHD. In contrast, deaths from CHD among nonsmokers were 1,008 compared to 1,674 among low T/N smokers ($p < .0001$).

In a more recent study, Benowitz et al. (1983) concluded that smokers of low T/N cigarettes do not consume less nicotine. These workers compared the amount of nicotine ingested by people who smoked low T/N cigarettes and by those who smoked high T/N brands. There was no difference. Apparently, the smoking machines that produce the smoke from which the tar and nicotine content is estimated, and the results of which are highly advertised, do not mimic the manner in which people smoke. The authors conclude, "Advertisements from cigarette manufacturers suggesting that smokers of low-yield cigarettes will be exposed to less tar and nicotine are misleading" (p. 141). These data demonstrate that smoking is a most unsafe habit. Young nonsmokers are advised not to start smoking, and older smokers are advised to quit.

In this section I have documented the effects of smoking cigarettes on coronary heart disease in some detail because I feel that this subject has not been sufficiently publicized compared to the effects of smoking on lung cancer. Actually, the mortality from smoking is considerably greater in heart disease. Another important point concerns the effects of quitting smoking on the incidence of the two diseases. The mortality of heart disease due to smoking falls much faster after quitting than the mortality of lung cancer.

In summary, I suggest that one of the most positive actions that a person can take towards health and wellness is to refrain from smoking.

Obesity and Heart Disease

Two large-scale surveys, the Build and Blood Pressure Study (Metropolitan Life Insurance Co., 1959) and the American Cancer Society (ACS) Survey (Lew & Garfinkel, 1979), both reported significant correlations between overweight/obesity and mortality from various diseases including heart disease in both men and women. The earlier study covered over 4.5 million insured Americans over the period 1935-1954. The ACS research was a long-term prospective study of over 750,000 men and women drawn from the general population over the period 1959-1972. It was the first weight–mortality study to take smoking habits into account. These valuable surveys on free-living subjects, although strongly suggesting a causative link between overweight and disease mortality, are more like ecological studies (Table 3.1) because of so many uncontrolled variables. The conclusions could suggest overweight/obesity as a risk factor for CHD, but their relative credibility is low.

Before obesity could be included with the accepted risk factors for coronary heart disease, data from a more controlled study were required. The 26-year follow-up from the Framingham Heart Study has provided such data (Hubert, Feinleib, McNamara, & Castelli, 1983). Sophisticated statistical analyses showed that the Metropolitan Relative Weight, or percentage of desirable weight on initial examination, predicted 26-year incidence of coronary heart disease in men independent of age, cholesterol, systolic blood pressure, cigarettes, left ventricular hypertrophy, and glucose intolerance. Relative weight in women was also demonstrated as an independent risk factor for a variety of coronary diseases. Any weight gain after the young adult years conveyed an increased risk of cardiovascular disease for both sexes. The folklore that it is natural and therefore healthy to gain weight as we age has been discredited by these studies. Insofar as heart disease and health-wellness are incompatible to some degree, avoidance of overweight/obesity is advisable.

The Framingham conclusions utilized the 1959 Metropolitan Weight Table in which the term *desirable body weight* is the weight associated with the lowest mortality (Build and Blood Pressure Study, 1959). Table 8.1A lists these weight ranges for men and women over 25. The Framingham calculations used the midpoint of the medium frame as their basis. Overweight is defined as 10%–20% above the median weight for a given height and obesity as over 20% above the median weight. Another Build Study was completed in 1979 and has led to a somewhat increased weight associated with the lowest mortality (Metropolitan Life Foundation, 1983). Based on the Framingham results, I think it advisable to stay with the 1959 table.

Apart from total obesity, the location of the fat depots have been found to correlate with the risks of heart disease. Having a pot belly is more dangerous than excess fat in the lower body. Measure the circumference of your waist and hips. The risk of heart disease increases if a woman's waist/hips ratio is over 0.8/1.0 and if a man's waist is bigger than his hips. There is little doubt that childhood obesity increases the chances of males' developing plaques early, to say nothing of the other complications of fatness that I mentioned in chapter 8. For these reasons, I have included a table of desirable weights for boys and girls as Table 8.1B.

Type A Behavior and Your Heart

Every affection of the mind that is attended with either pain or pleasure, hope or fear is the cause of an agitation whose influence extends to the heart.

> William Harvey, 1628
> De Motu Cordis

Type A behavior was discussed in chapter 7 as an example of stress mismanagement. I also discussed the importance of recognizing that form of behavior and learning to control it as an essential factor in achieving wellness. Type A behavior was originally suggested by Drs. Friedman and Rosenman (1974) as a risk factor for heart disease. In this section I'll present their original hypothesis and their experimental results to test the hypothesis, and show how it has been modified by subsequent research.

The Hypothesis: Personality Type as a Risk Factor

Friedman and Rosenman became dissatisfied with the results of their advising patients to avoid heart attacks according to the usual suggestions of cutting down on saturated fats, cholesterol, and salt in the diet; smoking less; exercising more; and keeping their weight in line. They were painfully aware that the predictive value of the four risk factors for an individual was almost nil. Blood cholesterol concentration, especially, although showing a significant correlation with heart disease when applied to populations, showed no correlation when applied to individuals. The two San Francisco cardiologists felt that something was missing in the standard medical approach to the prevention of heart disease.

Predictability was mentioned in chapter 3 as a critical procedure in evaluating hypotheses. One of the key tests of the risk factor concept was assessing the accuracy of predicting heart attacks in men in different populations and under different conditions than the one where the risk factors were originally measured. As we have seen, the four major risk factors passed this test with sufficiently high correlations to gain credibility. The accuracy of the predictions, however, was still low enough to allow the possibility that additional risk factors might be operating.

Friedman and Rosenman observed that many of their patients with heart disease had certain personality characteristics in common. These men were unconsciously stressing themselves, day in, day out, for years. The two cardiologists suspected that there might be a cause–effect relationship between the behavior of these men and their susceptibility to heart disease. This is another example of a clinical observation's serving as the basis of a hypothesis that could be tested in an experiment. The rest of this section will describe the first 25 years' history of the hypothesis and its development and evolution as more experimental data have become available from human epidemiological studies, as well as from animal experiments.

Testing the Type A Hypothesis

The first step in checking the hypothesis was to measure carefully the behavior characteristics of patients. To this end, Friedman and Rosenman devised the *structured interview*, a series of questions that probed a person's behavior under challenging (stress-inducing) conditions. Friedman and Rosenman postulate that it is the extreme Type A person who is most at risk of heart disease, and accordingly, they have focused on procedures to identify Type A.

In their first major report of assessing the effects of personality type on physiological measurements, Friedman and Rosenman selected three groups of men, aged 30-60 years. The first group consisted of 83 Type A men; the second of 83 Type B men; and the third, Type C, which was similar to Type B but included a chronic state of anxiety or insecurity. This last group consisted of 46 unemployed blind men. In addition to the psychological classification, the men were asked to keep a dietary diary that included alcohol consumption for 7 days. From these diaries, calculations were made of total calories, protein, carbohydrate, fat, animal fat, and percentage of total calories as fat. All the men were consuming a typical American high-fat diet of 46% of total calories as fat, most of which was animal (i.e., largely saturated fat).

Personal habits, such as number of cigarettes smoked per day, physical activities, hours worked per week, and hours of sleep per night were also recorded. Extreme Type A men smoked more than Type B men (26 cigarettes per day compared to 13), drank more alcohol (200 kcal per day compared to 144), and were more physically active (11 hours per week compared to 7). The kinds of physical activities were not specified and thus it is impossible to estimate whether the difference is significant. In any event, it tends to favor the Type A men.

Blood samples were analyzed for total cholesterol, and clotting time was also determined. Serum cholesterol in Type A men averaged 253 mg/dl, significantly higher than 215 mg/dl in Type B and 220 mg/dl in Type C. There was no significant difference in clotting time. The blood cholesterol results are very interesting in that they show a large difference that is independent of total fat and source of fat in the diet but does correlate with personality type.

As mentioned above, the Type A subjects were significantly higher in average blood cholesterol concentration and in smoking than either Types B or C. It is not surprising then that Friedman and Rosenman found clinical coronary disease 7 times more frequent in the Type A group than in the other two groups. They attribute these differences in risk factors and occurrence of coronary disease to the differences in behavior patterns.

In considering levels of blood cholesterol in individual Type A men in relation to incidence of heart disease, the investigators found that approximately the same percentage had heart disease with blood cholesterols below 250 mg/dl as those with blood cholesterols above 250 mg/dl. This lack of correlation between blood cholesterol concentration and predictable heart disease in individuals is well known (Stamler, 1978). A blood cholesterol in the range 200-300 mg/dl has no predictive value for an individual. It only holds for populations. In fact, it was this lack of correlation between risk factors and future incidence of heart disease in individuals that encouraged Friedman and Rosenman to attempt to identify other risk factors in the first place.

They also investigated familial tendency towards heart disease. If a man in the first group had heart disease, as had his father, their personalities and behaviors were recalled to be similar. However, the majority of Type A men with heart disease had no parental history of it. In the Type B group the lack of correlation of parental tendency for heart disease was even more impressive. None of the 23 men with positive parental history exhibited clinical CHD.

As might be expected, the Type A personality hypothesis of Friedman and Rosenman created quite a stir in heart disease research circles. Suddenly, there was a new risk factor to evaluate. But the hypothesis was far from proved. Even though the Friedman and Rosenman paper of 1959 appeared to be carefully planned and carried out, it did not include blood pressure measurements, and, more seriously, it was a retrospective study. In the work referred to above, the data were obtained from subjects who already had heart disease. As was mentioned in chapter 3, the conclusions of retrospective studies are necessarily weaker and less conclusive than prospective ones, because fewer variables are controlled. Accordingly, the San Francisco researchers set up a prospective study of over 3,000 men. It is known as the Western Cooperative Group Study. Rosenman, Brand, Sholtz, and Friedman (1976) presented their 8-year follow-up in 1976 and evaluated the data by the same sophisticated statistical method that the Framingham workers had used. The statistical analysis confirmed Type A behavior pattern as an independent risk factor for coronary disease.

Men classified as Type A by the structured interview, however, are not as coronary prone as might be imagined. In the Western Cooperative Group Study, for example, it was found that 65%–70% of Type A men were symptom free (Chesney and Rosenman et al., 1982). In other words, Type A classification tends to overestimate the numbers of men who will experience heart attacks. It is not selective enough. In technical parlance, its percentage of false positives is too high. Researchers are now attempting to identify and remove those components of the structured interview that have no predictive value for heart disease.

Other Assessments of Type A Behavior

The results I've summarized so far were all obtained under the supervision of Friedman and Rosenman using the structured interview as the means of distinguishing Type A from Type B men. The results were consistent and statistically significant. As I mentioned in chapter 3, however, an observation is not considered a fact in science until it has been confirmed in a second laboratory by other scientists. The reason for this caution is that it rules out personal bias or subjectivity in obtaining the results and interpreting them. I've already mentioned that the structured interview contains a large degree of subjectivity in the ways it is administered and in scoring the results.

The Friedman-Rosenman group recognized these limitations and collaborated in developing a second test called the Jenkins Activity Survey (Jenkins, Rosenman and Friedman, 1967), a self-reported written test of 50 questions about behavior. It provides a continuous range of scores in distinguishing Type A from Type B behavior. The test scores are based solely on content of the answers. The Jenkins survey differs from the structured interview in that the latter is based on the interviewer's evaluation of the actual behavior of the subject under stressful conditions whereas the Jenkins survey is scored according to how the subject thinks he would act under similar conditions.

The Jenkins Activity Survey has been applied to numerous groups to determine whether correlations exist between those subjects who experienced some type of heart disease and Type A classification. Positive associations were observed in many retrospective studies. The Chicago Heart Association sponsored a large-scale study of over 4,000 people aged 25–64, of both sexes, that compared the incidence of Type A to incidence of heart attacks (Shekelle, Schoenberger, & Stamler, 1976). When the risk factors of age, cholesterol, blood pressure, and cigarette smoking were controlled statistically, Type A score correlated significantly and positively with heart disease. In an important prospective study, Jenkins, Zynzanski, and Rosenman (1978) found that men scoring in the top third of the Type A scores experienced 1.7 times as many heart attacks as those in the lowest third.

A third test is called the Framingham Type A scale and consists of 10 questions that relate to time urgency and competitiveness (Haynes, Feinleib, & Kannel, 1980). In the Framingham study, the association of Type A behavior with heart disease in men occurred only in those holding white-collar jobs. Their risk of developing CHD was 2.5 times greater than Type B men ($p = .04$). The chances of Type A men developing other symptoms of coronary disease was also increased compared to Type B. Although the incidence of heart disease for women was lower than it was for men, CHD incidence was 2.5 times greater among Type A housewives aged 45-64 than for Type B housewives in the same age group ($p = .02$).

The authors also found that Type A behavior increased the risk of heart disease above that calculated on the basis of the other recognized risk factors. It appears that Type A behavior intensifies the effects of the usual coronary risk factors. In other words, a person with one or more of the identified risk factors for heart disease is at much greater risk than previous studies would predict if he or she also exhibits Type A behavior.

Correlations Among the Three Tests

Each of the three psychological tests mentioned above is self-consistent. By this I mean that, if the same population is tested more than once by the same test, consistent results are obtained. Unfortunately, if the three tests were to be administered to the same population, the results would not pick out the same individuals at risk. The Jenkins Activity Survey and the Framingham Type A test classifications agree with those of the structured interview in predicting types of heart disease in middle-class men at only 10%–20% above chance levels. These results suggest that the three tests are measuring different aspects of Type A behavior. Here, we have an interesting example of how a lack of a correlation in measuring a particular behavior by different procedures has led to a new understanding that certain kinds of behavior included in Type A may exert specific kinds of damage to the cardiovascular system. The structured interview is more accurate at predicting those subjects who will have myocardial infarction, and the Jenkins is more accurate at predicting those who will develop angina pectoris.

Control: External and/or Internal

Controlling their environment, which includes other people, is one of the outstanding characteristics of Type A behavior persons. There are certain situations, however, over which a person has no control. These psychosocial factors, such as death of a family member, divorce, loss of a job, and retirement, are recognized as stressful life events for many people. Recent studies suggest the Type A individuals respond to these events with more sickness and heart attacks than Type B individuals. According to Glass (1977), Type A subjects are engaged in a perpetual struggle to retain control. They attempt to avoid anxiety in coping with situations and people by gaining mastery over them. If these attempts to control their environment are unsuccessful, Type As give up and act helpless. Glass proposes that the cycle of active coping and controlling followed by giving up when their efforts are unsuccessful is correlated with large fluctuations in the secretion of catecholamines by the sympathetic nervous system. These on-off cycles of secretion are now thought to act as important factors in the development of atherosclerosis.

Even though one cannot control stressors in the environment, one can learn to control, or, better yet, to avoid the internal stress that they generate. These techniques, which fall under the general term of *stress management*, involve applying muscle relaxation procedures or types of meditation during or immediately after a strenuous session.

Self-Assessment of Behavior Type

Friedman and Rosenman (1974) devote a number of pages in their book to self-assessment techniques. How many of us go through life playing a role with no understanding of why we do the things we do, and no insight into the reasons behind people's reactions to us? The objective of self-assessment questionnaires is to increase self-awareness, give us insight into the motivations of our own actions, and help us seek other bases for ego-justification than the subjective rationalizations that we have relied on heretofore. Obviously, this objective is a very large order. A serious look into one's psyche may accomplish far more than preventing a heart attack.

Type As Recognize That They Are Type As

Herman, Blumenthal, Black, and Chesney (1981) investigated the question whether Type As recognize that they are Type As. A list of adjectives, both characteristic and uncharacteristic of Type A behavior, was submitted to Type A and Type B individuals, as determined by structured interview. The authors found a significant correlation between the Type A individuals' description of themselves and their characteristics, as described by interview. Interestingly, there was less agreement between the two assessments in the less socially acceptable behaviors. For example, many Type As are unaware of their hostility, drivenness , and egocentricity. These exceptions are important because, as we shall see, there is a closer relationship between hostility and subsequent risk of heart disease than any other single characteristic yet identified.

Correlations Between Specific Behaviors and Types of Damage to the Cardiovascular System

Recall that in the Framingham study and in most others heart disease was defined as any one of four conditions: sudden death, as confirmed by autopsy; acute myocardial infarction, a severe damage to a part of the heart muscle; silent infarction, a specific kind of heart arrhythmmia as measured by an electrocardiogram as the only symptom; and angina pectoris, a pain in the chest after exertion. Also recall that the original definition of Type A behavior contained about six factors, three or more of which placed a person at risk of a heart attack. It was soon realized that the three procedures of measuring Type A behavior could predict heart disease in the overall sense, but that they did not agree on how the individuals within the sample population would be affected. In an attempt to overcome this deficiency, Matthews, Glass, Rosenman, and Bortner (1977) ranked the different elements of Type A behavior and found that some were more accurate predictors of heart disease than others. The most accurate ones were competitive drive, impatience, vigorous voice characteristics, and free-floating hostility (quick to anger). It is now recognized that specific behaviors within the Type A behavior pattern were affecting types of heart disease to different extents.

In a large-scale, 4-year prospective study, Jenkins, Zynzanski, and Rosenman (1978) analyzed the behaviors of coronary-prone males using the Jenkins Activity Survey and related them to three types of heart disease: angina pectoris, silent myocardial infarction, and acute myocardial infarction. Future angina patients indicated by their answers that they had a low sense of time urgency and were openly competitive in many activities, including sports and games. They became highly upset when their favorite team lost. They reacted vigorously to environmental stimulation and frustration. They were irritated when interrupted while speaking but denied losing their temper. At work, they were active and responsible. Many of them held two or more jobs simultaneously for more than 4 years. They tended to take over a job they saw being done less well or more slowly than they could do it. Although not being late to appointments was important for them, they did not consider themselves as rushing or hurrying more than other men.

Apparently proneness to angina pectoris is easier to predict than future infarction. In a prospective Israeli study of 10,000 men, Goldbourt and Medalie (1977) found that future angina patients reported more life problems, were more anxious, and reacted more vigorously to environmental stressors than either a healthy control group, or a future myocardial infarction group. Similar results were obtained with the Framingham Type A scale. Haynes et al. (1980) could predict angina pectoris with much greater accuracy than infarction unless the infarction was accompanied by angina.

The potential candidates for an acute myocardial infarction (heart attack) in the Jenkins, Zynzanski, and Rosenman (1978) study exhibited quite different behavior. They found competition on the job stimulating. They were deeply involved in their jobs, often taking shorter vacations than permitted, but even so, looked forward to getting back to work. They were very time conscious. Besides never being late for appointments, they carried work with them so that they could keep busy while waiting for others who might be late. In another study, Ostfeld, Lebovits, Shekelle, and Paul (1964) found that infarction-prone men repressed their emotions and their anxieties more than those susceptible to angina pectoris.

The type of people who are subject to a silent infarction found realistic job deadlines pleasantly stimulating but seldom generated their own. They did not tend to work overtime on their own initiative, but they were often impatient for their vacation to end so that they could get back to work. They were impatient with long, slow talkers and did not hesitate to hurry them along. The characteristics of this behavior pattern are not as clear-cut as for the other two.

Many people have wondered whether Type A behavior is a peculiarity of the U.S. culture. Apparently it extends at least to Western Europe. Kornitzer, Kittel, DeBacker, and Dramaix (1981) interviewed over 19,000 Belgian blue-collar men aged 40–59 years. They found a high correlation between the overall Jenkins Activity Survey scores and the structured interview. Men with known heart disease, mostly angina pectoris, scored higher on the Jenkins total test and on the Jenkins-S (that portion measuring impatience and time urgency) than those with no symptoms of heart disease. Similarly, Appels, Jenkins, and Rosenman (1982) reported that Dutch angina patients scored higher on the total Jenkins questionnaire than normal controls. It is interesting that hard work by itself is not a predisposing factor for heart disease. Cohen (1978) and Simborg (1970) studied Japanese-Americans and reported that the hardworking characteristic unaccompanied by those of hard-driving and competitiveness, is not conducive to heart disease even in Type A subjects.

In summary, these studies definitely suggest that under the Type A umbrella some characteristic behaviors are predictive of an infarction, acute or silent, others of angina pectoris, and still others are not predictive of any type of heart disease. When these characteristics are identified more specifically and can be measured with some precision, a much higher accuracy in predicting heart attacks will have been attained. In this connection, it has already been found that Type B men are relatively immune to developing heart disease, no matter what their blood cholesterol concentrations may suggest.

Hostility: A Life-Shortening Personality Characteristic

Barefoot, Dahlstrom, and Williams (1983) correlated the incidence of heart disease and total mortality with the hostility exhibited by physicians 25 years previously when they were medical students. They found a fivefold higher incidence of heart disease in those with a hostility score above the median compared to those below it. This difference remained highly significant when corrected for smoking, age, family history, and hypertension. An unexpected result was the correlation between hostility and death from all causes. The death rate for physicians whose hostility scores were above the median while in medical school was 6.4 times greater than for those with scores below the median. In other words, the hostile men were dying sooner from other causes in addition to heart disease compared to the less hostile group. These results suggest that hostile students remain hostile as they age and become hostile adults, even when they are members of a high-income profession. In other words, financial success does not neutralize a deep-lying hostility.

Degrees of hostility were also correlated with subsequent heart disease in a prospective study of over 1,800 men employed at the Western Electric Company in Chicago (Shekelle, Gale, Ostfeld, & Paul, 1983). After 10 years, the incidence of heart disease, either an infarction or death, was significantly lower in those in the lowest fifth in hostility ranking compared to the middle fifth. Hostility remained as an independent risk factor when the data were corrected for the effects of smoking, age, blood pressure, cholesterol level in the blood, and intake of alcohol. In addition to heart disease, hostility had a significant correlation with death from all causes over a 20-year span. The men who scored in the highest fifth grouping of hostility had a 42% greater risk of death than those who scored in the lowest fifth.

Williams et al. (1980) at Duke University found that the behavioral characteristic of hostility correlated much higher with atherosclerosis than the overall Type A behavior pattern. Williams (1984) reviewed the work of the Duke University group on analyzing what the hostility questions were actually measuring. They carried out a factor analysis of the questions and came to the conclusion that the term cynicism, a mistrust of other people and their motives, was a more accurate description of the personality type than was hostility. They suggest that cynicism lies at the root of the hostile personality. This is an illustrative example of how hypotheses succeed each other in the course of research. Type A was followed by hostility as a major factor connecting behavior to heart disease, and this, in turn, may be succeeded by that of cynicism. And at the end of this succession of hypotheses is the question, what mechanism connects attitude-behavior to heart disease?

Correlations Between Type A Behavior and Occlusion of Coronary Arteries

Infarctions and sudden death are end results of the process of atherosclerosis. If there is a correlation between Type A behavior and heart disease, it should also be evident if the internal size (diameter) of the coronary arteries are measured. In fact, these measurements, which are obtained from *angiograms*, can be performed more than once, and the progression of the disease process can be followed directly on living people. This procedure is invasive and slightly dangerous; thus it is ordinarily only utilized on patients with known coronary atherosclerosis. Progression was defined as an increase of occlusion of 25% or more, or progression to total occlusion in any vessel.

The results obtained by Krantz, Sanmarco, Selvester, and Matthews (1979), relative to Type A behavior, were difficult to interpret. There was a significant, positive correlation between high scores on the Jenkins Activity Survey and progression of the disease, but not with assessment of Type A by structured interview. Occlusion-progression patients tended to score extremely high on the Jenkins survey and were very unlikely to score as Type Bs. For example, 86% of those whose occlusion progressed were classified as Type A, compared to 36% of the unchanged group ($p = .04$). Although the interview data were in the same direction, the correlation was too low to be statistically significant ($p = .21$). With regard to other factors, nonprogression patients (a desirable result) were rated more active in exercise ($p < .05$).

Five other studies have compared the extent of narrowing of these arteries with either the structured interview or with the Jenkins survey. Again the results were mixed. The interview produced a significant correlation in two studies and was negative in two, whereas the Jenkins survey was significant in one and nonsignificant in four. These negative results cannot be dismissed lightly. They are reported by competent, respected research scientists from well-known medical centers. Dimsdale,

Hackett, Hutter, and Block (1980) suggest that Type A pattern may not be as virulent for some populations as it is for others. For example, the Kaiser-Permanente study (G.D. Friedman et al., 1974) had a large black contingent, and the Dimsdale et al. (1980) report contained large numbers of Irish and Italian Catholics. Type A behavior may not be as damaging to the arteries in these groups compared to white Protestants due to the influence of factors as yet unknown.

In a very interesting study, Scherwitz et al. (1983) assessed 150 men for Type A behavior prior to coronary angiography. They found no relationship between Type A behavior and the extent of coronary artery disease. They did find, however, that the number of times a person used self-references (e.g., I, me, my) in answering the questions in the structured interview correlated positively with the extent of coronary artery disease and the number of previous heart attacks.

A more recent study by Kahn et al. (1982) used a noninvasive technique that utilized thallium-201 in myocardial perfusion studies. For patients without reported infarction, coronary artery disease severity was positively correlated with overall Type A as determined by structured interview. For patients with diagnosed coronary disease, severity was significantly correlated with job involvement only. Progression of occlusion was not estimated in this study.

Dembroski, MacDougall, Williams, Haney, and Blumenthal (1986) used the structured interview in a group of patients with various degrees of coronary artery disease to ascertain which components of the Type A pattern related to the severity of the disease as determined by angiographic methods. In contrast to Kahn et al. (1982), they found no correlation between global Type A and extent of disease. Of all Type A attributes measured, only potential for hostility (free-floating hostility) and anger-in (repressed anger) were significantly and positively associated with disease severity.

In recent years it has become evident that, although the Type A behavior hypothesis originally served a very valuable function in directing attention to this neglected area, it is being refined and extensively modified. The passing of the Type A behavior hypothesis as a global predictor of who will develop heart disease serves as another example that the only thing certain in scientific explanations is change, the continuation of uncertainty.

Reversing Type A Behavior Can Help Prevent a Subsequent Heart Attack

On reading M. Friedman and Rosenman's (1974) chapters on altering the Type A behavior pattern, I was impressed by the difficulties and length of time they implied it would take to produce a significant change. This conclusion was reinforced when I began looking at my own behavior from this standpoint and attempted to change some of my long-practiced habits. It is possible, even probable, that many Type A people will require professional help in achieving a significant change.

One of the few research studies on this subject was carried out by M. Friedman et al. (1982) on over 1,000 men, average age 53 ± 6.5 years, who already had experienced a myocardial infarction. More than 98% of the subjects were classed as moderate-to-severe Type A based on a structured interview. The subjects were divided into three groups: a control group that was examined and interviewed annually; a group that received cardiologic counseling on the usually accepted coronary risk factors; and a third group who, in addition to the cardiologic counseling, received advice and instruction on how to diminish the intensity of their Type A behavior.

The results at the end of the first year of a 5-year study suggested that behavioral counseling of postinfarction patients was effective in decreasing the number of subsequent heart attacks compared to the other two groups. There was significantly less ($p < .05$) nonfatal infarction in the behavioral-cardiologic counseled group than in either the group that was cardiologic counseled solely or the control group. The cardiovascular death rate was also significantly lower in the two counseled groups compared to the control group. The behavior-therapy patients showed significant changes away from Type A actions on both the structured interview and self-report measures. With regard to the specific Type A characteristic of hostility, patients who had a subsequent heart attack showed higher scores than those who had no recurrence. These results are very encouraging in showing that intervention programs are effective in decreasing subsequent heart attacks. The results also suggest that certain Type A behaviors, such as hostility, may be considered as definite risk factors for heart attacks, whereas other behaviors are not, or are much less so.

The 3-year cumulative results were reported by M. Friedman et al. (1984) in the American Heart Journal and showed even greater differences. The Type A behavior counseled group exhibited a 44% reduction in heart attacks compared to the control group ($p < .005$). These results indicate that significant components of Type A behavior can be altered in middle-aged men and that the effects of the behavior change are reflected in a decreased rate of heart attacks.

Skill at Coping Decreases Heart Attacks

It is obvious that, if a person is unaware of a negative behavior characteristic such as hostility or talking too much or too loudly, he or she will be unable to correct it. Those people who are aware of their behavioral faults will be in a much stronger position to cope and to correct the behavior if they choose. In addition to noting the practical aspects of getting along better with others, Vickers, Herrig, Rahe, and Rosenman (1981) found that skill at coping decreased the incidence of heart attacks.

The researchers measured coping and defense in 237 pairs of male twins (avg. age 48 years). Adequate coping depends on undistorted perceptions of the environment, feelings, and motives. These people analyze their problem-field accurately, and thus their actions are sensible. This description amounts to a definition of coping. Defenses, in contrast, result from inaccurate or distorted perceptions of what is happening in the environment. The decisions based on these distortions tend to be ineffectual and unsound. These people tend to misinterpret what is going on around them, and consequently actions are often inappropriate. If their decisions and/or actions affect someone besides themselves, or if they stick to a decision that others may have disagreed with, they may be questioned more or less critically as to why or how they reached such a decision. These questions may act as a signal for an increase in defense. They may respond angrily, leave in a huff, or at the other extreme attempt to shout down the opposition. Insecure persons may interpret criticisms of their judgments as a personal affront or insult. The problem is no longer the most logical interpretation of the data or facts that are available in reaching a decision, but what interpretation is most satisfying to the persons's self-esteem.

High defenses are like a high stone wall that protects the ego from the arrows of criticism. But the wall also shuts off other stimuli and makes an accurate reading of what is going on outside more difficult. We all differ in our perceptions of reality, but if one person maintains that he or she is right and others are wrong on a serious question and no discussion is allowed because it might hurt someone's feelings, anger and hostility can be predicted as a likely outcome.

Imagine driving a car with a malfunctioning speedometer, which indicates 50 mph when the car is actually traveling at 75 mph and comparably low at other speeds. On the freeway or straight road, the error may not be serious; but on a mountain road with many curves and hills, the error may result in a dangerous accident. Suppose you are the driver who believes that the speedometer readings are accurate, but your companion who is sitting in the passenger seat has another, and accurate, means of ascertaining the speed of the car. The argument could become quite heated before an accident occurred. People with high defenses are also living dangerously, for themselves as well as for their friends and associates.

Now we come to a watershed conclusion and a possible explanation of why all Type As are not subject to heart disease. Not all Type A behaviors may be defensive; some may imply adequate or even high coping. A high score on the Jenkins Activity Survey relating to job involvement indicates a high investment in work, concern about the job, motivation to do well, career planning, and so on. These characteristics add up to planning ahead to achieve goals and to finding the work challenging and interesting. In terms of coping and defense, a person with these characteristics would be considered to be coping adequately and well. He or she might be seldom exposed to unpleasant situations and his or her defenses would be low most of the time. Such people are not at high risk of heart attacks.

A high score on the speed and impatience questions implies a tendency to hurry, feel time pressure, and be annoyed with anything that distracts from achieving goals. These behavior characteristics reflect impulsiveness, poor reading of the environment, and thus high defensiveness. People suffering from hurry sickness are at a fairly high risk of heart attacks.

A major stressor may be handled with little or no stress by a person who is able to analyze it coolly, separate its key factors from the incidentals, and deal with the situation objectively. Individuals are like canoes. If an adult has not learned to paddle because "this is the way I am," has not learned to go with the flow, and cannot distinguish the main current from the back currents, he or she has not learned to cope. Even small waves (stressors) may endanger such a frail craft. Major ones may swamp it.

Other Approaches to Behavior Modification

It seems unrealistic to expect that a person can or will be able to change his or her behavior pattern *in toto*, even with professional counseling. However, if some components of Type A behavior could be shown to be more closely correlated with subsequent heart disease than others, the dangerous behavioral factors could be selected for change. This simplification could be expected to be more readily attainable than attempting to alter all the behavioral components.

Suppose a therapist was treating a woman with strong hostile feelings towards others. According to behavior management principles, the patient might be told to learn to control her hostility by thinking pleasant thoughts, making a conscious effort to relax when in the presence of hostile persons, or as Friedman and Rosenman (1974) suggest, be silent, say as little as possible which I interpret as, don't let your hostility show. These oversimplified suggestions and admonitions may not be very effective. The patient is trying to control her behavior without understanding why she has hostile feelings in the first place. This approach is comparable to fighting all fires with water. Water is commonly used, but there are some fires in which the fire spreads when water is applied. Similarly, my perception of what the media has emphasized about treating stress during the past 20 years is that relaxation is the secret to control. In my opinion, some forms of relaxation—such as TV watching—may help a tense person to relax when alone but are of little help in handling a situation in which the person usually has become angry and hostile.

Thoresen, Telch, and Eagleston (1981) divided the factors in Type A pattern into four mutually interactive categories: cognitive, behavioral, physiologic, and environmental. They call this approach the *cognitive social learning model*. The authors emphasize the cognitive model because they believe that a person's perception of reality, which includes his or her perceptions of himself or herself, are based on such cognition factors.

Therapy based on the cognitive social learning model is more ingenious in developing treatment strategies. The cognitive factors address why the patient feels he or she must vanquish the other person or be defeated himself or herself. Behavioral factors consider the role that angry, verbal outbursts play in achieving objectives. Physiologic factors are used to train the patient to become aware of his or her heart rate, breathing rate, and sweaty palms as predictors of a possible outburst. Through environmental factors the patient becomes aware of what conditions induce him or her to use hostility as a normal reaction to stress. In my opinion, there is no shortcut to controlling hostility, but the cognitive learning model appeals to me because it is based on an analysis of the major factors that comprise the foundation of an individual's behavior. I hope that, with the insight and understanding that is gained with this type of therapy, a person can learn to control his or her behavior. This objective is essential to wellness as well as to the prevention of heart attacks and other diseases.

Jenni and Wollersheim (1979) compared the effectiveness of cognitive therapy with stress management training for reducing the stress associated with Type A behavior. The subjects in this small-scale study were white-collar men and women (average age 42.5), of whom about a third were classified as high Type A and half as moderate Type A by structured interview.

Stress management training involved practice in progressive muscle relaxation. They were taught to recognize early tension cues and to respond with an immediate relaxation procedure. Cognitive therapy also involved recognition of tension cues, but, in addition, the subjects learned to identify the event responsible for the cues and become aware of their thought processes (beliefs or assumptions) in interpreting the event, and to distinguish the reasonable from the unreasonable beliefs. Finally, they learned to eliminate or modify their unreasonable beliefs and/or assumptions and to notice the decrease in tension that resulted. This program may sound difficult, but apparently the subjects learned the techniques of coping on a group basis in one 90-minute session a week for 6 weeks.

The subjects were asked to rate themselves twice: at the end of the experiment, and 6 weeks later by a self-administered rating questionnaire for Type A behavior. The cognitive therapy group was the only one that showed a significant decrease in Type A behavior. Both treatments reduced anxiety levels compared to controls, but neither treatment reduced cholesterol levels in the blood or affected blood pressure.

Holistic (Psychosomatic) Relationships

The effects of anger and hostility occur in more than the mind or the nervous system. These emotions affect the whole person. In this instance, the sympathetic nervous system activates the adrenal glands to secrete large amounts of epinephrine and norepinephrine into the blood. Long-term, chronic hostility can stimulate the secretion of other hormones like cortisol and ACTH. Although the mechanisms are not yet worked out, these hormones provide the linkages that will help explain the effects of stress on the development of atherosclerosis and heart attacks.

Scientists, as detectives, are now vigorously following these leads. What are the mechanisms by which hormones can influence the functioning of coronary arteries? Stimulation of the sympathetic-adrenal system in animals has shown that, as the blood pressure increases, the heart rate and oxygen consumption of the heart also go up, as does the concentration of free fatty acids in the blood. These same effects occur when catecholamines are injected directly into an animal. Thus, to extrapolate to humans, if a person is living under stressful conditions every day and the sympathetic nervous system–adrenal glands are overstimulated, the blood will contain an excess of free fatty acids as well as cholesterol, both of which are independent of diet (Dimsdale, Herd, & Hartley, 1983). The fatty acids may be taken up directly by cells in the arterial walls or converted to triglycerides, which may be deposited in the cells subsequently. These processes may result in the fatty streak, an early step in development of atherosclerosis.

Infarction can be induced by the formation of a *thrombus*, a small mass of clotted blood that can cut off the blood supply to a portion of the heart. Without oxygen and nutrients in the blood, that portion of the heart dies, which is the definition of an infarction. Catecholamine hormones may be involved in thrombus formation by stimulating the aggregation of small white cells in the blood, called platelets. This clump of cells may serve as the starting point of thrombus formation.

Type A Behavior Found Not Linked to Heart Disease

It is disappointing, but perhaps not surprising, that in an area of research as complicated as behavior measurement, inconsistent results would be obtained. A large-scale prospective study of Kaiser-Permanente clients in the San Francisco Bay area found no significant correlation between Type A behavior pattern and subsequent heart disease incidence (by G. Friedman, Ury, Klatsky and Siegelaub, 1974). The reasons for these negative findings are not clear. Shekelle et al. (1985) reported that a 7-year follow-up of 3,110 men participating in the Multiple Risk Factor Intervention Trial (MRFIT) found no difference in the incidence of heart attacks between those classified as Type A and those as near-Type B. The men in this study, however, were selected as a high-risk group, and this factor may have skewed the results towards a different outcome than that obtained when a random population was studied.

Another significant difference is the lack of correlation between the predictions of the structured interview and the Jenkins Activity Survey as to which individuals in a given population will develop heart disease as well as what type of heart disease they will have. These differences clearly indicate that the component characteristics of Type A behavior are not equal in inducing heart disease and that the two tests are not measuring the same components. Because the structured interview overpredicts the number of men who will develop heart disease, it would seem that certain questions are including characteristics that have little or no relationship to heart attacks. Their removal might improve the accuracy of the test.

Connections Between Insecurity, the Necessity for Control, and Living With Uncertainty

You may recall from chapter 3 that I discussed the necessity of scientists' learning to live with uncertainty, and suggested that the lay public should also. In that discussion I didn't specify to what type of uncertainty I was referring. Scientists face the continuing uncertainty about the accuracy of their interpretations of the data that they have obtained. They have concerns that their hypotheses probably will be ignored or refuted. They also face the possibility that some other scientist will beat them to an important discovery. Scientists learn to live with these uncertainties as part of the job.

Notice that I have not included the experiments themselves as part of the uncertainty. Scientists depend on the regularity of nature. A well-performed experiment is repeatable day after day and yields the same results, within experimental error. The expectations of being able to repeat an experiment and obtain the same results as yesterday amounts to a prediction. To predict a result means that the person knows and can control the important variables that are involved in the experiment. By the fifth time an experiment is repeated and yields the same result, the scientist has become confident; his or her insecurity has decreased. He or she has control of the situation.

Now, let's analyze the uncertainties in other human activities. Farmers realize that the weather is probably the most important variable in determining the size of their harvest, and they have no control at all over the weather. They recognize that there are good years and lean years, and if they do their job (that which is under their control) to the best of their ability, they will probably survive and may even prosper. Farmers, as a group, have learned to live with a great deal of uncertainty.

Consider investors who play the market. If they read the *Wall Street Journal*, they can find about six different opinions every day about why the averages are where they are and where they are going. I have often noticed that, when the market goes down, it is explained as being due to uncertainty about the Mideast situation, which way interest rates may go, or how long a major strike may last. I have the impression that uncertainty is the bane of the investment community.

Salespeople of many types have no way of predicting what the next day will bring. The fear of not making a sale for a day or a week could keep a person sleepless for many nights. Yet the successful salespeople whom I know seem to take this type of uncertainty in stride. Experience has given them the confidence that, while one day may be better than another, the market for their product will not suddenly disappear.

In these three examples the participants recognize that they are not in control of the situation. They also recognize that fretting about it will accomplish nothing, and they do not allow themselves to become stressed. In comparison to the others, scientists are lucky. They are finally able to exert control over the unknown. People need to develop enough self-confidence to deal with uncertainty on a continuing basis. This problem presents the most difficulty to the Type A personality.

In real life there are few situations in which one has such complete control as a scientist conducting an experiment. Real-life situations contain uncertainties of both events and people. In addition, real-life situations are usually unique in that they are not repeatable as an experiment. Yet many Type A people attempt to control the behavior and responses of others in real-life situations similarly to a scientist conducting an experiment.

Type As are competitive, achievement oriented, driven to win, and insecure. In this way they hope to influence the outcome to suit their own objectives. But unlike the scientist described above, whose security increases with repeated accurate predictions, Type As remain insecure no matter how many times they win. Their behavior seems independent of their success.

We may not understand or be able to relate Type A behavior or its component behaviors to disease until we can identify their underlying motivation and link them to mechanisms of atherosclerosis. We may continue to find discrepancies in the correlations between Type A behaviors and diseases until we can understand and reverse the insecurity that underlies the pathological behaviors. In my opinion, the search for coronary-prone behavior has just begun.

Physical Activity and Your Heart

Jogging is a fast-growing sport in America. A recent estimate found 20 million joggers, up from 5 million a few years ago. Most people who take up jogging have heard that it is healthy. Those who stay with it discover that it can be fun as well. Jogging has many advantages, such as lack of expensive equipment, convenience, ability to exercise alone, and relatively few hours per week necessary to stay in shape. Its devotees also claim many positive psychological effects: feelings of well-being, greater self-esteem, and less depression. These dividends alone would seem to justify participation in the activity.

But do jogging and other types of active physical activity actually help protect one against heart attacks? Should one assume that exercise promotes healthy hearts because it makes one sweat and is highly recommended by some members of the health professions? Or is the American Puritan tradition influencing behavior with the unconscious *assumption* that sloth and gluttony are bad and a person with enough willpower to avoid them should be rewarded with a longer, healthier life? Should we follow the lead of Robert Hutchins, former President of the University of Chicago? He is reported to have said, "Whenever I feel the urge to exercise, I lie down until it goes away." In this section I'll summarize a number of the studies that have been carried out to answer these questions.

First, I'll explain some of the complications and difficulties in this field. One complication stems from the difficulty of measuring physical activity in quantitative terms. Many studies have used physical activity at work as the prime variable. Others, assuming a sedentary population, have asked about leisure time activities only. The Framingham researchers set up a semiquantitative scale of activity, but they were well aware of its limitations.

In their first study of the effect of physical exercise on incidence of heart attacks, the Framingham group (Kannel, 1967) set up three criteria of lack of physical fitness: obesity, defined as over 20% above desirable weight; a rapid resting pulse of greater than 85/minute; vital capacity, less than 3 l for men and 2 l for women. With these criteria, they found that the most sedentary portion of the Framingham population, those with adverse values for two or more of the above traits, had a fivefold greater mortality from CHD over a 12-year period than those with no adverse traits who were most active.

In the second Framingham study, Kannel et al. (1971) classified each participant according to a *physical activity index*, and its relation to the incidence of CHD over the next 10 years was ascertained. Men classified as most sedentary in each age group had a coronary incidence almost twice that of those who were at least moderately active. Even so, the data were only marginally statistically significant. The authors admit that these studies were marred by an imprecise measure of physical activity. The conclusions are suggestive at best.

The fact that physical activity did not emerge as an independent risk factor for CHD in the studies mentioned above does not exclude the possibility that it may function as one. If physical activity was relatively constant in the Framingham population, it might not surface as a risk factor.

In contrast, the seven-country study of Keys (1970), which included Finnish farmers and lumberjacks who are very active physically, reported that these workers had one of the highest rates of CHD in the world. Can these contradictions be resolved? Subsequent work in Finland has helped to clarify the interdependence of risk factors.

Karvonen, Pekkarinen, Metsälä, and Rautanen (1961a) compared the diets of lumberjacks and farmers with those of less active workers in the county of North Karelia, East Finland. The lumberjacks consumed over 4,700 kcal per day, of which 45% was from fats, mostly saturated. The diet of the more sedentary workers in the same locale contained 2,700 kcal, of which 35% was from fats, mostly saturated. The serum cholesterol values of the two groups did not differ significantly, but both were high, varying from an average of 230 mg/dl in the 20-29 year group and gradually increasing to 280 mg/dl in the 50-59 year group. Despite their enormous fat consumption, the lumberjacks' serum cholesterol was in the same range as the less active men.

In a companion paper, Karvonen, Rautaharju, Orma, Punsar, and Takkunen (1961b) examined the electrocardiograms of the men in each group. They found that the main share of pathological ECGs came from the men in the lighter occupations. It is also interesting that particular waves of the electrocardiograms of the lumberjacks were similar to those of endurance athletes. The authors conclude that the data indicate that heavy exercise, which includes both strength and endurance activities, protects against heart attacks despite large amounts of a high-saturated fat diet.

In recent years, the HDL/LDL ratio has been found to correlate more closely to prevention of CHD than does overall total serum cholesterol level. Insofar as the present generation of lumberjacks works as hard and eats as much as its fathers, it would be interesting to measure its HDL/LDL ratios.

Unless the differences in physical activity at work are tremendous, as in the Finnish study, it is difficult to measure the amount, type, and intensity of exercise in large populations. The Framingham researchers took a first step in overcoming this difficulty by combining certain physiological attributes that have been established as being related to physical activity in a fitness index. Even so, correlating a fitness index directly to incidence of mortality of cardiovascular diseases involves too many *assumptions* to provide convincing conclusions. Measurements of such factors as diet, serum cholesterol level, smoking, blood pressure, height, weight, age, gender, and psychological attitudes are also necessary. If these variables have been measured, their effects on the fitness–disease relationship can be adjusted and estimated individually by statistical methods.

The first large-scale study in which risk factors were measured was conducted by Cooper et al. (1976). They ranked fitness on a scale of 5 based on a treadmill test time score for 3,000 middle-aged men. They found that fitness correlated directly to vital capacity and inversely to resting pulse rate. They also found significant negative correlations between fitness levels and the major CHD risk factors of serum cholesterol concentration and systolic blood pressure, adjusted for age, weight, and percent body fat. The data strongly support the hypothesis that higher levels of physical fitness confer protection against CHD by reducing risk factors.

I consider this work of Cooper et al. as a landmark. It focuses directly on the individual and relates physiological condition to level of risk factors. By measuring cardiovascular fitness directly, it obviates the difficult problem of estimating physical activity. Unfortunately, diet was not measured in this study. It is possible that the more fit men had lower serum cholesterol concentrations because they consumed less saturated fat and total fat than the less fit. However, it seems reasonable that people who work out regularly and whose body fat content is relatively low are oxidizing the fat in their diets, whether saturated or unsaturated, rather than depositing it in their arteries. This idea suggests that endurance-fit people have earned an extra degree of freedom with regard to the total fat and the saturated fat content of their diets.

More recently, the Cooper Clinic group (Gibbons, Blair, Cooper, and Smith, 1983) examined the associations between physical fitness and risk factors for CHD in healthy women 18-65 years. Endurance fitness was determined by a graded treadmill test. The effects of age and weight were adjusted by statistical calculations. The following risk factors were found to be independently associated with fitness: high-density lipoprotein cholesterol (HDL-C) ($p < .001$), total cholesterol/HDL-C ratio ($p \leqslant .001$), blood pressure ($p \leqslant .001$), and cigarette smoking ($p \leqslant .001$).

From these few examples we can see that pioneering work seeks to find correlations between variables. This approach often involves a large number of *assumptions*. As the area of research matures and the assumptions become recognized, they serve as hypotheses to be tested. When the number of untested assumptions becomes as low as the experimental situation allows, competent research work tends to confirm, rather than contradict each other. It will be interesting to see the Cooper approach, amplified to include dietary measurements, applied to other populations and age groups, and correlated to the incidence of cardiovascular diseases.

Calculating the Odds

If people know their serum cholesterol levels in mg/dl, systolic blood pressures, and smoking habits in number of cigarettes per day, they can calculate their relative risk of having a heart attack. The American Heart Association has devised a heart hazard appraisal called *Risko*, which evaluates the four risk factors (overweight, systolic blood pressure, blood cholesterol concentration, and cigarette smoking) for men and women in two age groups. The total score allows the calculation of relative risk for an individual (Appendix 10.A). Note that blood cholesterol is given less weight for males over age 55 but more for females over age 55. Because these four risk factors are largely under the control of each person, we are back to one of the major value judgments of this book: *each individual should take responsibility for his or her own health and take steps to lower the risk.*

Variations of Risk Factors With Age

The media have publicized the role of risk factors in the high incidence of CHD in America. Unfortunately, the publicity has usually omitted mentioning their relative effects on men of different ages. Smoking exerts the greatest influence up to age 50. In the years 50-54 the three factors are of approximately equal importance. In the range 55-59 hypertension becomes 2 1/2 times as important as smoking and about 4 times as important as serum cholesterol level (Pooling Project Research Group, 1978). These numbers suggest that younger men should not smoke and that older ones should control their blood pressure carefully.

How Sound Is the Diet–Heart Hypothesis?

Coronary heart disease is a recognized multifactorial disease, and three major risk factors (an elevated serum cholesterol, hypertension, and cigarette smoking) have been identified. According to the statistical analyses I have seen, they are independent and equal risk factors. However, some authorities believe that cholesterol level is more equal than the other two. Jeremiah Stamler (1978), an outstanding worker in this research area for many years, made the following statement to the American Heart Association in November, 1977:

> Since the data from both animal and human studies, e.g., the Japanese experience—indicate that high blood pressure and cigarette smoking are minimally significant for atherogenesis in the absence of the

nutritional-metabolic prerequisites, it is further reasonable and sound to designate "rich" diet as a *primary, essential, necessary cause* of the current epidemic of premature atherosclerotic disease raging in the Western industrialized countries. Cigarette smoking and hypertension are important secondary or complementary causes. (pp. 10, 11)

This statement is important because of Stamler's influence within the American Heart Association and on official government committees. But, like any scientific generalization, it needs to be critically examined. Does the evidence support his claims, or are they the opinion of an over-enthusiastic specialist?

By the "Japanese experience," Stamler is referring to the low rate of CHD in that country, even though heavy smoking and hypertension are common. The traditional Japanese diet, however, is low in saturated fats and cholesterol so that serum levels above 180 mg/dl are uncommon.

In addition, Stamler quotes data from studies of 47,000 Seventh-Day Adventists in California. The members of this sect are enjoined from drinking alcoholic beverages and smoking. The group contains a high proportion of vegetarians. Thus, by comparing the Adventist nonvegetarians with the general population, the risk of dying from CHD over a 6-year period was only 28% as much for Adventists in the age range 35-64 and 50% as much for Adventists over 65 (Phillips, Lemon, Beeson, & Kuzinaj, 1978). Recall that these impressive reductions in mortality are based on differences in smoking, drinking, and to some extent, diet. Diet itself was evaluated as a risk factor by comparing the CHD incidence rate of vegetarians to nonvegetarians in the Adventist population. They found that the risk of fatal CHD among nonvegetarian males aged 35-64 was 3 times greater than vegetarians in the same age group. The differential was much smaller for persons of either sex over age 65.

This large-scale prospective study seems to have been well conceived and executed. The conclusions support the Stamler position as strongly as epidemiological data can. Even though the data do not prove that a vegetarian diet, which essentially means a diet that is low in saturated fats and cholesterol, is more important than the other risk factors, this conclusion is strongly supported.

The effects of a vegetarian diet on serum cholesterol levels had been studied previously by West and Hayes (1968). Dietary constituents were estimated from a 25-hour food recall. The Adventists as a group showed significantly lower cholesterol values than a typical American population, which was matched as to age, sex, income, and so forth. Further, in the Adventist group itself, the complete vegetarians showed significantly lower serum cholesterol levels than nonvegetarians who consumed meat, fish, or fowl between 1 and 3 times a week. The dietary recall data showed some interesting differences in nutrient consumption. In comparing the vegetarians to the moderate nonvegetarians, the former consumed less total fat (33% vs 37% of total kcal), somewhat fewer calories from saturated fatty acids (11% vs 14%), and about one-half the cholesterol per day (193 mg vs 361 mg). For comparison, the typical U.S. diet has been reported to contain 42% of total kcal from fat, 18% of total kcal from saturated fatty acids, and cholesterol, over 500 mg/day (Gortner, 1975).

The effects of not smoking and drinking have also been estimated in a meat-eating group. In a 2-year retrospective study, Lyon, Wetzler, Gardner, Klauber and Williams (1978) found that the risk of fatal CHD among Mormons in the state of Utah was 35% lower than for non-Mormons.

What can we learn from these studies of two small sects whose lifestyles differ in significant ways from the average American? Because they both abstain from smoking and drinking alcohol, the lower incidence of CHD among the nonvegetarians can be attributed to the absence of these two habits.

In a study of Japanese men living in Hawaii, Yano et al. (1977) found a strong negative association between moderate alcohol consumption (equivalent to one or two highballs or one beer) and the risk of nonfatal heart attacks and death from CHD over a 6-year period. The protective effect of alcohol was correlated with an increase in the HDL/LDL ratio.

I want to emphasize the importance of volume of consumption when summarizing the effects of alcohol on the incidence of heart attacks. The equivalent of two drinks a day is considered protective. Three drinks neutralizes the protective effect of the first two, and as the numbers increase to four or more, the consumption of alcohol becomes a risk factor in itself.

In a follow-up of the Finnish studies mentioned previously, Puska et al. (1983) reported on community-based programs in North Karelia over the period 1972–1982. The objectives were to reduce the heart disease risk factors of smoking, serum cholesterol, and high blood pressure in the general population compared to a matched reference area. In middle-aged males (30-59 years) the effect of the program was estimated as a 28% reduction in smoking ($p < .001$), a 3% reduction in serum cholesterol ($p < .001$), a 3% reduction in systolic blood pressure ($p < .001$), and a 1% reduction in diastolic blood pressure ($p < .05$). In females, the reductions were, respectively, 14% (nonsignificant), 1% (nonsignificant), 5% ($p < .001$), and 2% ($p < .05$).

The effects of these reductions on cardiovascular mortality were reported by Tuomilehto et al. (1986). In North Karelia, the annual decline in mortality from all cardiovascular diseases was 2.9% in men, whereas it was 2.6% in the rest of Finland. In women, the decreases were 6.0% and 5.0%, respectively. The decline in mortality from cardiovascular disease in Finland is now one of the steepest in the world, similar to that found in the U.S. They attribute the greater decline in cardiovascular mortality in North Karelia to the community educational project mentioned above.

The Cholesterol Paradox

In distinction to the excellent correlations between blood cholesterol concentration and incidence of heart attacks in large populations, there is a lack of correlation between these two variables in individuals. Stamler (1978) referred to this situation as the *cholesterol paradox*. By this term he meant that cholesterol analyses of an individual's blood are of little value as predictors of heart attacks for that person. Unfortunately, this information is not widely known by the public or by many health workers.

Changes in blood cholesterol levels occur in individuals that seem independent of diet. Beynen and Katan (1984) have summarized their work on the effect of varying cholesterol in the diet on the levels of blood cholesterol in individuals. In one trial, dietary cholesterol was 120 mg/day, and in another it was 650 mg/day. Katan, Beynen, DeVries and Nobels (1986) found 17 hyper-responding subjects (average increase 22 ± 14 mg/dl) and 15 hypo-responding subjects (average increase 10 ± 12 mg/dl) to the increased amount of cholesterol. Jacobs, Anderson, Hannon, Keys and Blackburn (1983) and Katan and Beynen (1984) have measured similar individual variations in the cholesterolemic responses to changes in the type of dietary fat.

Wilkinson (1957) analyzed blood cholesterol in people over a 2-year period at weekly intervals and found variations as large as 100% within a period of some months. A recent review on measuring blood cholesterol (Roberts, 1987) mentions a study by Hegsted and Nicolosi (1987) that confirms the variations of the older reports. They found a variation as large as 50 mg/100 dl. Practically speaking, variations of this magnitude indicate that the result of any single test is unreliable. Two tests should be considered as routine, and if the results differ by more than 30 mg/dl, additional tests should be conducted until a reliable average is obtained.

On the other hand, if the serum of a male under age 70 contains over 260 mg/dl of total cholesterol, he should be concerned enough to place himself under the care of a physician or clinic for additional testing and follow-up.

Groover, Jernigan, and Martin (1960) measured the variations in blood cholesterol concentration in 177 individuals over a 5-year period. Only 38 subjects showed variations below 20%. Heart attacks occurred only in the group whose variation was 55% or greater. Of 16 heart attacks, 10 were observed in the 12 people with variations between 60% and 100% +. Groover et al. attributed much of the fluctuation to stress.

This interpretation of similar data was also reached by Friedman and Rosenman in their original study of Type A behavior (1959). From this viewpoint the cholesterol paradox is not a paradox at all. The data are telling us that blood cholesterol concentration in an individual is not an independent risk factor. Blood cholesterol level is influenced by stress and possibly by other personal idiosyncracies as well. Recall that in chapter

6 I mentioned the influence of stress on blood pressure. The effects of stress on other risk factors are obvious in individuals; the same effects are averaged out in populations.

On reading these conclusions you may wonder why I spent so much space discussing cholesterol as a risk factor when a blood analysis on a person will have little or no predictive value for heart disease. There are two reasons for my emphasis. In the first place, if you are a typical North American eating a typical North American diet, your blood cholesterol is probably too high. A change to the prudent diet can't hurt and may help you avoid a heart attack. Secondly, a low-fat high fiber diet serves as an excellent way to lose weight, and weight loss can add to wellness in many other ways than in the prevention of heart attacks. These benefits may occur with no change in blood cholesterol concentration.

In summary, I wish to repeat that none of the conclusions on stress and CHD are proved. But when numerous studies of thousands of people in different parts of the world at different times with quite different lifestyles confirm each other, the conclusions gain credibility. They may not be proved in the classical scientific sense, but they certainly seem reasonable. In my opinion, uncontrolled stress is the most damaging risk factor of all because of its secondary effects on increasing blood cholesterol concentration, on blood pressure, and often on cigarette smoking and alcohol consumption.

Animal Experiments Support the Stress–Heart Disease Connection

Do people's pets resemble their masters in personality and behavior? Does a Type B person acquire a Saint Bernard or collie, both of which are calm and self-possessed; and Type A people acquire a fox terrier, French poodle, Chihuahua or other nervous, excitable type? I have seen no studies on this question, but it does imply that animal behavior, in this instance that of dogs, varies widely. It should not be surprising then that animals have been used as experimental subjects in heart disease research in not only physiological studies but also psychological studies. It is obvious that the behavior of higher primates like monkeys resembles that of humans more than that of nonprimate species, but experiments with species as far removed from humans as rodents have provided interesting data on psycho-physiological reactions. Actually, the value of animal experiments should not be too surprising, because the nervous systems of all animals function by similar mechanisms. The major difference between the nervous system of a slug and us is one of complexity.

Measurement is the backbone of science. It is obviously difficult to measure aggression, hostility, impatience, and the other components of Type A behavior quantitatively. Yet, because dose-response curves are as essential with these factors as with the other risk factors, some attempt to quantitate them is necessary. Because the environment of animals is more easily regulated than that of free-living humans, some scientists have employed animals in psycho-social experiments and obtained some very interesting results.

Many of the components of Type A behavior are negative. It has been assumed that these psychological factors contribute to the stress that an individual generates. I have not seen studies in humans where positive factors like love and affection have been investigated. Presumably, positive factors should reduce stress. Nerem, Levesque, and Cornhill (1980) set up an experiment with young, male, New Zealand white rabbits. The experiment involved studying the effects of handling on diet-induced atherosclerosis.

The control animals received ordinary laboratory care. The experimental animals received "Cadillac" treatment. The same experimenter visited them for a half hour each morning during which time she handled, stroked, played with, and talked to them. In the course of an hour-long feeding period, each animal was also touched and talked to. During the day, a number of additional, short visits were made. In the course of the experiment, the rabbits learned to recognize the experimenter, and some sought her personal attention.

All the animals, controls and experimental alike, were fed ordinary rabbit chow laced with 2% cholesterol. This amount of cholesterol is known to be atherogenic to rabbits. Serum cholesterol concentration and blood pressure were measured weekly. Serum cholesterol was high in both groups. There was no significant difference in blood pressure or in heart rate. After 5 to 6 weeks, the animals were killed and the aortas were removed and stained for fat-containing plaques. The area of fatty plaques, however, was 60% less in the affectionately handled group compared to the controls (average p = approx. .02). The authors point out that lack of attention to socio-psychological factors may be responsible for the inconsistent results in published animal experiments. The implications for humans is obvious.

The other animal experiment was carried out with adult, male macaque monkeys (Kaplan et al., 1983). In contrast to the rabbit experiment, the monkeys were fed a prudent, low-cholesterol, low-saturated-fat diet. The experimental animals were stressed negatively by redistributing unfamiliar animals into the cages once every 12 weeks during the first year of the experiment and once every 4 weeks during the final 9 months. The control groups contained the same monkeys for the duration of the experiment. The rationale for this experiment comes from previous work that has demonstrated that the introduction of strangers fosters a high degree of social instability in macaques. The data obtained were both biochemical and behavioral.

Both groups were observed for aggressive behavior (e.g. biting, slapping, grasping) and for submission (e.g. fleeing, cowering, grimacing) over many separate periods. As in the rabbit experiment, the size of lesions in the coronary arteries were examined. The stressed animals had larger lesions in area and in thickness in their arteries compared to the controls ($p < .002$ and $p < .02$, respectively). The stressed animals showed significantly more severe aggression and severe submission than the controls ($p < .05$ in each category).

These interesting animal experiments on the relation of socio-psychological factors to a diet-independent development of atherosclerosis raise a variety of questions: What is the mechanism by which the handled rabbits are protected from plaque formation in their arteries even though their serum cholesterol is very high? What is the mechanism of plaque formation of stressed monkeys on a prudent diet? What is the relevance of these experiments to the human situation? Can a nonstressed person eat a high-saturated-fat diet safely? I, for one, do not believe that course would be prudent. I would guess that it takes far less to keep a rabbit content and happy than a human. Further, the *assumptions* involved in extrapolating from rabbits to humans on the diet-cholesterol-atheroma effects are too great, too untested, to encourage me to try it.

Other Suggested Dietary Modifications to Prevent CHD

So far in this chapter we have explored the medical research approach to cardiovascular diseases and their prevention. The dangers of a high serum cholesterol have been widely publicized. Many people seem quite familiar with the suggestions of popular authors on how to avoid heart attacks by dietary modification. Consequently, it may be valuable to look at their conclusions and to evaluate them using the same criteria I have employed in the previous section.

Lecithin Supplements for the Prevention of Heart Attacks

Lecithin is a popular item in health food stores. Much of its popularity is due to the writings of Adelle Davis. She discussed lecithin in her book *Let's Get Well* (1965), which is considered to be her most scientific book because it is thoroughly documented. I have chosen five sentences contained in one paragraph rather than isolated sentences so you can gain some idea of her style and how she connects ideas. I'll include her numbered references in my quotation so that readers who have access to the book can check her citations themselves if they choose. The following quote is from chapter 5, "Those Cholesterol Problems," under the heading "The importance of lecithin or phospholipids."

[a] All atherosclerosis is characterized by an increase of the blood cholesterol and a *decrease in lecithin*.[27] [b] As early as 1935 it was shown that experimental heart disease, produced by feeding cholesterol, could be prevented merely by giving a small amount of lecithin;[28] [c] and atherosclerosis has since been repeatedly produced in various species either by increasing the cholesterol or decreasing the lecithin.[19, 29] [d] If enough lecithin is given, the disease does not occur regardless of the amount of cholesterol which is fed.[30] [e] Even when atherosclerosis is far advanced, health is restored after lecithin is supplied in the diet.[29] [f] Furthermore, animals most resistant to atherosclerosis are those with the greatest ability to produce lecithin.[30] (p. 50)

These are important statements. Atherosclerosis and its common clinical resultant, coronary heart disease, are the leading causes of death of middle-aged men in America. If the secret to the prevention of this killer lies in a molecule called lecithin, the news should be proclaimed daily on every TV channel in the country.

A critical evaluation of the Davis paragraph is dependent on three questions: (a) Has she accurately summarized the references cited? (b) Has she referred to all literature that had been published at that time pertaining to the use of lecithin for the prevention or cure of atherosclerosis or only to the literature that supports her thesis? (c) If people followed Davis' recommendations, would they be endangering themselves? The book was written over 20 years ago, so a fair critique of her statements can be based only on knowledge available at that time. With this in mind, let's look at the documentation of the individual sentences of the Davis paragraph.

(a) This statement is based on an article published in 1943. It may have been accurate in 1943, but by 1965 when Davis wrote her book, many cases of atherosclerosis had been described in which blood cholesterol was not elevated (White et al., 1950; Kannel, Dawber, Kagan, Revotskie, & Stokes, 1961). She chose to ignore the data that did not support her position. In addition, lecithin was, and still is, seldom measured as a clinical determination. Her use of the word "all" to commence the sentence is a striking example of an invalid generalization.

(b) Davis refers to the production of atherosclerosis in rabbits, a species especially susceptible to diets that contain cholesterol. She implies that a similar generalization holds for humans. Here she is guilty of gross oversimplification and invalid extrapolation from one species to another. It was already known in 1965 that the situation was much more complicated than her remark indicates. Cholesterol in foods can certainly contribute to elevating blood cholesterol, but in humans, as the amount in the diet increases, the effect on the blood level decreases. By the time she wrote this sentence, the anticholesterolemic claims of effects of lecithin were already controversial. She cited one of the few papers in which positive results were reported. However, no quantitative data were presented in this article. It only contains qualitative descriptions of the appearance of the aortas of four rabbits, two in each group.

(c) In Davis' reference 29, cholesterol was fed to rabbits along with varying amounts of lecithin. Hypercholesterolemia was reduced, and the incidence of atherosclerosis was lowered. Score a point for Davis. However, she badly misquotes and misrepresents what was reported in reference 19 (Adlersberg, Bossak, Sher, & Sobotka, 1955). Their comment on humans with *hereditary hyperlipemia*: "The serum is clear and shows elevation of cholesterol and the phosphatides" (p. 30), that is, lecithin.

(d) It seems amazing that Davis (a natural food advocate) would refer to this excellent work, which included injecting rabbits with a synthetic detergent! Blood lecithin was elevated, and the incidence and severity of atherosclerosis was reduced in those animals that received the detergent called Tween 80. Plaques previously formed, however, were not reduced by the detergent. In her comment, Davis apparently confused lecithin with the synthetic detergent. In addition, the article referred to is not a scientific paper but an abstract. Abstracts are seldom, if ever, cited in scientific articles because the actual data are not presented and the details of the experiment are not included. As a final comment, injecting substances to avoid complications of the digestive system is not uncommon in medical research. But is it relevant as a therapy for hypercholesterolemia in humans? I suggest that there are easier, safer procedures for reducing blood cholesterol than injections twice a day with a synthetic detergent.

(e) This statement by Davis is just plain false. There is nothing in the reference she cites that says that atherosclerosis can be reversed by feeding lecithin.

(f) This comment, too, amounts to a gross misinterpretation. My first thought on reading this statement was that someone had measured lecithin synthesis in a number of animal species and showed a correlation between its rate of synthesis and resistance to atherosclerosis. But no experiments of this type were mentioned in the work to which Davis referred. Davis is apparently assuming that high levels of lecithin result from a high rate of synthesis. She ignores the possibility that the rate of degradation of lecithin may have been reduced.

Frankly, I found this exercise of really checking up on Adelle Davis an unpleasant experience. Previously, I had known of her unsound extrapolations from one species to another, her consistent usage of anecdotal observations, and her advocacy of raw milk and fertile eggs without supporting data; but I was unprepared to find a minefield of errors in one paragraph. Of the seven statements examined, one was accurate and the other six were false or misleading. Are you willing to trust your health and survival to this type of information?

It is unfortunate that people in general do not have the expertise (or the interest) to carry out exercises like the one I have just described for themselves. Are they trapped, to be exploited and misled by clever writers for years to come? I suggest that the public schools add courses on critical thinking and data evaluation of claims, not just in nutrition but on a variety of subjects, so that all young Americans become less gullible.

How Complete Is the Davis Paragraph?

There is a rhythm in Davis' writings, and this paragraph illustrates it well. She starts with a generalization ("All atherosclerosis is characterized by" . . .) and mentions an inverse correlation between cholesterol and lecithin levels in the blood. She then details how lecithin in the diet prevents elevated blood cholesterol. Davis follows that by stating that atherosclerosis can be produced not just by raising cholesterol but also by lowering lecithin. She hammers the point home by stating that lecithin in the diet will even reverse the plaques previously formed.

The reader is left with the definite impression that the way to avoid heart attacks is to go out and buy some lecithin and start eating it. She does not even hint that there are contrary data. How could one guess that she has carefully screened the literature and omitted almost everything that does not agree with her thesis?

Davis had the ability to take a complicated subject and oversimplify it to the point of absurdity. A layperson reading Davis would be led to think that she had explained how a disease process develops and how diet could contribute or help prevent it. Actually, she camouflaged her opinions by presenting them in the form of scientific references!

Some years ago Senator Muskie criticized what he called "one-armed" scientists. By this he meant experts who could not make simple declarative sentences. Instead, they would summarize a subject in terms of, "on the one hand," and present one side or viewpoint. Then they would say, "on the other hand," and discuss other views before drawing a conclusion or advocating a course of action. Is oversimplification of the Davis-type necessary for a writer to be popular in America? Does Senator Muskie's remark reveal the shallowness of congressional thinking? Those of us involved in public education realize the enormity of the challenge of presenting complex problems in an interesting way without being guilty of oversimplification. Somehow, the public must be educated to learn to cope with complexity and to realize that the prevention and cure for most diseases does not reside in a bottle of pills.

Another advocate of lecithin supplements was J.I. Rodale, the founder and long-term editor of *Prevention* magazine. In his book, *Your Diet and Your Heart* (1970), Rodale writes, "Lecithin is abundant in egg yolks and extremely important in cutting excess cholesterol in the blood stream. But whoever hears any strong publicity urging healthy people to eat . . . eggs to avoid heart disease?'' (p. 11). In asking this question, Rodale ignores the high cholesterol content of egg yolks and emphasizes their lecithin content. The idea that lecithin is able to form an emulsion with cholesterol and thus prevent its clogging up the arteries is at least 50 years old. Such emulsions can readily be formed in test tubes. It may seem like a reasonable thing to apply this conclusion to the blood, which also contains both cholesterol and lecithin. But anyone writing on medical matters for the public should know enough about blood chemistry to realize that neither cholesterol nor lecithin occurs freely in the blood. Both are bound to proteins. The lipoproteins I have mentioned earlier contain both of these lipids. These facts were well known to readers of the medical literature in the 1950s. Why did Rodale choose to ignore them?

The Wisdom of J.I. Rodale

The present editors of *Prevention* are republishing some of J.I. Rodale's articles under the heading, ''The Wisdom of J.I. Rodale.'' One of these articles was titled ''Lecithin for the Heart'' (Rodale, 1972). In it Rodale cites seven publications that report positive results of feeding lecithin supplements to animals and humans. The title of the article is somewhat misleading because only two of the references deal with lowering blood cholesterol. (Two dealt with its effects on diabetics, and two discuss the use of lecithin in skin diseases.) Rodale asks the sensible question, Why should we require lecithin in the diet when it can be made in the liver? He answers it as follows: ''One of the B-vitamins, choline, and the unsaturated fatty acids must be present for the liver to make lecithin. We have done our best to remove both of these substances from our national diet; so our supply of lecithin suffers'' (p. 195).

Now, to understand the fallacies in Rodale's statement, I need to mention that lecithin is composed of choline, fatty acids, glycerol, and phosphate, which are connected by chemical bonds to form one molecule. The first error comes from calling choline a B-vitamin, which, by definition, the body cannot make. Healthy people are perfectly capable of synthesizing all the choline they need provided they eat a sufficient amount of the essential amino acid methionine, which is widely distributed in proteins.

The second error is his *assumption* that the fatty acid composition of lecithin does not vary. For example, egg yolk lecithin, which Rodale advocated for the prevention of heart attacks, contains only 18% of its total fatty acids as PUFA. Egg yolk lecithin contains 2.3 times as much saturated fatty acids, those that tend to elevate blood cholesterol, than it does PUFA, those that tend to depress blood cholesterol (USDA, 1976). Soybean lecithin contains 52% of its total fatty acids as PUFA. These facts have been known for many years.

Does this reprinting of Rodale's "wisdom," without comment, tell you something about the acumen and knowledge of the present editors of *Prevention* magazine?

The April 1979 issue of *Prevention* magazine contains an update on lecithin. The article is titled "Winning Hearts and Minds with Lecithin" and was written by John Feltman. In the section in which he reviews recent work on lecithin in reducing blood cholesterol, Feltman states that "lecithin's well documented effects on the circulatory system are another matter. In this respect, lecithin has a long and proven track record as a practical, easy-to-use preventive agent." He then cites two recent reports and one older report of the efficacy of lecithin in reducing blood cholesterol concentration.

Now, soybean lecithin, as mentioned above, is an excellent source of linoleic acid, a polyunsaturated, essential fatty acid. A number of studies have demonstrated that the cholesterol-lowering effects of lecithin could be duplicated with corn oil or some other source of linoleic acid (Keys et al., 1957; Simons, Hickie, & Ruys, 1977). To my knowledge, no study has reported a beneficial effect of lecithin on people who were already ingesting an adequate amount of linoleic acid by use of corn, safflower, or soybean oil in their food. Why pay the premium price of lecithin capsules if you are using these vegetable oils in your kitchen?

Many people who have heard about lecithin or some other supplement may say to themselves, "Well, even if it doesn't live up to all the claims made for it, it's a natural substance and can't hurt me." This view is false and dangerous when applied to lecithin. Neither Davis, Rodale, nor Feltman addresses the question of whether lecithin is safe for everyone.

As we have seen, obese and overweight people are more likely to have a high level of blood cholesterol than normal-weight people. As a group, they are more likely to benefit from the cholesterol-lowering effects of lecithin. But we need to consider the energy content of lecithin. As a fat, lecithin contains about 9 kcal/g. A person adding 2 tablespoons a day to his or her diet (about 28 g) is thus increasing his or her intake by 250 kcal per day. In some of the experiments cited by Feltman (1979), 2 or 3 times as much lecithin was administered. Anyone will gain weight on this regimen unless an equal number of kcals are omitted from some other part of the diet. Of all the people in this world, the obese do not need a supplement that provides over 250 extra kcal per day!

None of the three authors mentioned that lecithin does not lower the cholesterol in all subjects to a significant degree. In fact, the effects of lecithin have been controversial in the medical literature for years (Davies

& Murdoch, 1959; Svanburg, Gustavson, & Ohlson, 1974). This means that your taking lecithin supplements is pretty much a gamble if you don't follow up with cholesterol determinations and find out if lecithin is really lowering your blood cholesterol. Self-medication, based on false claims for prevention or cure of a disease, may delay sound diagnosis and therapy for years. Such people actually increase their risk of developing the very disease they think they are avoiding.

Misguided attempts to prevent one disease may increase the possibility of promoting another. Overweight people who attempt to lower their blood cholesterol by taking large amounts of PUFA, either through extra lecithin or directly as a vegetable oil, greatly increase their risk of developing gallstones. Sturdevant, Pearce, and Dayton (1973) found that 58% of an obese group that took PUFA supplements developed gallstones. Because weight loss by itself often results in lower blood cholesterol, it would seem advisable that overweight persons lose extra pounds first, before ingesting extra lecithin or PUFA, if they wish to avoid the unpleasant pain of gallstones and the expense of a gallbladder operation.

Prevention *Magazine Advocates Use of Cod-Liver Oil to Prevent Heart Attacks*

The March 1979 issue of *Prevention* includes an article that is closely related to lecithin supplements, but you might not guess it from the title: "Cod-Liver Oil for Your Body Machinery." This article poses the interesting question: Why don't Eskimos, who eat a high-fat, animal diet, get heart attacks even though they eat large amounts of cholesterol?

The *Prevention* author quotes Dyerberg, Bang, Stoffersen, Moncada & Vane (1978) who have found a very unusual polyunsaturated fatty acid in cod-liver oil. It is named *eicosapentaenoic acid* or EPA for short. The source of EPA in the Eskimo diet is in the seal and walrus meat they eat. These polar-living, aquatic mammals do not synthesize EPA themselves but obtain it, in turn, from their food, which is species of fish, including the cod. Recent research now suggests that EPA is involved in at least three reactions that are closely related to heart diseases: its lowering of blood cholesterol concentrations; its anti-inflammatory, antiaggregating effects on white cells; and finally, its anticlotting properties.

Some years ago Kingsbury, Morgan, Aylott, & Emmerson (1961) showed that cod-liver oil was 2 times as effective as corn oil in reducing blood cholesterol concentrations in people. The difference can now be ascribed to the high-EPA and low-linoleic-acid content of cod-liver oil. Recall that plant oils, like corn and safflower, are rich in linoleic acid. The interesting work of Dyerberg et al. (1978) suggests that there may be differences in the effectiveness of specific polyunsaturated fatty acids as hypocholesterolemic agents.

In a well-controlled experiment by Phillipson, Rothrock, Connor, Harris, and Illingworth (1985), patients with hyperlipidemia were placed on three diets for 4 weeks each, differing primarily in fatty acid composition and fat content. The control diet was low in total fat and had a P/S ratio of 1.4. The fish-oil diet contained added EPA, and the vegetable-oil diet was rich in linoleic acid. The fish-oil diet resulted in average decreases of cholesterol (−36%) and triglycerides (−71%) compared to the control diet. The vegetable-oil diet had a much lesser effect.

Arachidonic acid is found in blood platelets. When an arterial wall is injured, platelets and other white blood cells respond by adhering to the injured area, aggregating, and forming a plug (a thrombus) that may block blood flow and result in a heart attack. Arachidonic acid, as mentioned in chapter 5, is a precursor of both prostaglandins and prostacyclins. The former promote platelet aggregation whereas the latter inhibit aggregation. EPA has been reported by Lee et al. (1985) at Harvard to form similar derivatives, which inhibit aggregation to a much greater extent than those formed from arachidonic acid.

Finally, the blood of Greenland Eskimos tends to clot slower than that of people eating conventional Western diets. Dyerberg et al. attribute the slow clotting to the formation of an anticlotting substance from EPA. This characteristic is of considerable value in preventing blood clots and helps to explain the low incidence of heart disease in these people. If a clot forms in a coronary artery, it can bring on a heart attack.

These specific effects resulting from consuming fish have been extended to the practical level of measuring its effects on heart disease directly. A number of ecological studies in Japan have correlated fish consumption with low incidence of heart disease. Kromhout, Bosschicter, and Coulander (1985) investigated the relationship of fish consumption to the incidence of coronary heart disease in men aged 40-59 years at outset, living in Zutphen, Netherlands, over a period of 20 years. Mortality from heart attacks was more than 50% lower among those who consumed an average of about an ounce of fish per day compared to those who did not. In this work, diet was not controlled but was estimated at intervals over the 20-year period.

The *Prevention* author ("Cod-liver oil," 1979) suggests that these effects of EPA may return cod- and other fish-liver oils to the popularity they enjoyed as early sources of vitamin D. Unfortunately, this article ends by misstating the vitamin D requirement for adults: "Unlike other vitamins, vitamin D is not present in significant amounts in the normal diet" (p. 71). The author has ignored the fact that most adults receive sufficient sunshine to manufacture their own vitamin D in their skin. According to the RDA booklet (National Research Council, 1980), the only people who may require supplementary vitamin D are those who are housebound or do not obtain it in fortified milk, margarine, or in eggs, liver, and butter.

After reading this article, a number of people probably purchased cod-liver oil either to lower their blood cholesterol or because they thought they might need extra vitamin D. Is there any danger in taking 2 tablespoons of cod-liver oil daily, as mentioned in the article? According to the *Merck Index* (Stecher, 1968), cod-liver oil contains a minimum of 85 USP units of vitamin D per gram. Two tablespoons at 14 g each equals 28 g, which calculates to an intake of 2,380 extra units per day. The RDA book (National Research Council, 1980) states, "Vitamin D is a potentially toxic substance, particularly in young children. . . . intakes should closely approximate the recommended allowance for both children and adults" (p. 62).

But I'm not yet finished with the dangers of supplementary cod-liver oil. It also contains vitamin A, which is not mentioned in the Prevention article. The *Merck Index* (Stecher, 1968) lists 850 USP units of vitamin A per gram. A consumption of 2 tablespoons per day (28 g) would furnish 23,800 units, which is equivalent to 7,140 ug (retinol equivalents). The RDA booklet cautions, "Excessive vitamin A is toxic to both children and adults and should be avoided. Regular ingestion of more than 7,500 retinol equivalents (25,000 IU) daily is not prudent" (p. 59). The quantities of vitamin A present in the suggested intake of cod-liver oil are close to the risk level.

This discussion on the vitamin content of cod-liver oil has certainly digressed from that of using it to depress one's blood cholesterol, but I believe it illustrates the care one should exercise before adding a supplement to one's diet for any purpose. Frankly, I am disappointed that the editors of *Prevention* published this article without including a caution on the dangers of excess fat-soluble vitamins. I further suggest that anyone who has been impressed with the fish-oil results mentioned above (as I have been) eat fish rather than fish-liver oils.

It pleases me to mention an article in the September 1985 issue of *Prevention* entitled "Feast on the Good Fish" by Denise Foley. In this article she reviews recent work on EPA and suggests eating fish one or two times a week. She does not suggest taking cod-liver oil as did the older articles.

Sugar and Heart Attacks

The role of common table sugar (sucrose) as an agent in cardiovascular disease was mentioned by J.I. Rodale (1970) in *Your Diet and Your Heart*. He wrote, "Only recently Dr. John Yudkin proved a direct relationship between the amount of refined sugar we eat and the incidence of heart diseases" (p. 11). It seems incredible that Rodale could have made such a remark if he read the nutrition literature and knew how Yudkin's work had been received by nutritionists who were working on the relations between diet and the prevention of heart disease. In the first place,

Yudkin, a respected scientist, did not claim to have proved such a relationship. As I explained in chapter 3, proof in dietary experiments is rare and elusive. Scientific proof is a small, wriggling, slippery catch, which usually eludes the nets of nutritionists. Careful scientists use the word cautiously. So should science popularizers.

In the second place, Yudkin and Roddy's (1964) conclusions were based on only 20 patients who retrospectively listed their sugar consumption. One of the benefits of their claims was that they stimulated a great deal of research on whether sugar intake was a risk factor for CHD that was comparable to that of saturated fats. A review of this work (Grande, Anderson, & Keys, 1972b) concluded that the ingestion of large amounts of sucrose does not result in a chronic increase of serum cholesterol. Yet Rodale continued his antisugar crusade until his death. Why?

Vitamin E and Your Heart

The second chapter of Rodale's book is entitled "A Cure for Heart Disease" and is written by W. E. Shute, M.D. This man published an account of their use of large amounts of vitamin E in the treatment of heart diseases in 1946 (Vogelsang and Shute). *Time* magazine publicized it in its issue of June 10, 1946, as follows:

> Out of Canada last week came news of a startling scientific discovery: a treatment of heart disease (the nation's No. 1 killer) which so far has succeeded against all common forms of the ailment. Large, concentrated doses of vitamin E . . . benefited four types of heart ailment (95% of the total): arteriosclerotic hypertensive, rheumatic, old and new coronary heart disease. The vitamin helps a failing heart. It eliminates anginal pain. It is non-toxic. (p. 45)

The following year Shute, Shute, and Vogelsang (1947) reported on 84 patients with angina pectoris who had been treated with vitamin E. A majority had responded positively to the vitamin E therapy.

Dr. Shute's enthusiasm for vitamin E has continued unabated for over 20 years, as is reflected in the following statements (Rodale, 1970).

> That the most dreadful single disease confronting mankind today, not tuberculosis, not cancer, but coronary heart disease, can be completely wiped out within the next 50 years is the major and most hopeful implication of our treatment of coronary heart disease by vitamin E. (p. 20)

> I would like to tell you about the workers who showed that deposition of cholesterol in the wall of the arteries in rabbits force-fed cholesterol could be prevented by vitamin E. (p. 24)

The Shute group has continued to publish their uncontrolled, positive observations over the years in books such as *Vitamin E for Ailing and Healthy Hearts* (Shute & Taub, 1969), and publicists like Adelle Davis, J.I. Rodale, and others have touted vitamin E for the prevention and cure of CHD. Why then is vitamin E not prescribed by physicians for their heart patients? Why do nutritionists not suggest that we all should be taking large amounts daily to prevent heart attacks?

The facts are that vitamin E was extensively tested by the medical profession in nine separate studies between 1948 and 1950 and found to be ineffective. In referring to this older work, Anderson (1974) comments that most of these studies were no better controlled than the original ones by the Shute group.

A pain in the chest (angina pectoris) is largely subjective in nature. Anxious patients are apt to feel better if their physicians tell them that their medication will relieve their pain. This well-recognized response (the placebo effect) is the main justification for double-blind trials of drugs, in which neither the patient nor the examining physician knows what drug or therapy the patient is receiving.

The work reported by Anderson (1974) is one of the few in which the double-blind procedure was followed. In addition, the dosages of vitamin E were approved in advance by Dr. Shute. With regard to controlling as many variables as possible in clinical studies of this type, the Anderson paper can be taken as a model. The results did not furnish statistically convincing evidence that vitamin E is of value in the treatment of angina, but a small beneficial effect could not be ruled out. Because of the small number of patients in this experiment, Anderson suggests that it be repeated. This situation provides another excellent example of how uncontrolled experiments can lead to controversy. The Anderson work has set standards by which to evaluate further work in this field.

The saddest facts are contributed by people with heart problems who dose themselves with large amounts of vitamin E for years instead of seeking sound medical advice. The vitamin E enthusiasts are more likely to become statistics in the coronary heart disease columns than those who attempt to lower their risk of an attack by reversing their risk factors.

Nicotinic Acid

Rodale's introduction to *Your Diet and Your Heart* is entitled, "Can Heart Disease Be Prevented?" In it he suggests following the steps outlined by Blakeslee and Stamler (1963). One of the steps is to choose a diet that reduces or maintains a low level of blood cholesterol. As we have seen, high blood cholesterol is presently recognized as a major risk factor for CHD. Rodale states that "researchers know that nicotinic acid, a B-vitamin, is an effective anti-cholesterol agent. But whoever hears any strong publicity urging healthy people to eat B-rich foods . . . to avoid heart disease'' (p. 11). The answer to Rodale's question can be found in Blakeslee and Stamler's book. They write,

The vitamin, nicotinic acid—the pellagra fighter—was one of the first agents shown to be effective in reducing blood cholesterol when taken in large daily doses. But the large amounts cause burning or flushing sensations, itchings and sometimes stomach upsets and liver damage. (p. 11)

Why did Rodale quote the first sentence above and ignore the second?

Dietary Fiber

Mark Bricklin (1979), Executive Editor of *Prevention*, wrote an article entitled, "Put Fiber to Work for Your Heart." He introduces the subject by referring to high-serum cholesterol resulting in clogged arteries. High-serum cholesterol can be reduced or avoided by eating a low-fat diet. But most Americans find such a diet unappetizing and won't stick to it. Is there any supplement, food or substance, that can be added to the diet that will reduce the blood cholesterol level?

Bricklin then refers to work in Oregon in which researchers made monkeys atherogenic by feeding them cholesterol. Alfalfa meal was then added to the atherogenic diet, and the arteries of these monkeys were compared with those that remained on the unmodified diet and those that received a low-cholesterol diet. The plaques in the arteries of those receiving alfalfa meal had disappeared! At this point Bricklin reveals the catch. Alfalfa meal had made up 50% of the food the one group of monkeys ate, an amount which is not feasible to include in human diets.

Bricklin asks two sensible questions about this research. Would alfalfa meal exert a similar effect in humans? How much alfalfa would be necessary in the diet to lower cholesterol in humans? The answers to these questions are not known at present. In the meantime, Bricklin is adding more alfalfa sprouts to his salads.

Bricklin also mentions an Italian study of elderly patients in which wheat bran (amount not stated) added to the diet decreased attacks of angina. This effect was attributed to less constipation and less straining at stool, a well-known effect of bran.

I do take exception, however, to Bricklin's summary of an article by Dr. J.N. Morris and colleagues "who suggest that lack of fiber in the diet may well be a *major cause* [italics added] of coronary thrombosis." As I have repeatedly emphasized, epidemiological data furnish us with correlations, not cause–effect relationships. I hope that popular authors on health and nutrition will help educate the public away from the oversimplification of cause and effect in studies of this type.

Bricklin concludes the article by referring to still another type of dietary fiber—pectin. This material, which is found in many fruits and vegetables, has been shown to lower blood cholesterol in humans when added to experimental low-fiber diets (Spiller & Shipley, 1977; Story & Kritchevsky, 1976).

Selenium

In recent years the element selenium has been demonstrated to be an essential nutrient for mammals (Sprinker, Harr, Newberne, Whanger, & Weswig, 1971). Like many other trace minerals, a specific selenium deficiency has not been identified in humans, but the probability that it is essential is very high. Selenium shares another property with a number of other essential nutrients; it's safety factor is quite low. (This term is explained in chapter 6). For this reason, its intake needs to be monitored carefully.

In *Prevention*, John Feltman (1979) has an article entitled, "Selenium, Double-Duty Protector," with the subtitle "The Same Mineral That Seems to Block Certain Types of Cancers Now Looks Like a Guardian of Heart Health as Well." Apart from the specific role that selenium may play in preventing cancer or heart disease, the article raises two general questions: Is the American public receiving an adequate amount in its diet? Are selenium supplements necessary or advisable? Here we encounter a situation in which expert opinions differ.

Feltman quotes Schrauzer and White, two of the well-known workers in this area of research, who recommend selenium supplementation for the entire American population. This conclusion is based on an analysis of selenium intake by 10 people in California. Schrauzer and White (1978) estimate that a selenium consumption of 300 mcg/day is adequate for humans. Their analyses of the intakes of Americans show a subnormal amount (only about 100 mcg/day). They recommend a supplement of 150 to 250 mcg/day, preferably in the form of a high-selenium yeast.

Shamberger, Gunsch, Willis, and McCormick (1978) at the Cleveland Clinic have been investigating the relationships between selenium ingestion and heart disease. They reported an epidemiological survey on the correlation between selenium in the diet and incidence of CHD in 25 countries. They found a high rate of CHD in those countries with a low average selenium intake, including the United States. Shamberger et al. believe that enough preliminary work has been done to warrant a large-scale clinical trial in the United States. In the meantime they are eating high-selenium foods such as mushrooms, asparagus, seafood, organ meats, and whole-wheat bread. In addition, they are taking a 50-mcg/day supplement.

Salonen, Alfthan, Huttunen, Pikkarainen, and Puska (1982) investigated the association between serum selenium and risk of death from acute heart disease and fatal and nonfatal myocardial infarction. The subjects were chosen on a case-control basis from a population of 11,000 people in two counties in East Finland with an exceptionally high mortality from cardiovascular diseases. The cases were aged 35-59 years and had died of CHD or had a definite myocardial infarction over a 7-year follow-up. Controls were matched for age, sex, tobacco consumption, serum cholesterol, diastolic blood pressure, and history of angina pectoris. Blood samples were drawn from all participants at the start of the experiment. As each case was identified, either by death or a nonfatal heart attack, a control was selected and matched as closely as possible for the six characteristics mentioned above. Selenium concentrations were then determined on both samples of blood.

The mean serum selenium concentration for all cases was 51.8 $\mu g/l$ and for all controls, 55.3 $\mu g/l$ ($p < .01$). A serum selenium of less than 45 $\mu g/l$ was associated with an adjusted relative risk of CHD death of 2.9; a relative risk of CVD death of 2.2 ($p < .01$); and relative risk of myocardial infarction of 2.1 ($p < .001$). Of the entire population studied, 22% of coronary deaths were attributable to low serum selenium. The soil of Finland, and therefore the grain grown on it, is known to be low in selenium content. A similar correlation has been reported from New Zealand (Shamberger et al., 1978). Conclusions from studies of this type must be interpreted cautiously. Case-control, retrospective studies fall under Category 4 of Table 3.1, and their degree of credibility is low.

In a more recent study of serum selenium levels, coronary heart disease and stroke, Virtamo et al. (1985) followed over 11,000 men aged 55-74 in a 5-year prospective cohort study in two rural areas of Finland. Men living in East Finland had a much higher rate of coronary disease than those living in the West. Yet the mean serum selenium concentration was higher in the West than in the East. In both populations, the associations between coronary deaths and myocardial infarctions with low serum selenium were nonsignificant. The authors point out that the lack of agreement between their results and that of Salonen et al. (1982) may be due to the differences in the age and sex of the populations, as well as differences in the design of the experiments. According to Table 3.1, this prospective study ranks higher in credibility than the retrospective one. I would conclude from this comparison that the burden of proof lies with those who maintain that serum selenium level below 45 $\mu g/l$ is a risk factor for heart disease.

The status of selenium as a general risk factor for heart disease is interesting but far from proved. A general recommendation for individuals is complicated by the variation in the selenium content of plant foods. The amount of selenium consumed is dependent on not only what is eaten but also where it was grown, which is often impossible to determine.

A special statement on "Selenium and Human Health" was published by the Food and Nutrition Board, Committee on Nutrition Misinformation

(1976). From animal experiments the committee estimated that the human requirement for selenium is in the range of 60-120 mcg/day. It stated further that "available evidence suggests that a well-balanced American diet furnishes this quantity of selenium. Therefore, there is no justification at this time for the use of selenium supplements by the general population" (p. 348). They do qualify their statement as follows: "Should selenium supplements eventually be considered desirable for those living in low-selenium areas or for those consuming vegetarian diets, a daily supplement of 50 to 100 mcg/day could probably be taken safely" (p. 348). Obviously, taking a supplement at present is controversial and may be dangerous if your selenium intake is already high.

Thus the main area of disagreement between the Schrauzer-Shamberger view and the committee's statement concerns the adequacy of the present American diet with regard to selenium. Because the safety factor for selenium is quite low, I would suggest that individuals who are concerned whether their intake is sufficient obtain a blood analysis before taking a supplement. The simplest, safest, solution is to include high-selenium foods in the diet as Shamberger suggests.

Vitamin B₆ (Pyridoxine)

The final article that I'll discuss concerns the possibility that a deficiency of vitamin B₆ may be involved as an underlying cause of arteriosclerosis (Kinderlehrer, 1979). Notice the use of the word cause in that sentence. *Prevention* editor Jane Kinderlehrer goes on to explain that the well-known risk factors, high serum cholesterol, smoking, high-fat diet, hypertension, and stress, play a role in the development of the disease but are not responsible for the initial injury to the arterial wall. This is an important and valid distinction. I discussed some aspects of this question earlier in this chapter.

Kinderlehrer interviewed Kilmer McCully, M.D., professor of pathology at Harvard Medical School, who has recently suggested that an excess of the amino acid homocysteine is the *cause* of atherosclerosis. McCully postulates that homocysteine is a toxic amino acid that causes the cells lining the artery to degenerate and slough off. To maintain itself, the artery synthesizes new cells and more connective tissue, which accumulates lipids such as cholesterol and triglycerides. These lipids serve as the focal point for an atheroma.

McCully believes that Western-type diets are high in meat and processed foods, and low in vitamin B₆. Such diets furnish an oversupply of the essential amino acid methionine, which is the precursor to homocysteine. When sufficient vitamin B₆ (pyridoxine) is present in the diet, a coenzyme is formed that assists in the conversion of the toxic homocysteine to a nontoxic amino acid called cystathionine. When vitamin B₆ is deficient, toxic amounts of homocysteine build up, and the pathological process commences. McCully suggests a diet that is lower in meat and higher in grains than Americans have been consuming. A predominantly vegetarian diet would furnish us with more vitamin B_6 and with less methionine.

It is unfortunate that Kinderlehrer ends the interview with McCully with no further comments. Many people might be stimulated to head for the nearest health food store or supermarket and load up on vitamin B_6. As with so many other areas of disease-related nutritional research, a review of the literature reveals that this hypothesis is controversial. There seems to be general agreement that homocysteine acts as a toxic substance on arterial cells, but there is no agreement on the concentrations necessary to cause lesions. To speak of homocysteine's causing the lesion in a scientific sense implies that no other substances are involved. The available data are far from being conclusive on this question. In addition, there is no physiological basis for thinking that all arteriosclerosis must develop from one cause.

For McCully's hypothesis to be given serious consideration, supporting data, like demonstrating an excess of homocysteine in experimental animals with growing atheromas or showing that patients with arteriosclerosis are deficient in vitamin B_6, will be required.

The Soft Water-Heart Attack Hypothesis

Ordinarily, one doesn't think of drinking water as a source of essential nutrients, at least those nutrients that are required in amounts above the microgram range. Thus it was surprising to find that Kobayashi (cited in Neri & Johansen, 1978) related the chemical composition of river water to the incidence of apoplexy and that Schroeder in the U.S. (1960, 1966) correlated the hardness of water to cardiovascular diseases. Soft water contains a preponderance of monovalent cations and is often slightly acid in reaction. Hard water contains a preponderance of calcium and magnesium ions, which are divalent. Calcium is usually present in larger amounts than magnesium. These studies are examples of the ecological type mentioned in Table 3.1 and thus, by themselves, have a low degree of credibility.

Subsequent work in this area, as reviewed by Seelig and Heggtveit (1974), has definitely placed the possibility of subacute magnesium deficiency as a risk factor for coronary heart disease (Allen, 1960; Neri & Johansen, 1978) in soft water regions of the U. S. and Canada. Anderson, Neri, and Schreiber (1975) determined the magnesium content of the heart muscles of accident victims in towns of high and low magnesium content in their water supplies. They found 918 mcg magnesium in the hearts of those who had lived in an area that furnished 3 mg/liter of magnesium in the water. In contrast, those consuming water that contained 29 mg/liter of magnesium had a content of 982 mcg in their heart muscles. This difference is statistically significant and the data support the idea that people living in soft water areas should supplement their diets with magnesium, or eat high-magnesium foods regularly.

As mentioned in chapter 5, magnesium is a well-recognized essential element. Its RDA for the U.S. is listed as being in the range 300-400 mg/day for adults. Its known functions include suppression of arrhythmias in the hearts of experimental animals. These results support the clinical hypothesis of Bajusz (1967) and Anderson, LeRiche, and MacKay (1969) that magnesium protects against the often fatal arrhythmias that occur after a myocardial infarction.

According to Seelig and Heggtveit (1974), magnesium therapy for prevention of arrhythmias in heart disease is widely used in Europe; but, unfortunately, the lack of well-controlled clinical trials has delayed its use for this purpose in the U.S. These authors also mention that animal experiments have demonstrated high intakes of vitamin D_2 or fat increase magnesium requirements. Thus the high-fat, North American diet may result in a relative magnesium deficiency and contribute to the high incidence of heart disease in the U.S. This possibility deserves further study. The following are two suggestions for people who live in soft-water areas or those who drink commercial soft water:

1. Have a blood analysis for magnesium. Are you within the normal range?
2. Eat good sources of magnesium-containing foods regularly, such as nuts, legumes, grains, dark-green vegetables, and seafoods.

Should Dietary Changes for Everyone Be Included in Government Recommendations?

It is but a small step from Stamler's (1978) statement concerning "the current epidemic of premature atherosclerosis raging in Western industrialized countries" (p. 11) and his view that diet is the most important cause of the epidemic, to the position that government should do something about it. In fact, the U.S. Senate Select Committee on Nutrition and Human Needs (1977) has emphasized dietary changes for the American people over the other risk factors in the prevention of CHD. Is this position justified?

I recognize that few of you will influence government policy. Yet you will be affected by it and should know how to respond to it. Let me translate a few statistics into comments. In the seven-country study the total incidence rate per year of CHD (death, myocardial infarct, and angina pectoris) in men aged 40-59 was 17.1/1,000 in the U.S. compared with 2/1,000 in Japan, 3.0/1,000 in Greece, and 5.0/1,000 in Yugoslavia. The

U.S. rate is 8 times that of Japan and 6 times that in Greece. These numbers define what is meant by an epidemic of premature atherosclerosis. Yet, if we look at the absolute number for the U.S., it amounts to less than 2% per year. From the risk factor data that I have already reviewed, we know that most of these men exhibited one or more risk factors. This means that they were living at higher risk of incurring CHD than a similar population that did not exhibit any risk factors. Yet, with present techniques, it is impossible to identify individuals in advance of a coronary attack.

Epidemiologists and nutritionists are divided on a policy of action. Some are in favor of the federal government's publicizing the risk factors and advocating that adults reduce the fat and cholesterol content of their diets, that smokers stop smoking, and that everyone reduce the salt content of their diets, and learn to relax. There are four major reasons that support this policy. First, as a blanket recommendation, it would include the 2% of middle-aged men at the most risk. Second, the recommendations are not considered harmful if carried out by those adults who do not need them. Third, it is relatively inexpensive. It requires no identification of individuals at risk through expensive blood analyses and visits to physicians or clinics. Handouts to the media and interviews with well-known medical personalities are relatively cheap. Fourth, it leaves the primary responsibility with the individual, where many health authorities believe it belongs.

Those opposing this policy have a quiver full of arrows to shoot it down. They state that the diet risk factor CHD linkage is not sufficiently proved to warrant a government-sponsored publicity campaign. The credibility of many federal agencies is already low: Why risk lowering it further? A publicity campaign would needlessly frighten many people; and it would disrupt the cattle, dairy, and egg-producing industries. A federally sponsored publicity campaign would fail because most people exclude themselves from the population at risk ("It always happens to the other fellow").

What action do I advocate to readers of this book? I consider you as a select group. No one would have read this far if he or she were not more interested than the average person in the prevention of CHD. As a consequence, your knowledge is sounder and deeper than that of most of the lay public. My suggestions follow.

Summary

At the end of this long chapter I feel like the walrus who has talked of many things. Perhaps too many. Perhaps you are wondering how to put it all together without becoming a yogi. I'll suggest a 3-point program as a means of getting started. In my opinion, a very important factor in a person's life is how stressors are handled. So my first general suggestion is to inventory this area of your life. For starters, take the stress tests in the Appendix of chapter 4. Your ranking will determine the next step.

If your stress index is high, you need to consider the important question of whether to try to manage it yourself or to seek professional help. If you have been aware of your stresses for some years and haven't made much progress in dealing with them, you may wish to enroll in a stress management class as a first step. From the work of M. Friedman et al. (1984) mentioned above, stress management should include Type A behavior modification. Contact your state health department or a nearby university or college for a list of such classes. Another option is to read a good book on stress control if you think this is all you need. Talking things over with a friend with whom you can be open, frank, and honest is often very helpful.

An important characteristic of well people is their positive self-image. They recognize their weaknesses, of course, but they know their strengths and utilize them. The overall balance is positive. I suggest this objective for your improvement in stressor management. If you have been running yourself down for the past 10 or 20 years, it will take time for you to develop your negative image into a positive one. Just assume that it can be done and make a start! Remember, you are not alone. Others will help you, and you will help others.

My second suggestion is to start an endurance exercise program as soon as possible. If you are over 35 and out of shape, walking is an excellent way to start. Follow the suggestions outlined in chapter 7. If you have another preference, do it! The main thing is not to overextend yourself at the start and to incorporate exercise into your life as a regular habit. It is now recognized that endurance exercise promotes somato-psychological health. Once established, aerobics will aid you in managing stressors and developing a positive self-image.

When you feel ready for it, you may consider quitting smoking. At some point in smokers' progression towards wellness, they view it as a self-destructive habit. Quitting smoking is no longer viewed as a tremendous self-sacrifice to attain a vague objective called health or wellness, but as another step towards making your life more enjoyable. There are a number of programs sponsored by state health departments and lung associations that are effective in aiding long-time smokers to stop. A hypnosis session, followed by use of a relaxation tape as needed at home, has worked well for many people.

I recommend that everybody learn or improve these three skills: stressor management, endurance exercise, and not smoking. They form a trio that reinforce each other. An occasional slipup in one of them won't derail the whole enterprise. These recommendations are not controversial. In following them you are electing a course of action that has increased health–wellness for millions of people. You, too, can soon begin to enjoy the positive benefits.

Despite the tremendous publicity given to diet composition and its effect on blood concentrations of cholesterol, I am placing it last on my list of interventions. My reasons are as follows. In distinction to the three interventions mentioned above, in which the desirable effects on the individual follow directly from the suggested lifestyle changes, significant lowering of blood cholesterol by dietary alterations cannot be predicted for individuals unless the changes are truly major and the person follows the diet faithfully. Also, the effects of a decreased blood cholesterol on subsequent heart disease on individuals are not as clear-cut as might be desired. Finally, a number of sports medicine experts believe that the HDL/total cholesterol ratio is a more valid indicator for avoiding a heart attack than the total cholesterol. This ratio is increased in the desirable direction by endurance exercise, not by diet.

Not all people with hypercholesterolemia respond to dietary changes. If you have a fasting total cholesterol of > 260 mg/dl, you may find the following personal experiment interesting and valuable. Change to the prudent diet and stick with it faithfully for 6 months. Alter your other habits as little as possible. Have your serum cholesterol remeasured monthly. If it has dropped to < 250 mg/dl, stay with the diet and have serum cholesterol checked once or twice a year. If it hasn't dropped, you may want to try the Connors' alternative diet (Conner & Conner, 1986) or the Pritikin program (Pritikin & McGrady, 1979), although I have reservations about high-carbohydrate, low-fat diets.

Recent work has found that the low-fat (30% of calories), high-carbohydrate (55% of calories) diet decreased HDL levels as well as that of total cholesterol. Monounsaturated fatty acids as substitutes for carbohydrates did not have this effect. The most recent recommendation for fatty acid ratios is PUFA to MUFA to SFA = 1:3:2 (Grundy, 1986).

Similarly, the dietary factors responsible for hypertension are also controversial. A portion of the population responds to salt restriction, but the majority do not. McCarron, Morris, Henry, and Stanton (1984), in a provocative article based on survey data, conclude that hypertension is more likely to result from a deficiency of an essential nutrient such as calcium than from an excess of salt. My impression is that, although weight loss would result in lower blood pressure for many, the widespread decreases in hypertension that have occurred in the large epidemiological intervention experiments have been accomplished with drugs.

The effect of overeating (e.g., overweight and obesity) has finally come into its own as an independent risk factor for heart disease. It is also recognized as a factor contributing to a higher incidence of cancer, diabetes, and high blood pressure. Obesity is the most common form of malnutrition present in developed countries and the most difficult for people to control on a long-term basis. The average overweight person will buy the latest fad diet book, follow it for a few weeks, and then return to former habits. Yet, if people have been successful in controlling stressors and starting an exercise regime, they have a much better chance of also being successful in regulating food intake than if they started dieting first. The change in metabolism initiated by aerobics also helps lower the set point.

For many people, overeating can be considered as a form of self-generated stress mismanagement. The futility of suggesting to overweight people that they should eat fewer calories has been reported over and over again. Caloric restriction is acknowledged to be an unpleasant experience, and most people who diet under close supervision return to their old habits when unsupervised. I interpret this behavior as being due to treating the symptom of overweight and not attempting to discover the reasons why the overweight person eats too much.

In my opinion, obese people are as sick as alcoholics. Both groups suffer from low self-esteem. They hate themselves for their excesses but are unable to control them because their basic feelings about themselves are so negative. They suffer from the impostor syndrome. Even when they do something well, they can't accept compliments on a job well done, but make deprecating remarks about themselves. They can't imagine themselves as being successful. Adult support groups like Alcoholics Anonymous, Overeaters Anonymous, and Weight Watchers have helped millions who were close enough to the positive shore to get a foothold on their lives. For those other millions further out, professional psychological help may be their only hope of gaining the necessary self-esteem to begin a wellness program.

A person who has begun to identify and control his or her stressors and to engage in endurance exercise will, at some point, begin to understand for what reasons he or she was overeating. Long-term personal diet management now becomes possible. I consider stressor identifications and their management as the key for not only the control of risk factors in the prevention of disease but also the development of wellness.

Appendix 10A
RISKO

Men

		54 or Younger	55 or Older
Find the column for your age group. Everyone starts with a score of 10 points. Work down the page *adding* points to your score or *subtracting* points from your score.		Starting Score [10]	Starting Score [10]

1. Weight

Locate your weight category in the table below. If you are in . .

	54 or Younger	55 or Older
weight category A	Subtract 2	Subtract 2
weight category B	Subtract 1	Add 0
weight category C	Add 1	Add 1
weight category D	Add 2	Add 3
	Equals [ ]	Equals [ ]

2. Systolic Blood Pressure

Use the "first" or "higher" number from your most recent blood pressure measurement. If you do not know your blood pressure, estimate it by using the letter for your weight category. If your blood pressure is . . .

		54 or Younger	55 or Older
A	119 or less	Subtract 1	Subtract 5
B	between 120 and 139	Add 0	Subtract 2
C	between 140 and 159	Add 0	Add 1
D	160 or greater	Add 1	Add 4
		Equals [ ]	Equals [ ]

3. Blood Cholesterol Level

Use the number from your most recent blood cholesterol test. If you do not know your blood cholesterol, estimate it by using the letter for your weight category. If your blood cholesterol is . . .

		54 or Younger	55 or Older
A	199 or less	Subtract 2	Subtract 1
B	between 200 and 224	Subtract 1	Subtract 1
C	between 225 and 249	Add 0	Add 0
D	250 or higher	Add 1	Add 0
		Equals [ ]	Equals [ ]

4. Cigarette Smoking

If you . . .

(If you smoke a pipe, but not cigarettes, use the same score adjustment as those cigarette smokers who smoke less than a pack a day.)

	54 or Younger	55 or Older
do not smoke	Subtract 1	Subtract 2
smoke less than a pack a day	Add 0	Subtract 1
smoke a pack a day	Add 1	Add 0
smoke more than a pack a day	Add 2	Add 3
	Final Score Equals [ ]	Final Score Equals [ ]

Your Height		Weight Category (lbs.)				
Ft	In	A	B	C	D	
5	1	up to 123	124-148	149-173	174 plus	Because both blood pressure
5	2	up to 126	127-152	153-178	179 plus	and blood cholesterol are re-
5	3	up to 129	130-156	157-182	183 plus	lated to weight, an estimate
5	4	up to 132	133-160	161-186	187 plus	of these risk factors for each
5	5	up to 135	136-163	164-190	191 plus	weight category is printed
5	6	up to 139	140-168	169-196	197 plus	at the bottom of the table.
5	7	up to 144	145-174	175-203	204 plus	
5	8	up to 148	149-179	180-209	210 plus	
5	9	up to 152	153-184	185-214	215 plus	
5	10	up to 157	158-190	191-221	222 plus	
5	11	up to 161	162-194	195-227	228 plus	
6	0	up to 165	166-199	200-232	233 plus	
6	1	up to 170	171-205	206-239	240 plus	
6	2	up to 175	176-211	212-246	247 plus	
6	3	up to 180	181-217	218-253	254 plus	
6	4	up to 185	186-223	224-260	261 plus	
6	5	up to 190	191-229	230-267	268 plus	
6	6	up to 195	196-235	236-274	275 plus	

Weight Table for Men Look for your height (without shoes) in the far left column and then read across to find the category into which your weight (in indoor clothing) would fall.

	A	B	C	D
Estimate of Systolic Blood Pressure	119 or less	120 to 139	140 to 159	160 or more
Estimate of Blood Cholesterol	199 or less	200 to 224	225 to 249	250 or more

Women

Find the column for your age group. Every-one starts with a score of 10 points. Work down the page *adding* points to your score or *subtracting* points from your score.

	54 or Younger	55 or Older
	Starting Score **10**	Starting Score **10**

1. Weight
Locate your weight category in the table below. If you are in . .

		54 or Younger	55 or Older
	weight category A	Subtract 2	Subtract 2
	weight category B	Subtract 1	Subtract 1
	weight category C	Add 1	Add 0
	weight category D	Add 2	Add 1
		Equals ☐	Equals ☐

2. Systolic Blood Pressure
Use the "first" or "higher" number from your most recent blood pressure measurement. If you do not know your blood pressure, estimate it by using the letter for your weight category. If your blood pressure is . . .

		54 or Younger	55 or Older
A	119 or less	Subtract 2	Subtract 3
B	between 120 and 139	Subtract 1	Add 0
C	between 140 and 159	Add 0	Add 3
D	160 or greater	Add 1	Add 6
		Equals ☐	Equals ☐

3. Blood Cholesterol Level
Use the number from your most recent blood cholesterol test. If you do not know your blood cholesterol, estimate it by using the letter for your weight category. If your blood cholesterol is . . .

		54 or Younger	55 or Older
A	199 or less	Subtract 1	Subtract 3
B	between 200 and 224	Add 0	Subtract 1
C	between 225 and 249	Add 0	Add 1
D	250 or higher	Add 1	Add 3
		Equals ☐	Equals ☐

4. Cigarette Smoking
If you . . .

		54 or Younger	55 or Older
	do not smoke	Subtract 1	Subtract 2
	smoke less than a pack a day	Add 0	Subtract 1
	smoke a pack a day	Add 1	Add 1
	smoke more than a pack a day	Add 2	Add 4
		Equals ☐	Equals ☐

5. Estrogen Use
Birth control pills and hormone drugs contain estrogen. A few examples are: • Premarin • Ogan • Menstranol • Provera • Evex • Menest • Estinyl • Meurium

• Have your ever taken estrogen for five or more years in a row?
• Are you age 35 years or older and are now taking estrogen?

		54 or Younger	55 or Older
	No to both questions	Add 0	Add 0
	Yes to one or both questions	Add 1	Add 3
		Final Score Equals ☐	Final Score Equals ☐

Weight Table for Women
Look for your height (with-out shoes) in the far left column and then read across to find the category into which your weight (in indoor clothing) would fall.

Because both blood pressure and blood cholesterol are re-lated to weight, an estimate of these risk factors for each weight category is printed at the bottom of the table.

Your Height	Weight Category (lbs.)								
Ft In	A	B	C	D	Ft In	A	B	C	D
4 8	up to 101	102-122	123-143	144 plus	5 3	up to 122	123-148	149-172	173 plus
4 9	up to 103	104-125	126-146	147 plus	5 4	up to 127	128-154	155-179	180 plus
4 10	up to 106	107-128	129-150	151 plus	5 5	up to 131	132-158	159-185	186 plus
4 11	up to 109	110-132	133-154	155 plus	5 6	up to 135	136-163	164-190	191 plus
5 0	up to 112	113-136	137-158	159 plus	5 7	up to 139	140-168	169-196	197 plus
5 1	up to 115	116-139	140-162	163 plus	5 8	up to 143	144-173	174-202	203 plus
5 2	up to 119	120-144	145-168	169 plus	5 9	up to 147	148-178	179-207	208 plus
					5 10	up to 151	152-182	183-213	214 plus
					5 11	up to 155	156-187	188-218	219 plus
					6 0	up to 159	160-191	192-224	225 plus
					6 1	up to 163	164-196	197-229	230 plus

	A	B	C	D
Estimate of Systolic Blood Pressure	119 or less	120 to 139	140 to 159	160 or more
Estimate of Blood Cholesterol	199 or less	200 to 224	225 to 249	250 or more

What Your
Score Means

| 0-4 | You have one of the lowest risks of Heart Disease for your age and sex. |

Warning
- If you have diabetes, gout or a family history of heart disease, your actual risk will be greater than indicated by this appraisal.

| 5-9 | You have a low to moderate risk of Heart Disease for your age and sex but there is some room for improvement. |

- If you do not know your current blood pressure or blood cholesterol level, you should visit your physician or health center to have them measured. Then figure your score again for a more accurate determination of your risk.

| 10-14 | You have a moderate to high risk of Heart Disease for your age and sex, with considerable room for improvement on some factors. |

| 15-19 | You have a high risk of developing Heart Disease for your age and sex with a great deal of room for improvement on all factors. |

- If you are overweight, have high blood pressure or high blood cholesterol, or smoke cigarettes, your long-term risk of heart disease is increased even if your risk in the next several years is low.

| 20 & over | You have a very high risk of developing Heart Disease for your age and sex and should take immediate action on all risk factors. |

How to
Reduce Your Risk

- Try to quit smoking permanently. There are many programs available.
- Have your blood pressure checked regularly, preferably every twelve months after age 40. If your blood pressure is high, see your physician. Remember blood pressure medicine is only effective if taken regularly.
- Consider your daily exercise (or lack of it). A half hour of brisk walking, swimming or other enjoyable activity should not be difficult to fit into your day.
- Give some serious thought to your diet. If you are over-weight, or eat a lot of foods high in saturated fat or cholesterol (whole milk, cheese, eggs, butter, fatty foods, fried foods) then changes should be made in your diet. Look for the American Heart Association Cookbook at your local bookstore.
- Visit or write your local Heart Association for further information and copies of free pamphlets on many related subjects including:
  - Reducing your risk of heart attack.
  - Controlling high blood pressure.
  - Eating to keep your heart healthy.
  - How to stop smoking.
  - Exercising for good health.

Some Words
of Caution

- If you have diabetes, gout, or a family history of heart disease, your real risk of developing heart disease will be greater than indicated by your RISKO score. If your score is high and you have one or more of these additional problems, you should give particular attention to reducing your risk.
- If you are a woman under 45 years or a man under 35 years of age, your RISKO score represents an upper limit on your real risk of developing heart disease. In this case your real risk is probably lower than indicated by your score.
- If you are a woman whose use of estrogen has contributed to a high RISKO score, you may want to consult your physican. Do not automatically discontinue your prescription.
- Using your weight category to estimate your systolic blood pressure or your blood cholesterol level makes your RISKO score less accurate.
  - Your score will tend to overestimate your risk if your actual values on these two important factors are average for someone of your height and weight.
  - Your score will underestimate your risk if your actual blood pressure or cholesterol level is above average for someone of your height or weight.

Note. From *RISKO. A Dietary Approach to the Prevention of Coronary Heart Disease* (pp. 1-4) by The American Heart Association, 1981, Dallas, TX: Author. Copyright 1981 by The American Heart Association.

Chapter

11

Wellness and the Quality of Life

Who well lives, long lives, for this age of
ours
Should not be numbered by years, days,
and hours.
Guillaume de Salluste
Seigneur de Bartas, 1544-1590

This chapter will help you

- understand that a positive (wellness) attitude is difficult to maintain unless you regularly engage in some form of endurance exercise;
- realize that exercise probably becomes more important for wellness as you age;
- undertake self-experiments to obtain maximum benefits at minimum danger; and
- enjoy the game of Wellness Index.

Wellness and Feedback

The diagram we began with in chapter 1 is really an outline of feedback systems. Our behavior, either personal or interpersonal (social), provides the central nervous system with many feedback signals. We can adjust our behavior in accordance with these signals if we choose and thereby accomplish a wide variety of objectives. Some of these may maintain or increase wellness; others may decrease it.

Physical activity stimulates the muscles to produce feedback signals that have a positive effect on the nervous system and which tend to increase wellness. If the exercises have been general and involved most of the muscles, the signals, too, arise from all over the person, and a general feeling of well-being (i.e., wellness) prevails.

For years the term *psychosomatic* has been used to refer to communication between body and mind with the implication that the mind controlled the body. To emphasize the importance of the inverse relation of the body on the mind, the term *somatopsychic* has been created. This term also suffers from the mind-body dualism but draws attention to the effects of muscle activity on the nervous system.

The time relations of feedback also strongly affect behavior. When we really feel good, we know it. Can you imagine anyone saying, "I felt on top of the world yesterday but didn't realize it"? That all-too-rare feeling comes when our minds and our bodies seem to be in tune, coordinated, and reinforcing each other. Feedback from behavior can be very slow, however, requiring months or even years. Occasionally I receive an insight, a new meaning or interpretation of a happening that occurred years ago, that completely changes my reaction to it. I might add that not all of these are ego boosting. I accept them as contributing to my wellness. Part of my interpretation of wellness is learning to live with myself as a human being and to accept myself with all my faults and not berate myself for not being a god. I rationalize my failures by thinking that wellness feelings are based more on intent and attempts to act as a model human being than on achieving demi-god status.

Roadblocks to Wellness

Actually, premature death might be considered the greatest roadblock to wellness. Recent figures on the three major chronic diseases ranked in terms of years of potential life lost before age 65 in the U.S., and recently released by the Centers for Disease Control (1986), are sobering.

The first is malignant neoplasms (cancer) at 1,800,000 years lost; the second is heart diseases at 1,563,000; and the third is cerebrovascular diseases at 266,000. When ranked by deaths per 100,000 people, the order is slightly different: heart diseases, 324/100,000; cancer, 192/100,000; and cerebrovascular, 66/100,000 (Centers for Disease Control, 1986).

This ranking is not new. These diseases have been the biggest killers since the 1950s. I reproduce them here, not because I expect reading them will change people's behavior, especially children's, but to show the size of the problem and what might be accomplished. In fact, the incidence of both heart diseases and hypertension has been significantly reduced in the U.S. and Finland in recent years. This research, and the attendant publicity, has demonstrated not only that many people are voluntarily altering their health habits, but also that these changes by adults can affect the subsequent incidence of these diseases.

All three of these diseases have long latent periods. Overweight/obesity has been identified as a risk factor in all three. Symptoms generally don't develop before middle age or even later. With all three, it is now considered advisable to postpone the onset of symptoms as long as possible rather than to attempt to reverse them after they have appeared.

The feelings of wellness have been lost by many civilized people. The tensions, frustrations, and discontents of civilization have banished feelings of wellness. To many people, relaxation means being entertained by sitting in a chair sipping a drink, looking at a sitcom, or attending a movie or a ball game. These are pleasurable activities, but they are not tension-relieving on a long-term basis. People return from vacations as tense as ever. Even gambling has become a passive sport as witnessed by the popularity of slot machines and bingo. Macho people play poker and bridge where ability still affects the outcome.

How does one overcome a roadblock? How do you break out of a downward spiral? In my opinion, too many people in America are choosing alcohol and hard drugs as their way out. The way I am suggesting is admittedly more difficult, but it has been achieved by enough people to make me optimistic that other millions can also do it. It amounts to generating desires and satisfactions from within rather than attempting to buy them as though they were consumer items.

The question becomes: How can people who have not felt well since they were ten, who have been living a life of ease and inactivity, and who are stuck in a boring job or are unemployed be convinced of the relationship between physical activity and wellness sufficiently strongly for them to change their lifestyle? It requires making an *assumption* that it will work for them. It amounts to an act of faith in themselves.

Quality of Life: Quality of Health

The activities that we use to describe quality of life are very different for different people. To me, quality of life means considerable physical activity, not just for health's sake but because I enjoy it. To someone else, quality of life may mean being able to read for hours each day. Others may prefer gambling casinos and one-armed bandits. Still others may engage in spiritual/religious activities. I make no value judgments on other peoples' quality of life.

I do assume, however, that whatever your type of work and whatever you like to do in your spare time, you will enjoy your activities more and be able to participate in them for many more years if you maintain your health. I also assume that good nutrition and a certain amount of physical activity are essential to the long-term goal of health maintenance and wellness. In other words, your quality of life is affected in large part by your quality of health.

What if a person's quality of life includes such bad habits as smoking a pack of cigarettes a day, habitual overeating, and occasional overdrinking? It is obvious that some people live for the moment only, whereas others may think that "it can't happen to me." Some people keep their cars in better shape than they do their bodies. Would you ride in a car that had smooth tires or worn brake linings, or that stalled unpredictably, without being concerned? Overweight, hypertensive smokers are taking even greater chances with their lives.

The wellness helix in Figure 11.1 shows attitude as one of its three strands. In my opinion, your attitude is the key to all of your actions. Many people may agree intellectually with the statements that I make

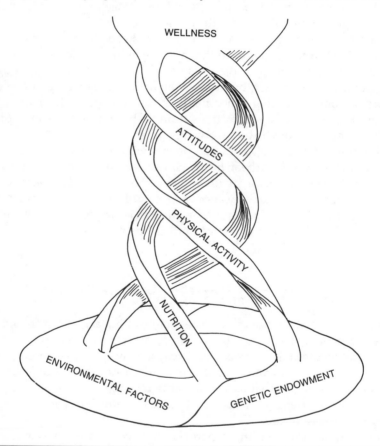

Figure 11.1 Wellness helix.

in this chapter, but if they are not motivated sufficiently to do something they will have missed the whole point. Although action without knowledge is foolhardy, knowledge without action is sterile.

Living dangerously is, of course, each individual's right. If people are aware of the risks they are taking and are willing to take the consequences, all we can do is wish them luck. This book is not for such people, at least for now. Others with the same habits may not be satisfied and may be looking for ways to change their lifestyles but may not know where to begin. For them, this chapter may be helpful. I would suggest, first, a gradual increase in physical activity.

Fitness Feedback

If we are physically fit, our bodies not only are in shape but send signals to the nervous system that tend to stimulate a positive self-image. This type of feedback is rapid and almost continuous. When our joints feel lubricated and our muscles are in tone, we tend to feel positive in a general sense. We are on target. These effects should not be surprising in view of the history of human development.

The evolution of the human species, starting with the early hominids, is thought to cover about 5 million years. Throughout most of this period, survival was dependent on physical activity. Hunting-gathering, agriculture, construction, war: All required coordinated effort between the muscular system and the nervous system. Up until recently, this connection was taken for granted. With few exceptions, all of mankind had no choice but to earn a living by physical activity. In this connection it is interesting that the word *work* is derived from the Greek *wergon* meaning action. Exercise psychologists and physiologists are working out the pathways and mechanisms by which the nervous and muscular systems interact. This interaction is essential to the coordinated behavior on which individual survival depends.

The evolutionary view of man's development leads to the conclusion that considerable physical activity is not only desirable for health maintenance, but is probably essential. Next, I will refer to some of the studies that correlate wellness with physical activity. The results are sufficiently consistent to warrant the suggestion that a certain minimum of physical activity is probably as necessary for long-term wellness as an adequate diet.

Psychological Benefits From Physical Activity

The reasons behind this suggestion are based on the psychological effects of physical activity. The literature is filled with statements about the positive psychological effects of exercise. Susan Edmiston (1978) in *Woman's Day* wrote the following:

> During a period of severe depression I began to study jujitsu. My purpose was to feel safer on the streets of New York City. The immediate results were completely unexpected. Within two weeks, the training began to have a dramatic effect on my life. My posture and mood changed markedly as passivity and depression gave way to energy and euphoria.
>
> Many other women have had similar experiences. One friend of mine took up running and discovered a new sense of calm and ease. Margo Lawrence, a TV producer, took up ballet three years ago and now goes to class four or five times a week. Although she has changed physically, it's the psychological change that's dramatic. Her image of herself is so improved that she recently auditioned to appear on camera. (p. 99)

At a symposium on exercise and health, Hales (1979) reported that Dr. William Haskell at Stanford Medical School outlined five major contributions of exercise, one of which was psychological factors. These psychological factors are described in terms of the layperson: "Most active people speak of improved mood, less tension, even a certain euphoria" (p. 23). Haskell quoted a 1978 Harris Poll in which active exercisers cited such psychological benefits as sleeping better, feeling more relaxed, having more concentration and discipline, and having an improved self-confidence and self-esteem.

This conclusion is echoed in a Surgeon General's Report (1979): "People who exercise regularly report that they feel better, have more energy . . . often lose excess weight as well as improve muscular strength and flexibility. Many also experience psychological benefits including enhanced self-esteem, greater self-reliance, decreased anxiety, and relief from mild depression" (p. 133).

I want to emphasize that exercise is not just for the young. It can be commenced at any age. Edmiston (1978) mentions a 64-year-old woman who had begun swimming 7 years earlier after the removal of a spinal disc left one leg paralyzed. Swimming helped her in regaining use of the leg and also has aided her psychologically.

De Vries (1981) has reported that tranquilizer effects can be readily achieved in people by moderate amounts of aerobic exercise. Cooper (1978) summarized the effects of an exercise program as follows:

> Improve your physical fitness category. Start one of the programs of aerobic exercise you'll find in our chart pack. As you get more fit you'll gradually find your other risk factors are coming into line. Dieting will be easier and won't have to be so extreme. Your willpower,

bolstered by regular exercise, will help you cope with urges for tobacco and alcohol. And the strength you feel, coupled with your decreases in adrenal hormone levels, will help you ride out stress situations with more calm and more confidence. (p. 43)

Wilson, Morley, and Bird (1980) examined the psychological effects of varying degrees of exercise of 30 men, 20-45 years, living in a large city. Each person was asked to complete a profile of his mood states the previous week. The subjects were divided into three groups: 10 marathon runners who regularly ran 6 to 20 miles on 6 or 7 days a week for the previous 2 years; 10 joggers who averaged 1 or 2 miles on 3 to 5 days a week for the previous 2 years; and 10 nonexercisers from the same socioeconomic stratum as the joggers and runners.

The consistency of the results is impressive. The marathoners and joggers reported less depression ($p < .003$), less anger ($p < .001$), less confusion ($p < .001$), and more vigor ($p < .001$) than the nonexercisers. The marathoners also reported less fatigue and tension than the nonexercisers. In a comparison of the marathoners to the joggers, the former came out better in reporting less depression, less anger, less confusion, and more vigor.

This work raises the interesting possibility that, although jogging short distances 3 to 5 days a week may be sufficient to maintain cardiovascular fitness and to elevate mood somewhat, running longer distances has even greater psychological benefits. The results obtained in this study confirm and extend those from other laboratories (Cureton, 1963; Folkins & Sime, 1981; Ismail & Young, 1973; Lion, 1978; Morgan, 1979).

A general objection to this type of study is that despite the impressive p values, such a survey proves nothing. The type of person who takes up running, especially marathon running, is quite different from those who prefer not to exercise that vigorously. Thus the psychological differences may have been inherent in the two groups. The criticism is justified, but consider the difficulties in obtaining subjects for a more rigorous experiment.

Suppose a scientist had available 1,000 men or women chosen at random in a specified age group, say 25 to 35 years, all in good health and with no serious psychological or physical problems. Collecting a group of this size would be no mean task. The researcher would than randomly assign each person to one of three groups: nonexercisers, joggers, and marathoners. They would all be given a personality mood profile check list. No differences would be expected among the groups. Each subject's mood profile would be measured after 1, 2, or more years.

I would guess that the dropout rate in the marathon group would be very high, whereas that among the joggers would be appreciable. These changes would seriously affect the statistical significance of the measurements. Thus even this ideal experiment would not furnish as conclusive results as might be imagined. In other words, it will probably be a long time, if ever, before there are more conclusive data on mood changes of runners/joggers than those mentioned above.

In an interesting small-scale, short-term experiment, Sinyor, Schwartz, Perronnet, Brisson, and Seraganian (1983) placed 15 fit and 15 unfit persons in psychosocial stressful situations and measured their emotional responses. Heart rate and subjective arousal level increased markedly during the stressors in both groups. Aerobically fit subjects showed more rapid heart rate recovery following the stressors, and lower levels of anxiety at the conclusion of the session. The results suggest that trained subjects may be capable of faster recovery in both physiological and subjective aspects of emotionality.

Collingwood, Douds, Williams and Wilson (1978) have described a very interesting and valuable experiment on the effect of fitness training on young (18- to 26-year-old) male rehabilitation clients. One person from each of 25 matched pairs was randomly selected for the physical training program, which required participation for an hour a day, 5 days a week for 4 weeks (20 hours total). The workouts included calisthenics, aerobics, and agility exercises. The subjects were tested before and after the training by various fitness measurements and for body attitude and self-concept. The subjects were also rated by their counselors for physical, intellectual, and interpersonal behavior before and after the training program.

As might be expected, the experimental subjects increased significantly in physical fitness. In addition, they also demonstrated greater positive changes on body attitudes ($p = .001$); self-concept ($p = .05$); and self-acceptance ($p = .05$). The counselors' evaluations, although not as quantitative, also showed improvement by the experimental subjects in physical functioning, intellectual functioning, and emotional-interpersonal functioning. The control subjects showed no significant changes in either physical, intellectual, or emotional-interpersonal behaviors. The results were considered significant enough by the rehabilitation facility administration to adopt the physical fitness program on a regular basis for the clients. The results of this study confirm similar experiments by others on the positive effects of fitness training on behavior and self-attitude of clients as well as of normal people.

The reports I have mentioned vary from anecdotal to semicontrolled scientific experiments. The impressive thing about them is their consistency. A person is quite unusual who doesn't benefit psychologically from some type of regular exercise. In fact, many health experts suggest exercise as the first step toward wellness.

The question that needs to be raised at this point concerns whether these reports are sufficiently conclusive to warrant a general recommendation to the readers of this book. Will adopting an aerobic exercise program help you to cope? This question can be considered from either an empirical or a theoretical point of view. Folkins and Sime (1981) have critically reviewed over 100 experimental studies that attempt to answer some aspect of this question. They divided the experimental designs into three categories. Pre-experimental designs are studies of one group before and after the exercise program. Also included are case studies with a similar testing design. The second are quasi-experimental designs, in which both experimental and control groups receive both pre- and post-tests. Unfortunately, the experimental group was seldom assigned on a random basis. The third are true experimental designs, in which the groups are truly equivalent at the start and sufficient environmental variables have been controlled so that one may infer with some assurance that the results are due to the difference in exercise between the two groups and not to some other variable like changes in diet, motivation, and so forth.

The results suggest that physical fitness training leads to improved mood, self-concept, and work behavior. Other aspects of personality, as measured by Cattell's Sixteen Personality Factor questionnaire (Ismail & Young, 1973) or the Minnesota Multiphasic Personality Inventory (Naughton, Bruhn, & Lategola, 1968), did not change significantly from fitness training. The important question raised above cannot be answered at this time with the assurance that it deserves. Insofar as an improved self-concept helps a person to cope, the answer is yes. The other studies, although consistent among themselves, do not warrant a high degree of confidence in their conclusions. I might add that no study reported a decrease in desirable psychological traits. Folkins and Sime (1981) suggest that this field of research is ripe for well-designed, long-term experimental studies from which definite conclusions can be drawn.

I'll briefly summarize two experiments that approached this subject in different ways. Roth and Holmes (1985) asked 112 subjects to report their stressful life changes for the previous 12 months, and then to have their fitness evaluated by a submaximal bicycle ergometer test. A high level of stress the preceding year correlated with poorer physical health for subjects with a low level of endurance fitness than for fit people. In addition, fit subjects reported less depression resulted from previous stressful events than the less fit. Goldwater and Collis (1985) randomly assigned college students to a cardiovascular fitness program or to a control program for 6 weeks. The cardiovascular group showed a greater reduction of anxiety and a greater increase in well-being than the control group. From a theoretical standpoint, the *proprioceptive receptor system* provides a pathway by which signals can flow from the skeletal muscles to the nervous system. These signals result in the positive somatopsychic effects mentioned previously.

Don't misunderstand me. The people I know who exercise, including myself, do not float on cloud nine sipping nectar all the time. We are subject to depression, anxiety, and frustrations like anyone else. But my impression is that as a group we weather stresses better than nonactive people. Often when people get down in the dumps they cut down or give up exercising altogether. The remedy is just the opposite. A long brisk walk in a park or in the woods, jogging, or whatever aerobic exercise you like to do, just do it, and there is a good chance that you'll feel better. I don't apologize for this anecdotal paragraph. It's on my list of things that can't hurt and may help.

Effects of Fitness Loss

Friends have told me that they have not started an exercise program because once they start, they'll have to continue with it. In one sense they are correct. There is no question that becoming fit and maintaining it requires an aerobics program for a minimum time each session and a minimum of three sessions per week. The implication that something dreadful will befall a person who stops exercising, however, is quite inaccurate. A person who stops exercising becomes gradually unfit. That is all. The positive signals that they have been receiving from their muscle-nervous system feedback also stop. Some people who are used to daily physical activity suffer withdrawal symptoms within a day or two if they stop the activity. These symptoms affect mood and even behavior. Baekeland (1970) asked a group of students who exercised regularly to stop it for 30 days and to report any consistent psychological effects that they noticed. The effects were all negative and included insomnia, increased anxiety, and increased sexual tension.

These psychological states are not uncommon in the nonexercising population. It is possible, perhaps even probable, that the surfacing of these unpleasant effects were not withdrawal symptoms but merely a return to what is considered normal in the general population. I suspect that relatively unfit people become inured to these unpleasant states and tend to accept them as stresses of modern living.

Many people seem unaware of the close connection between their physical and mental states. In our culture the former is often ignored and negative psychological feelings like anxiety, tension, and insomnia are treated with over-the-counter or prescribed drugs. The holistic approach suggests that the whole person be examined first. If the body is unfit, steps to improve it should be undertaken before drugs are prescribed. This approach is now being applied by some psychiatrists who are treating depressed patients with aerobic training.

Fitness Training and Psychic Therapy

Greist et al. (1979), at the University of Wisconsin, divided 28 depressed patients into three groups: the first was treated with short-term therapy, a second with unlimited therapy, and the third ran 3 times a week with no therapy. At the end of the 10-week study, the runners and those who received short-term therapy were greatly improved. Greist et al. concluded that ". . . as treatment for moderate depression, running was at least as effective in alleviating depression symptoms and target complaints as either time-limited or time-unlimited psychotherapy" (p. 47). Depression, of course, can range from mild to severe, and from short- to long-term. Although it is likely that patients who can be induced to become physically active will become less depressed, there are many others for whom such activity would be out of the question.

In another experimental study, Hanson (1970) cited by Folkins and Sime (1981) reported that 30 minutes of movement training, 5 times a week, helped decrease anxiety in 4-year-olds enrolled at the UCLA elementary school.

Psychiatrist T. Kostroluba (1980) as cited by Drake (1980) treats patients by encouraging them to run. He speaks of running as "fending off the demons of the soul" and of fulfilling three ultimate delusions of mankind. The first delusion is that running makes people think that they can control their environment and their health. The second delusion of running is that it brings people into contact with other like-minded persons. Feelings of elitism are fostered, which are satisfying to the ego. The third delusion of runners is their belief in the generation of personal magic that produces a feeling of power. This delusion likewise "strengthens the ego in its eternal battle with the super-ego" (p. 11).

The reports of Greist et al. (1979) and of Hanson (1970) deserve special comment because they are among the few studies in this subject area in which the participants have been assigned to a group on a random basis. These studies approach one-variable experiments and thus are entitled to a much higher degree of confidence than those in which the participants served as their own controls, or in which the participants were volunteers. These two reports will gain in stature if and when they are confirmed by other scientists with even larger groups.

I have written this section as if everyone would benefit from aerobic exercise. This *assumption* may be too general because it ignores the attitudes, beliefs, and expectations of people with regard to physical activity. Individual differences must be recognized in working out an activity program.

Attitude and behavior form a tight couple. A pessimistic, defeatist-type of person is less apt to try new things and less likely to become involved in community affairs, for example, than an optimistic, outgoing person. Our attitudes, however, are not the maypole around which we dance. Psychologists now assign that role to our value systems and *assumptions*. These form the central pivot of our lives and determine how we interpret experiences. In fact, the only reality we know is filtered through the screen of our value judgments and assumptions.

For example, fat people may be depressed (an attitude) because they think (assume) that is the reason they are not more popular (a value). Their attitude influences whether they suffer in silence and do nothing, go on a diet, or join a weight loss group. They may lose 50 lb, but if the desired result (popularity) is not achieved, they are likely to gain weight again. In other words, therapy that does not probe into and make people aware of their value systems and the effects that these have on their attitudes and behavior is often unsuccessful.

This limitation also applies to physical activity's effect on attitude. Although physical activity may improve attitude, unless the activity meshes with the person's value system—by which I mean that the chosen activities are truly enjoyable—they will not survive the usual flush of original enthusiasm. The unknown mechanism by which physical activity influences attitude is probably different from that of psychotherapy. The holistic view expressed in this book suggests that the two supplement and reinforce each other.

Aging Gracefully Equals Aging Aerobically

Earlier I enviously mentioned the enormous energy of a 5-year-old child. What about that of a 10-year-old? In these 5 years a person develops a bigger body and is better coordinated. A 10-year-old should be able to do more and do it better than a 5-year-old. But what do we find? We find them sitting in front of a TV set an average of over 4 hours per day! Gilliam, Katch, Thorland, and Weltman (1977) found close to half of Michigan elementary school children showed one or more coronary risk factors. Fortunately, they also found that high blood lipids (cholesterol) could be reduced in a 12-week program of vigorous physical activity for 25 minutes per day, 4 days a week. In other words, children need and benefit from aerobic exercise as much as adults. It is likely that much of the teenage obesity, self-consciousness, and clumsiness could be avoided by programs of aerobic exercises. The art of aging gracefully should be practiced by everyone at as young an age as possible.

Fortunate are the people who reach 50 both fit and competent. They need merely to continue on a wellness program with allowances for aging. Such people, unfortunately, are all too rare in America. The majority of Americans are fat at 50. It is still widely believed that weekend activity is sufficient to keep a person in shape. It isn't. In fact, it is safer to do nothing than to exercise vigorously once a week. Serious injuries, stiffness, and fatigue may be the reward, and the danger of a heart attack is increased (Brooks & Fahey, 1984, p. 518).

Many people who are not fit may attend an aerobics dance class or attempt to jog with a friend and decide that the effort is too great. They may conclude that they have passed the age when fitness was a feasible goal. This conclusion is most unfortunate because it needn't be accepted. The walking program presented in Table 7.6 can be used as a specific means of trailblazing. It applies to anyone who is well enough to walk. It suggests daily walking at a comfortable pace, with gradually increasing speed as the person becomes able. Even obese people soon begin to benefit from the training effect. If walking with a partner helps, do it. If you prefer to walk when and where you want by yourself, do that. At the beginning, make it as easy as possible for yourself to open your door and get out. Later on, when the regular activity becomes enjoyable and you look forward to it, you may want to set goals for yourself.

Many people are suspicious of self-experimentation. It smacks of being too scientific, too introspective. If you number yourself in this group and want to let your feelings be the sole guide to your actions, go right ahead. The main thing is to do something active each day. Other people may enjoy self-experimentation and get a kick out of watching their progress or improvement in whatever program they have mapped out for themselves. For this group, I suggest choosing objective measurements whenever possible and recording the results.

De Vries (1970) studied the effects of an exercise program on men aged 52 to 88 (average age 69.5). Volunteers were solicited from the Leisure World retirement community in Laguna Hills, California. Each subject was examined by a physician, and only those who were medically free of diagnosable cardiovascular, pulmonary, or other disorders that would contraindicate vigorous exercise were admitted to the training regimen. The program began with an easy run-walk exercise that gradually increased in aerobic intensity. The regimen also included a calisthenics warm-up period and a cool-down to prevent soreness and improve joint mobility.

After 42 weeks of training, the oxygen volume per pulse increased 29% ($p = .05$), vital capacity increased 20% ($p = .01$), minute volume of respired air increased 35% ($p = .01$), strength increased 12% ($p = .01$), and muscle girth increased 1% ($p = .05$). There were no statistically significant changes in blood pressure, muscle relaxation, physical work capacity, weight, or percent body fat. The control group, who did not exercise, showed no significant changes in any parameter. De Vries concluded that overall fitness improved significantly in the exercise group under conditions that were both safe and effective.

From the standpoint of wellness, it is as desirable for 75-year-old people to maintain their fitness as it is for 25-year-olds. In this connection, it is significant that the U.S. Tennis Association in 1977 established singles and doubles championships for men 80 and over. One occasionally reads about octogenerians or even centenarians who climb mountains, swim, run long distances, or accomplish other feats of physical prowess. I look forward to the day when such accomplishments will no longer be newsworthy.

Kraus (1972) suggests that much of the back pain suffered by Americans is due to muscle tension. He mentions that a group of physicians examined over 3,000 patients and found that 83% of those with back pain had no pathological disorder. Pain was due to weakness or stiffness of key muscles. Tension and lack of physical activity contributed to the disabilities. Relaxation and stretching exercises of tight muscles was effective in decreasing back pain. Exercise even helped patients with advanced osteoarthritic changes.

Outwitting Freud

As you may recall, Freud suggested that the three common responses to the diseases of civilization were withdrawal, pleasurable activities, and anesthesia (i.e., alcohol and drugs). It is interesting that two pleasurable activities that he didn't mention were overeating and smoking cigarettes. At that time the pathological consequences of chronic overeating and inhaling tobacco smoke were relatively unknown. Medical research in recent years has conclusively demonstrated the serious effects of these two habits. The self-destructive effects of both have been widely publicized so that anyone who continues to smoke or overeat is publicly admitting that he or she has a psychological problem that is unresolved. There are two major differences between these two habits and excessive drinking. Smoking and overeating are not as rapidly debilitating as alcoholism or as devastating on personal relationships. Also, a person's ability to keep a job is not impaired to the same extent. For these reasons, and possibly others, the two habits are less socially unacceptable than alcoholism.

Many people are well enough so that when the consequences of smoking or overeating are pointed out to them (as I have attempted to do in this book), they can quit. These people should keep the following suggestions in mind: Don't look at controlling appetite or quitting smoking as giving up something you enjoy for a pie-in-the-sky reward that you may collect 20 or 40 years from now; look at it as giving up one set of habits that have been demonstrated to restrict living activities for another set that are life-enhancing, here and now. For those other people who can't quit, I suggest that they start seeking help immediately and continue experimenting with different methods until they find one that works.

Minding the Minutes of Everyday Existence

Are you overworked, harried, and generally too busy?

If the answer to this question is yes, ask yourself another:

Are you aware of your priorities?

If the answer to this question is also yes, then you may need to inquire what satisfactions you are receiving from being overworked and harried. Perhaps you really like it, but hesitate to admit it. However, if your priorities seem in opposition to your actions and attitude, you may find playing the living game fun, as well as useful in working your way out of your predicament. Any person can play, and the only requirement is being honest with yourself. Playing involves making up personal questions, answering them, and basing future behavior on rational choices.

If you don't know your long-term priorities, or are not clear about them, now is the time to find out. On a relaxed, nonwork morning, go back over the week's activities hour by hour, from getting up to going to bed. If you can't recall details, keep a list first so that you can review it later. Separate your actions into two categories: those you need to do or have to do, such as your job, your responsibilities to other people, shopping, food preparation, eating, sleeping, and the like; and those you do voluntarily because you want to. Now look critically at both lists.

Score each activity from 1 to 5, with the highest number representing the most satisfactory on a long-term basis. What are the trade-offs? Is your job boring and leading you to a dead-end? Do you stay with it only because it pays well? Try to imagine how you'll feel about your job in 5 years. Which means more to you: a challenging but lower-paying job with a future, or the extra money that you're earning now, which allows you to buy nice clothes, a handsome car, or a VCR?

Consider your relationships with others. Is being a spouse and a lover as delightful as you had imagined it? Or is the shine wearing off the veneer? Is the relationship deepening? How do you see your role in improving the relationship? After the first serious fight in marriage, how do you recapture the romantic feeling? Should you take the initiative or wait for your lover to make the first move? How do you learn to forgive? Is everything forgivable? If not, where do you draw the line?

Consider communication. How many of your thoughts can you tell your friends? Have you any idea how many they can tell you? Do you become angry at criticism of any kind? Can you make suggestions to your lover without making him or her angry? If you feel inept at these interchanges, do you wish to improve? Is it what you say, or how you say it? Do you know where you can obtain expert assistance?

Types of Voluntary Activities

- Having fun (immediate enjoyment)
- Learning
- Cultivating personal relationships
- Exercising for fitness maintenance
- Pursuing wellness

These activities can be judged on two scales: time and satisfaction. All five categories should be represented by a significant amount of time per week or month, although the amount of time that is significant may vary from one category to another or from year to year. Satisfaction should be high in all voluntary activities, although it need not be immediate.

Practices That Probably Won't Hurt, and May Help

The advances in medical sciences since 1950 are truly awe inspiring. Most of them are due to applications of technology to medical problems. We may expect such advances to continue. Despite this progress, one hears and reads about dozens or hundreds of patients who have sought medical advice and therapy for their problems, but have received little or no benefit. In fact, a sufficient number of people have been injured by physicians that malpractice insurance rates are at an all-time high. These sad incidents are the result of human errors, and, unfortunately, they will probably continue. What alternatives are available to people who have not been helped by the medical system either as a result of poor medical practice or because no therapy is known?

Left to their own devices, people will, and have, tried almost anything and everything. Such trials—I cannot call them experiments—are probably the basis of folk medicine. The results are strictly empirical. Someone has a pimple on his face and, for whatever reason, takes "X" and the pimple goes away. He tells his friends with pimples about it; they take "X" and are likewise cured. In a few years enough people have tried it and reported success that it is written up in *Prevention* magazine or in a Sunday supplement, and it becomes available to millions. There is no way of stopping such trials, and I am not even convinced that it would be desirable if it could be done. However, the public should be aware that certain cautions are essential so that people don't injure themselves in carrying out these practices. These cautions have been mentioned previously but, because of their importance, are worth repeating.

Caution One: Dosage

Remember that anything can be injurious if taken in large enough amounts. If the remedy you have heard about is an essential nutrient, check its safety factor in Table 6A.1. It is dangerous to exceed the highest listed safe amount for an extended period of time. If the substance does not appear in this table, try to find information on its safe range in the latest edition of the Merck Index, a textbook in nutrition, or other reliable source. State agricultural experiment stations and state universities have human nutrition departments and/or poison control centers that may be called or written for information. In addition, some pharmacists are knowledgeable on nutrition matters.

Caution Two: Time

Ask yourself this question: Is the remedy or change going to last a week, a month, a year, or for the rest of my life? The longer it is to last, the more careful you should be about dosage. One meal of polar bear liver, which contains 13,000 to 18,000 IU of vitamin A per gram (approximately 409,000 IU per ounce), can be fatal to a human.

Caution Three: Side Effects

In addition to the desirable changes that you are expecting, other effects may also occur. Remain aware of this possibility. If some undesirable effect happens, it is probably advisable to cut down on the dosage or stop completely.

Here are some practices that may not hurt and may help:

1. Decrease total fat content of diet from 40% to 30%.
2. Increase fiber content of diet by eating whole wheat bread, other whole grains, brown rice, and fresh fruits and vegetables daily.
3. Try whole-body relaxation techniques: meditation, massage, stress management. Relax your tongue before going to sleep.
4. Learn exercise techniques for endurance, exercise for 20 minutes, a minimum of 3 times per week. These should include adequate warm-up and cool-down periods. For strength, exercise for 15 minutes, 1-2 times per week.
5. Read food labels and use their information in food planning.
6. Swallow 1 mg fluoride per day (2.2 mg NaF) if your tap water is not fluoridated. Pills require a prescription.
7. Don't add salt to foods.
8. Consume processed foods minimally.
9. Take extra calcium (400-800 mg/day) if you don't drink much milk or eat dairy products.
10. Take extra vitamin C (250 mg/day) and total dietary fiber (25-40 g/day), preferably in food.
11. If confronted with a medical problem or condition, such as an allergy, hay fever, hyperactivity, headache, or other pain, and traditional medicine has been given a fair chance and has not helped, try something unconventional such as massage, acupuncture, no-additives diet, or extra vitamins. Check with knowledgeable people

or read reliable books in advance that the practice is neither harmful nor dangerous on a long-term basis.
12. Take time to enjoy something each day.

This list could be extended almost indefinitely, especially if curative
therapies were to be included. The ones included here are primarily for
wellness maintenance.

Children Are Parents of Adults

Kannell and Dawber (1972), in a paper entitled "Atherosclerosis as a Pediatric Problem," discussed the means by which the incidence of coronary
heart disease could be lowered. At present, one out of five males will
develop heart disease by age 60. They suggest that pediatricians look for
risk factors such as hypercholesterolemia and hypertension in children.
Early detection and control have a good chance of lowering the percentage of people who will develop heart disease in later life. They emphasize the role of diet and physical activity in controlling and avoiding risk
factors.

Williams, Arnold, and Wynder (1977) have begun a *Know Your Body*
program in New York and suburban schools. They examined over 3,000
children from 11 to 14 years old and found that 17% had blood cholesterol
over 180 mg/dl, 12% were classed as obese, and 10% smoked cigarettes.
Other studies have found that 40% of high school seniors smoke. Williams
et al. instituted a health intervention program that included both dietary
and physical activity components. It will be interesting to see how long-
term compliance and benefits compare in this age group with intervention programs with adults.

At what age should protective, life-enhancing measures be commenced?
For the first few years of life, diet is under the complete control of adults.
Is it important to monitor a child's diet? If so, at what age should it begin? Is it important to monitor a child's physical activities? If so, at what
age should it begin? Some pediatricians recommend that the prudent diet
be commenced at age 2 (Kwiterovich, 1986; National Institutes of Health
Consensus Conference, 1985). Admittedly, this recommendation is far
from proved and is controversial.

Dietz and Gordon (1981) reviewed the studies on infant, childhood,
and adolescent obesity and concluded that both heredity and environment contribute. They consider that family relationships are the most important factors, especially in young children. As children age, peer group
and cultural factors become more important. TV viewing, for example
cuts down on physical activity as well as encourages children to consume
high energy foods. Metabolic differences, i.e., heredity, undoubtedly account for differences in susceptibility to obesity.

Rather than picking a number out of a hat, I feel more comfortable suggesting a three-point plan as a basis for deciding when to initiate dietary control. This plan is based on the principle that children require the RDAs of essential nutrients and, like adults, should avoid overweight/ obesity. Point 1: Adults should insure that infants/children eat a varied, high-nutrient density diet. Point 2: Calories should be monitored in relation to physical activity. Obviously, calories need be sufficient for adequate growth and development. Beyond that requirement, calories should not be in excess to result in obesity/overweight (above the 75th percentile of the weight charts). Because most children like milk and drink lots of it, fat content can be regulated as a first measure of weight control. A thin and/or active child can be given whole milk; a stocky child, 2% milk; and one verging on overweight, 1% or even skim milk. If this tactic is insufficient to keep weight in the healthy range, other fats, as in spreads, meats, and rich desserts should be monitored. Point 3: Sweets should be regulated, but not prohibited for all children. If a child prefers a high-sugar cereal, he or she should be allowed less or no jam on the toast, and so on.

As soon as a child is old enough to understand the connection between eating and health, the idea of moderation should be introduced. Moderation includes quantity of calories as well as adequacy of nutrients. Another general guideline is that of responsibility. Again, as soon as the child learns that a stove or a pot is hot and can burn if one isn't careful, the idea of health can be introduced and the child made aware that ultimately his or her health is under her or his control. Notice that this recommendation combines the objectives of the Food and Nutrition Board with some of the dietary guidelines of the prudent diet advocates. In addition, it emphasizes the roles of physical activity as a nondietary means of weight control and personal responsibility as a lifelong guiding principle.

Healthful nutritional behavior of children has also been achieved by programs in the public schools. Douglas Fisk (1979) initiated a massive effort in the California public schools in *A Successful Program for Changing Children's Eating Habits*. Evaluation of the program was based both on knowledge gained and behavioral changes. Among teenagers, for example, 48% met the minimum requirements in each of the four food groups before instruction, whereas 69% did after instruction. This program has been successfully introduced in the nutrition teaching in the public schools of 11 other states, as well as for medical and dental students and the general public.

From Fisk's report and recent updates (Shortridge, personal communication, 1987) that detail successful mass nutrition educational programs, I conclude that it is not essential to start at age 2 or thereabouts. However, I think that it is advisable to identify children at risk as early on as possible. This group includes children from families in which parents or grandparents have had heart attacks, strokes, or diabetes at relatively young ages. The checkup should include analysis of blood lipids, glucose, and blood pressure. If any of these are out of line, a physician should be consulted.

A Wellness Index and Its Use

Using the three major strands that contribute to the wellness helix as a basis, I have divided each into smaller categories that readers can look at and grade themselves on a scale of their own choosing. Although I have placed percentages on the three major subdivisions of the Wellness Index, I have reservations about the advisability of attempting to quantify them. My objective is merely to indicate that attitude is the most important of the three in that it affects the other two more than they affect it. Because of these reservations, I have not quantified the subdivisions but suggest that each person place some percentages by each of the headings that will add up to the total. In doing this evaluation, your own value judgments will be utilized. In addition, you may want to add one or more categories of your own.

Your scores on the stress tests (Appendix 4A) will give you some idea of your coping capabilities in the different areas. No matter what the score, you may be pleased or dissatisfied with them. The comments on the scores are to help you decide whether you need help. Your evaluation of your personal relationships and personal satisfactions are very subjective. In thinking about these questions, you should strive to become aware of your inner feelings and not just make excuses for your inadequacies or pretend that your adequacies excuse your inadequacies. How many times have you acted boorishly and felt sorry about it later? How many times have you acted boorishly and have not been aware of it? What is responsible for the difference? What is your definition of boorish?

In my opinion, the distinction between active participation (A) and passive spectating (P) is an important one, with my bias favoring the former. You can get some idea of their ratio by clocking the hours you spend at each over a couple of average weeks. I suggest that A/P should be greater than 1. Voluntary mental stimulation is classed as an active activity. I would place the time you spend thinking about this index as active.

Lifestyle habits may be either positive or negative. I classify smoking, using mind-altering drugs, and overusing alcohol as negative; and blood pressure control, by whatever means, as positive. Both nutrition and exercise might be classed as lifestyle habits, but I have placed them in distinct categories because of their importance.

As was mentioned in chapters 7 and 8, fatness is related to both diet and endurance exercise. I suggest any value below 20% fat for men, and

25% for women as positive, and above those figures as negative. These percentages would be almost impossible of attainment by diet alone, aerobic activity is also needed. For this reason, I have placed it under "Exercise" rather than "Nutrition." Consumption of dietary fiber should total about 25 g/day (1 oz/day) from all the six types. Because these components are difficult to measure, suggested foods and amounts are included in Table 6A.

I credit all types of physical exercise as positive, with endurance classified as the most valuable. By voluntary physical stresses I mean such activities as long-distance running (10 kilometers and further), rock climbing, mountaineering, white-water rafting and kayaking, gliding, parachute jumping, long-distance swimming, and bicycling. Obviously, these activities will vary with age and previous experience.

Finally, I suggest that looking at the index will be interesting and perhaps useful on an annual basis. If you keep notes each time, I predict the results will be quite amusing, and possibly valuable, over a period of years.

A Wellness Index

Attitude   40%
  Spirituality
    Your value judgments, assumptions, reverence, and responsibilities to the unknowable, cosmos, Planet Earth, and their contents
  Stress management evaluation
    Questionnaire
    Personal Opinion
  Personal relationships
    At work
    Family
    Friends
  Personal satisfactions
    At work
    Enjoyment-of-life activities (hours/week)
  Active—Participant (+)   Passive—Spectator (−)
    Sports   Sports
    Arts   TV
    Hobbies
  Voluntary mental stimulation (+)
    Reading   Leading discussions
    Writing   Giving talks
    Helping others
    Relaxation—meditation

    Lifestyle habits (+)
    Smoking (−)
    Use of mind-altering drugs (−)
    Blood pressure control (+)
    Consumption of alcoholic beverages in excess of two
    drinks/day (−)

Nutrition   30%
    Consumption of the RDA for all the essential nutrients
    25 g of mixed dietary fiber per day
    A low-fat (about 30% kcal) diet
    Determine, as objectively as possible, if you are sensitive to par-
       ticular dietary constituents such as cholesterol, salt, lactose,
       gluten, and caffeine; if so, modify your diet accordingly.

Exercise   30%
    A minimum of 45 minutes of endurance exercises 3 times per
       week, including warm-up and cool-down
    Strength exercises, 1-2 times per week
    Percentage of body fat (±)
    Voluntary physical stresses (+)
    Fun activities (hiking, sports, etc.); may include any or all of
       the above

In the "Nutrition" and "Exercise" sections, I have included specific goals as desirable, but in the "Attitude" section, there are habits and behaviors that have a negative impact on wellness, as well as those that have positive effects. Basically, this index is just a starting point for learning something about yourself in the areas of improvement that might be most valuable.

Summary

Good health during the middle years (35-70) is not an automatic condition. Some habits promote it, others demote it. Each person should be educated to recognize the consequences of each kind of habit and motivated to practice the healthful and avoid the unhealthful, or his or her health may be endangered. Each person should also recognize that the basic decisions are private. An adult in a free society is expected to make these decisions based on his or her own self-interest. Even though the costs of lifesaving medical care are being borne to a greater extent by the public, the person who becomes a patient pays in coin other than money. Medicine may contribute to health and may prolong life; it cannot furnish wellness.

The pursuit of wellness is more demanding than for health. Achieving and maintaining wellness requires even more awareness and motivation than for health. The pursuit of wellness is a lifelong activity and represents the ultimate in individual responsibility. In distinction to health, where people continue to hope that poor health "won't happen to me," the pursuit of wellness is positive, and people think, "It can happen to me."

With beauty before me, I walk.
With beauty behind me, I walk.
With beauty above me, I walk.
With beauty below me, I walk.
With beauty all around me, I walk.
In old age, the beautiful trail, I walk.
In beauty it is finished.
In beauty it is finished.
In beauty it is finished.
In beauty it is finished.
(from The Night Chant, A Navajo Prayer)

References

Abraham, S., & Carroll, M.D. (1981). *Fats, cholesterol and sodium intake in diet of persons 1-74 years: United States* (Advance data No. 54. DHHS Publication No. PHS 81-1250). Hyattsville, MD: National Center for Health Statistics.

Abraham, W.M. (1979). Factors in delayed muscle soreness. *Medicine and Science in Sports, 9*, 11-20.

Adams, C., & Richardson, M. (1981). *Nutritive value of foods* (Home and Garden Bulletin No. 72). Washington, DC: U.S. Government Printing Office.

Adlersberg, D., Bossak, E.T., Sher, I., & Sobotka, H. (1955). Effects of electrophoresis and monomolecular layer studies with scrum lipoproteins. *Clinical Chemistry, 1*, 18-33.

Alchman, V.D. (1983). *Stress management—A manual for nurses.* New York: Grune and Stratton.

Alderman, J.D., et al. (1986). *A modified well-tolerated niacin regimen markedly lowers cholesterol HDL ratio.* Unpublished manuscript.

Alexander, M.V. (1956). *Relationship between muscular fitness of well-adjusted child and non-well-adjusted child.* Unpublished doctoral dissertation, University of Michigan.

Allen, H.A.J. (1960). *An investigation of water hardness, calcium, and magnesium in relation to mortality in Ontario.* Unpublished doctoral dissertation, University of Waterloo, Ontario, Canada.

Allen, L.H., & Solomons, N.W. (1984). Copper. In N.W. Solomons & I.H. Rosenberg (Eds.), *Absorption and malabsorption of mineral nutrients* (pp. 199-230). New York: Alan R. Liss.

Allen, R.J., & Leahy, J.S. (1966). Some effects of dietary dextrose, fructose, liquid glucose and sucrose in adult, male rat. *British Journal of Nutrition, 20*, 339-347.

American College of Sports Medicine. (1986). *Guidelines for graded exercise testing and exercise prescription* (3rd ed.). Philadelphia: Lea and Febiger.

American Heart Association. (1978). *Cooking without your salt shaker.* Cleveland, OH: Author.

American Heart Association. (1981). *RISKO. A dietary approach to the prevention of coronary heart disease.* Dallas, TX: Author.

American Medical Association Council on Scientific Affairs. (1979). American Medical Association concepts of nutrition and health. *Journal of the American Medical Association, 242,* 2335-2338.

Anderson, J.W., Story, L., Sieling, B., Chen, W.J.L., Petro, M.S., & Story, J. (1984). Hypocholesterolemic effects of oat-bran or bean intake for hypercholesterolemic men. *American Journal of Clinical Nutrition, 40,* 1146-1155.

Anderson, T.W. (1974). Vitamin E in angina pectoris. *Canadian Medical Association Journal, 110,* 401-405.

Anderson, T.W., LeRiche, W.H., & MacKay, J.S. (1969). Sudden death and ischemic heart disease. *New England Journal of Medicine, 280,* 805-807.

Anderson, T.W., Neri, L.C., & Schreiber, G.B. (1975). Ischemic heart disease, water hardness and myocardial magnesium. *Canadian Medical Association Journal, 113,* 199-203.

Anderson, T.W., Reid, D.B.W., & Beaton, G.H. (1972). Vitamin C and the common cold: A double blind trial. *Canadian Medical Association Journal, 107,* 503-508.

Annest, J.L., & Mahaffey, K. (1984). *Blood lead levels for persons ages 6 months–74 years: U.S. 1976-1890* (National Center for Health Statistics, Vital and Health Statistics Series No. 233, DHHS Publication No. PHS 84-1683). Washington, DC: U.S. Government Printing Office.

Antonovsky, A. (1979). *Health, stress and coping.* San Francisco: Jossey-Bass.

Appel, J.A., & Briggs, G.M. (1980). Biotin. In R.S. Goodhart & M.E. Shils (Eds.), *Modern nutrition in health and disease.* Philadelphia: Lea & Febiger.

Appels, A., Jenkins, C.D., & Rosenman, R.H. (1982). Coronary-prone behavior in the Netherlands: A cross-cultural validation study. *Journal of Behavioral Medicine, 5,* 83-90.

Appleton, L. (1949). *Relationship between physical ability and success at U.S. military academy.* Unpublished doctoral dissertation, New York University.

Aristotle. (1928). *The works of Aristotle* (Vol. 8, 2nd ed.). Clarendon Press.

Åstrand, I., Åstrand, P.O., Christensen, E.H., & Hedman, R. (1960). Intermittent muscular work. *Acta Physiological Scandinavica, 48,* 448-453.

Atkins, R. (1977). *Dr. Atkins' superenergy diet.* New York: Bantam Books.

Atkins, R.C., & Linde, S. (1978). *Dr. Atkins' superenergy diet.* New York: Bantam Books.

Baekeland, F. (1970). Exercise deprivation. *Archives of General Psychiatry*, **22**, 365-369.

Bagchi, N., Brown, T.R., Urdanivia, E., & Sundick, R.S. (1985). Induction of autoimmune thyroiditis in chickens by dietary iodine. *Science*, **230**, 325-327.

Bahnson, C.B. (1980). Stress and cancer: State of the art (Part 1). *Psychosomatics*, **21**, 975-981.

Bahnson, C.B. (1981). Stress and cancer: State of the art (Part 2). *Psychosomatics*, **22**, 207-220.

Bahnson, C.B., & Bahnson, M.B. (1969). Ego defenses in cancer patients. *Annals of the New York Academy of Sciences*, **164**, 346-359.

Bailey, C. (1978). *Fit or fat?* Boston: Houghton Mifflin.

Bajusz, E. (1967). Heart disease and soft and hard water. *Lancet*, **1**, 726.

Barbezat, G.O., Casey, C.E., Reasbeck, P.G., Robinson, M.F., & Thomson, C.C. (1984). Selenium. In N.W. Solomons & I.H. Rosenberg (Eds.), *Absorption and malabsorption of mineral nutrients* (pp. 231-258). New York: Alan R. Liss.

Barefoot, J.C., Dahlstrom, W.G., & Williams, R.B., Jr. (1983). Hostility, CHD incidence, and total mortality: A 25-year follow-up study of 255 physicians. *Psychosomatic Medicine*, **45**, 59-63.

Bayless, T.M. (1976, October). Recognition of lactose intolerance. *Hospital Practice*, pp. 97-102.

Beach, R.S., Gershwin, M.E., & Hurley, L.S. (1982). Zinc, copper and manganese in immune function and experimental oncogenesis. *Nutrition and Cancer*, **3**, 172-191.

Beauchamp, G.K., Berzino, M., & Engelman, K. (1983). Modification of salt taste. *Annals of Internal Medicine*, **98**, 763-769.

Beech, H.R., Burns, L.E., & Sheffield, B.F. (1982). *A behavioral approach to the management of stress.* New York: Wiley.

Benditt, E.P. (1977, February). The origin of atherosclerosis. *Scientific American*, pp. 74-85.

Bennett, I., & Simon, M. (1973). *The prudent diet.* New York: D. White.

Benowitz, N.L., Hall, S.M., Herning, R.I., Jacob, P., III, Jones, R.T., & Osman, A.L. (1983). Smokers of low-yield cigarettes do not consume less nicotine. *New England Journal of Medicine*, **309**, 139-142.

Benson, H. (1975). *The relaxation response.* New York: Avon Books.

Benson, H. (1984). *Beyond the relaxation response.* New York: Time Books.

Berger, R.A. (1962). Optimum repetitions for the development of strength. *Research Quarterly*, **33**, 334-338.

Bergh, U., & Ekblom, B. (1979). Physical performance and peak aerobics power at different body temperatures. *Journal of Applied Physiology*, **46**, 885-889.

Bergstrom, J. (1967). Local changes of ATP and phosphoryl creatine in human muscle tissue in connection with exercise. *Physiology of muscular exercise* (American Heart Association Monograph, No. 15, pp. 191-196). New York: American Heart Association.

Beutler, E. (1980). Iron. In R.S. Goodhart & M.E. Shils (Eds.), *Modern nutrition in health and disease* (pp. 350-352). Philadelphia: Lea & Febiger.

Beynen, A.C., & Katan, M.B. (1984). [Letter to the editor]. *Nutrition Reviews, 42*, 201-202.

Bhussry, B.R. (1970). Chronic toxic effects on enamel organ. In *Fluorides and human health* (WHO Monograph Series, No. 59, pp. 230-238). Geneva: World Health Organization.

Black, H. (Ed.). (1980). *The Berkeley Co-op food book.* Palo Alto, CA: Bull.

Blakeslee, A., & Stamler, J. (1963). *Your heart has nine lives.* Englewood Cliffs, NJ: Prentice-Hall.

Blaxter, K.L. (1971). Methods of measuring the energy metabolism of animals and interpretation of results. *Federation Proceedings, 30*, 1436-1443.

Blumenthal, J.A., Williams, R.S., Needels, T.L., & Wallace, A.G. (1982). Psychological changes accompany aerobic exercise in healthy middle-aged adults. *Psychosomatic Medicine, 44*, 529-536.

Bogardus, D., LaGrange, B.M., Horton, E.S., & Sims, E.A.H. (1981). Comparison of carbohydrate-containing and carbohydrate-restricted hypocaloric diets in the treatment of obesity. *Journal of Clinical Investigation, 68*, 399-404.

Bonen, A., & Belcastro, A. N. (1976). Comparison of self-selected recovery methods on lactic acid removal rates. *Medicine and Science in Sports, 8*, 176-178.

Brady, D.M. (1980). Running injuries. *Clinical Symposia, 32*, 2-36.

Brandfonbrener, M., Landowne, M., & Shockin, W. (1955). Changes in cardiac output with age. *Circulation, 12*, 557-566.

Brandon, R.N. (1979). Science, senators, and uncertainty. *Federation Proceedings, 38*, 2564-2566.

Brewster, L., & Jacobson, M. (1978). *The changing American diet.* Washington, DC: Center for Science in the Public Interest.

Bricklin, M. (1979, January). Put fiber to work for your heart. *Prevention,* pp. 28-34.

Briggs, M.H. (1974). Vitamin E supplements and fatigue. *New England Journal of Medicine, 290*, 579.

Brodsky, G. (1974). *From Eden to aquarius.* New York: Bantam Books.

Brody, J. (1981). *Jane Brody's nutrition book.* New York: W.W. Norton.

Brooks, G.A., and Fahey, T.D. (1984). *Exercise physiology.* New York: John Wiley & Sons.

Brown, B. (1974). *New mind, new body.* New York: Harper and Row.

Bulpitt, C.J. (1982, March/April). Is there a new member in the high blood pressure mafia? *Nutrition Today*, pp. 6-11.

Bulpitt, C.J. (1985). Blood pressure and potassium consumption. In C.J. Bulpitt (Ed.), *Handbook of hypertension: Vol. 6. Epidemiology of hypertension* (pp. 191-205). New York: Elsevier Science Publishers.

Burkitt, D.P., & Trowell, H.C. (Eds.). (1975). *Refined carbohydrate foods and disease*. New York: Academic Press.

Burton, B.T., Foster, W.R., Hirsch, J., & Van Itallie, T.B. (1985). Health implications of obesity: An NIH consensus development conference. *International Journal of Obesity*, **9**, 155-170.

Burton, G.W., & Ingold, K.U. (1984). Beta carotene: An unusual type of lipid antioxidant. *Science*, **224**, 569-573.

Cade, R., Mars, D., Wagemaker, H., Zauner, C., Packer, D., Privette, M., Cade, M., Peterson, J., & Hood-Lewis, D. (1984). Effect of aerobic exercise training on patients with systemic arterial hypertension. *American Journal of Medicine*, **77**, 785-790.

Cairns, J. (1978). *Cancer, science and society*. San Francisco: Freeman.

Caldwell, G., & Zanfagna, P.E. (1974). *Fluoridination and truth decay*. Reseda, CA: Top-Ecol Press.

Cannon, W.B. (1939). *The wisdom of the body*. New York: W.W. Norton.

Carlisle, E.M. (1984). Silicon. In E. Frieden (Ed.), *Biochemistry of essential ultratrace elements*. New York: Plenum Press.

Carlisle, H.J., & Stellar, E. (1969). Caloric regulation and food preference in normal, hyperphagic and aphagic rats. *Journal of Comparative and Physiological Psychology*, **69**, 107-114.

Carpenter, K.J. (1981). Effects of different methods of processing maize on its pellagrenic activity. *Federation Proceedings*, **40**, 1531-1537.

Carr, D.B., Bullen, B.A., Skrinar, G.S., Arnold, M.A., Rosenblatt, M., Beitins, I.Z., Martin, J.B., & McArthur, J.W. (1981). Physical conditioning facilitates exercise-induced secretion of beta-endorphin and beta-lipotropin in women. *New England Journal of Medicine*, **305**, 560-563.

Castelli, W.P., Garrison, R.S., Dawber, T.R., McNamara, P.M., Feinleib, M., & Kannel, W.B. (1981). The filter cigarette and coronary heart disease: The Framingham story. *Lancet*, **2**, 109-113.

Castelli, W.P., & Levitas, I.M. (1977, June). New look at lipids: Why they're not all bad. *Current Prescribing*, pp. 39-43.

Centers for Disease Control. (1986). *Morbidity Mortality Weekly Report*, **35**, 457.

Charlesworth, E.A., & Nathan, R.G. (1984). *Stress management—A comprehensive guide to wellness*. New York: Atheneum.

Chesney, M.A., & Rosenman, R.H. (1982). Type A behavior: Observations on the past decade. *Heart and Lung*, **11**, 12-19.

Chopra, J.G., Forbes, A.C., & Habicht, J.P. (1978). Protein in the U.S. diet. *Journal of the American Dietetic Association, 72,* 253-258.

Christakis, G., Ringler, S., Archer, M.S., Winslow, S., Jampel, S., Stephenson, J., Friedman, G., Fein, H., Kraus, H., & James, G. (1966). Anti-coronary club: A seven year report. *American Journal of Public Health, 56,* 299-314.

Clark, L. (1969). *Secrets of health and beauty.* New York: Pyramid Communications.

Cleave, T.L., Campbell, G.D., & Painter, N.S. (1969). *Diabetes, coronary thrombosis and the saccharine disease* (2nd ed.). Bristol, England: John Wright.

Cochran, J.W., & Cochran, A. (1984). Monosodium glutamania: Chinese restaurant syndrome revisited. *Journal of the American Medical Association, 252,* 899.

Cod liver oil for your body machinery. (1979, March). *Prevention,* pp. 69-71.

Cohen, V.B. (1978). The influence of culture on coronary-prone behavior. In T.M. Dembroski, S.M. Weiss, S.G. Haynes, & M. Feinleib (Eds.), *Coronary-prone behavior* (pp. 191-198). New York: Springer-Verlag.

Collingwood, T.R., Douds, A., Williams, H., & Wilson, R.D. (1978). Effects of a police-based diversion program upon youth resource development. *Carkhuff Institute of Human Technology Research Reports, 2,* 1-27.

Combs, G.F., Jr., & Combs, S.B. (1986). *The role of selenium in nutrition.* New York: Academic Press.

Comfort, A., & Comfort, J. (1979). *The facts of love. Living, loving and growing up.* New York: Ballantine Books.

Committee on Dietary Allowances—Food and Nutrition Board. (1980). *Recommended dietary allowances.* Washington, DC: National Academy of Sciences.

Connor, S.L., & Connor, W.E. (1986). *The new American diet: The lifetime family eating plan for good health.* New York: Simon & Schuster.

Consumers Union. (1979). Blood pressure kits. *Consumer Reports, 44,* 142-146.

Consumers Union. (1982, September). Breads. *Consumer Reports,* 438-443.

Consumers Union. (1984). Salt and your health. *Consumer Reports, 49,* 17-22.

Consumers Union. (1985, May). Food, drugs or frauds? *Consumer Reports,* 275-281.

Cook, J.D., & Monsen, E.R. (1977). Vitamin C, the common cold, and iron absorption. *American Journal of Clinical Nutrition, 30,* 235-241.

Cooper, K.H. (1968). *Aerobics.* New York: Bantam Books.

Cooper, K.H. (1983). *The aerobics program for total well being.* New York: Bantam Books.

Cooper, K.H., Pollock, M.L., Martin, R.P., White, S.R., Linnerud, A.C., & Jackson, A. (1976). Physical fitness vs. selected coronary risk factors. *Journal of the American Medical Association, 236*, 166-169.

Coronary Drug Project Research Group. (1975). Clofibrate and niacin in coronary heart disease. *Journal of the American Medical Association, 231*, 360-379.

Costill, D. L. (1985). Carbohydrate nutrition before, during and after exercise. *Federation Proceedings, 44*, 364-368.

Cousins, N. (1979). *Anatomy of an illness.* New York: Norton.

Cousins, N. (1983). *The healing heart.* New York: Norton.

Crew, M.B., & Hopkins, L.L. (1981). Metabolism and toxicity of vanadium. In D.F. Williams (Ed.), *Systematic aspects of biocompatability* (Vol. I, pp. 179-186). Boca Raton, FL: CRC Press.

Crosby, L. (1980). Fiber—standardized sources. *Nutrition and Cancer, 1*, 15-26.

Cureton, T.K. (1963). Improvements of psychological states by means of exercise-fitness programs. *Journal of the Association for Physical and Mental Rehabilitation, 17*, 14-25.

Curley, J. (1983, December 22). Swamped state utility regulators now try to cope with AT&T split. *Wall Street Journal,* Section 2, p. 21.

Dahl, L.K. (1972). Salt and hypertension. *American Journal of Clinical Nutrition, 25*, 231-242.

Dahlkoetter, J., Callahan, E.J., & Linton, J. (1979). Obesity and the unbalanced energy equation: Exercise vs eating habit changes. *Journal of Counseling and Clinical Psychology, 47*, 898-905.

Dalton, K. (1983). *Once a month* (2nd ed.). Claremont, CA: Hunter House.

Daugherty, S.A., & Entwisle, G. (Eds.). (1983). Hypertension detection and follow-up program. In *Baseline characteristics of the enumerated, screened and hypertensive participants: Part 2. Hypertension* (Vol. 5). Bethesda, MD: American Heart Association.

Davies, L.G.G., & Murdoch, L.M. (1959). Lipostabil: A pilot study. *British Medical Journal, 2*, 619-620.

Davis, A. (1965). *Let's get well.* New York: Harcourt, Brace and World.

Davis, J.T. (1979). *Walking!* Kansas City, MO: Andrews and McMeel.

Dayton, S. (1970). Cholesterol, atherosclerosis, ischemic heart disease and stroke. *Annals of Internal Medicine, 72*, 97-109.

De Vries, H.A. (1970). Physiological effects of an exercise training regimen upon men age 52 to 88. *Journal of Gerontology, 25*, 325-336.

De Vries, H.A. (1981). Tranquilizer effect of exercise: A critical review. *The Physician and Sports Medicine, 9*, 47-55.

De Vries, H.A. (1986). *Physiology of exercise* (4th ed.). Dubuque, IA: William C. Brown.

DeLorme, T.L., & Watkins, A.L. (1951). *Progressive resistance exercise.* New York: Appleton-Century-Crofts.

Dembroski, T.M., MacDougall, J.M., Williams, R.B., Haney, T.L., & Blumenthal, J.A. (1986). Components of type A, hostility and anger in relationship to angiographic findings. *Psychosomatic Medicine, 47,* 219-233.

Dempsey, J. (1964). Anthropometrical observations on obese and non-obese young men undergoing a program of vigorous physical exercise. *Research Quarterly, 35,* 275-289.

Department of National Health and Welfare. (1975). *Dietary standards for Canada.* Ottawa: Department of Public Printing and Stationery.

Deutsch, R. (1976). *Realities of nutrition.* Palo Alto, CA: Bull.

Dill, D.B., Talbot, J.H., & Edwards, H.T. (1930). Studies in muscular activity: VI. Response of several individuals to a fixed task. *Journal of Physiology, 69,* 267-305.

Dimsdale, J.E., Hackett, E.P., Hutter, A.M., & Block, P.C. (1980). The risk of type A mediated coronary disease in different populations. *Psychosomatic Medicine, 42,* 55-62.

Dimsdale, J., Hartley, H., Gurney, T., Ruskin, J.N., & Greenblatt, D. (1984). Postexercise peril. *Journal of the American Medical Association, 251,* 630-632.

Dimsdale, J.E., Herd, J.A., & Hartley, L.H. (1983). Epinephrine mediated increases in plasma cholesterol. *Psychosomatic Medicine, 45,* 227-232.

Do lowered lipids diet really reduce coronary risk? (1979, January 3). *Medical Tribune,* p. 3.

Dominquez, R.H., & Gajda, R. (1982). *Total body training.* New York: Warner Books.

Donnison, C.P. (1929). Blood pressure in the African native. *Lancet, 1,* 6-7.

Donsbach, K. (1976). *Preventive organic medicine.* New Canaan, CT: Keats.

Drake, C. (1980, August 3). Jogging can fend off demons of the soul. *Salt Lake Tribune,* p. W11.

Draper, H.H., & Robison, G.A. (1986). Controversy in pharmacology: Calcium and hypertension. *Federation Proceedings, 45,* 2732-2762.

Duncan, K., Baron, J.A., & Weinsier, R.L. (1983). Effects of high and low energy density diets on satiety, energy intake and eating time of obese and nonobese subjects. *American Journal of Clinical Nutrition, 37,* 763-767.

Dustman, R., et al. (1984). Aerobic exercise training and improved neuropsychological function of older individuals. *Neurobiology of Aging, 5,* 35-41.

Dyerberg, J., Bang, H., Stoffersen, E., Moncada, S., & Vane, J.R. (1978). Eicosapentaenoic acid (EPA) and the prevention of thrombosis and atherosclerosis. *Lancet, 2,* 117-119.

Eastwood, M., & Mowbray, L. (1976). Binding of components of mixed micelle to dietary fiber. *American Journal of Clinical Nutrition, 29,* 1461-1467.

Edmiston, S. (1978, November). Surprising rewards of strenuous exercise. *Woman's Day,* pp. 98-104.

Edwards, R.H.T. (1981). Human muscle function and fatigue. In R. Porter & J. Whelan (Eds.), *CIBA Foundation Symposium 82 on human muscle fatigue* (pp. 1-18). London: Pitman Medical.

Edwards, R.H.T., Wilkie, D.R., Dawson, M.J., Gordon, R.E., & Shaw, D. (1982). Clinical use of nuclear magnetic resonance in the investigation of myopathy. *Lancet, 1,* 725-731.

Ellis, A. (1978). *Sex without guilt.* North Hollywood, CA: Wiltshire.

Endicott, J., Halbreich, U., Schacht, S., & Nee, J. (1981). Premenstrual changes and affective disorders. *Psychosomatic Medicine, 43,* 519.

Engel, B.T., Glasgow, M.S., & Gaarder, K.R. (1983). Behavioral treatment of high blood pressure: III. Follow-up results and treatment recommendations. *Psychosomatic Medicine, 45,* 12.

Enger, S.C., Herbjornsen, H.K., Erikssen, J., & Fretland, A. (1977). High density lipoproteins (HDL) and physical activity: The influence of physical exercise, age, and smoking on HDL-cholesterol and the HDL total cholesterol ratio. *Scandinavian Journal of Laboratory and Clinical Investigation, 37,* 251-255.

Enoka, R.M., & Stuart, D.G. (1985). Contribution of neuroscience to exercise studies. *Federation Proceedings, 44,* 2279-2285.

Enstrom, J.E. (1984). Smoking and longevity studies. *Science, 225,* 878.

Entmacher, D.S. (1983, July/August). Those new height and weight tables. *Nutrition Today,* pp. 16-26.

Erickson, H., & Swain, M.A. (1982). Model for assessing potential adaptation to stress. *Research in Nursing and Health, 5*(2), 93-101.

Evans, C.L. (1949). *Principles of human physiology* (10th ed.). Philadelphia: Lea and Febiger.

Ewald, E.B. (1975). *Recipes for a small planet.* New York: Ballantine.

Ewing, L., Irving, J.B., Kerr, F., & Kirby, B.J. (1973). Static exercise in untreated systemic hypertension. *English Heart Journal, 35,* 413-421.

Falkner, B. (1981). Cardiovascular responses to stress in adolescents. In G. Onesti & K.E. Kim (Eds.), *Phasic pressor mechanisms: Hypertension in young and old* (pp. 11-17). New York: Greene & Stratton.

Feingold, B. (1975). *Why your child is hyperactive.* New York: Random House.

Feldenkreis, M. (1972). *Awareness through movement.* New York: Harper and Row.

Feltman, J. (1979, April). Winning hearts and minds with lecithin. *Prevention.*

Feltman, J. (1979, June). Selenium, the double-duty protector. *Prevention*, pp. 46-51.

Festinger, L. (1954). A theory of social comparison processes. *Human Relations*, **7**, 111-140.

Finberg, L., Landis, J.R., & Harlan, W.R. (1976). Fast foods for adolescents. *American Journal of Diseases of Children*, **130**, 362-363.

Fisk, D.A. (1979). Successful program for changing children's eating habits. *Nutrition Today*, **14**(3), 6-34.

Fleischman, A.I., Bierenbaum, M.L., Raichelson, R., Hayton, T., & Watson, P. (1970). Vitamin D and hypercholesterolemia in adult humans. In R.D. Jones (Ed.), *Atherosclerosis* (pp. 468-472). New York: Springer-Verlag.

Folkers, K., Shizukuishi, S., Willis, R., Scudder, S.L., Takernara, K., & Longenecker, J.B. (1984). The biochemistry of vitamin B_6 is basic to the cause of Chinese restaurant syndrome. *Zeitschrift fur Physiolgische Chemie*, **365**, 405-414.

Folkins, C.H., & Sime, W.E. (1981). Physical fitness training and mental health. *American Psychologist*, **36**, 373-389.

Foley, D. (1985, September). Feast on the good fish. *Prevention*, pp. 40-44.

Food and Nutrition Board. (1974). *Hazards of overuse of vitamin D*. Washington, DC: National Research Council.

Food and Nutrition Board. (1976). Selenium and human health. *Nutrition Reviews*, **34**, 347-348.

Food and Nutrition Board, National Academy of Sciences. (1980). Toward healthful diets. *Nutrition Today*, pp. 7-11.

Food and Nutrition Board. (1980). *Toward healthful diets*. Washington, DC: The National Research Council.

Fox, E.L., & Mathews, D.K. (1981). *Physiological basis of physical education and athletics* (3rd ed.). Philadelphia: Saunders College.

Fredericks, C. (1965). *Carlton Fredericks' low carbohydrate diet*. New York: Award Books.

Freud, S. (1962). *Civilization and its discontents* (J. Strachey, Trans.). New York: W.W. Norton. (Original work published 1930)

Friedman, D., Rarno, B.W., & Gray, G.J. (1984). Tennis and cardiovascular fitness in middle-aged men. *Physician and Sports Medicine*, **12**, 87-91.

Friedman, G.D., Ury, H.K., Klatsky, A.I., & Siegelaub, A.G. (1974). A psychological questionnaire predictive of myocardial infarction results from the Kaiser-Permanente epidemiological study of myocardial infarction. *Psychosomatic Medicine*, **36**, 327-343.

Friedman, M., & Rosenman, R.H. (1959). Association of specific overt behavior pattern with blood and cardiovascular findings. *Journal of the American Medical Association*, **169**, 1286-1296.

Friedman, M., & Rosenman, R. (1974). *Type A behavior and your heart*. New York: Ballantine Books.

Friedman, M., Thoresen, C.E., Gill, J.J., Powell, L.H., Ulmer, D., Thompson, L., Price, V.A., Rabin, D.D., Breall, W.S., Dixon, T., Levy, R., & Bourg, E. (1984). Alteration of type A behavior and reduction in cardiac recurrences in postmyocardial infarction patients. *American Heart Journal, 108,* 237-248.

Friedman, M., Thoresen, C.E., Gill, J.J., Ulmer, D., Thompson, L., Powell, L., Price, V., Elek, S.R., Rabin, D.D., Breall, W.S., Piaget, G., Dixon, T., Bourg, E., Levy, R.A., & Tasto, D.L. (1982). Feasibility of altering type A behavior pattern after myocardial infarction. Recurrent coronary prevention project study: Methods, baseline results and preliminary findings. *Circulation, 66,* 83-92.

Friedman, M., & Ulmer, D. (1984). *Treating type A behavior and your heart*. New York: Ballantine Books.

Gaarder, K.R., & Montgomery, P.S. (1981). *Clinical biofeedback* (2nd ed.). Baltimore: Williams and Wilkins.

Gallwey, W.T. (1974). *The inner game of tennis*. New York: Random House.

Garrison, R.J., Feinleib, M., Castelli, W.P., & McNamara, P.M. (1983). Cigarette smoking as a confounder of the relationship between relative weight and long-term mortality. *Journal of the American Medical Association, 249,* 2199-2203.

Gelman, E., Hager, M., Thomas, R., & Canin, E. (1985, July 29). The president's case. *Newsweek,* pp. 16-18.

Gerras, C. (Ed.). (1977). Bioflavonoids: The "useless" vitamin we need. In *The complete book of vitamins* (pp. 363-375). Emmaus, PA: Rodale Press.

Gettman, L.R., Ward, P., & Hagan, R.D. (1982). A comparison of combined running and weight training with circuit weight training. *Medicine and Science in Sports and Exercise, 14,* 229-357.

Gibbons, L.W., Blair, S.N., Cooper, K.H., & Smith, M. (1983). Association between coronary heart disease risk factors and physical fitness in healthy adult women. *Circulation, 67,* 977.

Gilfillan, S.C. (1965). Lead poisoning and the fall of Rome. *Journal of Occupational Medicine, 7,* 53-60.

Gilliam, T.B., Katch, V.L., Thorland, W., & Weltman, A. (1977). Prevalance of CHD risk factors in active children 7-12 years of age. *Medicine and Science in Sports, 9,* 21-25.

Ginter, E. (1976). Ascorbic acid synthesis in certain guinea pigs. *International Journal for Vitamin and Nutrition Research, 46,* 173-179.

Girdano, D.A., & Everly, G.S., Jr. (1986). *Controlling stress and tension* (2nd ed.). Englewood Cliffs, NJ: Prentice-Hall.

Glass, D. (1977). *Behavior patterns, stress, and coronary disease*. Hillsdale, NJ: Lawrence Albaum.

Glass, D.C. (1977). Stress, behavior patterns and coronary disease. *American Scientist*, **65**, 177-187.

Glueck, C.J., & Stein, E.A. (1979). Treatment and management of hyperlipoproteinemia in childhood. In R. Lery, B.M. Rifkind, B.H. Dennis, & N.D. Einst (Eds.), *Nutrition lipids and coronary heart disease* (pp. 285-307). New York: Raven Press.

Goldbourt, U., & Medalie, J.H. (1977). Characteristics of smokers, nonsmokers and ex-smokers among 10,000 adult males in Israel. *American Journal of Epidemiology*, **105**, 75-86.

Goldwater, B.C., & Collis, M.L. (1985). Psychological effects of cardiovascular conditioning: A controlled experiment. *Psychosomatic Medicine*, **47**, 174-181.

Gollnick, P.D. (1985). Metabolism of substrates: Energy substrate metabolism during exercise and as modified by training. *Federation Proceedings*, **44**, 353-357.

Gordon, G.S., & Genant, H.K. (1985). The aging skeleton. *Clinics in Geriatric Medicine*, **1**, 95-118.

Gordon, G.S., & Vaughn, C. (1986). Calcium and osteoporosis. *Journal of Nutrition*, **116**, 319-322.

Gordon, T., Castelli, W.P., Hjortland, M.C., Kannel, W.B., & Dawber, T.R. (1977). Predicting coronary heart disease in middle-aged and older persons: The Framingham Study. *Journal of the American Medical Association*, **238**, 497-499.

Gore, M. (1982). Chinese restaurant syndrome. In E.F.P. Jelliffe & D.B. Jelliffe (Eds.), *Adverse effects of food* (pp. 211-223). New York: Plenum Press.

Gortner, W.A. (1975). Nutrition in the U.S. (1900-1974). *Cancer Research*, **35**, 3246-3253.

Gotto, A.M., Jr. (1986). Treatment of hyperlipidemia. *American Journal of Cardiology*, **57**, 11G-16G.

Graham, S., Snell, I.M., Graham, J.B., & Ford, L. (1971). Social trauma in the epidemiology of cancer of the cervix. *Journal of Chronic Diseases*, **24**, 711-725.

Grande, F., Anderson, J.T., & Keys, A. (1972a). Diets of different fatty acid composition producing identical serum cholesterol levels in man. *American Journal of Clinical Nutrition*, **25**, 53-60.

Grande, F., Anderson, J.T., & Keys, A. (1972b). Sucrose and various carbohydrate containing foods and serum lipids in man. *American Journal of Clinical Nutrition*, **27**, 1043-1051.

Gray, I.E., & Gray, L.K. (1983). Diet and juvenile delinquency. *Nutrition Today*, **18**, 14-22.

Green, W. (1966). Psychosocial setting of the development of leukemia and lymphoma. *Annals of the New York Academy of Sciences*, **125**, 794-801.

Greer, S., & Morris, T. (1975). Psychological attributes of women who develop breast cancer. A controlled study. *Journal of Psychosomatic Research*, **19**, 147-153.

Greer, S., & Morris, T. (1978). Study of psychological factors in breast cancer. *Social Science and Medicine*, **12**, 129-138.

Greist, J.H., Klein, M.H., Eischens, R.R., Faris, J.W., Gurman, A.G., & Morgan, W.P. (1979). Running as a treatment for depression. *Comprehensive Psychiatry*, **20**, 41-54.

Grim, C.E., Luft, F.C., Miller, J.Z., Meneely, G.R., Battarbee, H.D., Hames, C.G., & Dahl, L.K. (1980). Racial differences in blood pressure in Evans County, Georgia: Relationship to sodium and potassium intake and plasma renin activity. *Journal of Chronic Diseases*, **33**, 87-94.

Grinker, R., & Spiegel, J.P. (1945). *War neuroses*. Philadelphia: Blakiston.

Groover, M.E., Jr., Jernigan, J.A., & Martin, C.D. (1960). Variations in serum lipid concentration and clinical coronary disease. *American Journal of Medical Science*, **239**, 133-139.

Grundy, S.M. (1986). Cholesterol and coronary heart disease. *Journal of the American Medical Association*, **256**, 2849-2850.

Guerard, M. (1977). *Cuisine minceur*. New York: W. Morrow.

Guthrie, H.A. (1975). *Introductory nutrition* (3rd ed.). St. Louis: C.V. Mosby.

Guthrie, H. (1977). Concept of a nutritious food. *Journal of the American Dietetics Association*, **71**, 14-19.

Guy, R. (1759). *An essay on schrirrus tumors and cancers*. London: J & A Churchill.

Guyon, J. (1981, September 29). Now, for the start-and-stop dieter, there's a fork with a traffic light. *Wall Street Journal*, p. 35.

Gwinup, G. (1975). Effect of exercise alone on weight of obese women. *Archives of Internal Medicine*, **135**, 676-680.

Habicht, J.P. (Chair). (1979). American Institute of Nutrition symposium. Translation of scientific and nutrition findings to social policy. *Federation Proceedings*, **38**, 2551-2569.

Hagberg, J.M., Goldring, D., Ehsani, A.A., Heath, G.W., Hernandez, A., Schechtman, K., & Holloszy, J.O. (1983). Effect of exercise training on the blood pressure and hemodynamic features of hypertensive adolescents. *American Journal of Cardiology*, **52**, 763-768.

Haglund, K. (1986, March 3). Aerobic exercise spells difference. *Medical News*, p. 3.

Hagnell, O. (1966). Premorbid personality of persons who develop cancer in a total population investigated in 1947 and 1957. *Annals of the New York Academy of Sciences*, **125**, 846-855.

Halbreich, U., Endicott, J., & Nee, J. (1983). Premenstrual depressive changes. *Archives of General Psychiatry*, **40**, 535-542.

Hales, D.R. (1979, October). Prescription for life includes 90-day plan for "addictive" aerobic exercise. *Medical News*, p. 23.

Hall, R.H. (1974). *Food for nought*. Hagerstown, MD: Harper and Row.

Hall, Y., Stamler, J., Cohen, D.B., Monjonnier, L., Epstein, M.B., Berkson, D.M., Whipple, I.T., & Catchings, S. (1972). Effectiveness of a low saturated fat, low cholesterol, weight-reducing diet for the control of hypertriglyceridemia. *Atherosclerosis*, **16**, 389-403.

Halsted, C.H. (1976). Nutritional implication of alcohol. In D.M. Hegsted et al. (Eds.), *Present knowledge in nutrition* (4th ed., pp. 467-477). Washington, DC: Nutrition Foundation.

Hamilton, C.L. (1964). Rat's preference for high fat diets. *Journal of Comparative Physiological Psychology*, **58**, 459-460.

Hamilton, E.M.N., Whitney, E.N., & Sizer, F.S. (1985). *Nutrition: Concepts and controversies* (3rd ed.). St. Paul, MN: West.

Hammond, E.C., Garfinkel, L., Seidman, H., & Lew, E.A. (1976). Tar and nicotine content of cigarette smoke in relation to death rates. *Environmental Research*, **12**, 263-274.

Hannon, B.M., & Lohman, T.G. (1978). Energy cost of overweight in the U.S. *American Journal of Public Health*, **68**, 765-767.

Hansen, R.G. (1973). An index of food quality. *Nutrition Reviews*, **31**, 1-7.

Hansen, R.G., Sorenson, A.W., Witwer, A.J., & Wyse, B.W. (1979). *Nutritional quality index of foods*. Westport, CT: Avi.

Hanson, D.J. (1982, March 29). Effects of foam insulation ban far reaching. *Chemical Engineering News*, pp. 34-37.

Hanson, P.S. (1970). The effect of a concentrated program in movement behavior on the affective behavior of four year old children at university elementary school. *Dissertation Abstracts International*, **31**, 3319A. (University Microfilms No. 71-00629)

Harburg, E., Schull, W.J., Erfurt, J.C., & Schork, M.A. (1970). A family set method for estimating heredity and stress: I. A pilot survey of blood pressure among negroes in high and low stress areas, Detroit, 1966-1967. *Journal of Chronic Diseases*, **23**, 69-81.

Harlan, W.R., Hull, A.L., Schmouder, R.L., Landin, J.R., Thompson, R.E., & Larkin, F.A. (1984). Blood pressure and nutrition in adults. The national health and nutrition examination survey. *American Journal of Epidemiology*, **120**, 17-28.

Harper, A. (1974). Recommended dietary allowances: Are they what we think they are? *Journal of the American Dietetic Association*, **64**, 151-156.

Harper, A.E. (1979). Dietary goals: A skeptical view. *American Journal of Clinical Nutrition*, **38**, 310-321.

Harris, R., & Karmas, E. (1975). *Nutritional evaluation of food processing* (2nd ed.). Westport, CT: Avi.

Harris, T.G. (1986, June). At your best on the job? *American Health,* pp. 48-53.

Hartung, G.H., Foreyt, J.P., Mitchell, R.E., Vlasek, I., & Gotto, A.M., Jr. (1980). Relation of diet to high-density-lipoprotein cholesterol in middle-aged marathon runners, joggers, and inactive men. *New England Journal of Medicine,* **302,** 357-361.

Hawkins, M.O. (1956). Exercise and emotional stability. *Child Study,* **33,** 7-10.

Hayes, K.C., & Hegsted, D.M. (1973). Toxicity of vitamins. In *Toxicants occurring naturally in foods.* Washington, DC: National Academy of Sciences.

Haynes, S.G., Feinleib, M., & Kannel, W.B. (1980). The relationship of psychosocial factors to coronary heart disease in the Framingham Study: III. Eight-year incidence of coronary heart disease. *American Journal of Epidemiology,* **111,** 37-58.

Heaton, K.H. (1976). Fiber, blood lipids, and heart disease. *American Journal of Clinical Nutrition,* **29,** 125-126.

Hegsted, D.M. (1978). Dietary goals—a progessive view. *American Journal of Clinical Nutrition,* **31,** 1504-1509.

Hegsted, D.M. (1979). Evidence and proof in making policy decisions. *Federation Proceedings,* **38,** 2560-2563.

Hegsted, D.M., & Nicolosi, R.J. (1987). Individual variation in serum cholesterol levels. *Proceedings of the National Academy of Science* (US), **84,** 6259-6261.

Helyar, J. (1981, October 16). Talking to your dog can help to lower your blood pressure. *The Wall Street Journal,* p. 1.

Herberg, L., Doppen, W., & Major, E. (1974). Dietary-induced hypertrophic-hyperplastic obesity in mice. *Journal of Lipid Research,* **15,** 580-585.

Herbert, V., Colman, N., & Jacob, E. (1980). Folic acid and vitamin B_{12}. In R.S. Goodhart & M.E. Shils (Eds.), *Modern nutrition in health and disease.* Philadelphia: Lea & Febiger.

Herman, S., Blumenthal, J.A., Black, G.M., & Chesney, M.A. (1981). Self-ratings of Type A (coronary prone) adults: Do Type A's know they are Type A's? *Psychosomatic Medicine,* **43,** 405.

Hess, J., & Hess, K. (1979). *The taste of America.* New York: Grossman.

Hettinger, T., & Mueller, E.A. (1953). Muskelleistung und Muskeltraining. *Arbeitsphysiologie,* **15,** 111-126.

Higgins, M.W., Keller, J.B., Metzner, H.L., Moore, F.E., & Ostrander, D. (1980). Studies of blood pressure in Tecumseh, Michigan: II. Antecedents in childhood of high blood pressure in young adults. *Hypertension,* **2,** I117-I123.

High protein diets and bone homeostasis. (1981). *Nutrition Review*, **39**, 11-13.

Hirao, Y., & Patterson, C.C. (1974). Lead aerosol high pollution in the High Sierra overrides natural mechanisms which exclude lead from a food chain. *Science*, **184**, 989-992.

Hiss, T. (1987, June 22). Reflections: Experiencing places. *New Yorker*, pp. 45-68.

Hjermann, I., Holme, I., Velve Byre, K., & Leren P. (1981). Effect of diet and smoking intervention on the incidence of coronary heart disease. *Lancet*, **12**, 1303-1310.

Hobbes, T. (1976). *Leviathan, 1651*. London: J.M. Dent & Sons.

Hoeg, J.M., Gregg, R.E., & Brewer, B., Jr. (1986). An approach to the management of hyperlipoproteinemia. *Journal of the American Medical Association*, **255**, 512-521.

Hokanson, J.E., & Burgess, M. (1962). Effects of three types of aggression on vascular processes. *Journal of Abnormal and Social Psychology*, **64**, 446-449.

Holick, M.F., MacLaughlin, J.A., & Doppelt, S.H. (1981). Regulation of cutaneous previtamin D_3 photosynthesis in man: Skin pigment is not an essential regulator. *Science*, **211**, 590-592.

Holloszy, J.O., & Booth, F.W. (1976). Biochemical adaptations to endurance exercise in muscle. *Annual Review of Physiology*, **38**, 293-314.

Holloszy, J.O., Skinner, J.S., Toro, G., & Cureton, T.K. (1964). Effect of six months training program of endurance exercise on serum lipids of middle aged men. *American Journal of Cardiology*, **14**, 753-760.

Holman, R.T., Johnson, S.B., & Hatch, T.F. (1982). A case of human linolenic acid deficiency involving neurological abnormalities. *American Journal of Clinical Nutrition*, **35**, 617-623.

Holmes, T.H., & Masuda, M. (1974). Life changes and illness susceptibility. In B.S. Dohrenwend & B.P. Dohrenwend (Eds.), *Stressful life events* (pp. 45-72). New York: Wiley.

Hopkins, F.G. (1949). The analyst and the medical man. In *Hopkins and biochemistry* (p. 134). Cambridge, MA: Heffer and Sons. (Original work published 1906)

Hopkins, P.N., & Williams, R.R. (1986). Identification and relative weight of cardiovascular risk factors. *Cardiology Clinics*, **4**, 3-31.

Hopkins, P.N., Williams, R.R., & Hunt, S.C. (1984). Magnified risks from cigarette smoking for coronary prone families in Utah. *Western Journal of Medicine*, **141**, 196-202.

Hormann, I., Velvebyre, K., Holme, I., & Leren, P. (1981). Effect of diet and smoking intervention on the incidence of coronary heart disease. *Lancet*, **2**, 1303-1310.

Hubert, H.B., Feinleib, M., McNamara, P.M., & Castelli, W.P. (1983). Obesity as an independent risk factor for cardiovascular disease: A 26-year follow-up of participants in the Framingham heart study. *Circulation*, **67**, 968-976.

Hughes, R.E., & Wilson, H.K. (1977). Flavonoids: Some physiological and nutritional considerations. *Progress in Medicinal Chemistry*, **14**, 285-301.

Hulley, S.B., Cohen, R., & Widdowson, G. (1977). Plasma high-density lipoprotein cholesterol level. *Journal of the American Medical Association*, **238**, 2269-2271.

Hurley, B.F., Seals, D.R., Ehsani, A.A., Cartier, L.J., Dalsky, G.P., Hagberg, J.M., & Holloszy, J.O. (1984). Effects of high intensity strength training on cardiovascular function. *Medicine and Science in Sports and Exercise*, **16**, 483-488.

Huxley, H. (1969). The mechanism of muscular contraction. *Science, 164*, 1256-1366.

Hypertension Detection and Follow-Up Program Cooperative Group. (1979). Five year findings of the hypertension detection and follow-up program. *Journal of the American Medical Association*, **242**, 2562-2571.

Iacono, J.M., & Dougherty, R.M. (1983). The role of dietary polyunsaturated fatty acids and prostaglandins in reducing blood pressure and improving thrombogenic indices. *Preventive Medicine*, **12**, 60-69.

Iber, F. (1971). Alcoholism, the liver sets the pace. *Nutrition Today, 6*, 2.

Ingjer, F.C. (1978). Capillary supply and mitochondrial content of different muscle fiber types in untrained and endurance-training men. *European Journal of Applied Physiology*, **104**, 238-240.

Irwin, M.I. (1980). *Nutritional requirements of man*. Washington, DC: Nutrition Foundation.

Ismail, A.H., & Young, R.J. (1973). Effect of chronic exercise on the personality of middle aged men by univariate and multivariate approaches. *Journal of Human Ergology, 2*, 47-57.

Itallie, T.B. van, Wegal, K.R., Yang, M.U., & Funk, R.C. (1985). Clinical assessment of body fat content in adults: Potential role of electrical impedence methods. In A.E. Roche (Chair), *Body-composition assessments in youth and adults*. Report of Sixth Ross Conference on Medical Research. Columbus, OH: Ross Labs.

Jacobs, D.R., Jr., Anderson, J.T., Hannan, P., Keys, A., & Blackburn, H. (1983). Variability in individual serum cholesterol response to change in diet. *Arteriosclerosis, 3*, 349-356.

Jacobson, E. (1983). *Progressive relaxation* (2nd ed.). Chicago: University of Chicago Press.

Jacobson, H. (1980). *Racewalk to fitness*. New York: Simon and Schuster.

Jacobson, M. (1975). *Nutrition scoreboard*. New York: Avon Books.

Jackson, R.L., Kashyap, M.L., Barnhart, R.L., Allen, C., Hogg, E., & Glueck, C.J. (1984). Influence of polyunsaturated and saturated fats on plasma lipids and lipoproteins in man. *American Journal of Clinical Nutrition, 39,* 589-597.

Jemmott, J.B., et al. (1983). Academic stress, power motivation and decrease in secretion rate of salivary secretory immunoglobulin A. *Lancet, 1,* 1400-1402.

Jencks, B. (1979). *Your body* (2nd ed.). Chicago: Nelson-Hall.

Jenkins, C.D., Rosenman, R.H., & Friedman, M. (1967). Development of an objective psychological test for the determination of the coronary-prone behavior pattern in employed men. *Journal of Chronic Diseases, 20,* 371-379.

Jenkins, C.D., Zyzanski, S.J., & Rosenman, R.H. (1971). Progress toward validation of a computer-scored test for the type-A coronary prone behavior pattern. *Psychosomatic Medicine, 33,* 193-202.

Jenkins, C.D., Zyzanski, S.J., & Rosenman, R.H. (1978). Coronary-prone behavior: One pattern or several? *Psychosomatic Medicine, 40,* 25-43.

Jenkins, R.J., & Guthrie, H. (1984). Identification of index nutrients for dietary assessment. *Journal of Nutrition Education, 16,* 15-18.

Jenni, M.A., & Wollersheim, J.P. (1979). Cognitive therapy, stress management training, and the type A behavior pattern. *Cognitive Therapy Research, 3,* 61-72.

Johnson, M.A., Polgar, J., Weightman, D., & Appleton, D. (1973). Data on distribution of fiber types in thirty-six human muscles. *Journal of Neurological Science, 18,* 111-129.

Joint Committee on Nomenclature. (1950). Term "vitamin P" recommended to be discontinued. *Science, 112,* 628.

Joint National Committee on Detection, Evaluation and Treatment of High Blood Pressure. (1984). The 1984 report of the Joint National Committee on Detection, Evaluation and Treatment of High Blood Pressure. *Archives of Internal Medicine, 144,* 1045-1057.

Kahn, J.P., Kornfeld, D.S., Blood, D.K., Lynn, R.B., Heller, S.S., & Frank, A. (1982). Type A behavior and the thallium stress test. *Psychosomatic Medicine, 44,* 431-436.

Kanareck, R.B., & Hirsch, E. (1977). Dietary induced overeating in experimental animals. *Federation Proceedings, 36,* 154-158.

Kannel, W.B. (1967). Habitual level of physical activity and risk of CHD. *Canadian Medical Association Journal, 96,* 811-812.

Kannel, W.B. (1983). High density lipoproteins: Epidemiological profile and risks of coronary artery disease. *American Journal of Cardiology, 22,* 9B-12B.

Kannel, W.B., & Dawber, T.R. (1972). Atherosclerosis as a pediatric problem. *Journal of Pediatrics, 80,* 544-554.

Kannel, W.B., Dawber, Y.R., Kagan, A., Revotskie, N., & Stokes, J., III. (1961). Factors of risk in the development of coronary heart disease—six-year follow-up experience. *Annals of Internal Medicine, 55,* 33-50.

Kannel, W.B., Gordon, T., Sorlie, P., & McNamara, P.M. (1971). Physical activity and coronary vulnerability: Framingham study. *Cardiology Digest, 6,* 28-40.

Kannel, W.B., & Sorlie, P. (1975). Hypertension in Framingham. In O. Paul (Ed.), *Epidemiology and control of hypertension* (pp. 553-593). Miami, FL: Miami Symposia Specialists.

Kaplan, J.R., Manuck, S.B., Clarson, T.B., Lusso, F.M., Taub, D.M., & Miller, E.W. (1983). Social stress and atherosclerosis in normocholesterolemic monkeys. *Science, 220,* 733-735.

Kaplan, N.M. (1980). The control of hypertension: A therapeutic breakthrough. *American Scientist, 68,* 537-545.

Karvonen, M., Kentala, K., & Musta, O. (1957). Determination of maximum heart rate reserve. *Annals of Medical Experimental Biology Fenn, 35,* 307-315.

Karvonen, M.J., Pekkarinen, J., Metsala, P., & Rautanen, Y. (1961). Diet and serum cholesterol of lumberjacks. *British Journal of Nutrition, 52,* 157-163.

Karvonen, M.J., Rautaharju, P.M., Orma, E., Punsar, S., & Takkunen, J. (1961, February). Cardiovascular studies on lumberjacks. *Journal of Occupational Medicine,* 49-53.

Katan, M.B., Beynen, A.C., DeVries, J.H.M., & Nobels, A. (1986). Existance of consistent hypo- and hyperresponders to dietary cholesterol in man. *American Journal of Epidemiology, 123,* 221-234.

Kato, H., et al. (1973). Epidemiological studies of coronary heart disease and stroke in Japanese men living in Japan, Hawaii, and California. *American Journal of Epidemiology, 97,* 372-380.

Kay, R.H., & Truswell, A. (1977). Effect of citrus pectin on blood lipids and fecal steroid excretion in man. *American Journal of Clinical Nutrition, 30,* 171.

Kenney, R.A. (1980). Chinese restaurant syndrome. *Lancet, 1,* 311-312.

Kerr, W. (1962). *Decline of pleasure.* New York: Simon and Schuster.

Keye, W.R., Jr. (1983). Update: Premenstrual syndrome. *Endocrine and Fertility Forum, 6,* 1-3.

Keye, W.R., Jr., & Strong, T. (1983). Premenstrual syndrome: An enigma. *Continuing Education for the Family Physician, 18,* 913-918.

Keys, A. (1970). Coronary heart disease in seven countries. *Circulation, 41* (Suppl. 1), 1-211.

Keys, A. (1980, July/August). Overweight, obesity, coronary heart disease, and mortality. *Nutrition Today,* pp. 16-22.

Keys, A. (1984). Serum cholesterol response to dietary cholesterol. *American Journal of Clinical Nutrition, 40,* 351-359.

Keys, A., Anderson, J.T., & Grande, F.J. (1957). Serum cholesterol response to dietary fat. *Lancet*, 1, 787.

Keys, A., Aravanis, C., Blackburn, H., Van Buchem, F.S.P., Buzina, R., Djordjevic, B.S., Fidanza, F., Karvonen, M.J., Menotti, A., Puddu, V., & Taylor, H.L. (1972). Coronary heart disease: Overweight and obesity as risk factors. *Annals of Internal Medicine*, 77, 15-27.

Khaw, K.T., & Rose, G. (1982). Population study of blood pressure and associated factors in St. Lucia, West Indies. *International Journal of Epidemiology*, 11, 371-377.

Kies, C., & Fox, H.M. (1977). Dietary hemicellulose interactions influencing serum lipid patterns and protein nutritional status of adult men. *Journal of Food Science*, 42, 440-443.

Kimura, N. (1956). Analysis of 10,000 post-mortem examinations in Japan. In A. Keys & P.D. White (Eds.), *World trends in cardiology: Vol 1. Cardiovascular epidemiology* (pp. 22-23). New York: Hoeber-Harper.

Kinderlehrer, J. (1979, September). B₆ may be the answer to heart disease. *Prevention*, pp. 138-146.

King, J.C., Cohenour, S.H., Coruccini, C.G., & Schneeman, P. (1978). Evaluation and modification of the basic four food guide. *Journal of Nutrition Education*, 10, 27-29

Kingsbury, K.J., Morgan, O.M., Aylott, L., & Emmerson, R. (1961). Effects of ethyl arachidonate, cod liver oil and corn oil on plasma cholesterol level. *Lancet*, 1, 739-741.

Kjellberg, S.R., Rudke, V., & Sjostrand, J. (1949). Increase of the amount of hemoglobin and blood volume in connection with physical training. *Acta Physiologica Scandinavica*, 19, 146-151.

Klatsky, A.L., Friedman, G.D., Siegelaub, A.B., & Gerard, M.J. (1979). Alcohol consumption and blood pressure. *New England Journal of Medicine*, 296, 1194-1200.

Knochel, J.P. (1982). Neuromuscular manifestations of electrolyte disorders. *American Journal of Medicine*, 72, 521.

Kolars, J.C., Levitt, M.D., Aougi, M., & Savaiano, D.A. (1984). Yogurt—An autodigesting source of lactose. *New England Journal of Medicine*, 310, 1-3.

Kolata, B. (1985a). Obesity declared a disease. *Science*, 227, 1019-1020.

Kolata, B. (1985b). Why do people get fat? *Science*, 227, 1327-1328

Kolata, G.B. (1979). Treatment reduces deaths from hypertension. *Science*, 206, 1386-1387.

Kolata, G. (1982). Heart study produces a surprise result. *Science*, 218, 31-32.

Kolata, G. (1983). Cholesterol-heart disease link illuminated. *Science*, 221, 1164-1166.

Kolata, G. (1985). Debate over colon cancer screening. *Science,* **229,** 636-637.

Kornitzer, M., Kittel, F., DeBacker, G., & Dramaix, M. (1981). The Belgian heart disease prevention project: Type "A" behavior pattern and the prevalence of coronary heart disease. *Psychosomatic Medicine,* **43,** 133-146.

Krantz, D.S., Sanmarco, M.I., Selvester, R.H., & Matthews, K.A. (1979). Psychological correlates of progression of atherosclerosis in men. *Psychosomatic Medicine,* **41,** 467-475.

Kraus, B. (1984). *The Barbara Kraus sodium guide to brand names & basic foods.* Brooklyn, NY: Parade Publication.

Kraus, H. (1972). Evaluation of muscular and cardiovascular fitness. *Preventive Medicine,* **1,** 178-184.

Kraus, H., & Raab, W. (1961). *Hypokinetic diseases.* Springfield, IL: Charles C Thomas.

Krebs, H.A. (1966). The regulation of the release of ketone bodies by the liver. In G. Weber (Ed.), *Advances in enzyme regulation* (Vol. 4, pp. 339-353). New York: Pergamon Press.

Kromhout, D., Bosschieter, E.B., & Coulander, C., de L. (1985). The inverse relation between fish consumption and 20-year mortality from coronary heart disease. *New England Journal of Medicine,* **312,** 1.

Krotkiewski, M. (1984). Effect of guar gum on body weight, hunger ratings, and metabolism in obese subjects. *British Journal of Nutrition,* **52,** 97-105.

Kuo, P.T., Kostis, J.B., Moreyra, A.E., & Hayes, J.A. (1979). *American Journal of Clinical Nutrition,* **32,** 941.

Kurland, H.L. (1981, December). Medical benefits of Tai Chi Chuan. *Inside Kung Fu,* pp. 33-36.

Kurtz, T.W., & Morris, R.C., Jr. (1983). Dietary chloride as a determinant of "sodium-dependent" hypertension. *Science,* **222,** 1139-1141.

Kwiterovich, P.O. (1986). Biochemical, clinical, epidemiologic, genetic, and pathologic data in the pediatric group relevant to the cholesterol hypothesis. *Pediatrics,* **78,** 349-362.

Kwok, R.H.M. (1968). Chinese restaurant syndrome. *New England Journal of Medicine,* **278,** 796.

Langford, H.G., and Watson, R.L. (1975). Electrolytes and hypertension. In P. Oglesby (Ed.), *Epidemiology and control of hypertension* (p. 119). New York: Stratton Intercontinental Bookcorp.

Lappe, F.M. (1971). *Diet for a small planet.* New York: Friends of the Earth/Ballantine.

Laskarzewski, P.M., Glueck, C.J., & Rao, D.C. (1984). Family resemblance for plasma lipids and lipoprotein concentrations in blacks. *Arteriosclerosis,* **4,** 65-69.

Latin, R.W., Johnson, S.C., & Ruhling, R.O. (1987). Anthropometric estimation of body composition of older men. *Journal of Gerontology*, **42**, 24-28.

Lazarus, R.S. (1966). *Psychological stress and the coping process*. New York: McGraw-Hill.

Lazarus, R.S., & Folkman, S. (1984). *Stress, appraisal and coping*. New York: Springer.

Lecos, C. (1986, May 19). New regulation to help sodium-conscious consumers. *FDA Consumer*, 17-19.

Lee, R.H., Hoover, R.L., Williams, J.D., Sperling, R.I., Ravalese, J., III, Spur, B.W., Robinson, D.R., Corey, E.J., Lewis, R.A, & Austen, K.F. (1985). Effect of dietary enrichment with eicosapentaenoic and docosehexaenoic acids on in vitro neutrophil and monocyte leukotriene generation and neutrophil function. *New England Journal of Medicine*, **312**, 1217-1223.

Lehtonen, A., & Vicari, J. (1978). Serum triglycerides and cholesterol and serum high-density lipoprotein cholesterol in highly physically active men. *Acta Medica Scandinavica*, **204**, 111-114.

LeShan, L. (1959). Psychological states of factors in malignant disease. *Journal of the National Cancer Institute*, **22**, 1-18.

Lew, E.A., & Garfinkel, L. (1979). Variations in mortality by weight among 750,000 men amd women. *American Journal of Public Health*, **69**, 782-783.

Light, K.C., Koepke, J.P., Obrist, P.A., & Willis, P.W. (1983). Psychological stress induces sodium and fluid retention in men at high risk of hypertension. *Science*, **220**, 429-431.

Lind, A.R., & McNichol, G.W. (1967). Muscular factors which determine the cardiovascular response to sustained rhythm exercise. *Canadian Medical Association Journal*, **96**, 706-713.

Linden, V. (1977). Correlation of vitamin D intake to ischemic heart disease, hypercholesterolemia and renal caltinosis. In M. Seelig (Ed.), *Nutritional imbalances in infant and adult disease* (pp. 23-42). New York: SP Books.

Lion, L.S. (1978). Psychological effects of jogging. *Perceptual Motor Skills*, **47**, 1215-1218.

Lipid Research Clinics Program. (1984a). The lipid research clinics coronary primary prevention trial results: I. Reduction in incidence of coronary heart disease. *Journal of the American Medical Association*, **251**, 351-364.

Lipid Research Clinics Program. (1984b). The lipid research clinics coronary primary prevention trial results: II. The relationship of reduction in incidence of coronary heart disease to cholesterol lowering. *Journal of the American Medical Association*, **251**, 365-374.

Loftus, E. (1975). Leading questions and the eyewitness report. *Cognitive Psychology*, **7**, 560-565.

Lund-Johansen, P. (1980). Haemodynamics in essential hypertension. *Clinical Science, 59,* 343-354

Lyon, J.L., Wetzler, H.P., Gardner, J.W., Klauber, M.R., & Williams, R.R. (1978). Cardiovascular mortality in Mormons and non-Mormons in Utah, 1969-1971. *American Journal of Epidemiology, 108,* 357-365.

MacLaughlin, J.A., Anderson, R.R., & Holick, M.F. (1982). Spectral character of sunlight modulates photosynthesis of previtamin D_3 and its photoisomers in human skin. *Science, 216,* 1001-1003.

MacMahon, B., & Pugh, T.F. (1970). *Epidemiology, principles and methods.* Boston: Little Brown.

Madans, J., Kleinman, J.C., & Cornoni-Huntley, J. (1983). Relationship between hip fracture and water fluoridation: An analysis of national data. *American Journal of Public Health, 73,* 296-298.

Malmros, H. (1950). The relation of nutrition to health: A statistical study of the relation of wartime on arteriosclerosis, cardiosclerosis, tuberculosis, and diabetes. *Acta Medica Scandinavica, 138*(Suppl. 246), 137-153.

Marshall, C.W. (1983). *Vitamins and minerals. Help or harm?* Philadelphia: George F. Stickely.

Marshall, E. (1985). The academy kills a nutrition report. *Science, 230,* 420-421.

Martin, G.M., & Sprague, C.A. (1973). Symposium on *in vitro* studies related to atherogenesis: Life histories of hyperplastoid cells from aorta and skin. *Experimental Molecular Pathology, 18,* 125-141.

Mathur, K.S., Khan, M.A., & Sharma, R.D. (1968). Hypocholesterolemic effect of Bengal gram: A long-term study in man. *British Journal of Medicine, 1,* 30-31.

Matthews, K.A., Glass, D.C., Rosenman, R.H., & Bortner, R. (1977). Competitive drive, pattern A, and coronary heart disease: A further analysis of some data from the Western Collaborative Group Study. *Journal of Chronic Diseases, 30,* 489-498.

Matthews, K.A., & Siegel, J.M. (1983). Type A behavior pattern in children and adolescents. In A.R. Baum & J.E. Singer (Eds.), *Handbook of health and medical psychology* (Vol. 2). Hillsdale, NJ: Erlbaum.

Mattson, F.H., Erickson, B.A., & Kligman, A.M. (1972). Effect of dietary cholesterol on serum cholesterol in man. *American Journal of Clinical Nutrition, 25,* 589-594.

Mayer, J., Roy, P., & Mitra, K.P. (1956). Body weight and caloric intake as function of physical activity. *American Journal of Clinical Nutrition, 4,* 169-175.

McCarron, D.A. (1982). Low serum concentration of ionized calcium in patients with hypertension. *New England Journal of Medicine, 307,* 226-228.

McCarron, D.A., Morris, C.D., & Cole, C. (1982). Dietary calcium in human hypertension. *Science, 217*, 267-269.

McCarron, D.A., Morris, C.D., Henry, H.J., & Stanton, J.L. (1984). Blood pressure and nutrient intake in the United States. *Science, 24*, 1392-1397.

McCay, C.M., Drowell, M.F., & Maynard, L.A. (1935). The effect of retarded growth upon the length of life span and upon the ultimate body size. *Journal of Nutrition, 10*, 63-79.

McDonald, J.B. (1979). Not by alcohol alone. *Nutrition Today, 14*, 14-19.

McLaren, D.S. (1984). Vitamin A deficiency and toxicity. In *Present knowledge in nutrition*. Washington, DC: Nutrition Foundation.

Meares, A. (1985). *A way of doctoring*. Melbourne: Hill of Content.

Meneely, G.R. (1973). Toxic effects of dietary sodium chloride and the protective effect of potassium. In F. Strong (Chair), *Toxicants occurring naturally in foods* (pp. 26-42). Washington, DC: National Academy of Science.

Mertz, W. (1981). Essential trace elements. *Science, 213*, 1332-1338.

Mertz, W. (1984). Chromium. In N.W. Solomons & I.W. Rosenberg (Eds.), *Absorption and malabsorption of mineral nutrients* (pp. 259-288). New York: Alan R. Liss.

Metivier, G. (1983). Effect of an acute exercise bout on serum level of testosterone and luteinizing hormone in male subjects above 40 years of age. In H.B. Knittgen, J.A. Vogel, & J. Poortmans (Eds.), *International series on sport sciences: Biochemistry of exercise* (Vol. 13, pp. 667-671). Champaign, IL: Human Kinetics.

Metropolitan Life Foundation. (1983). 1983 Metropolitan height and weight tables. *Statistical Bulletin, 64*(1), 2-5.

Metropolitan Life Insurance Company. (1959). New weight standards for men and women. Build and blood pressure study. *Statistical Bulletin, 40*, 1-4.

Metropolitan Life Insurance Company. (1960). *How to control your weight*. New York: Author.

Miettinen, M., Turpeinen, O., Karvonen, M.J., Elosuo, R., & Paavilainen, E. (1972). Effect of cholesterol-lowering diet on mortality from coronary heart disease and other causes. *Lancet, 2*, 835-838.

Miller, D.R., & Hayes, K.C. (1982). Vitamin excess and toxicity. In J.N. Hathcock (Ed.), *Nutritional toxicology* (Vol. I). New York: Academic Press.

Miller, G.H., & Gerstein, D.R. (1984). Smoking and longevity. *Science, 227*, 1412.

Miller, G.R., & Hayes, K.C. (1982). Vitamin excess and toxicity. *Nutritional Toxicology, 1*, 81-133.

Miller, J.A. (1973). Naturally occurring substances that can induce tumors. In F. Strong (Chair and Ed.), *Toxicants occurring naturally in foods* (2nd ed., pp. 508-549). Washington, DC: National Academy of Sciences.

Miller, N.E., Thelle, D.S., Forde, O.H., & Mjos, O.D. (1977). Tromso heart study. HDL and CHD: A prospective case control study. *Lancet, 1,* 965-968.

Mindell, E. (1979). *Vitamin bible.* New York: Warner Books.

Mooney, J. (1983, December 18). Meet Wayne Cook. *Salt Lake Tribune,* Section D, p. 1.

Morgan, W.P. (1979). Anxiety reduction following acute physical activity. *Psychiatric Annals, 9,* 141-147.

Morrison, F.R., & Paffenbarger, R.S., Jr. (1981). Epidemiological aspects of biobehavior in the etiology of cancer: A critical review. In S. Weiss, J. Herd, & B. Fox (Eds.), *Perspectives on behavioral medicine* (pp. 135-161). New York: Academic Press.

Multiple Risk Factor Intervention Trial Research Group. (1982). Risk factor changes and mortality results. *Journal of the American Medical Association, 248,* 1465-1477.

Multiple Risk Factor Intervention Trial Research Group. (1983, January/February). The multiple risk factor intervention trial report released. *Nutrition Today,* pp. 20-26.

Muslin, H.L., Gyarfas, K., & Pieper, W.J. (1966). Separation experience and cancer of the breast. *Annals of the New York Academy of Sciences, 125,* 802-806.

National Institutes of Health. (1983). Consensus development conference statement: Defined diets and childhood hyperactivity. *American Journal of Clinical Nutrition, 37,* 161-165.

National Institutes of Health Consensus Conference. (1983). Defined diets and childhood hyperactivity. *Journal of the American Medical Association, 248,* 290-292.

National Institutes of Health Consensus Conference. (1985). Lowering blood cholesterol to prevent heart disease. *Journal of the American Medical Association, 253,* 2080-2086.

National Research Council. (1980). *Recommended dietary allowances* (9th ed.). Washington, DC: National Academy of Sciences.

Naughton, J., Bruhn, J.G., & Lategola, M.T. (1968). Effects of physical training on physiologic and behavioral characteristics of cardiac patients. *Archives of Physical Medicine and Rehabilitation, 49,* 131-137.

Nerem, R.M., Levesque, M.J., & Cornhill, J.F. (1980). Social environment as a factor in diet-induced atherosclerosis. *Science, 208,* 1475-1476.

Neri, L.C., & Johansen, H.L. (1978). Water hardness and cardiovascular mortality. *Annals of the New York Academy of Science, 304,* 203-219.

Nesheim, R. O. (1974). Nutrient changes in food processing. *Federation Proceedings, 33,* 2367-2369.

Nessim, S.A., Chin, H.P., Alaupovic, P., & Blankenhorn, D.H. (1983). Combined therapy of niacin, colestipol, and fat-controlled diet in men with coronary bypass. Effect on blood lipids and apolipoproteins. *Arteriosclerosis, 3,* 568-573.

Newbold, H.L. (1973). *Meganutrients for your nerves.* New York: Berkley.

Nielsen, F.H. (1984). Nickel. In E. Frieden (Ed.), *Biochemistry of essential ultratrace elements.* New York: Plenum Press.

Nielsen, F.H., & Mertz, W. (1984). Other trace elements. In *Present knowledge of nutrition* (5th ed.). Washington, DC: Nutrition Foundation.

Nielsen, F.H., & Uthus, E.O. (1984). Arsenic. In E. Frieden (Ed.), *Biochemistry of essential ultratrace elements* (pp. 319-340). New York: Plenum Press.

Nriagu, J.O. (1983). Saturnine gout among Roman aristocrats. *New England Journal of Medicine, 308,* 660-661.

Olson, J.A. (1987). Recommended dietary intakes (RDI) of vitamin A in humans. *American Journal of Clinical Nutrition, 45,* 704-714.

Olson, J.A., & Hodges, R.E. (1987). Recommended dietary intakes (RDI) of vitamin C in humans. *American Journal of Clinical Nutrition, 45,* 693-703.

Olson, R.E. (1980). Statement to House subcommittee on domestic marketing, consumer relations and nutrition. *Nutrition Today,* pp. 12-19.

Olson, R.E. (1985). Dietary fat recommendations. *Science, 227,* 1154.

Orlans, H. (1979). On knowledge, policy, practice and fate. *Federation Proceedings, 38,* 2553-2556.

Oscai, L.B. (1982). Dietary induced severe obesity: A rat model. *American Journal of Physiology, 242,* R212-R215.

Ostfeld, H.M., Lebovits, B.Z., Shekelle, R.B., & Paul, O. (1964). A prospective study of the relationship between personality and coronary heart disease. *Journal of Chronic Diseases, 17,* 265-276.

Pachter, H.M. (1951). *Magic into science.* Scranton, PA: Henry Schuman.

Page, I.H. (1983, March/April). The MRFIT study: A commentary by a maverick. *Nutrition Today,* p. 12.

Parker, W. (1885). *A study of 397 cases of cancer of the female breast.* New York: G.P. Putnam & Sons.

Pauling, L. (1974). Are recommended daily allowances for vitamin C adequate? *Proceedings of the National Academy of Science, 71,* 4442-4446.

Pell, S., & Fayerweather, W.E. (1985). Trends in the incidence of myocardial infarction and in associated mortality and morbidity in a large employed population, 1957-1983. *New England Journal of Medicine, 312,* 1005-1011.

Pennington, J.A., & Church, H.N. (1985). *Food values of portions commonly used* (14th ed.). Philadelphia: J.B. Lippincott.

Perera, F., & Petito, C. (1982). Formaldehyde: A question of cancer policy? *Science*, **216**, 1285-1291.

Phillips, R.L., Lemon, F.R., Beeson, L., and Kuzinaj, N. (1978). Coronary heart disease mortality among Seventh Day Adventists with differing dietary habits: Preliminary report. *American Journal of Clinical Nutrition*, **31**, S191-S198.

Phillipson, B.E., Rothrock, D.W., Connor, W.E., Harris, W.S., & Illingworth, D.R. (1985). Reduction of plasma lipids, lipoproteins, and apoproteins by dietary fish oils in patients with hypertriglyceridemia. *New England Journal of Medicine*, **312**, 1210-1216.

Pike, R.L., & Brown, M.L. (1975). FAO/WHO energy and protein requirements. FAO/WHO requirements of vitamin A, thiamin, riboflavin and niacin. In *Nutrition: An integrated approach*. New York: Wiley.

Pirkle, J., Schwartz, J., Landis, J.R., & Harland, W.R. (1985). The relationship between blood lead levels and blood pressure and its cardiovascular risk implications. *American Journal of Epidemiology*, **121**, 246-258.

Pollock, M.L., Dawson, G.A., Miller, H.S., Jr., Ward, A., Cooper, D., Headley, W., Linnerad, A.C., & Nomeir, M.M. (1976). Physiologic responses of men 49 to 65 years of age to endurance training. *Journal of the American Geriatrics Society*, **24**, 97-110.

Pollock, M.L., Wilmore, V.H., & Fox, S.M. (1978). *Health and fitness through physical activity*. New York: John Wiley & Sons.

Pollock, M.L., Wilmore, J., & Fox, S.M. (1985). *Exercise in health and disease*. Philadelphia: W.B. Saunders.

Pooling Project Research Group. (1978). Relationship of blood pressure, serum cholesterol, smoking habit, relative weight and ECG abnormalities to incidence of major coronary events. *Journal of Chronic Disease*, **31**, 201-306.

Popper, K. (1968). *The logic of scientific discovery* (3rd ed.). London: Hutchinson.

Prince, F. (1981). *Diet for life*. New York: Simon and Schuster.

Pritikin, N., & McGrady, P. (1979). *The Pritikin program for diet and exercise*. New York: Bantam Books

Puska, P., Salonen, J.T., Nissinen, A., Tuomilehto, J., Vartianen E., Korhonen, H., Tanskanen, A., Ronnqvist, P., Koskela, K., & Huttenen, J. (1983). Change in risk factors for coronary heart disease during 10 years of a community intervention programme (North Karelia project). *British Medical Journal*, **287**, 1840-1841.

Rahe, R.H., Herrig, L., & Rosenman, R.H. (1978). Heritability of Type A behavior. *Psychosomatic Medicine*, **40**, 478-486.

Rahe, R.H., Hervig, L., Romo, M., Siltanen, P., Punsar, S., Karvonen, M.J., & Rissanen, V. (1978). Coronary behavior in three regions of Finland. *Journal of Psychosomatic Research*, **22**, 455-450.

Rapp, J. (1983). Paradigm for identification of primary genetic causes of hypertension in rats. *Journal of Chromic Diseases*, **31**, 201-306.

Reuben, D. (1976). *The save your life diet*. New York: Ballantine Books.

Roberts, L. (1987). Measuring cholesterol is as tricky as lowering it. *Science*, **238**, 482-483.

Robertson, L., Flinders, C., & Godfrey, B. (1976). *Laurel's kitchen*. Berkeley, CA: Nilgiri Press.

Rodahl, K. (1966). *Be fit for life*. New York: Harper and Row.

Rodale, J.I. (Ed.). (1961). *Complete book of food and nutrition*. Emmaus, PA: Rodale Books.

Rodale, J.I. (Ed.). (1970). *Your diet and your heart*. Emmaus, PA: Rodale Books.

Rodale, J.I. (1972, August). Lecithin for the heart. *Prevention*, pp. 191-196.

Rombauer, I.S., & Becker, M.R. (1974). *Joy of cooking*. New York: New American Library.

Rosenman, R.H., Brand, R.J., Sholtz, R.I., & Friedman, M. (1976). Multivariate prediction of coronary heart disease during 8.5 year follow-up in the Western Collaborative Group Study. *American Journal of Cardiology*, **37**, 903-909.

Ross, R., & Glomset, J.A. (1976). The pathogenesis of atherosclerosis. *New England Journal of Medicine*, **295**, 369-377.

Ross, R., & Harker, L. (1976). Hyperlipidemia and atherosclerosis. *Science*, **193**, 1094-1100.

Roth, D.L., & Holmes, D.S. (1985). Influence of physical fitness in determining the impact of stressful life events on physical and psychologic health. *Psychosomatic Medicine*, **47**, 164-173.

Russell, B. (1948). *Human knowledge*. London: George Allen and Unwin.

Rusznyak, S., & Szent-Gyorgyi, A. (1936). Vitamin P: Flavonols as vitamins. *Nature*, **138**, 27.

Sahlin, K. (1982). Effect of acidosis on energy metabolism and force generation in skeletal muscle. In H.B. Knuttgen, J.A. Vogel, & J. Porrtmans (Eds.), *International series on sport sciences: Vol 13. Biochemistry of exercise* (pp. 151-160). Champaign, IL: Human Kinetics.

Salonen, J.T., Alfthan, G., Huttunen, J.K., Pikkarainen, J., & Puska, P. (1982). Association between cardiovascular death and myocardial infarction and serum selenium in a matched-pair longitudinal study. *Lancet*, **2**, 175-179.

Saltin, B. (1981). Muscle fiber recruitment and metabolism in exhaustive dynamic exercise. In R.H.T. Edwards (Chair), *Human muscle fatigue: Physiological mechanisms*. Ciba Foundation Symposium 82. London: Pitman Medical.

Saltin, B., Henriksson, J., Nygaard, E., Andersen, P., & Jansson, E. (1977). Fiber types and metabolic potentials of skeletal muscles in sedentary man and endurance runners. *Annals of the New York Academy of Sciences*, **301**, 3-29.

Sarason, I.G., & Johnson, J.H. (1976). *Report on life stress and coping in relation to performance and organizational effectiveness* (Tech. Rep.). Arlington, VA: Office of Naval Research.

Sasaki, N. (1962). High blood pressure and the salt intake of the Japanese. *Japanese Heart Journal*, **3**, 313-324.

Sauberlich, H.E. (1980). Pantothenic acid. In R.S. Goodhart & M.E. Shils (Eds.), *Modern nutrition in health and disease*. Philadelphia: Lea & Febiger.

Schaumburg, H., Byck, R., Gerstl, R., & Mashman, M.H. (1969). Monosodium L-glutamate: Its pharmacology and role in the Chinese restaurant syndrome. *Science*, **163**, 826-828.

Schaumburg, H., Kaplan, J., Windebank, A., Vick, N., Rasmus, S., Pleasure, D., & Brown, M.J. (1983). Sensory neuropathy from pyridoxine abuse. *New England Journal of Medicine*, **309**, 445-448.

Schemmel, R. (1976). Physiological consideration of food storage and utilization. *American Zoologist*, **16**, 661-670.

Schemmel, R., & Mickelsen, O. (1974). Influence of diet, strain, age and sex on fat depot mass and body composition of the nutritionally obese rat. In J. Vague & J. Boyer (Eds.), *The regulation of the adipose tissue mass* (Proceedings of the 4th International Meeting of Endocrinology, pp. 238-253). New York: Elsevier.

Scherwitz, L., McIlvain, R., Laman, C., Patteron, J., Dutton, L., Yusim, S., Lester, J., Kraft, I., Rochelle, D., & Leacham, R. (1983). Type A behavior, self-involvement and coronary atherosclerosis. *Psychosomatic Medicine*, **45**, 47-57.

Schmale, A., & Iker, H. (1966). Psychological setting of uterine cervical cancer. *Annals of the New York Academy of Sciences*, **125**, 807-813.

Schrauzer, G.N., & White, D.A. (1978). Selenium in human nutrition: Dietary intakes and effects of supplementation. *Bioinorganic Chemistry*, **8**, 303-318.

Schroeder, H.A. (1960). Relations between hardness of water and death rates from certain chronic and degenerative diseases in the U.S. *Journal of Chronic Diseases*, **23**, 586.

Schroeder, H.A. (1966). Municipal drinking water and cardiovascular death rates. *Journal of the American Medical Association*, **95**, 115.

Schuette, S.A., & Lenkiwiles, H.M. (1984). Calcium. In *Present knowledge in nutrition* (5th ed). Washington, DC: Nutrition Foundation.

Schultz, J.H. (1932). *Das autogene training*. Leipzig: G. Thieme Verlag.

Schultz, J.H., & Luthe, W. (1959). *Autogenic training*. New York: Grune and Stratton.

Schwartz, C.C., Halloran, L.G., Vlahcevic, Z.R., Gregory, D.H., & Swell, L. (1978). Preferred utilization of free cholesterol from HDL for biliary cholesterol secretion in man. *Science, 200*, 62-64.

Sclafani, A., & Springer, D. (1976) Dietary obesity in adult rats: Similarities to hypothalamic and human obesity syndromes. *Physiological Behavior, 17*, 461-471.

Sebrell, W.H., Jr. (1981). History of pellagra. *Federation Proceedings, 40*, 1520-1522.

Seelig, M.S., & Heggtveit, H.A. (1974). Magnesium relationships in ischemic heart disease: A review. *American Journal of Clinical Nutrition, 27*, 59-79.

Select Committee on GRAS Substances. (1977). Evaluation of health aspects of GRAS food ingredients: Lessons learned and questions unanswered. *Federation Proceedings, 37*, 2525-2561.

Selver, C. (1957). Sensory awareness and total functioning. *General Semantics Bulletin, 20 & 21*, 5-17.

Selye, H. (1956). *The stress of life.* New York: McGraw-Hill.

Senate Select Committee on Nutrition and Human Needs. (1977). *Dietary goals for the United States.* Washington, DC: U.S. Government Printing Office.

Shamberger, R.J., Gunsch, M.S., Willis, E., & McCormick, L.J. (1978). Selenium in heart disease: II. Selenium and other trace metal intakes and heart disease in 25 countries. In D.D. Hempill (Ed.), *Trace substances in environmental health* (Vol. 12, pp. 48-52). Columbia, MO: University of Missouri Press.

Shangold, M., Gatz, M., & Thysen, B. (1981) Acute effects of exercise on plasma concentration of prolactin and testosterone in recreational women runners. *Fertility & Sterility, 35*, 699-702.

Sharkey, B.J. (1984). *Physiology of fitness* (2nd ed.). Champaign, IL: Human Kinetics.

Sharkey, B.J., Simpson, C., Washbarn, R., & Confessore, R. (1980). HDL-cholesterol. *Running, 5*, 38-41.

Shekelle, R.B., et al. (1981). Psychological depression and 17-year risk of death from cancer. *Psychosomatics, 43*, 117-126.

Shekelle, R.B., Gale, M., Ostfeld, A.M., & Paul, O. (1976). Correlates of the JAS type A behavior pattern score. *Journal of Chronic Diseases, 29*, 381-394.

Shekelle, R.B., Gale, M., Ostfeld, A.M., & Paul, O. (1983). Hostility, risk of coronary heart disease, and mortality. *Psychosomatic Medicine, 45*, 109-114.

Shekelle, R.B., Hulley, S.B., Neaton, J.D., Billings, J.H., Borhani, N.O., Gerace, T.A., Jacobs, D.R., Lasser, N.L., Mittlemark, M.B., & Stamler, J. (1985). The MRFIT behavior pattern study: II. Type A behavior and incidence of coronary disease. *American Journal of Epidemiology, 122*, 559-570.

Shekelle, R.B., Schoenberger, J.B., & Stamler, J. (1976). Correlates of the JAS type A behavior pattern score. *Journal of Chronic Diseases*, **29**, 381-394.

Shute, W., & Taub, H. (1969). *Vitamin E for ailing and healthy hearts*. New York: Pyramid Books.

Shute, W., Shute, E., & Vogelsang, A. (1947). Vitamin E in heart disease. *Medical Record*, **160**, 91-96.

Simborg, D.W. (1970). The status of risk factors and coronary heart disease (a review). *Journal of Chronic Diseases*, **22**, 515.

Simons, L.A., Hickie, J.B., & Ruys, J. (1977). Treatment of hypercholesterolemia with oral lecithin. *Australian and New Zealand Journal of Medicine*, **7**, 22-26.

Simonson, E. (1957). Change of physical fitness and cardiovascular functions with age. *Geriatrics*, **12**, 28-39.

Simopoulos, A.P. (1985). Health implications of overweight and obesity. *Nutrition Reviews*, **43**, 33-40.

Sims, E.A.H. (1976). Experimental obesity, dietary-induced thermogenesis, and their clinical implications. *Clinics in Endocrinology and Metabolism*, **5**, 377-395.

Sims, E.A.H., Danforth, E., Horton, E.S., Bray, G.A., Glennon, J.A., & Salans, L.B. (1973). Endocrine and metabolic effects of experimental obesity in man. *Recent Progress in Hormone Research*, **29**, 457-486.

Sinyor, D., Schwartz, S.G., Perronnet, F., Brisson, G., & Seraganian, P. (1983). Aerobic fitness level and reactivity to psychosocial stress: Physiological, biochemical, and subjective measures. *Psychosomatic Medicine*, **45**, 205-217.

Sjostrom, M., & Friden, J. (1982). Morphological studies of muscle fatigue. In H.G. Knuttgen, J.A. Vogel, & J. Poortmans (Eds.), *International series on sport sciences: Vol 13. Biochemistry of exercise*. Champaign, IL: Human Kinetics.

Skinner, J.S., Holloszy, J.O., & Cureton, T.K. (1964). Effects of a program of endurance exercises on physical work capacity and anthropometric measurements of fifteen middle-aged men. *American Journal of Cardiology*, **14**, 747-752.

Smith, M. (1978, November 10). Don't bring stress home. *Salt Lake Tribune*, Section C, p. 5

Solomon, N. (1976). *Doctor Soloman's easy no-risk diet*. New York: Warner Books.

Solomons, N.W. (1984). Other trace minerals: Manganese, molybdenum, vanadium, nickel, silicon, and arsenic. In N.W. Solomons & I.H. Rosenberg (Eds.), *Absorption and malabsorption of mineral nutrients* (pp. 269-296). New York: Alan R. Liss.

Solomons, N.W., & Cousins, R.J. (1984). Zinc. In N.W. Solomons & I.H. Rosenberg (Eds.), *Absorption and malabsorption of mineral nutrients* (pp. 125-198). New York: Alan R. Liss.

Sorenson, A.W., & Lyon, J.I. (1979). Nutritional epidemiology: A research approach. *Family and Community Health*, 1, 69-82.

Souchek, J., Stamler, J., Dyer, A., Paul, O., & Lepper, M. (1979). The value of two or three versus a single reading of blood pressure at a first visit. *Journal of Chronic Disease*, 32, 197-210.

Southgate, D.A.T., Baily, B., Collinson, E., & Walker, A.F. (1976). A guide to calculating intakes of dietary fiber. *Journal of Human Nutrition*, 30, 303-312.

Spencer, H., Kramer, L., Norris, C., & Osis, D. (1982). Effect of small doses of aluminum containing antacids on calcium and phosphorus metabolism. *American Journal of Clinical Nutrition*, 36, 32-40.

Spiller, G., & Shipley, E. (1977). Perspectives in dietary fiber in human nutrition. *World Review of Nutrition and Dietetics*, 27, 105-131.

Sprinker, L.H., Harr, J.H., Newberne, P.M., Whanger, P.D., & Weswig, P.H. (1971). Selenium deficiency symptoms in rats fed vitamin E supplemented rations. *Nutrition Reports International*, 4, 335-340.

Stamler, J. (1978). Lifestyles, major risk factors, proof, and public policy. *Circulation*, 58(1), 1-19.

Stamler, J., Farinaro, E., Mojonnier, L.M., Hall, Y., Moss, D., & Stamler, R. (1980). Prevention and control of hypertension by nutritional-hygienic means. *Journal of the American Medical Association*, 243, 1819-1823.

Stamler, R., Stamler, J., Riedlinger, W.F., Algera, G., & Roberts, R.H. (1978). Weight and blood pressure. Findings in hypertension screening of 1 million Americans. *Journal of the American Medical Association*, 240, 1607-1610.

Stecher, P.G. (Ed.). (1968). *Merck index*. Rahway, NJ: Merck & Co.

Steinfeld, J.L. (1984). Smoking and health. *Western Journal of Medicine*, 141, 878-883.

Stern, R.M., & Ray, W.J. (1980). *Biofeedback*. Lincoln, NE: University of Nebraska Press.

Story, J.A., & Kritchevsky, D. (1976). Dietary fiber and lipid metabolism. In G.A. Spiller & R.J. Amen (Eds.), *Fiber in human nutrition* (pp. 171-184). New York: Plenum Press.

Stuart, R.B. (1985). *Act thin, stay thin*. New York: Jove.

Sturdevant, R.A.L., Pearce, M.L., & Dayton, S. (1973). Increased prevalence of cholelithiasis in man ingesting a serum cholesterol lowering diet. *New England Journal of Medicine*, 288, 24-27.

Sulloway, F. (1979). *Freud—Biologist of the mind*. New York: Basic Books.

Suls, J., & Fletcher, B. (1985). Self-attention, life stress, and illness: A prospective study. *Psychosomatic Medicine*, 47, 469-481.

Sun, M. (1984). Renewed interest in food irradiation. *Science*, 223, 667-668.

Sun, M. (1985). EPA accelerates ban on leaded gas. *Science*, 227, 1448.

Surgeon General of the U.S. (1979a). *Report on health promotion and disease prevention* (HEW Publication No. 79-55071). Washington, DC: U.S. Government Printing Office.

Surgeon General of the U.S. (1979b). *Smoking and health: A report of the Surgeon General* (DHEW Publication No. PHS 79-50066). Washington, DC: U.S. Government Printing Office.

Svanberg, U., Gustafson, A., & Ohlson, R. (1974). Polyunsaturated fatty acids in hyperlipoproteinemia: II. Administration of the essential phospholipids in hypertriglyceridemia. *Nutrition and Metabolism, 17*, 338-346.

Swami, A. (1946). *Hindu psychology.* New York: Harper.

Syster, B., & Stull, G. (1970). Muscular endurance retention as a function of length of detraining. *Research Quarterly, 41*, 105-109.

Taller, H. (1961). *Calories don't count.* New York: Simon and Schuster.

Tannahill, R. (1973). *Food in history.* New York: Stein and Day.

Taves, D.R. (1979). Continuing evaluation in the use of flourides. In E. Johansen, D.R. Taves, & T.O. Olsen (Eds.), *AAAS Selected Symposium 11.* Boulder, CO: Westview Press.

Taylor, F. (1981). Iodine: Going from hypo- to hyper-. *FDA Consumer, 15*, 15-18.

Taylor, W.F. (1972). Renal calculi and self-medication with multivitamin preparations containing vitamin D. *Clinical Science, 42*, 515-522.

Thiebaud, D., Acheson, K., Schutz, Y., Felber, J.P., Golay, A., Defronzo, R.A., & Jequier, E. (1983). Stimulation of thermogenesis in men after combined glucose—long chain—triglyceride infusion. *American Journal of Clinical Nutrition, 37*, 603-611.

Thomas, A., McKay, D., & Cutlip, M. (1976). A nomograph method for assessing body weight. *American Journal of Clinical Nutrition.*

Thomas, C.B. (1976). Precursors of premature disease and death: The predictive potential of habits and family attitudes. *Annals of Internal Medicine, 85*, 653-658.

Thomas, C.B. (1977). *Habits of nervous tension: Clues to the nervous condition. The precursors study.* Baltimore, MD: Johns Hopkins School of Medicine.

Thomas, C.B., & Duszynski, K.R. (1974). Closeness to parents and the family constellation in a prospective study of five disease states: Suicide, mental illness, malignant tumor, hypertension and coronary heart disease. *Johns Hopkins Medical Journal, 134*, 251-270.

Thomas, C.B., Duszynski, K.R., & Schaffer, J.W. (1979). Family attitudes reported in youth as potential predictors of cancer. *Psychosomatic Medicine, 41*, 287-302.

Thoresen, C.E., Telch, M.J., & Eagleston, J.R. (1981). Approaches to altering the type A behavior pattern. *Psychosomatics, 22*, 472-482.

Tillotson, J.L. (1973). Epidemiology of coronary heart disease and stroke in Japanese men living in Japan, Hawaii, and California: Methodology for comparison of diet. *American Journal of Clinical Nutrition, 26,* 177-184.

Too much sugar. (1978, March). *Consumer Reports,* pp. 1136-1142.

Tsai, A.C., Kelley, J.J., Peng, B., & Cook, N. (1978). Study on effect of megavitamin E in man. *American Journal of Clinical Nutrition, 31,* 831-837.

Tuomilehto, J., Geboers, J., Salonen, J.T., Nissinen, A., Kuulasmaa, K., & Puska, P. (1986). Decline in cardiovascular mortality in N. Karelia and other parts of Finland. *British Medical Journal, 293,* 1068-1071.

Turpeinen, O. (1979). Effect of cholesterol-lowering diet on mortality from CHD and other causes. *Circulation, 59,* 1-7.

U.S. Department of Agriculture. (1976). *Composition of foods: Fats and oils* (Handbook No. 8-4). Washington, DC: U.S. Government Printing Office.

U.S. Senate Select Committee on Nutrition and Human Needs. (1977a). *Dietary goals for the United States.* Washington, DC: U.S. Government Printing Office.

U.S. Senate Select Committee on Nutrition and Human Needs. (1977b). *Dietary goals for the United States* (2nd ed.). Washington, DC: U.S. Government Printing Office.

Vallee, B.L., Ulmer, D.D., & Wacker,W.E.C. (1960). Arsenic toxicology and biochemistry. *American Medical Association Archives of Industrial Health, 21,* 132-151.

Vickers, R.R., Hervig, L.K., Rahe, R.H., & Rosenman, R.H. (1981). Type A behavior pattern and coping and defense. *Psychosomatic Medicine, 43,* 381.

Vik, T., Try, K., Thelle, P., & Forde, O. (1979). Tromso heart study: Vitamin D metabolism and myocardial infarction. *British Medical Journal, 2,* 176.

Virtamo, J., Valkeila, E., Alfthan, G., Punsar, S., Huttunen, J.K., & Karvonen, M.J. (1985). Serum selenium and the risk of coronary heart disease and stroke. *American Journal of Epidemiology, 122,* 276-282.

Vitale, J.J. (1976). *Vitamins.* Kalamazoo, MI: Upjohn.

Vitamin C toxicity. (1976). *Nutrition Review, 34,* 236-237.

Vogelsang, A., & Shute, E.V. (1946). Effect of vitamin E in coronary heart disease. *Nature, 157,* 772.

Wahren, J. (1977). Glucose turnover during exercise in man. *Annals of the New York Academy of Science, 301,* 45-54.

Waitz, G. (1985). Grete's great for warm-up. *Health and Fitness Magazine,* pp. 36-42.

Waldman, R., & Stull, G.A. (1969). Effects of various periods of inactivity on retention of newly acquired levels of muscular endurance. *The Research Quarterly*, **40**, 396-401.

Wallace, R.K., Silver, J., Mills, P.J., Dillbeck, M.C., & Wagoner, D.E. (1983). Systolic blood pressure and long-term practice of the transcendental meditation and TM-Sidhi program: Effects of TM and systolic blood pressure. *Psychosomatic Medicine*, **45**, 41-46.

Watkins, L.O. (1984). Worldwide experience: Coronary artery disease and hypertension in black populations. *Urban Health*, **13**, 30-35.

Weinberger, M.H., Luft, F.C., Bloch, R., Henry, D.P., Pratt, J.H., Weyman, A.E., Rankin, L.I., Murray, R.H., Willis, L.R., & Grim, C.E. (1982). The blood pressure-raising effects of high dietary sodium intake: Racial differences and the role of potassium. *Journal of American College of Nutrition*, **1**, 139-148.

Weindruch, R., & Walford, R.L. (1982). Dietary restriction in mice beginning at 1 year of age: Effect on life span and spontaneous cancer incidence. *Science*, **215**, 1415-1417.

West, R.O., & Hayes, O.B. (1968). Diet and serum cholesterol levels: A comparison between vegetarians and non-vegetarians in the Seventh Day Adventist Group. *American Journal of Clinical Nutrition*, **21**, 853-862.

Whatmore, G.B., & Kohli, D.R. (1974). *Physiopathology and treatment of functional disorders*. New York: Grune and Stratton.

White, N.K., Edwards, J.E., & Dry, T.J. (1950). Correlations in coronary artery disease. *Circulation*, **1**, 645.

Whitescarver, S.A., Guthrie, G.P., Jr., & Kotchen, T.A. (1984). Salt-sensitive hypertension: Contribution of chloride. *Science*, **223**, 1430-1432.

Whyte, H.M., & Havenstein, N. (1976). A perspective view of dieting to lower the blood cholesterol. *American Journal of Clinical Nutrition*, **29**, 784-790.

Wilkinson, C.F., Jr. (1957). Drugs other than anticoagulants in treatment of arteriosclerotic heart disease. *Journal of the American Medical Association*, **163**, 927-930.

Williams, C.L., Arnold, C.B., & Wynder, E.L. (1977). Primary prevention of chronic disease beginning in childhood. The "Know Your Body" program. *Preventive Medicine*, **6**, 344-357.

Williams, R., & Kalita, D.K. (Eds.). (1979). *Physicians handbook of orthomolecular medicine*. New Canaan, CT: Keats.

Williams, R.B., Jr. (1984, September/October). An untrusting heart. *The Sciences*, pp. 30.

Williams, R.B., Haney, T.L., Lee, K.L., Kong, Y.H., Blumenthal, J.A., & Whalen, R.E. (1980). Type A behavior, hostility, and coronary atherosclerosis. *Psychosomatic Medicine, 42,* 539-549.

Williams, R.J. (1975). *Physicians' handbook of nutritional science.* Springfield, IL: Charles C Thomas.

Williams, R.J., Heffley, J.D., Yew, M., & Bode, C.R. (1972). A renaissance of nutritional science is imminent. *Perspectives in Biology and Medicine, 17,* 1-15.

Wilmore, J. (1974). Alterations in strength, body composition and anthropometric measurements consequent to a 10-week training program. *Medicine and Science in Sports, 6,* 133-138.

Wilson, B. (1984). Toxicants occurring naturally in foods. In R.E. Olsen (Chair and Ed.), *Present knowledge in nutrition* (5th ed., pp. 819-839). Washington, DC: Nutrition Foundation.

Wilson, V.E., Morley, N.C., & Bird, E.I. (1980). Mood profiles of marathon runners, joggers, and non-exercisers. *Perceptual Motor Skills, 50,* 117-118.

Winston, M., & Eshleman, R. (Eds.).(1984). *American Heart Association cookbook.* New York: McKay.

Wolfe, T. (1968). *The electric kool-aid acid test.* New York: Farrar, Straus and Giroux.

Wolff, J. (1969). Iodide goiter and the pharmacological effects of excess iodide. *American Journal of Medicine, 47,* 101-103.

Wolpe, J. (1973). *The practice of behavior therapy* (2nd ed.). New York: Pergamon Press.

Woo, R., Garrow, J.S., & Pi-Sunyer. F.X. (1982a). Effect of exercise on spontaneous calorie intake in obesity. *American Journal of Clinical Nutrition, 36,* 470-477.

Woo, R., Garrow, J.S., & Pi-Sunyer, F.X. (1982b). Voluntary food intake during prolonged exercise in obese women. *American Journal of Clinical Nutrition, 36,* 478-484.

Wurtman, J. (1979). *Eating your way through life.* New York: Raven Press.

Wynder, E.L. (1976). Nutrition and cancer. *Federation Proceedings, 35,* 1309-1315.

Wyse, B.W., Sorenson, A.W., Wittwer, A.J., & Hansen, R.G. (1976). Nutritional quality index identifies consumer nutrient needs. *Food Technology, 30,* 22-40.

Yano, K., Rhoads, G.G., & Kugan, A. (1977). Coffee, alcohol and risk of CHD among Japanese men living in Hawaii. *New England Journal of Medicine, 297,* 405-409.

Yiamouyiannis, J., & Burk, D. (1977). Fluoridation and cancer age-dependence of cancer mortality related to artificial fluoridation. *Fluoride, 10,* 102-123.

Yudkin, J. (1972). *Sweet and dangerous*. New York: Peter Wyden.

Yudkin, J., & Roddy, J. (1964). Levels of dietary sucrose in patients with occlusive atherosclerotic disease. *Lancet, 2*, 6-8.

Zimbardo, P. (1979). *Psychology and life* (10th ed.). Glenview, IL: Scott, Foresman.

Zonana, V.F. (1982, August 18). Don't move a muscle till you're wired in on "passive exercise." *Wall Street Journal*.

Zurer, P.S. (1986). Food irradiation. *Chemical and Engineering News, 64*, 46-56.

Author Index

Subject Index